Surgical Techniques of the Foot and Ankle

Maneesh Bhatia
Editor

Surgical Techniques of the Foot and Ankle

Springer

Editor
Maneesh Bhatia
Consultant Orthopaedic Foot Ankle Surgeon
University Hospitals Leicester, Spire Hospital
Leicester and Nuffield Health Leicester
Leicester, UK

Associate Professor
University of Leicester
Leicester, UK

Professor
DeMontfort University Leicester
Leicester, UK

ISBN 978-3-031-93741-5 ISBN 978-3-031-93742-2 (eBook)
https://doi.org/10.1007/978-3-031-93742-2

This Springer imprint is published by the registered company Springer Nature Switzerland AG
The registered company address is: Gewerbestrasse 11, 6330 Cham, Switzerland

Preface

The foot and ankle remain one of the most intricate and fascinating regions in orthopaedic surgery. Each operation in this field demands not only precision and skill but also a deep appreciation of anatomy, balance, and biomechanics. Over the years, I have come to realise that true mastery lies not only in knowing what to do but in understanding why and how every decision in the operating theatre matters.

The idea for this book, *Surgical Techniques of the Foot and Ankle*, grew out of countless conversations with colleagues, trainees, and mentors around the world. Many of us have shared the same questions—how can we make complex procedures reproducible, how can we communicate surgical 'feel' through words and images, and how can we ensure that the next generation inherits not just our techniques but our reasoning and philosophy? This book aims to answer those questions in a structured, stepwise, and visually guided format.

Each chapter represents the collective experience of expert surgeons who have dedicated their careers to improving patient outcomes. Their willingness to share their techniques, insights, and even their mistakes is what makes this volume special. I am deeply grateful for their contributions and generosity of spirit.

I have always believed that surgical education thrives on collaboration. As educators, we are merely custodians of knowledge—tasked with refining, recording, and passing it forward. My hope is that this book will serve not only as a reference for surgical technique but also as an inspiration to innovate responsibly, teach openly, and never stop learning.

Finally, I owe immense gratitude to my colleagues, mentors, and trainees who continue to challenge and inspire me every day, and to my family for their constant support and understanding throughout this demanding yet deeply fulfilling journey.

Leicester, UK Maneesh Bhatia

Contents

Chapter 1
Hallux Valgus and Bunionette

Pascal Rippstein and Philipp Friederichsen

Introduction

Over the course of evolution, the human foot has transformed from a tree-dwelling primate structure into a highly complex system that supports bipedal walking. The first ray, once a highly mobile grasping unit with an opposable thumb, has evolved into a more rigid structure to provide better support during locomotion. The stabilization of the first ray seems not to be yet complete. Its remaining mobility can cause it to deviate from its normal alignment, resulting in a condition known as metatarsus primus varus accompanied by hallux valgus deformity. The goal of surgery is to realign and stabilize the deviated first ray, thereby restoring its supporting function.

Surgical Techniques

Understanding the Problem

In hallux valgus, the first metatarsal gradually shifts and rotates medially—a condition known as metatarsus primus varus—resulting in a loss of its normal position above the sesamoids [1]. As this happens, the great toe deviates laterally into a valgus deformity which progressively worsens over time. The soft tissues surrounding the metatarso-phalangeal joint become increasingly loose on the medial side while contracting on the lateral side.

P. Rippstein (✉) · P. Friederichsen
Department of Foot and Ankle Surgery, Schulthess Clinic, Zürich, Switzerland
e-mail: Pascal.rippstein@kws.ch; Philipp.friederichsen@kws.ch

M. Bhatia (ed.), *Surgical Techniques of the Foot and Ankle*,
https://doi.org/10.1007/978-3-031-93742-2_1

Addressing the Problem

Surgery is the only effective treatment to correct hallux valgus [2]. Goal of surgery is to restore normal anatomy by repositioning the first metatarsal from its varus alignment back to its proper location, and by simultaneously reducing the laterally subluxed great toe on its metatarsal head [3]. To correctly achieve this realignment, additional procedures are required on the soft tissues around the metatarso-phalangeal joint, particularly addressing the contracted lateral structures. Whether performed using an open or minimally invasive technique, the success of the procedure largely depends on the surgeon's expertise rather than the chosen approach.

Choosing the Right Procedure for Each Deformity

Various surgical techniques have been developed to correct hallux valgus, and these can be categorized based on where along the metatarsal the correction is made (Table 1.1).

Distal Procedures

Distal procedures (chevron osteotomy, short scarf osteotomy….) are located at the distal metatarsal metaphysis, often extending into the metatarsal head. Distal procedures have the advantages of being relatively easy to perform and of healing well. Surgery time is short, and patients recover usually quickly. On the other hand, the correction capability is limited since contact area between distal and proximal metatarsal fragments is rather small and the distance for the needed lateral translation of the distal fragment is bigger than proximal procedures.

Proximal Procedures

Proximal procedures (base metatarsal osteotomy, Lapidus) are located at the proximal metaphysis or at the first tarso-metatarsal joint. As they address the apex of the metatarsus primus deformity, they can correct any degree of deformity. However, they are technically more challenging, they have a higher risk of complications, and a more demanding recovery process.

Table 1.1 Different types of procedures with their correction and healing potential

Procedures	Correction potential	Healing potential
Distal	+	+++
Diaphyseal	++	++
Proximal	+++	+
"Full metatarsal"	++(+)	+++

Diaphyseal Procedures

Diaphyseal procedures (Ludloff, Mau osteotomies) are located in the middle of the metatarsus and offer a compromise by allowing more correction than distal procedures with better healing potential than proximal one. Although they improve on healing compared to proximal techniques, their corrective power is more limited.

"Full Metatarsal" Procedures

Some procedures (long scarf osteotomy) are extending from the proximal to the distal metaphysis of the first metatarsal and we classify them therefore as "full metatarsal" procedures (Fig. 1.1). They combine the benefits of both distal (good healing potential) and proximal (high corrective capability) techniques, allowing for correction of almost all degrees of hallux deformity with high success rate. In our clinic, over 90% of all hallux valgus requiring surgery are treated with scarf osteotomy, using the long scarf for severe deformities.

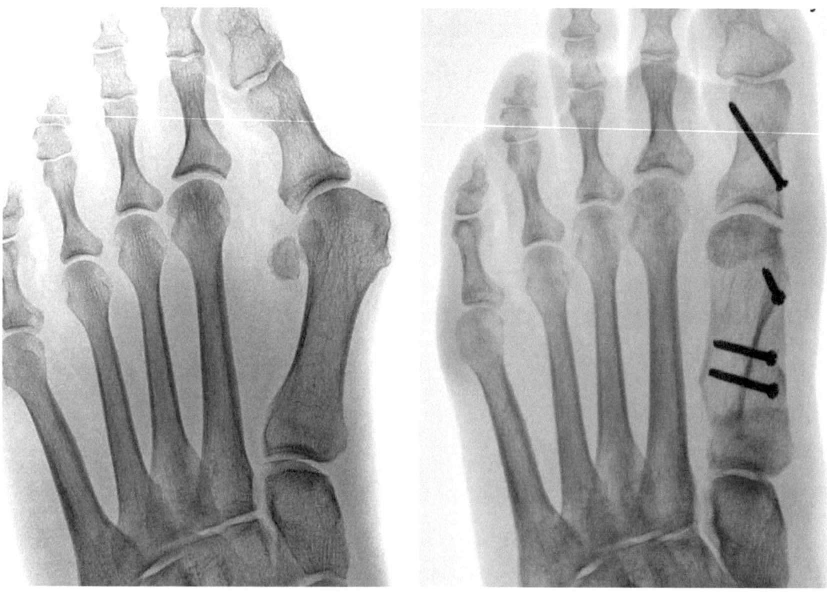

Fig. 1.1 Long scarf as a "full metatarsal" osteotomy. Three reasons explain why this severe deformity could be reduced with scarf. First, the metatarsal is quite wide and allowed therefore more lateral translation of the distal metatarsal fragment. Second, the contact surface between both metatarsal fragments has been increased thanks metatarsal shortening. And third, the long scarf as a "full metatarsal" osteotomy provides more contact surface for fixation and stability between both metatarsal fragments

First Metatarsophalangeal (MP1) Fusion

For certain hallux valgus deformities, MP1 fusion offers the best and safest treatment option. This is especially true when the MP1 joint is affected by painful arthritis [4]. In patients with rheumatoid arthritis, even if the joint does not yet show arthritic changes, MP1 fusion should be considered because the medial capsule is often weak, which increases the risk of bunion recurrence [5]. Additionally, due to the underlying disease, arthritis may develop over time.

MP1 fusion is also a valuable option for revision surgery after multiple unsuccessful procedures. In such cases, the bone and medial soft tissues are often significantly compromised, making conventional corrective techniques less reliable for long-lasting results.

Because the lateral soft tissues around the MP1 joint are typically contracted, reducing the great toe from its pathological valgus position and stabilizing it with an arthrodesis usually results in an automatic reduction of the metatarsus primus varus. It is important not to release these contracted lateral tissues when treating a bunion with MP1 fusion, as they help achieve the correction. However, the amount of varus reduction that can be achieved is limited; the more severe the deformity, the less effective the correction will be. If the correction proves insufficient, an additional proximal procedure—such as a Mau osteotomy, base osteotomy, or Lapidus procedure—may be required to properly realign the first metatarsal [6].

Resection of the Base of the Great Toe Phalanx

Known as the Keller-Brandes procedure, this technique was widely used in the past but often resulted in poor functional outcomes. It is no longer recommended for active patients. However, for older, less active individuals, this procedure remains a good option because it is straightforward, fast, and safe, allowing for immediate weight-bearing with a low complication rate and effective pain relief [7].

Additional Bony Procedures

Even when the MP1 joint is successfully realigned, a residual valgus deformity may persist at the proximal phalanx of the big toe—a condition known as hallux interphalangeus. This residual deformity can cause mechanical conflicts with the second toe. Moreover, the extensor and flexor hallucis longus tendons remain misaligned, exerting deforming forces around the MP1 joint and eventually contributing to bunion recurrence. In these cases, performing an Akin osteotomy (a varisation procedure on the proximal phalanx) is recommended to achieve complete realignment of the first ray [8].

The distal articular surface of the first metatarsal may be abnormally oriented laterally, a condition referred to as a pathological Distal Metatarsal Articular Angle (DMAA). This is common in juvenile hallux valgus deformities and can also occur after metatarsal base osteotomies that involve significant correction (Fig. 1.2). A pathological DMAA can lead to joint incongruity when the great toe is realigned to the first metatarsal axis, thereby increasing the risk of bunion recurrence and potentially leading to MP1 arthrosis over time. To correct this, the articular surface of the metatarsal head must be repositioned to a physiological orientation. This can be achieved together with a distal or midshaft osteotomy or, if the metatarsus primus varus correction needs to be performed more proximally, through an additional retrocapital varisation osteotomy (commonly known as the Reverdin osteotomy) [9].

Soft Tissue Procedures

The soft tissues around the MP1 joint play an integral role in the bunion deformity and must be addressed along with the bony corrections. Over time, due to the long-standing hallux valgus deformity, the lateral MP1 soft tissues become progressively

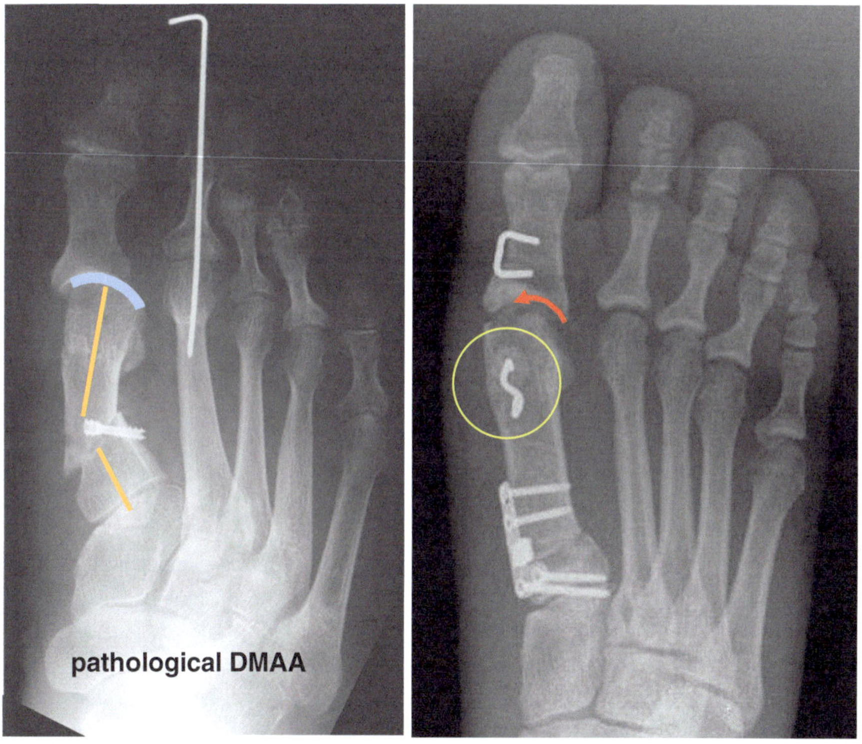

Fig. 1.2 Due to the angulation created within the metatarsus with the base osteotomy, the DMAA increases (**a**) and might need a correction with a distal retrocapital osteotomy (Reverdin osteotomy) (**b**)

retracted, forming a stiff "wall" that prevents the metatarsal head from returning to its proper position over the sesamoids. To allow the metatarsal head to move laterally back into place, this "wall" must be opened. A longitudinal incision in the MP1 capsule—just dorsal to the lateral sesamoid—is usually sufficient, eliminating the need for a more extensive lateral release in most cases.

Achieving a long-lasting correction requires more than just realigning the first ray and great toe; a balanced tension between the lateral and medial soft tissues around the MP1 joint is essential. This balance should be achieved and confirmed intraoperatively using the "push up" test (Fig. 1.17b). During this test, the forefoot is held in a simulated weight-bearing position by lifting it from the plantar side. The great toe should remain well-aligned on the metatarsal head, without a tendency to drift into valgus or varus, and the medial sesamoid should be positioned directly beneath the medial aspect of the metatarsal head.

In severe cases where the lateral soft tissues are very contracted, merely opening the lateral MP1 capsule might not allow for adequate reduction. High residual lateral tension can leave the first metatarsal inadequately reduced over the sesamoids, with the hallux still deviating in a valgus position during the "push up" test. In these instances, shortening the first metatarsal by 3–5 mm can effectively release the lateral tension and allow a stable, physiological correction of the deformity. However, caution is needed: shortening the first metatarsal may cause the lesser metatarsals—especially the second—to become relatively longer, which can lead to metatarsalgia. If necessary, additional shortening procedures on the second and even the third metatarsals should be considered. For subluxed lesser MP joints, an intra articular shortening Weil osteotomy is preferred, while a diaphyseal shortening osteotomy (with plate fixation) is recommended if the joint is healthy to avoid iatrogenic stiffness.

If these measures still do not allow for tension-free reduction of the MP1 joint, a tenotomy of the lateral branch of the flexor hallucis brevis tendon at its distal attachment on the lateral sesamoid may be performed. In very rare cases where even this does not suffice, a salvage procedure can be considered: reattaching the plantar portion of the incised MP1 capsule to the metatarsus with a non-resorbable suture. This fixation must be tensioned carefully to maintain the metatarsal head over the sesamoids and counteract the lateral pull while still allowing full range of motion of the MP1 joint. Such an approach, however, increases overall joint tension and should only be used as a last resort when all other attempts to correct the deformity have failed.

All these soft tissue procedures should be performed in a stepwise manner until a satisfactory reduction is achieved. Simply tightening the medial capsule in an attempt to correct any residual deformity—when the metatarsal head is not properly positioned over the sesamoids and lateral tension remains high—may provide temporary improvement, but it is likely to fail over time and should not be considered as a solution.

Location of Deformity Correction: Distal Versus Proximal

Deciding where to correct a bunion deformity—distally or proximally—is commonly based on the intermetatarsal and metatarsophalangeal angles. However, in our opinion, the width of the first metatarsal is the most reliable indicator for determining the level of correction.

Distal Procedures

With distal procedures, the osteotomized fragment of the first metatarsal is shifted laterally until it forms a physiological angle with the second metatarsal. Preoperative weight-bearing radiographs help estimate how much translation is needed. If this lateral shift still leaves enough overlapping bone for stable fixation with the proximal metatarsal, a distal osteotomy is viable. If not, the fragment cannot be securely fixed, and a more proximal correction becomes necessary.

The potential for lateral translation depends not only on the intermetatarsal angle between the first and second metatarsals but also on the width of the first metatarsal. A wider metatarsal allows for greater translation while maintaining sufficient bone overlap for stable fixation. For instance, a bunion with only a slight increase in the intermetatarsal angle may not be suitable for distal correction if the first metatarsal is narrow. Conversely, even severe deformities might be corrected distally if the first metatarsal is wide enough (Fig. 1.3). Additionally, the type of distal procedure (with the scarf osteotomy offering more correction than the classical chevron, for example) and the surgeon's expertise are critical factors.

Proximal Correction: Base Osteotomy Versus TMT1 Fusion

When distal procedures cannot achieve adequate realignment, proximal corrections are indicated. These techniques address the deformity at its apex and are powerful enough to correct even the most severe cases of metatarsus primus varus. Since hallux valgus is marked by a medial shift/rotation of the first metatarsal—originating at its base at the TMT1 joint—the most logical correction is at or near this joint (Fig. 1.4).

Proximal metatarsal osteotomies, however, are performed slightly distal to the true apex. This can result in less physiological alignment and may lead to pathological angulation at the osteotomy site, along with an increased distal metatarsal articular angle (DMAA) (Fig. 1.2). In severe cases, an additional retrocapital osteotomy (such as the Reverdin osteotomy) might be necessary. In contrast, TMT1 fusion provides a larger surface for bone healing, offers more room for stable osteosynthesis with screws or plates and doesn't have an influence on the DMMA.

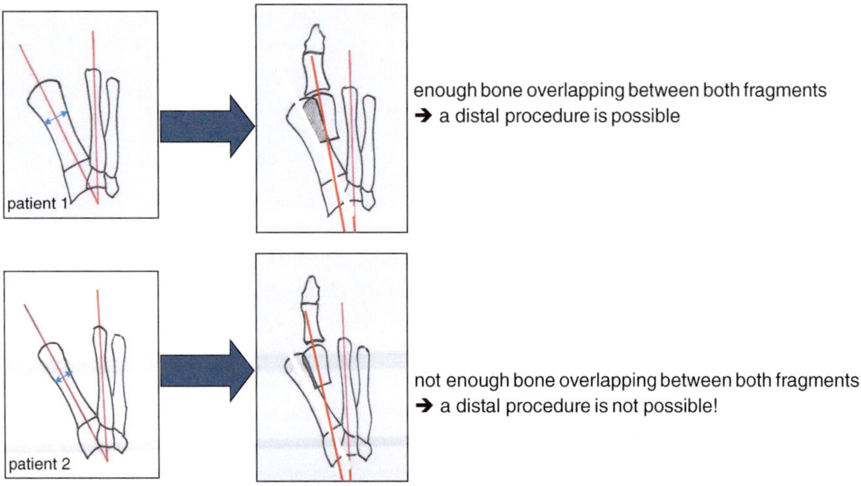

Fig. 1.3 The first metatarsus of patient 1 is wide enough to provide a sufficient overlapping surface between both metatarsal fragments once the distal fragment has been translate to a position which brings the IM 1-2 angle back to a normal value. A distal procedure is therefore possible for him. Patients 2 exhibits exactly the same IM 1-2 angle than patient 1 but his first metatarsal is narrower and leaves not enough bone overlapping between both fragments after reduction of the IM angle 1-2. A distal procedure is for him not possible

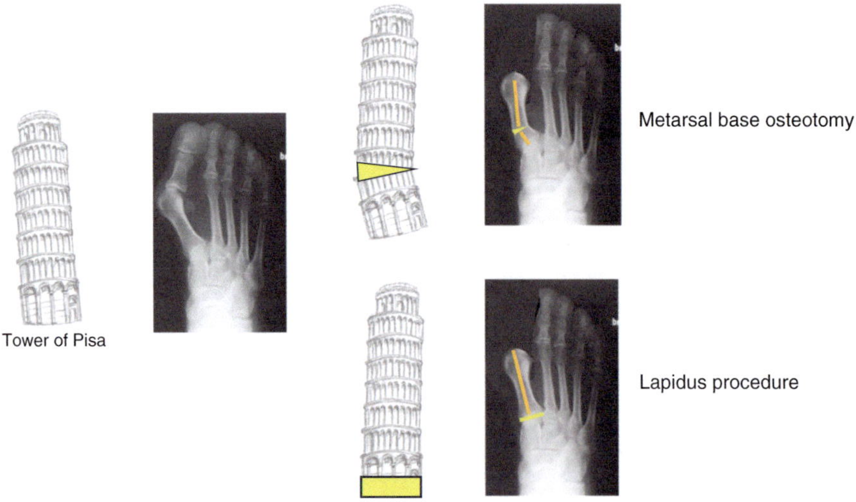

Fig. 1.4 The metatarsus primus correction is more pyhsiological if performed at the first metatarsophalangeal joint

Hallux Valgus Surgery and Hindfoot Valgus

When planning hallux valgus surgery, it is essential to consider the alignment of the hindfoot. A significant hindfoot valgus may need to be addressed alongside the bunion correction. The first metatarsal acts as a long medial "arm" that supports the foot. Repositioning this "arm" without correcting an associated pes plano-valgus (flatfoot) can weaken medial support and exacerbate the flatfoot deformity. Even if the pes plano-valgus is asymptomatic, correcting it—with a medial slide, calcaneal osteotomy or other appropriate measures—should be considered to ensure a balanced and long-lasting surgical outcome.

Scarf Osteotomy

Principle

The scarf osteotomy, first described 1991 [10], is a Z-shaped cut through the first metatarsal that creates two bone fragments—a distal and a proximal fragment. The distal fragment is shifted laterally until the metatarsus primus varus deformity is fully corrected (Fig. 1.5). For stable fixation, there must be sufficient overlap between the fragments; if the overlap is insufficient, a more proximal procedure is required as described above. Depending on its length, the scarf osteotomy may be classified either as a distal osteotomy or as a "full metatarsal" osteotomy.

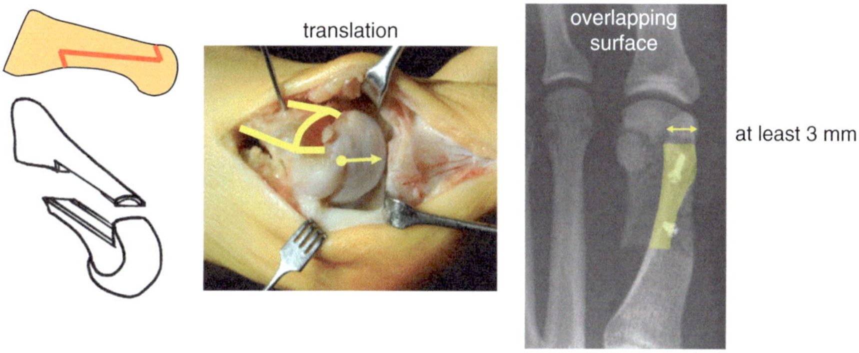

Fig. 1.5 Scarf is a Z shaped osteotomy which distal fragment is translated laterally to correct metatarsus primus deformity. The size of the resulting overlapping surface between both metatarsal fragments after full correction of the deformity determines if a scarf osteotomy is possible or not for a given deformity

Advantages

Stable Osteotomy

The Z-shape of the cut creates a "self-locking" effect at both the proximal and distal transverse cuts, forming a "three-points fixation" system along with the diaphysis (Fig. 1.6). The osteotomy's length can be adjusted to increase the overlapping surface area, thereby enhancing stability and healing. Additionally, the longitudinal cut typically extends into the dense cancellous bone of the metatarsal head, providing robust fixation that allows for full weight-bearing in a postoperative shoe with minimal risk of secondary displacement.

Preserved Blood Supply

Because the procedure leaves the plantar soft tissues attached to the distal fragment, the blood supply to this fragment and especially to the metatarsal head remains largely intact. This significantly reduces the risk of complications such as head necrosis and pseudarthrosis.

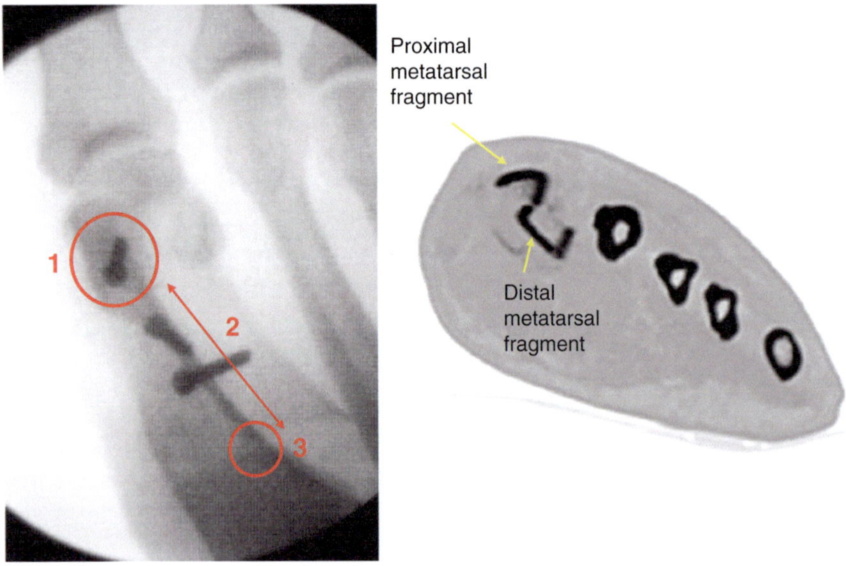

Fig. 1.6 The "3 points of fixation" system of the scarf: (1) distal self-locking z shaped transverse osteotomy in dense cancellous bone of the metatarsal head, (2) long diaphyseal support and (3) proximal self-locking z shaped transverse osteotomy. The CT shows the overlapping between proximal and distal metatarsal fragments in a case with maximal lateral translation of the distal metatarsal fragment

Powerful Correction

When performed as a long osteotomy, the scarf technique becomes a "full metatarsal" osteotomy capable of correcting even severe deformities (Fig. 1.1). Its length also facilitates metatarsal shortening when needed. Furthermore, with metatarsal shortening, the overlapping surface between the proximal and the distal fragment increases (Fig. 1.7), allowing for greater lateral translation.

Indications

A scarf osteotomy is indicated when at least 3 mm of overlapping bone can be achieved between the distal and proximal fragments at the level of the distal transverse osteotomy (Fig. 1.5). The longer the osteotomy, the greater the overlap surface and subsequent stability. In our experience, over 90% of hallux valgus deformities can be effectively corrected with a scarf osteotomy—using the long version for more severe cases.

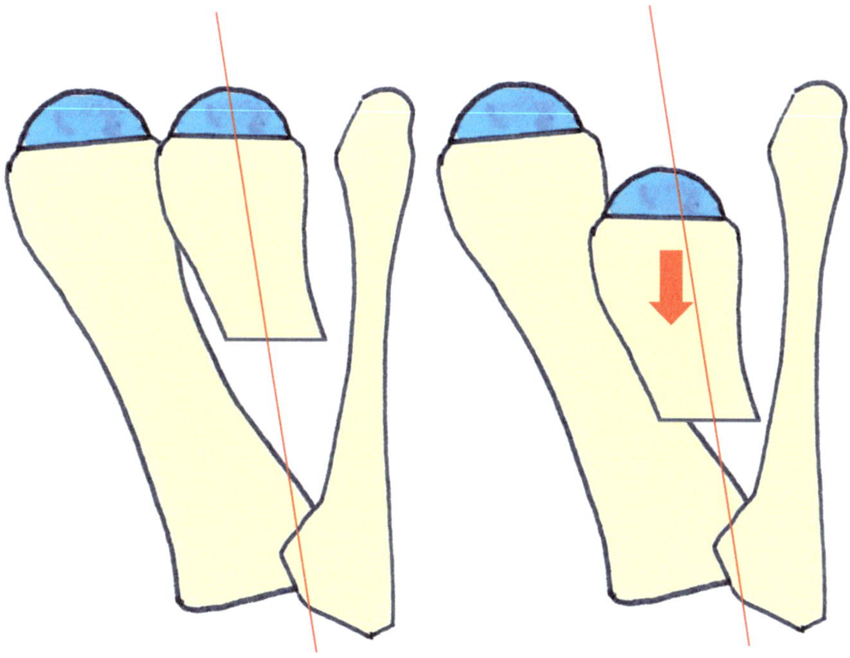

Fig. 1.7 Metatarsal shortening increases the overlapping surface between proximal and distal metatarsal fragments for a same amount of lateral translation of the distal fragment and increases therefore even more the correction potential of scarf osteotomy

Surgical Technique

Set-Up

The patient is positioned supine and after receiving an ankle block the procedure is performed under a supramalleolar tourniquet, which is usually well tolerated.

Approach

Incise the skin longitudinally along the medial side of the MP1 joint. Dissect carefully soft tissues off the articular capsule—taking care to avoid injury to the dorso-medial sensory nerve of the big toe. Incise the capsule in line with the skin incision and detach soft tissues from the dorso-medial aspect of the metatarsus along the planned osteotomy length. Preserve the plantar soft tissues to maintain the blood supply to the distal metatarsal fragment (Fig. 1.8). Pay special attention to the artery running from the plantar-medial posterior metatarsal neck into the metatarsal head to prevent metatarsal head necrosis.

Lateral Soft Tissue Release

Detach extensively soft tissues from the dorsal aspect of the proximal phalanx to be able to sublux the proximal phalanx plantar and gain a good access to the lateral-plantar part of the MP1 joint (Fig. 1.9). Introduce a knife blade between the metatarsal head and the sesamoids to reach the lateral part of the joint (Fig. 1.10). Incise then longitudinally the lateral capsule, just dorsal from the lateral sesamoid. Since it is not always possible to completely visualize the lateral MP1 joint, this step must sometimes be performed blindly, by knife palpation. This step “opens” the MP1 joint at the lateral side, enabling the metatarsal head to return to its physiological position over the sesamoids.

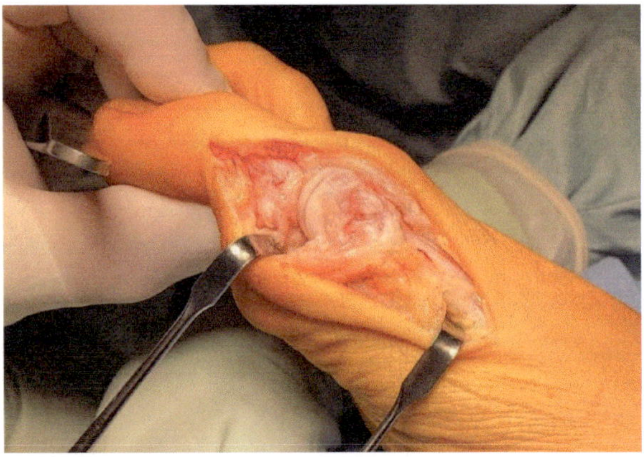

Fig. 1.8 Plantar soft tissues are left attached to the plantar aspect of the distal metatarsal fragment to keep its blood supply as intact as possible

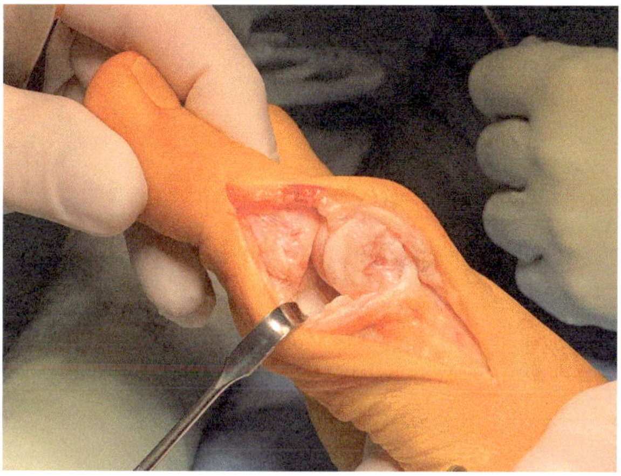

Fig. 1.9 The dorsal soft tissues of the proximal phalanx base have been extensively detached to allow plantar subluxation of the big toe and give access to the latero-plantar part of the MP1 joint for the lateral release

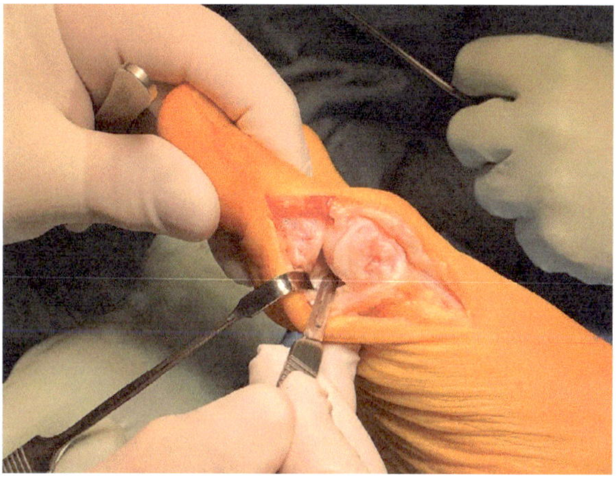

Fig. 1.10 The lateral MP1 joint is longitudinally incised, just over the lateral border of the lateral sesamoid

Osteotomy

Longitudinal Cut (Figs. 1.11a, b)

Using an oscillating saw, begin by cutting only the medial cortex to verify the direction of the osteotomy before completing it.

Start at the junction where the dorsal one-third meets the plantar two-thirds of the metatarsal head. This will leave more bone distal from the osteotomy and provide more hold for the distal screw.

Extended the osteotomy proximally to the point where the dorsal two-thirds meet the plantar one-third. This will leave a larger bone bridge on the proximal fragment dorsal from the transverse cut, at the potential breaking point.

Complete the cut through the lateral cortex, keeping the saw blade parallel to the floor to maintain the metatarsal head's level (Fig. 1.11b). If a slight plantar

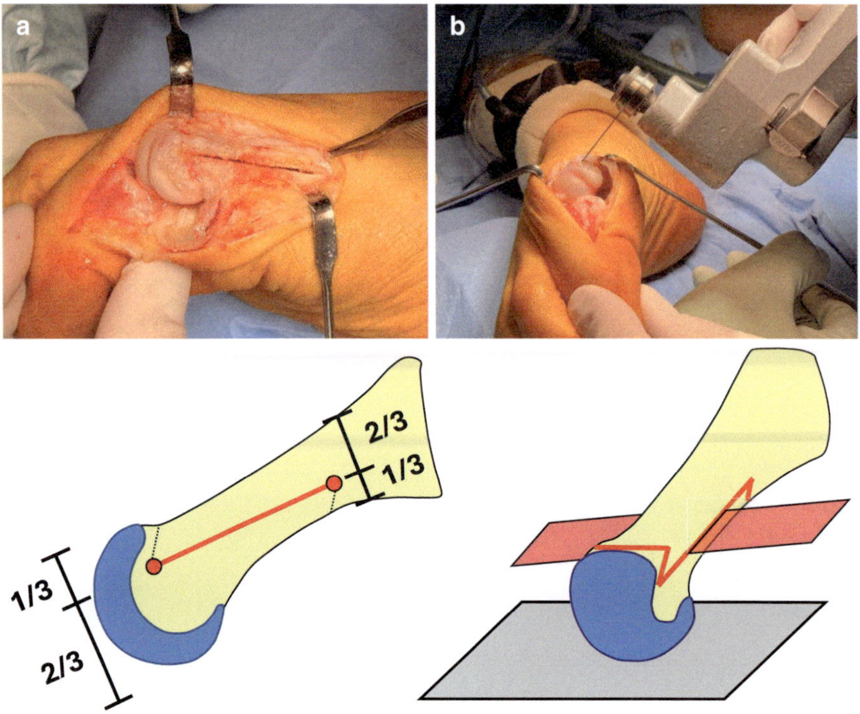

Fig. 1.11 (**a**, **b**) Longitudinal cut. The plane of the cut is parallel to the plane of the ground or slightly inclinated from medio-dorsal to lateroplantar if some degree of metatarsal head plantarisation is required

displacement is needed to correct an elevated head and increase the load on the metatarsal head, then the cut can be inclined from medial-dorsal to plantar-lateral. Remember that the amount of plantar displacement is proportional to the osteotomy's inclination and to the amount of translation. Avoid a too pronounced osteotomy's inclination which will create a significant bony step distal between both fragments.

Transverse Cuts (Figs. 1.12a–c)

The orientation of the transverse cuts affects the final length of the metatarsal. Cuts made perpendicular to the axis of the second metatarsal maintain length (Fig. 1.12c), whereas cuts angled distally (the angle with the longitudinal cut is greater than 90°) lengthen, and those angled proximally (the angle with the longitudinal cut is smaller than 90°) shorten the metatarsal.

If the transverse cuts are not perpendicular to the 2nd metatarsal long axis, the length variation depends not only on the angle formed by the transversal and the longitudinal cuts directions but also on the amount of translation. The more the distal metatarsal fragment is laterally translated, the bigger the impact will be on the

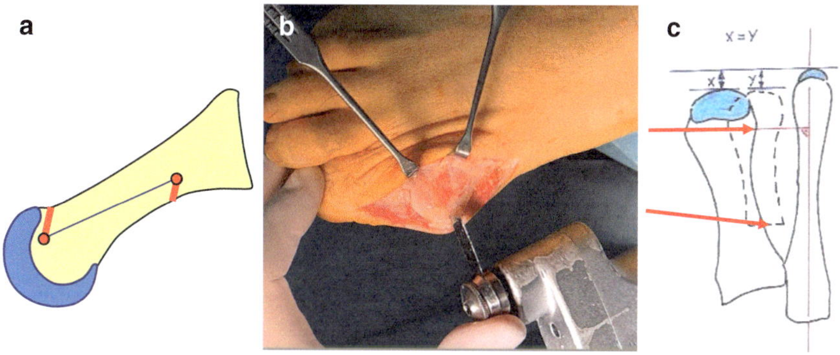

Fig. 1.12 (**a–c**) Tranverse cuts. The distal cut is running perpendicular to the axis of the second metatarsus if first metatarsal length should remain identical. This cut's direction is usually following the border of the cartilage. The proximal cut is performed stricly parallel or slightly divergent to the distal one. It should never be performed convergent to the distal one, since this would block the lateral translation of the distal fragment

metatarsal length. Since the effective amount of translation performed to achieve the needed bunion correction is only exactly known during the surgery, it is not possible to determine precisely in advance the amount of metatarsal shortening which will be achieved with a given oblique transverse cut. To shorten the metatarsus, it is therefore preferable to perform the transverse cuts perpendicular to the second metatarsus long axis and to perform parallel cuts some millimeters away from the first cuts, leaving two equal wide bone segments to be removed (Fig. 1.13). Some 1–2 mm should be added to the bone segments width because of the bone loss resulting from the saw cuts to determine the exact amount of metatarsal shortening resulting from this procedure.

In most cases, the metatarsal length should not be changed. Never lengthen the first metatarsal since lengthening increases the pressure at the metatarso-phalangeal joint, causes potential joint pain and increases the risk of valgus- and varus deformity. Consider a first metatarsal shortening when the lateral metatarso-phalangeal tension is too high, preventing the great toe from being reduced with a well-balanced tension around the MP1 joint.

Perform first the distal transverse cut. Place the osteotomy just behind the dorsal metatarsal head cartilage (Fig. 1.12a–c) and orientate it perpendicularly to the long axis of the second metatarsal. This direction usually follows the border of the metatarsal head cartilage (Fig. 1.12b, c). If you don't feel confident with the direction of your cut, place a K-wire into the first metatarsal and check with fluoroscopy its perpendicularity to the second metatarsal long axis. Perform then the transverse cut parallel to the direction of the K-wire (Fig. 1.12c).

Perform then the proximal transverse cut, after having detached the plantar soft tissues at the level of the cut. Make sure to perform this second transverse osteotomy at least perfectly parallel or better slightly divergent from the first one (Fig. 1.12c), since a convergent cut would block the lateral translation of the distal metatarsal fragment.

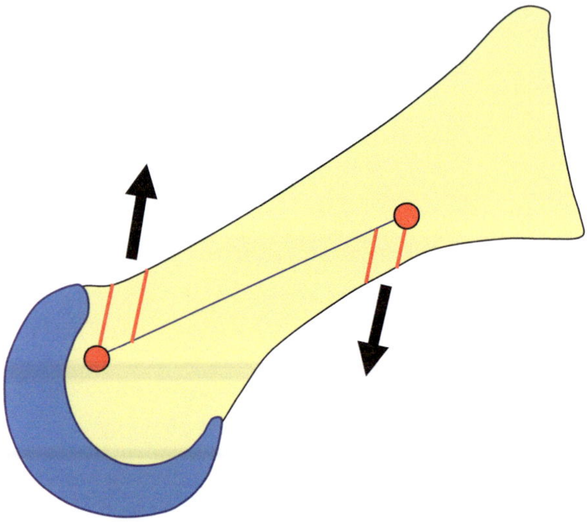

Fig. 1.13 Metatarsal shortening by removal of 2 bone segments on each transverse cut. The width of those segments which of some 1–2 mm should be added (bone loss due to the saw blade) gives the amount of metatarsal shortening

Distal Metatarsal Fragment Translation and Temporary Fixation

The distal metatarsal fragment is now totally separated from the proximal one and ready to be translated laterally. However, to be able to translate it freely, it is important to release also the soft tissues attached on the lateral side of the metatarsal. Introduce a knife blade through the longitudinal osteotomy and run it through laterally the soft tissues along the osteotomy from proximal to distal (Fig. 1.14a). Once you have reached the distal point of the longitudinal osteotomy, turn the blade towards dorsal and cut vertically the soft tissues ("L-shape" cut) to achieve this release (Fig. 1.14b). Without performing this release, you might have difficulty translating the distal metatarsal fragment laterally at the place you need to have it.

Translate the distal fragment by pushing it laterally while pulling at the same time the proximal fragment with a clamp in the opposite direction ("pull and push" maneuver, Fig. 1.15). Push the distal fragment as much as needed, making sure to leave an overlapping surface between both fragments of at least some 3 mm at the level of the distal cut (Fig. 1.5). Make sure to translate the distal fragment without rotating it to ensure bone contact with the proximal fragment all along the osteotomy, especially at the level of the proximal transverse cut.

Temporarily fix both metatarsal fragments with a 1.25 mm K-wire. Place the K-wire some 10 mm proximal from the distal transverse cut and introduce it from the proximal fragment into the distal fragment in a way which will leave enough room for the distal screw to be introduced later (Fig. 1.16a–c). Clamps are better not used for this temporary fixation since they need to be pushed through the plantar soft tissues and contribute to devitalization of the distal metatarsal fragment.

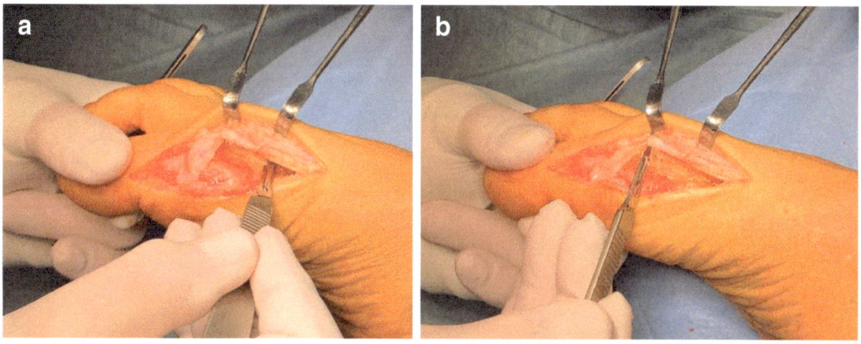

Fig. 1.14 (**a**, **b**) Additional lateral soft tissue release to allow free lateral translation of the distal metatarsal fragment

Fig. 1.15 The "pull and push" maneuver to translate laterally the distal metatarsal fragment

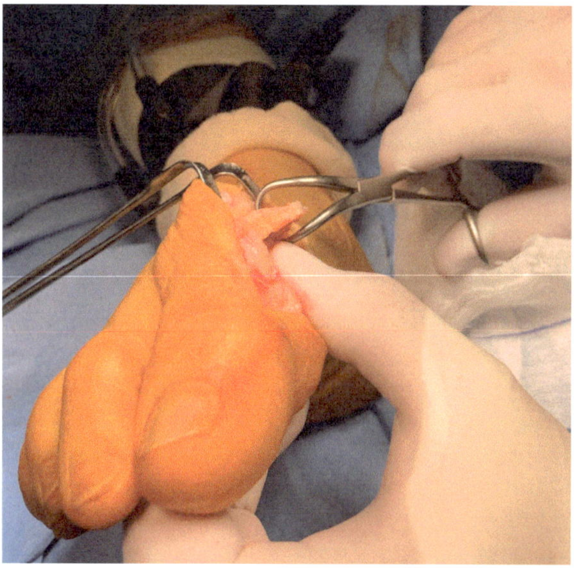

Check the reduction with the "push up" test: hold the forefoot in a simulated weight-bearing situation by pushing it from the plantar aspect with one hand in the position it would have if it stood on the floor (Fig. 1.17a, b). The metatarsophalangeal joint should be reduced, the metatarsal head should be centered on both sesamoids—the medial sesamoid is seen under the medial part of the metatarsal head (Fig. 1.17c)—and the tension around the MP1 joint should be well balanced, without the tendency for the great toe to shift in a valgus or varus position. The achieved reduction should always be checked clinically (Fig. 1.17b, c) as well as radiologically (Fig. 1.18a, b) before proceeding to the definitive osteosynthesis with screws.

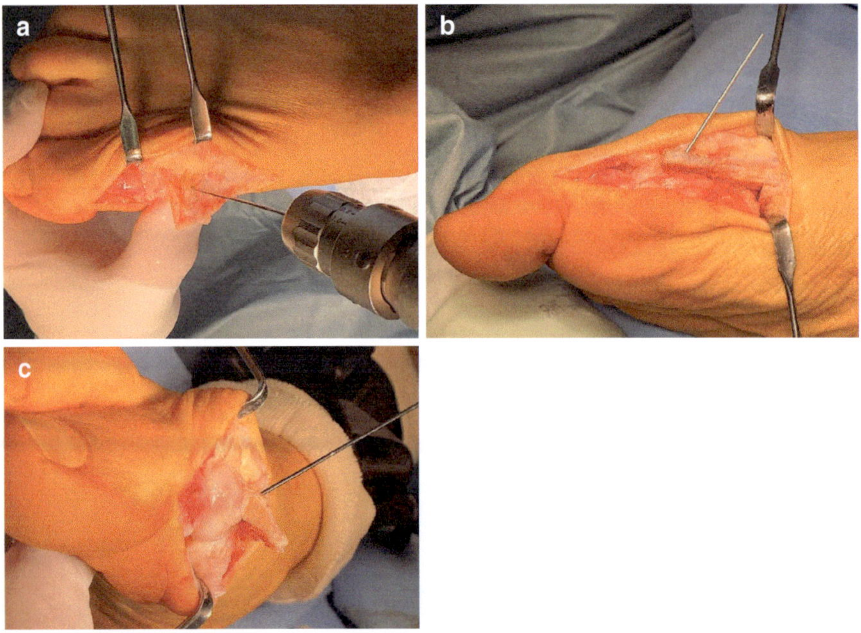

Fig. 1.16 (**a–c**) Temporary fixation of lateraly translated distal metatarsal fragment with a 1.25 mm K-wire. Enough room should be left lateral from the K-wire to place later the distal screw

If the metatarsal head is not reduced on the sesamoids, work again on the lateral soft tissues to allow it to move over the sesamoids to its physiological position. If the metatarso-phalangeal joint tension is too high laterally and the great toe tends to shift back into a valgus deformity, consider shortening the first metatarsal by some millimeters (Fig. 1.13). Metatarsal shortening allows in most cases to balance the lateral-medial forces around the metatarso-phalangeal joint. If this is still not sufficient and if additional shortening would be excessive, then consider a tenotomy of the flexor hallucis brevis lateralis at its attachment at the distal sesamoid pole. If the reduction is still not achieved, consider then the tenotomy of the adductor tendon.

As a rule, don't expect anything from tensioning the medial MP1 capsule on itself to complete an insufficient reduction. If forces around the MP1 joint are left unbalanced before closing the articular capsule medially, medial capsule tensioning will not solve the problem, and the valgus deformity will most probably recur.

Osteosynthesis

Fix the distal fragment with two 2.0 mm cortical screws (Figs. 1.19 and 1.20). Place the first screw into the proximal metatarsal fragment laterally, some 5–10 mm proximal from the distal transverse cut. Aim the metatarsal head, staying as medial as

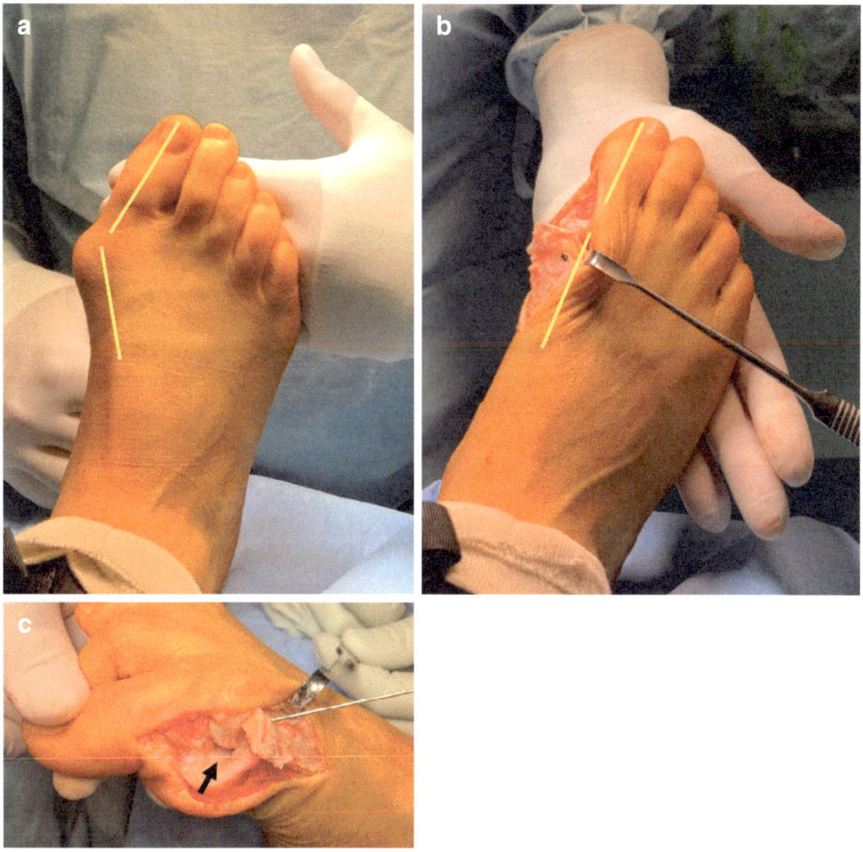

Fig. 1.17 (**a–c**) After lateral soft tissue release and lateral translation of the distal metatarsal fragment, under simulated weight bearing condition ("push up" test), the great toe should be reduced on the metatarsal head, without tendency to shift back into valgus position (**b**). The metatarsal head is perfectly reduced on both sesamoids, the medial sesamoid is seen just under the medial part of the metatarsal head (**c**)

possible but being far enough from the medial pseudo-exostosis for its later resection.

If the lateral translation of the distal fragment has been maximal, the overlapping surface between both fragments will be small and it might be difficult and risky to place a screw too distal where the bone bridge on the proximal metatarsal fragment will be very narrow (after later medial resection). Insert therefore the screw more proximal and aim for a bi-cortical fixation, proximal from the plantar aspect of the metatarsal head. Make sure to be far enough from the metatarsal head to avoid any conflict between the screw and the sesamoid, since bi-cortical screws usually go over the cortex.

Place the second screw some 5–10 mm distal from the proximal transverse cut, orientating it relatively obliquely to reach the laterally displaced distal fragment

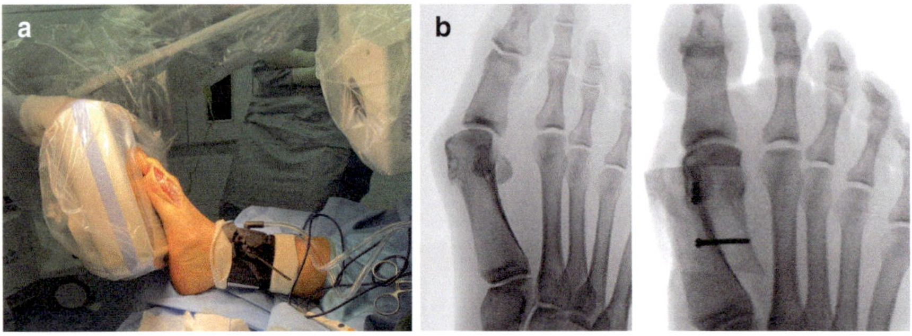

Fig. 1.18 The reduction is also checked with fluoroscopy before proceeding to the definitive osteosynthesis with screws (**a**, **b**) (which as been taken in this picture after the screw fixation) show what should be achieved if the correction has been successfully achieved: the metatarso-phalangeal joint is reduced, the metatarsus primus varus has been completely corrected with a physiological intermetatarsal angle 1-2 and the metatarsal head lying well centered on both sesamoids. Notice that the capsule is medially still open at this stage, attesting that a good balances of forces has been achieved around the MP1 joint

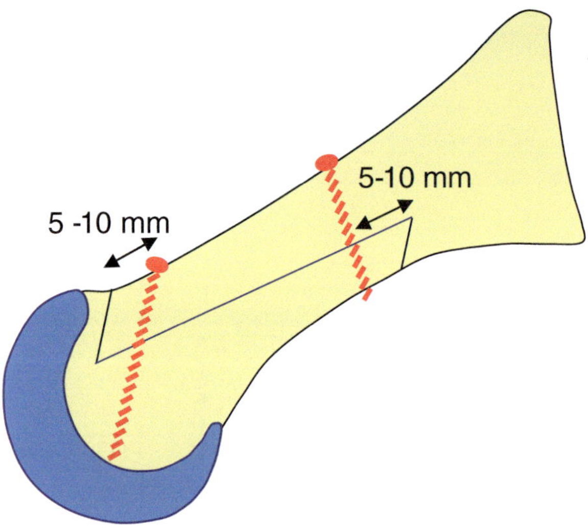

Fig. 1.19 Osteosynthesis with 2 compression screws

(Figs. 1.19 and 1.20). Remove the K-wire. If the fixation appears to be not strong enough (osteoporotic bone quality), place a third screw in-between the first two screws (Fig. 1.1). If the fixation is exceptionally still not strong enough or if you get into trouble with the screw fixation, use a long T-shaped plate and place it on the medial side of the metatarsus. Fix the one end on the metatarsal head, and the other one on the metatarsal base, at least some 20 mm more proximal than the proximal transverse cut.

Resect the medial metatarsal part with an oscillating saw. Start distally to resect the medial pseudo-exostosis. Extend the cut proximally through the proximal fragment by aiming the most medial point of the proximal transverse cut (Fig. 1.21a).

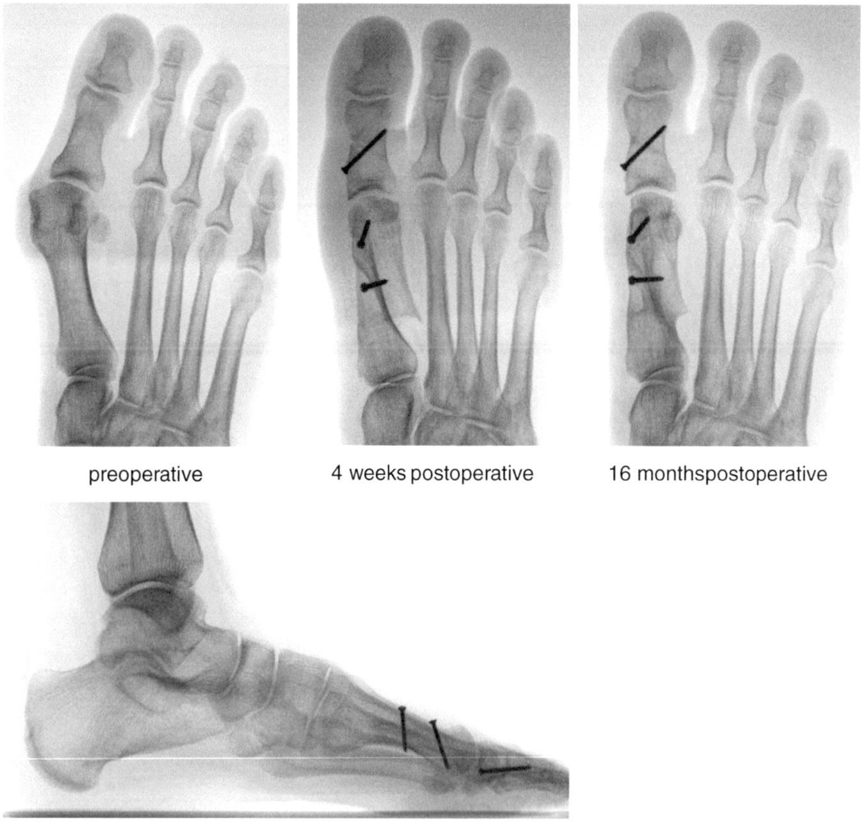

Fig. 1.20 Scarf osteotomy. Note the relative important first metatarsal width, which allows large lateral translation of the distal metatarsal fragment while still leaving a good overlapping contact area with the proximal metatarsal fragment. The radiographs 16 months postoperative show a nice remodelling of the first metatarsal with good first ray realignment

Resect the extra-articular medial part of the base of the great toe's phalanx, in line with the previously performed cut on the metatarsal head and obtain one single resection plane (Fig. 1.21b).

Resect the dorso-medial corner on the metatarsal head since it is sometimes a little prominent and subject to cause some pain in narrow shoes (Fig. 1.21c).

Akin Osteotomy

A significant residual valgus deformity can be observed even if the metatarso-phalangeal joint is perfectly reduced. The deformity is located within the proximal phalanx of the great toe, distal from the now reduced metatarso-phalangeal joint ("hallux interphalangeus"). This extra articular deformity should also be addressed to obtain a better balance of the forces acting on the great toe, to prevent potential

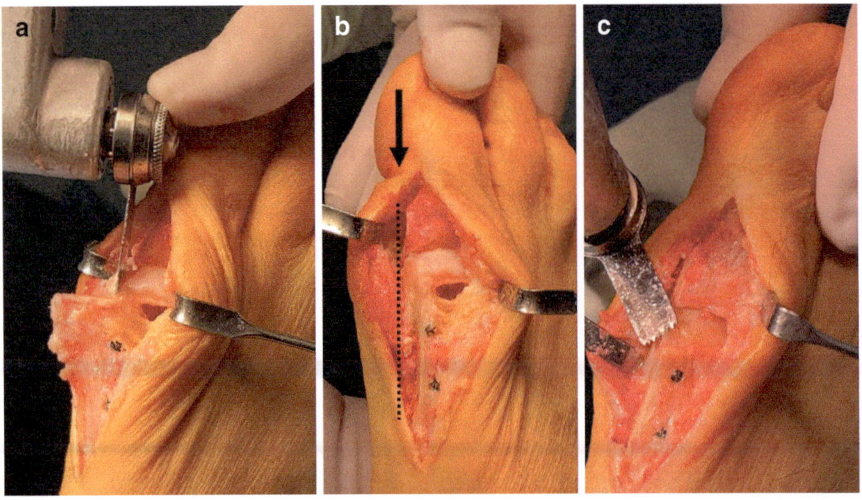

Fig. 1.21 (**a–c**) Medial bone resection. The osteotomy starts distal and runs from the medial pseudo-exostosis to the most medial point of the proximal transverse cut (**a**). The extra-articular part of the base of the proximal phalanx is then resected in line with the plane of the previously performed osteotomy on the metatarsus (**b**). The dorso-medial corner on the metatarsal head is also resected to prevent any mechanical conflict with narrow shoes (**c**)

painful conflict between the great toe and the second toe and to improve the cosmetic result of the surgery. Leave however a minimal residual interphalangeal valgus which corresponds to normal anatomy.

Extend the medial incision distally. Detach soft tissues from the dorsal and from the plantar aspect of the proximal phalanx. Protect flexor and extensor longus tendons with two retractors. Perform an oblique osteotomy running from distal medial to proximal lateral, taking care of leaving the lateral cortex intact (Fig. 1.22a). The lateral end of the osteotomy should be placed just distal from the base of the phalanx to allow soft closing of the osteotomy. Perform a second cut to obtain a medial based wedge (Fig. 1.22a, b). The width's wedge is determined according to the needed correction. Close the osteotomy, weakening the lateral cortical bridge with the oscillating saw if needed.

Place a screw starting at the cortico-cancellous junction (Fig. 1.22c) and aim it as perpendicular as possible to the osteotomy line. The cortical border will provide a good support to the head of the screw. Check the correction and adapt it if needed. If the correction is excessive, just open the osteotomy as much as needed. The gap resulting from this opening can be filled with part of the resected bone or even left open if the gap is not exceeding 2–3 mm. If the correction is insufficient, proceed to an additional resection to increase the size of the wedge.

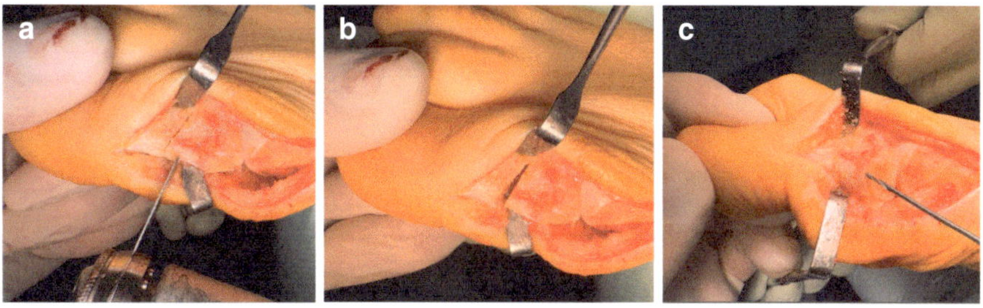

Fig. 1.22 (**a**–**c**) Akin osteotomy. The apex of the wedge is located just distal from the lateral base of the proximal phalanx (**a**, **b**). The cortex on the border of the previously resected area of the proximal phalanx provides a good support for the screw's head (**c**)

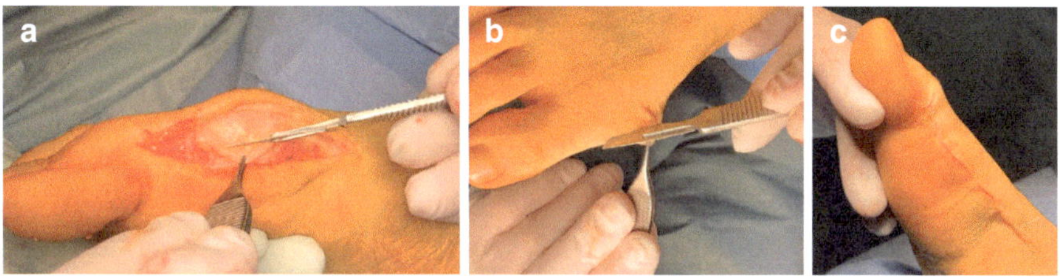

Fig. 1.23 Resection of the excesss of joint capsule (**a**) and skin (**b**) and skin closure with intracutaneous resorbable suture (**c**)

Closure

Because the medial soft tissues have been chronically stretched, simply suturing them end-to-end may leave a gap that fills with hematoma and edema. Therefore, resect any excess capsule and skin to allow for a tight closure (Fig. 1.23a, b). If the capsule is thin, consider reinforcing it by suturing the dorsal capsule flap on the plantar one to reinforce the medial capsule.

Don't rely on capsule reefing on itself to complete an unsatisfactory reduction of the first metatarsal on the sesamoid and/or to correct an unbalanced lateral-medial tension around the metatarso-phalangeal joint. The capsule is not able to keep this "forced" reduction over time and hallux valgus deformity will mostly recur. A long-lasting reduction needs imperatively anatomical reduction and balanced forces around the great toe. If this has not been achieved before closing the capsule, work again on the reduction and/or soft tissue tension.

Close the skin with an intracutaneous resorbable suture which will give the best cosmetic results (Figs. 1.23c and 1.24b). Since a good balance of forces around the great toe has been yet achieved, the bandage should be applied in a way which keeps the great toe in its correct position, leaning against the second toe (Fig. 1.25).

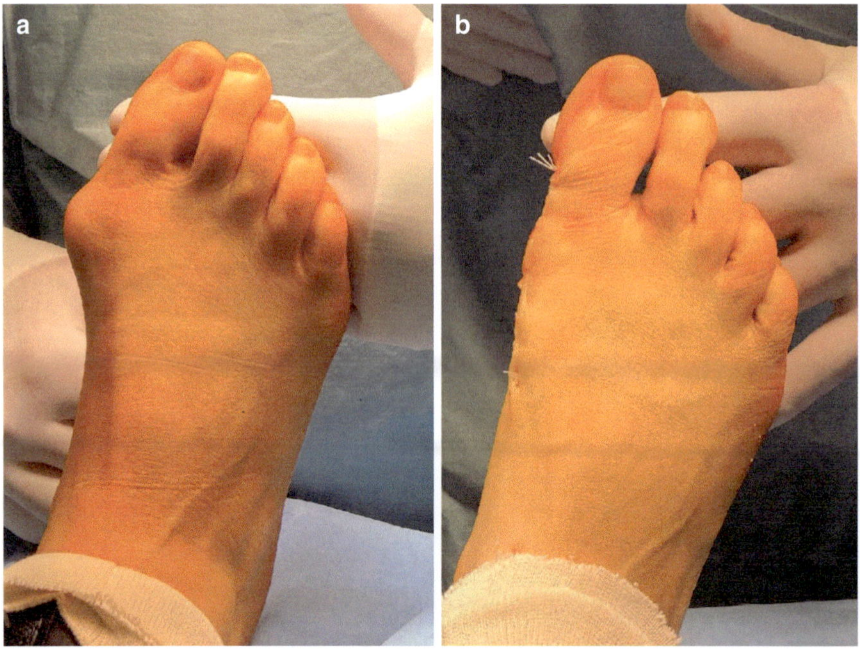

Fig. 1.24 Forefoot immediatly before (**a**) and after surgery (**b**)

Fig. 1.25 The bandage is applied with slight compression on the big toe which should lean against the second toe

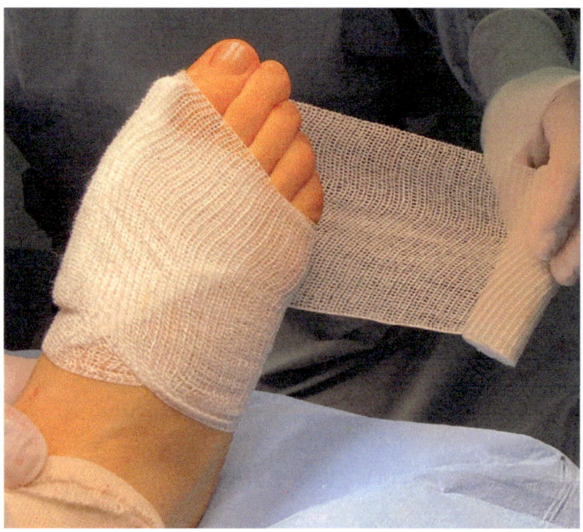

Bandages holding the big toe in a varus position (so called "Hohmann bandage") are contra-indicated since they keep the great toe out of the balance in a varus direction and are generally the expression of the surgeon's inability to have achieved a good hallux valgus correction.

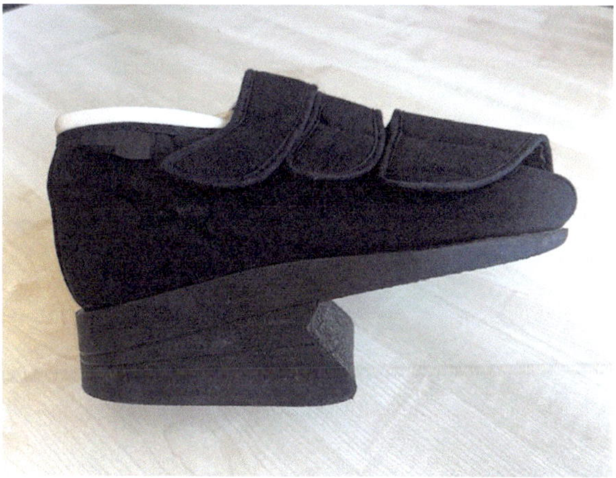

Fig. 1.26 Postoperative shoe with negative heel ("Barouk Type 1" shoe, Romans Industrie)

Postoperative Care

Patients are allowed full weight-bearing on the operated foot from the first postoperative day, provided they use a special postoperative shoe with a heel wedge that shifts load to the hindfoot (Fig. 1.26). A radiographic evaluation is performed at 4 weeks to verify osteosynthesis stability before transitioning to regular footwear. Physiotherapy is prescribed only if needed to improve the range of motion or if the patient experiences insecurity during ambulation.

Lapidus Procedure

First Ray Instability

First ray instability in hallux valgus surgery is often a subject of debate [11]. There are two versions of the Lapidus procedure—the "original" (Fig. 1.27a) and the "modified" (Fig. 1.27b)—and the choice between them depends largely on the stability of the first ray.

Functional Instability

Forefoot stability during gait is partly maintained by the "windlass mechanism" (Fig. 1.28) [12]. Here, the strong plantar fascia, which originates at the calcaneus and inserts into the flexor tendons, wraps around the metatarsal head as the big toe dorsiflexes during toe-off. This wrapping action pulls the calcaneus toward the toes, raising the midtarsal arch and stabilizing the first ray.

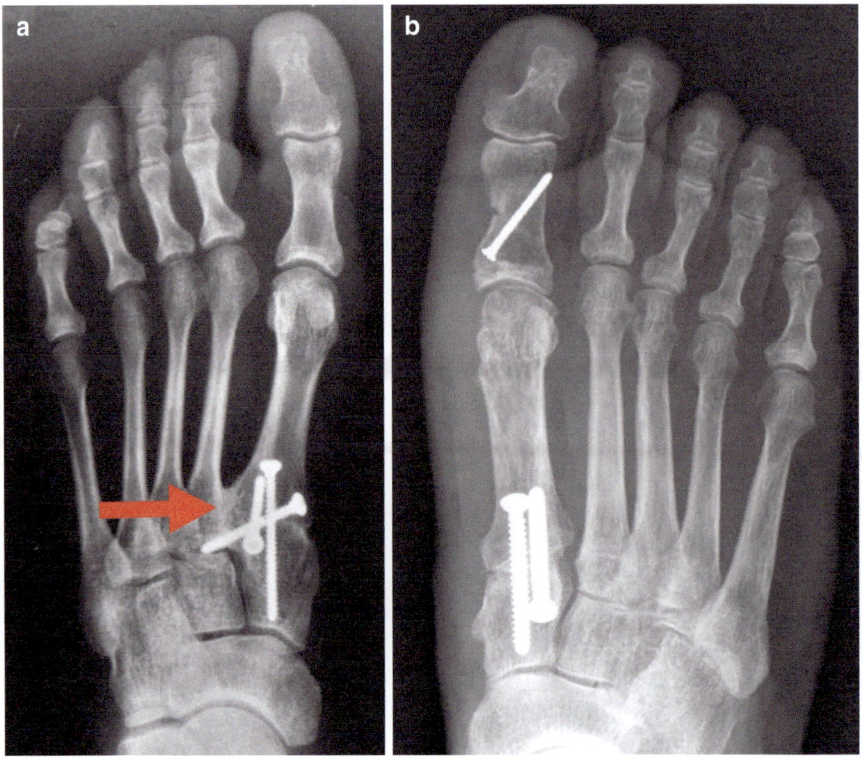

Fig. 1.27 The 2 Lapdidus procedures: the “original” one which fixes the first tarso-metatarsal and the first ray with the second one (**a**) and the “modified” Lapidus which fuses only the tarso-metatarsal joint (**b**)

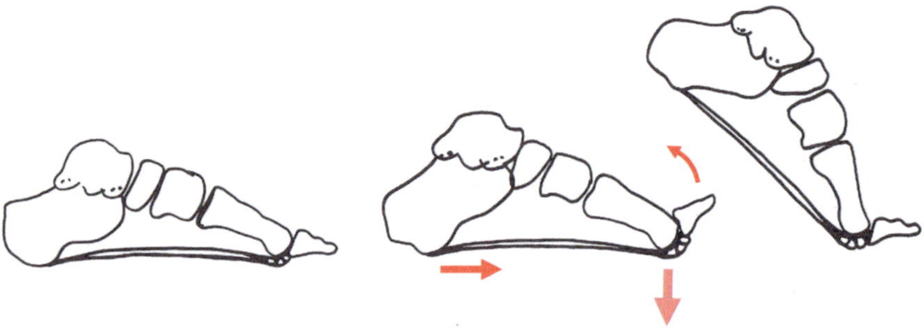

Fig. 1.28 The windlass mechanism

In hallux valgus, however, the portion of the plantar fascia under the first ray is malpositioned relative to the MP1 joint. It fails to wrap properly around the metatarsal head during toe-off, and the windlass mechanism fails, resulting in a functional instability of the first ray [13]. Realigning the first ray through hallux valgus surgery—regardless with what kind of procedure—typically restores the windlass mechanism and thus stabilizes the ray without the need for stabilizing arthrodesis at the Lisfranc.

Structural Instability

In some patients—especially those with joint hyperlaxity or severe pes planovalgus—a true, or "structural," instability exists around the first tarsometatarsal (TMT1) joint. This instability is not solely due to an isolated TMT1 issue (often evidenced by a plantar gap on lateral weight-bearing radiographs) but is frequently associated with failure of the Lisfranc ligaments connecting the first and second rays [14]. In these cases, TMT1 fusion alone is typically insufficient, and additional arthrodesis between the first and second rays (the "original" Lapidus) is required.

Distinguishing between functional and structural instability is key, as isolated TMT1 fusion (the modified Lapidus) may not adequately stabilize a structurally unstable first ray.

Principle

The Lapidus procedure addresses the metatarsus primus varus deformity at its origin—the TMT1 (first tarso-metatarsal or first Lisfranc) joint. Due to the nature of the Lapidus procedure, addressing the deformity at its base, it allows for correction of any degree of deformity. In cases of "functional" instability, realigning the first ray with a TMT1 fusion (modified Lapidus) is generally sufficient. However, when "structural" instability is present, additional bony fixation between the first and second rays ("original" Lapidus) is necessary to achieve lasting stability.

Indications

Because the Lapidus procedure is technically more demanding and poses greater challenges for recovery than distal procedures, it is primarily indicated for severe metatarsus primus varus deformities that cannot be adequately corrected by distal procedures and for cases with true, structural first ray instability.

Surgical Procedure

MP1 Joint

Begin the procedure at the MP joint with an approach similar to that used in the scarf osteotomy. Resect the medial pseudo-exostosis early at this step to better control metatarsal rotation after resection of the TMT1 joint.

TMT1 Joint

Make a dorsal incision over the TMT1 joint while carefully protecting the medial branch of the superficial peroneal nerve (Fig. 1.29a). Incise the retinaculum lateral to the extensor hallucis longus tendon (Fig. 1.29b) to expose the joint (Fig. 1.29c). When performing a modified Lapidus, preserve the Lisfranc ligaments between the first and second rays to avoid inducing instability.

Resection cuts should be made obliquely—from dorsal-distal to plantar-proximal—mirroring the natural inclination of the joint (Fig. 1.30a). Except in cases with a long first metatarsal, minimize resection to prevent excessive shortening that could lead to transfer metatarsalgia, while ensuring enough bone is removed to permit secure fusion.

Using a long saw blade (the TMT1 joint is approximately 30 mm deep (Fig. 1.30c)), start the cut on the first metatarsal base. The cut should remain perpendicular to its long axis, and should follow its joint plan (Fig. 1.30b).

Resect the articular surface of the first cuneiform. The cut should be perpendicular to the second metatarsal axis, leaving a lateral based wedge. To minimize the metatarsal shortening, start the cut medially on the cartilage (Fig. 1.30b).

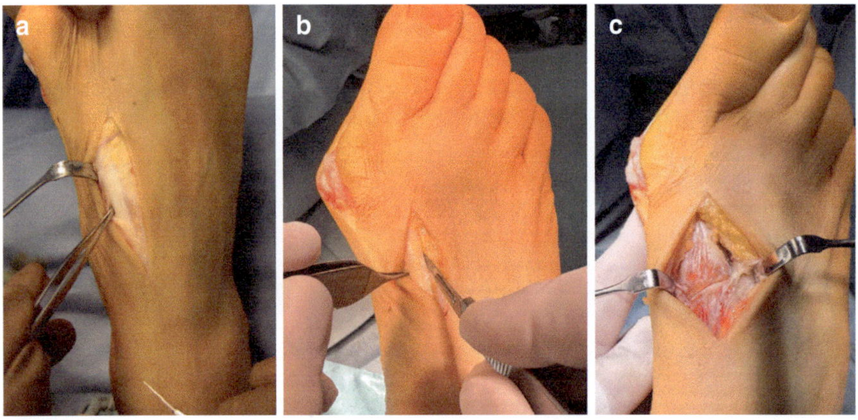

Fig. 1.29 Surgical approach to the first metatarso-phalangeal joint. The ramus medialis of nervus peroneus superficialis is identified and medially retracted (**a**). Retinaculum is incised lateral from extensor hallucis longus tendon (**b**). The TMT1 joint is exposed (**c**)

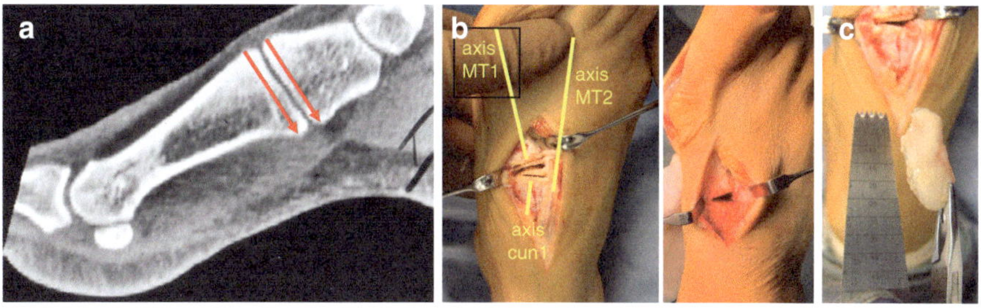

Fig. 1.30 First metatarso-phalangeal joint resection. The dorso-plantar joint resection is performed obliquely, following the joint inclination (**a**). The cuts on first metatarsal basis and first cuneiforme are orientated perpendicular to their axis (**b**). The first metatarso-cuneiform joint is some 30 mm deep and ist resection needs therefore a long saw blade (**c**)

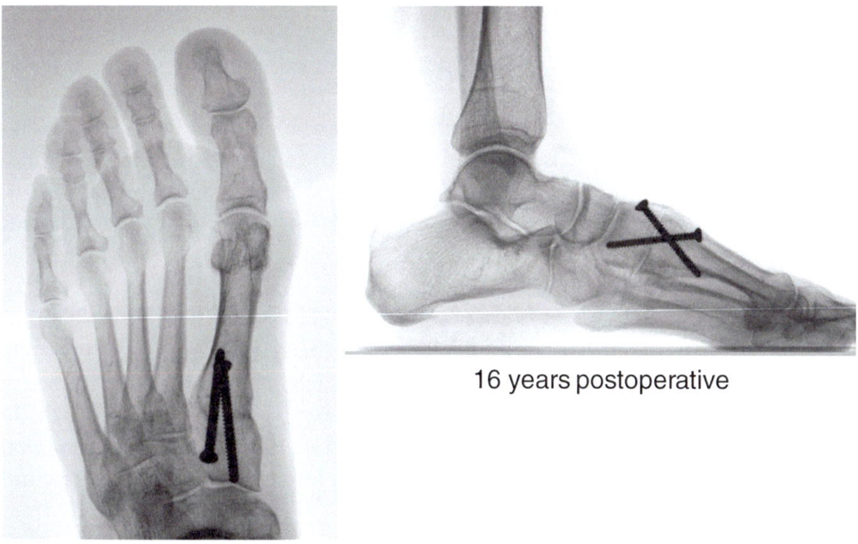

Fig. 1.31 Screw position for "modified" Lapidus. Both compression screws are inserted some 20 mm away from the joint. The lateral screw is bicortical and reaches the lateral part of the metatarsal basis. The medial screw runs medial from the lateral one and is positioned as horizontal as possible for optimal joint compression

Fixation for "Modified" Lapidus

After the classical Lapidus technique became popular in the 1990s, various advanced fixation methods (screws, plates, aiming devices…) emerged. However, using two well-placed compression screws remains an effective and safe method (Fig. 1.31).

Manually reduce the first metatarsal to the cuneiform by squeezing the forefoot and gently pushing the first metatarsal laterally using your thumb on the medial aspect of the first metatarsal head (where the pseudo-exostosis has been resected) (Fig. 1.32a). Make sure that the very plantar part of the resected joint has been

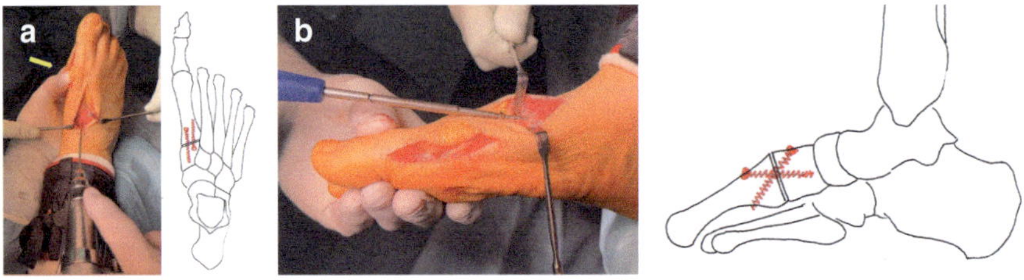

Fig. 1.32 (**a**, **b**) TMT1 is reduced by pushing the metatarsal head laterally while the first compression screw is inserted laterally into the cuneiform, some 20 mm proximal to the joint and directed distally to the plantar part of the metatarsal base. The second compression screw is inserted medial from the first screw, as horizontal as possible, some 20 mm distal to the joint

completely removed to ensure that the resected articular surfaces will be well opposed. If the lateral portion of the first metatarsal base impinges on the second metatarsal, resect 2–3 mm of its lateral aspect to achieve proper centering. Maintain correct rotational alignment by using the resected medial pseudo-exostosis under your thumb as a reference (Fig. 1.32a).

With the first metatarsal held in position, insert a 3.5 mm cortical compression screw from the dorso-lateral aspect of the first cuneiform, approximately 15–20 mm proximal to the joint, into the plantar part of the first metatarsal base (Fig. 1.32a). This screw compresses more specifically the lateral and plantar joint surfaces. Next, insert a second 3.5 mm cortical compression screw from the dorsal midpoint of the first metatarsal base, about 15–20 mm distal from the joint, aimed medially from the first screw into the first cuneiform. This screw should be placed as horizontally as possible (Fig. 1.32b), almost perpendicular to the resected joint surface, to provide best possible compression. This screw will also provide rotational stability. In weak osteoporotic bones, it may extend through the first naviculo-cuneiform joint (totally stiff and therefore not a problem) into the navicular bone to ensure stability. Countersink deeply the holes for the screws heads to prevent longitudinal fracture when tightening the screws (Fig. 1.33).

Check clinically and radiologically the achieved reduction as for the scarf. With the "push up" test, the intermetatarsal 1-2 angle should be reduced, the first metatarsal head should be centered on both sesamoids, the great toe should rest on the metatarsal head without tendency to drift into valgus or varus (Fig. 1.34).

If TMT-1 joint resection leads to significant shortening of the first metatarsal relative to the second metatarsal, consider a shortening procedure on the second metatarsal. For subluxed second MP joint, a Weil osteotomy is preferred; if the joint is healthy, a midshaft osteotomy is advised to avoid destabilization and stiffening of the metatarsophalangeal joint.

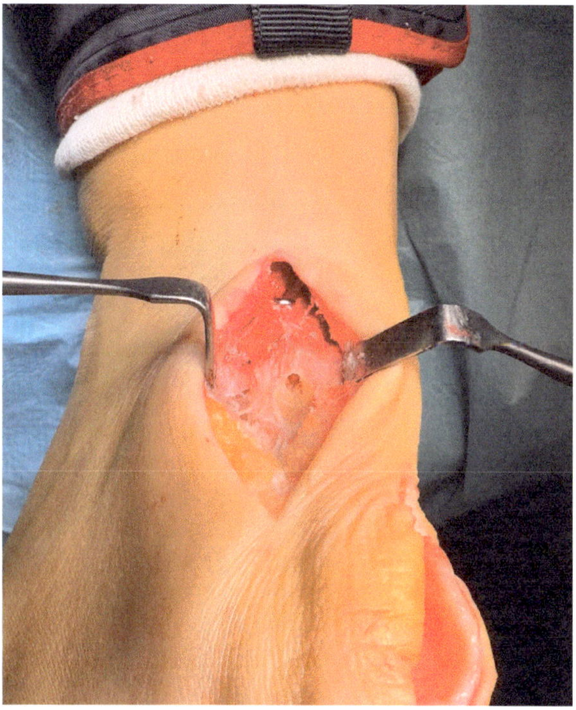

Fig. 1.33 Generous countersink to leave enough room for the screws heads and prevent longitudinal fractures when tightening the screws. Well countersinked screw's head also prevent potential mechanical conflict with shoes

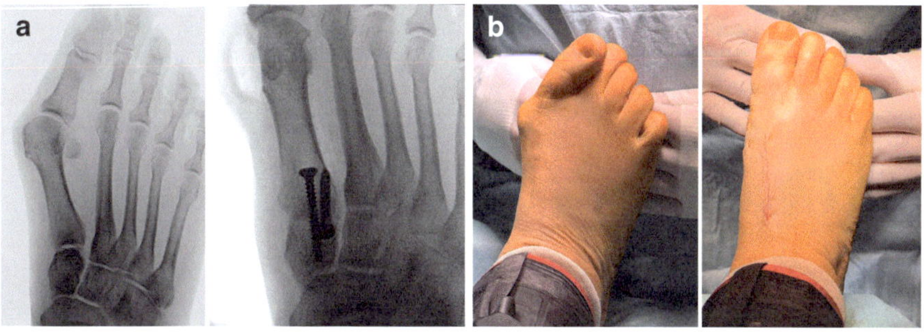

Fig. 1.34 The foot is brought on the plateform of the C-arm to check under simulated weight-bearing (s. Fig. 1.16) the reduction of the first metatarsal on both sesamoids with corresponding reduction of the intermetatarsal angle 1-2. Screw position and length is checked simultaneously (**a**). On the right side, corresponding clinical finding immediatly pre- and postopertive (**b**)

Fixation for "Original" Lapidus

The original Lapidus extends the modified technique by additionally fixing the first ray to the second ray (Figs. 1.27a and 1.35). This approach requires meticulous positioning in the sagittal plane because, once fixed, the first ray becomes rigid. Overcorrection in plantar flexion may cause metatarsalgia under the first metatarsal head, while excessive dorsal extension could lead to transfer metatarsalgia under the second or third metatarsals.

After preparing the TMT1 joint as described above, remove the cortex from the lateral surface of the first metatarsal base and the corresponding surface of the second metatarsal. Because achieving bone consolidation is more challenging at this level, extend the fixation to include the joint between the first and second cuneiforms. Preparation of this joint usually leaves a small gap (typically about 2 mm) which should be filled with cancellous bone, best harvested from the calcaneus.

Insert the first compression screw into the metatarso-cuneiform joint as described previously (running from proximal to distal). If this osteosynthesis is not yet stable enough, you may insert the second screw from the metatarsal into the cuneiform, as described previously. However, be aware that this second screw might make the placement of the screw which will fix the first metatarsal to the second ray difficult as it might be in its way.

Position now the first ray correctly in the sagittal plane (extension-flexion). Place yourself in front of the foot and hold the lesser metatarsals with one hand, as your other hand is holding the first metatarsal. Bring the first metatarsal head in the same plane as the second and third metatarsal heads. This adjustment is purely clinical. Once the first metatarsal position is felt as correctly placed, ask your assistant to insert a 1.4 mm K-wire from the medial cuneiform perpendicular into the second metatarsal base or into the intermediate cuneiform. Check again clinically the position of the first metatarsal in the sagittal plane, making sure that the first metatarsal head is lying in the same plane as the second and third metatarsal heads.

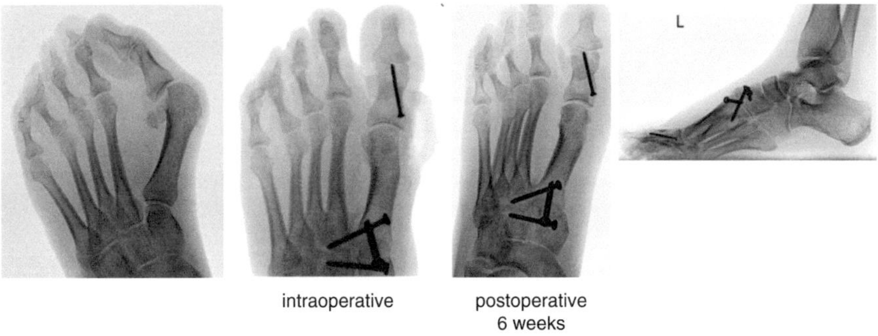

Fig. 1.35 "Original" Lapidus. Down Syndrom patient with severe "structural" first ray hypermobility. Two screws fixate the first to the second ray (metatarsus 1–2 and cuneiforme 1–2). Note the cancellous bone graft in-between both rays

Harvest some cancellous bone from the calcaneus through a small lateral approach and place it into the prepared areas in-between both metatarsals and both cuneiforms.

Squeeze the forefoot to abduct the first metatarsal in its correct position and drill the bone, starting from the metatarsal base some 15–20 mm distal from the joint line and ending into the second metatarsal base. Use a position screw technique which will allow you to control and maintain accurately the first metatarsal position regarding its angle with the second metatarsus (IM 1-2 angle). Check the intermetatarsal angle 1-2 with fluoroscopy. If this angle needs to be changed, remove the position screw from the second metatarsal, adapt the amount of abduction of the first metatarsal and reinsert the position screw into the second metatarsal in the new position. Repeat this step until you have reached a perfect first metatarsal alignment. Remove the K-wire.

Place now a 3.5 mm compression screw from the first cuneiform into the second one. Check with fluoroscopy the length of the screw which should stop at the second cuneiform.

Any additional procedures, such as an Akin osteotomy or further soft tissue management, are performed as previously described for the scarf osteotomy.

Postoperative Care

Traditionally, patients are advised to partially weight-bear with a walker for 6 weeks after a Lapidus procedure. However, the modified Lapidus—preserving mobility of the first ray in the sagittal plane—tolerates weight-bearing forces better. In cases of good bone quality and stable fixation, immediate full weight-bearing in a postoperative shoe with a heel wedge may be permitted for 6 weeks.

Radiographic evaluation is performed at 6 weeks postoperatively. Patients who undergo the modified Lapidus can transition from the walker or specialized shoe to comfortable full-weight-bearing footwear. In contrast, those who have the more rigid original Lapidus are advised to continue using a walker for an additional 2 weeks, gradually increasing the load on the operated leg until full weight-bearing is achieved.

Bunionette Deformity

Introduction

A bunionette is a deformity of the fifth ray similar to a bunion of the first ray. While both bone and soft tissue corrections might be considered in theory, the bunionette deformity is typically less severe in soft tissue contracture, making a bony procedure alone sufficient in most cases.

Bunionettes are classified into three types [15]:

- **Type 1:** Characterized by an enlarged lateral aspect of the fifth metatarsal head.
- **Type 2:** Marked by a lateral bowing of the distal metatarsal diaphysis.
- **Type 3:** Involves increased abduction of the fifth metatarsal, corresponding to an increased intermetatarsal angle between the fourth and fifth metatarsals.

Each type is addressed surgically with a tailored approach. Patients may also experience metatarsalgia beneath the fifth metatarsal head, often accompanied by hyperkeratosis, which should be evaluated and managed during the same procedure.

Surgical Technique

Set Up

The patient is placed in a supine position and receives an ankle block with light sedation. A supramalleolar tourniquet is applied.

Approach

Make a longitudinal skin incision along the axis of the fifth metatarsal, starting at the base of the proximal phalanx of the fifth toe. For a Type 1 deformity, extend the incision proximally up to the metatarsal head, whereas for Type 2 and Type 3 deformities, the incision is continued further to the proximal diaphysis.

Incise the metatarsophalangeal joint capsule longitudinally to expose the metatarsal head, and if the medial capsule is contracted, release it in a manner similar to that used in hallux valgus surgery.

Osteotomies

Resection of the Lateral Exostosis

Since metatarsal axes are physiological in bunionette type 1, resection of the lateral exostosis alone efficiently solves the problem. The resection is best performed with an oscillating saw and should be aligned to the lateral border of the metatarsal. Excise excess capsule and skin before closing the approach.

Medial Closing Osteotomy

This osteotomy is particularly adapted for the correction of bunionette type 2 since it corrects the deformity at its apex. However, rotational osteotomy can alternatively also be used for this purpose.

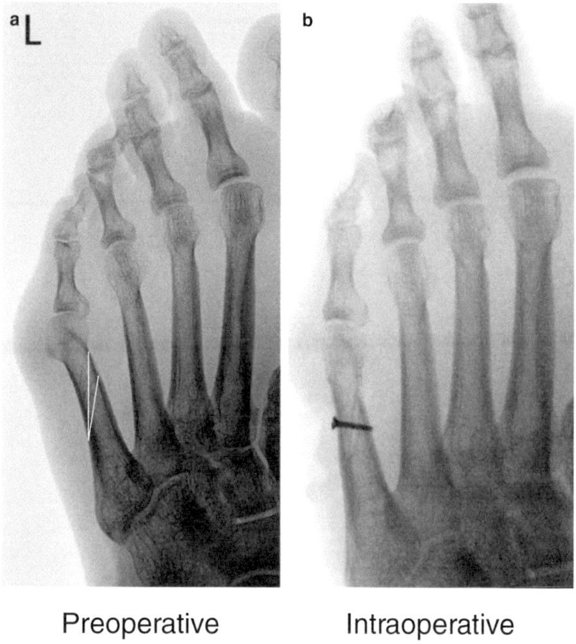

Fig. 1.36 (**a**, **b**) Bunionette deformity type 2. The correction is achieved by a medial closing wedge osteotomy centered on the bow of the deformity

Expose the dorsal surface of the metatarsal and remove from there a bone wedge. This wedge is placed in the bowing, it is oblique to the long metatarsal axis and its base is located medial distal (Fig. 1.36a). It is crucial to preserve the lateral cortex and to fashion the wedge long enough to improve stability and healing potential. Stabilize the osteotomy with one or two 2.0 mm cortical compression screws inserted from lateral to medial (Fig. 1.36b). Resect the lateral pseudo-exostosis of the metatarsal head. Excise excess capsule and skin before closing.

Rotational Osteotomy

This osteotomy is classically used to correct bunionette 3 deformities. Since this osteotomy also can allow dorsiflexion of the fifth metatarsal head if needed, it is also indicated for bunionette deformities associated with metatarsalgia.

Perform a long oblique osteotomy with an oscillating saw, starting just behind the articular cartilage at the top of the metatarsal head and extending to the plantar cortex at the level where the metatarsal begins to widen to form its base (Fig. 1.37a). Care must be taken not to extend the osteotomy too proximally (Fig. 1.37b), as the cut must exit through the plantar cortex.

Approximately 5–10 mm of the medial cortex is preserved proximally to maintain the stability of the distal fragment; cutting this cortex prematurely would lead to instability and complicate both the correction and fixation. If fifth metatarsal metatarsalgia is present, perform a second cut to remove a small distal based wedge

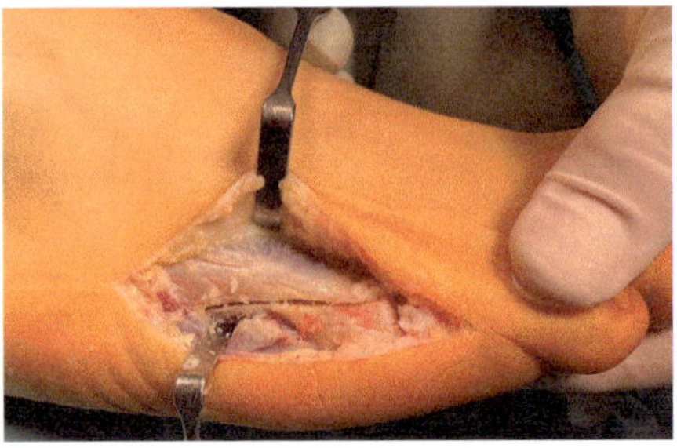

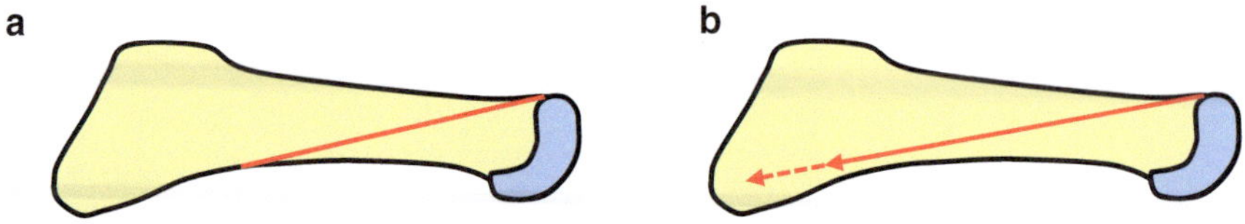

Fig. 1.37 Rotational osteotomy running from retrocapital dorsal through the cortex plantar proximal where the metatarsus begins to widen to build its base (**a**). The osteotomy should not run too proximal since it will not perforate the plantar cortex to be completed (**b**)

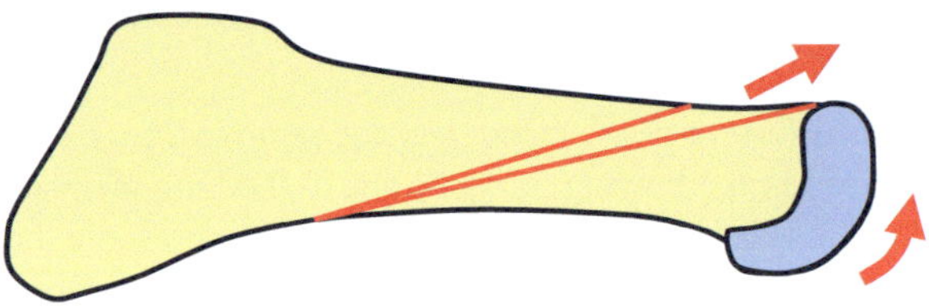

Fig. 1.38 Rotational osteotomy: to relief metatarsalgia, a second cut is performed to build a wedge which is removed, allowing extension of the metatarsal head

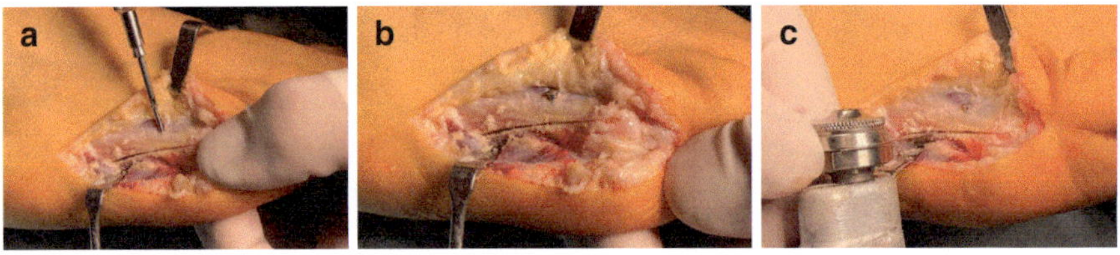

Fig. 1.39 Rotational osteotomy: fixation with a cortical compression screw inserted at the osteotomy midpoint, as perpendicular as possible to the osteotomy (**a**). The screw is not tighten (**b**) to allow to complete the osteotomy proximal on the medial aspect of the metatarsal (**c**)

(Fig. 1.38), thereby allowing dorsiflexion of the metatarsal head when the osteotomy is closed.

Insert a 2.0 mm cortical compression screw dorsally at about the midpoint of the osteotomy, running perpendicular to the cut (Fig. 1.39a). Don't tighten it yet (Fig. 1.39b) and subsequently cut the remaining medial cortex to complete the

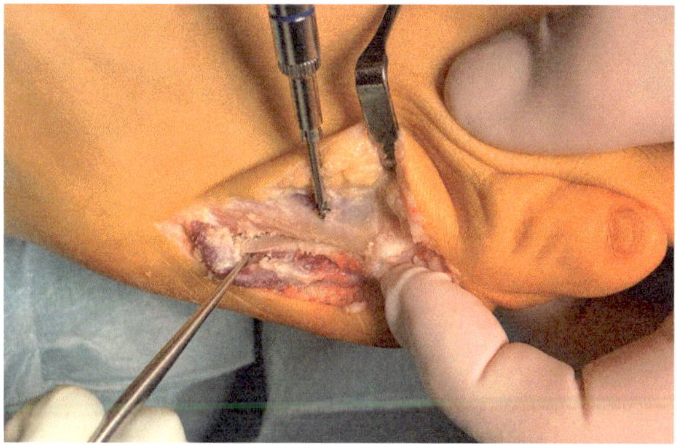

Fig. 1.40 Rotational osteotomy: the distal fragment is rotated around the untightened screw by pulling the distal fragment proximally with a small hook and by pushing at the same time the head medially

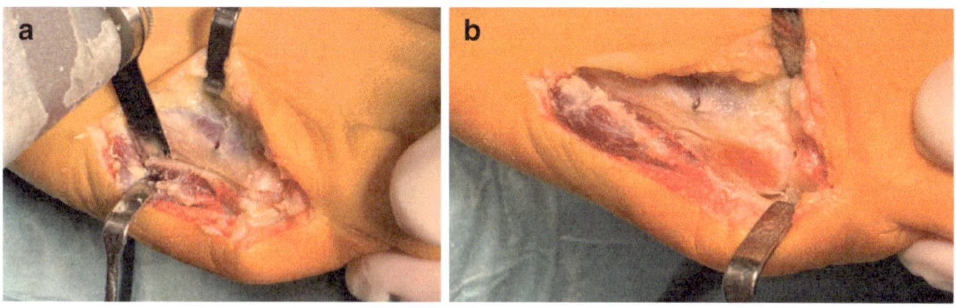

Fig. 1.41 Rotational osteotomy: after having tightened the screw, lateral bone excess is resected proximally (**a**) as well as the lateral pseudoexostosis of the metatarsal head (**b**)

osteotomy (Fig. 1.39c). Rotate the distal fragment medially around the screw until full correction of the bunionette is achieved. This rotation can be facilitated by grasping the proximal portion of the distal fragment on the plantar side with a small hook, pulling it laterally while pushing the metatarsal head medially (Fig. 1.40). Once proper alignment is confirmed, the compression screw is tightened, and if necessary, a second compression screw is added for increased stability. Resect the lateral protrusions from both the distal fragment (on its proximal aspect) (Fig. 1.41a) and the proximal fragment (on its distal aspect) as well as the lateral pseudo-exostosis of the metatarsal head with an oscillating saw (Fig. 1.41b).

Closure

Excise excess capsule and skin (Fig. 1.42a) and close the capsule without tension. Close the skin best with an intracutaneous suture to optimize the cosmetic result (Fig. 1.42b).

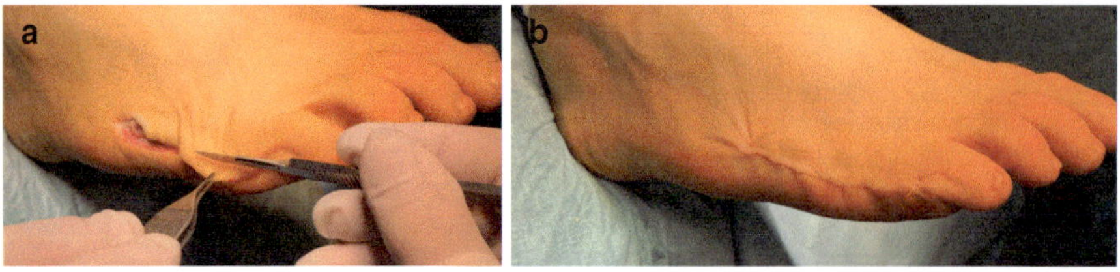

Fig. 1.42 Rotational osteotomy: the skin excess is resected (**a**) and the closure is performed with an intracutaneous suture for optimal cosmetic result (**b**)

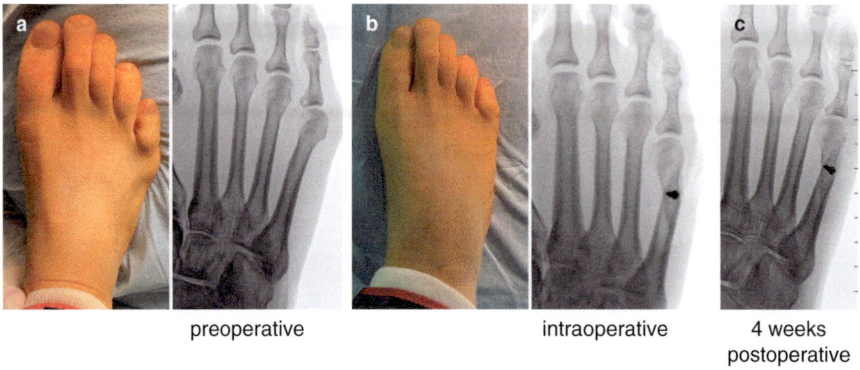

Fig. 1.43 (**a**–**c**) Rotational osteotomy: radiographs are taken preoperatively, intraoperatively and at 4 weeks postoperatively

Postoperative Care

Postoperatively, patients are allowed to bear full weight immediately in specialized shoes with heel wedge. A radiographic evaluation is performed at 4 weeks (Figs. 1.43a–c), after which patients may transition to standard, comfortable footwear, and physiotherapy is generally not required unless specifically indicated.

References

1. Lee HY, Lalevee M, Mansur NSB, Vandelune CA, Dibbern KN, Barg A, et al. Multiplanar instability of the first tarsometatarsal joint in hallux valgus and hallux rigidus patients: a case–control study. Int Orthop. 2022;46(2):255–63.
2. Fraissler L, Konrads C, Hoberg M, Rudert M, Walcher M. Treatment of hallux valgus deformity. EFORT Open Rev. 2016;1(8):295–302.
3. Robinson A, Limbers J. Modern concepts in the treatment of hallux valgus. J Bone Joint Surg Br. 2005;87(8):1038–45.

4. Agoropoulos Z, Efstathopoulos N, Mataliotakis J, Kokoroghiannis C, Karachalios G, Karras K, et al. Long-term results of first metatarsophalangeal joint fusion for severe hallux valgus deformity. Foot Ankle Surg. 2001;7(1):9–13.
5. Stevens BW, Anderson JG, Bohay DR. Hallux metatarsophalangeal joint fusion for the rheumatoid forefoot. Foot Ankle Clin. 2007;12(3):395–404.
6. Rippstein PF, Park Y-U, Naal FD. Combination of first metatarsophalangeal joint arthrodesis and proximal correction for severe hallux valgus deformity. Foot Ankle Int. 2012;33(5):400–5.
7. Axt M, Wildner M, Reichelt A. Late results of the Keller-Brandes operation for hallux valgus. Arch Orthop Trauma Surg. 1993;112:266–9.
8. Arnold H. The Akin procedure as closing wedge osteotomy for the correction of a hallux valgus interphalangeus deformity. Oper Orthop Traumatol. 2008;20:477–83.
9. Isham SA. The Reverdin-Isham procedure for the correction of hallux abducto valgus: a distal metatarsal osteotomy procedure. Clin Podiatr Med Surg. 1991;8(1):81–94.
10. B AII. Modified scarf bunionectomy: our experience in more than 1000 cases. J Foot Surg. 1991;30:609.
11. Symeonidis PD, Anderson JG. Original and modified Lapidus procedures: proposals for a new terminology. JBJS. 2021;103(4):e15.
12. Bolgla LA, Malone TR. Plantar fasciitis and the windlass mechanism: a biomechanical link to clinical practice. J Athl Train. 2004;39(1):77–82.
13. Fuller EA. The windlass mechanism of the foot. A mechanical model to explain pathology. J Am Podiatr Med Assoc. 2000;90(1):35–46.
14. Solomou G, Bilyy A, Tadikonda P, Gurdas B, Pasapula C. Diagnostic accuracy of clinical, radiological and device-driven tests for the detection of First Ray Instability: a systematic review. Foot. 2024;59:102080.
15. Shi GG, Humayun A, Whalen JL, Kitaoka HB. Management of bunionette deformity. J Am Acad Orthop Surg. 2018;26(19):e396–404.

Chapter 2
Surgery of the Lesser Toes

Karan Malhotra and Alexander Beer

Introduction

Lesser toe deformities are a common, yet deceptively complex pathology: almost a quarter of patients undergoing forefoot surgery will have some procedure performed on the lesser toes. [1] Despite the prevalence of lesser toe surgery, there is a surprising paucity of published outcomes data. Perhaps this is on account of the significant heterogeneity in presenting pathologies, and the myriad treatment options available. Until recently there were also few randomised controlled trials comparing techniques long considered established practice. As with much of foot and ankle surgery, there are a few pathologies which are encountered frequently, for which surgical treatment is relatively straightforward. In this chapter we discuss some of the surgical techniques available to the foot and ankle surgeon to treat deformities of lesser toes and present a strategy for assessing and managing pathology of the lesser toes.

Importance of Functional Anatomy of the Lesser Toes

In humans, the role of the toes is to share load with the metatarsal heads during gait [2, 3]. In a normal foot, this contact of the toes with the ground is a passive process, brought about by the plantar fascia [4]. In a well-functioning foot, there is also a harmony to the relative lengths of the metatarsals, which is often termed a metatarsal cascade or parabola [5–8]. Surgeons need to respect this parabola and the

K. Malhotra (✉) · A. Beer
Royal National Orthopaedic Hospital, Stanmore, London, UK
e-mail: a.beer@nhs.net

M. Bhatia (ed.), *Surgical Techniques of the Foot and Ankle*,
https://doi.org/10.1007/978-3-031-93742-2_2

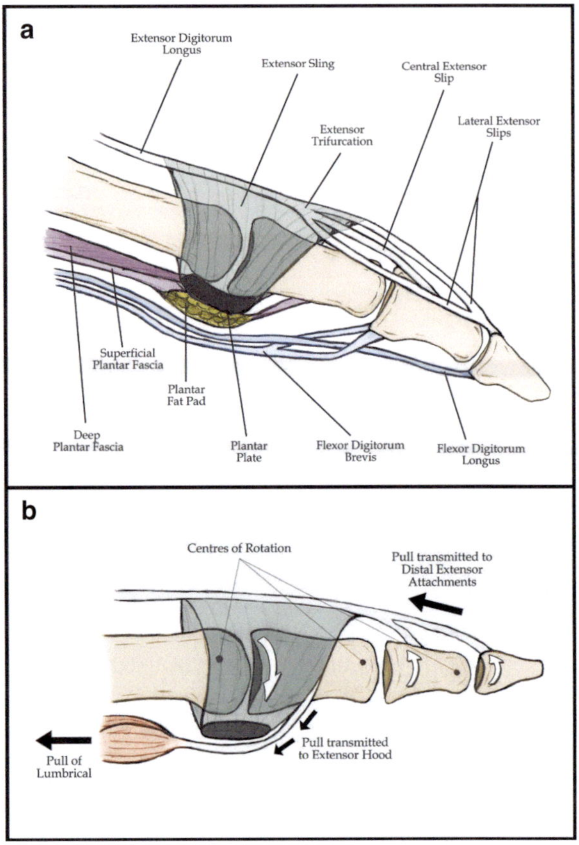

Fig. 2.1 The basic anatomy of the plantar plate, and extrinsic muscles of the lesser toes (**a**), and the anatomy and function of the intrinsic muscles (**b**). *Modified with permissions from Malhotra et al.* [9] *Creative Commons Licence 4.0 (CC BY-NC).* https://creativecommons.org/licenses/by-nc/4.0/

delicate balance between intrinsic and extrinsic muscles, ligaments constraining movements, and the plantar fascia in order to restore function. Figure 2.1 illustrates the key anatomical features of the structures supporting the lesser toes.

Pathology

Any pathology which interferes with the balance of the lesser toes will result in increased load to the metatarsal heads and consequent metatarsalgia. Although trauma can be a cause of acute failure of any of the supportive structures described, most often failure occurs over time due to abnormal load. This may be attributed to ill-fitting footwear, defunctioning of the first ray (such as with hallux valgus), inflammatory disorders, or neuromuscular disorders. Regardless of the cause, once an imbalance occurs, it does not self-correct, and it is inevitable that the deformity will progress. Although deformities often occur at multiple levels, the authors find it helpful to consider the pathology at discrete levels.

Deformity at the metatarsophalangeal joint (MTPJ) commonly occurs in the sagittal or axial plane. Sagittal plane deformity may be associated with plantar plate tears [10–12]. In some cases dorsal subluxation may occur with a tendency to deviate into varus / valgus (axial plane)—a **crossover toe** [10]. Common deformities at the interphalangeal joints (IPJs) are often associated with MTPJ deformity, and can be at the distal interphalangeal joint (DIPJ)—**mallet toe**, or at the proximal interphalangeal joint (PIPJ)—**hammer toe/claw toe**. We prefer to use the term 'claw toe' when the primary pathology is at the MTPJ, often due to neuromuscular imbalance [9, 13, 14].

A thorough history and examination should be performed, identifying all components of the deformity in the sagittal, axial, and coronal planes. Investigations should be aimed at confirming (rather than making) the diagnoses.

Operative Treatment

It is important to acknowledge that non-operative management is effective in a significant proportion of patients and should always be explored prior to surgery. Where this has been ineffective, surgery may be considered.

The aims of surgery are to restore the biomechanics and balance of the toes. This may involve correcting a hallux valgus or other foot deformities. There remains little high-quality evidence to guide management as most papers are retrospective case-series. However, the operative strategy will depend on the degree of deformity and whether the deformities are reducible. We suggest a proximal to distal approach, with stabilisation of the MTPJ a key step. We present a stepwise algorithm for treatment, previously described by Malhotra et al. [9]; other authors have described similar algorithms [15]. Although there are a multitude of procedures to address each of the pathologies highlighted, the principles and order of correction are more important than the specific surgical technique used.

General Operative Considerations

The authors prefer to perform forefoot surgery in the supine position with a calf tourniquet inflated to a maximum of 250 mm Hg. Perioperative antibiotics are given when metal implants are left *in situ*. A small sandbag is used to counteract any excessive hip external rotation. Patients receive an ankle block and the surgery is done with fluoroscopic guidance with a mini C-Arm image intensifier. The tourniquet is released prior to skin closure to assess the vascularity of the toes before the application of dressings. Cases are performed as a day case procedure. In all cases patients are permitted immediate unrestricted weight bearing in a flat, although they are advised elevation for the first two weeks post surgery.

Addressing the MTPJ

As discussed previously, it is important to reduce and stabilise any deformities of the MTPJ prior to correcting distal deformities. Figures 2.2 and 2.3 demonstrate our recommended treatment algorithm for dealing with deformities in the sagittal and axial planes respectively.

Soft Tissue Releases

The first step is often a dorsal release of the MTPJ. This is a stepwise process which may be done open or percutaneously [15]. The first part of this procedure is an extensor release—traditionally this was done as an open z-lengthening through a longitudinal incision. However, a percutaneous tenotomy has similar outcomes and can be done through a single stab incision just medial or lateral to the tendon using a Beaver blade [16–19]. Should this prove insufficient a further dorsal capsulotomy

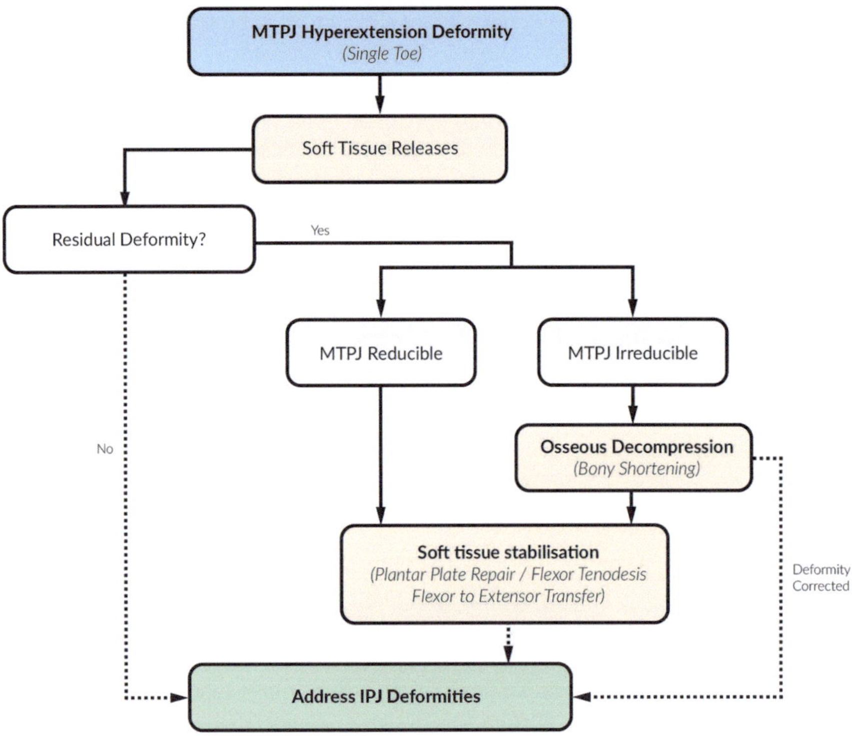

Fig. 2.2 Surgical algorithm for the management of sagittal plane deformities of the MTPJ. The proposed algorithm is for a single toe, although other concurrent deformities in the hallux or other toes should also be addressed. *Modified with permissions from Malhotra et al.* [9] *Creative Commons Licence 4.0 (CC BY-NC).* https://creativecommons.org/licenses/by-nc/4.0/

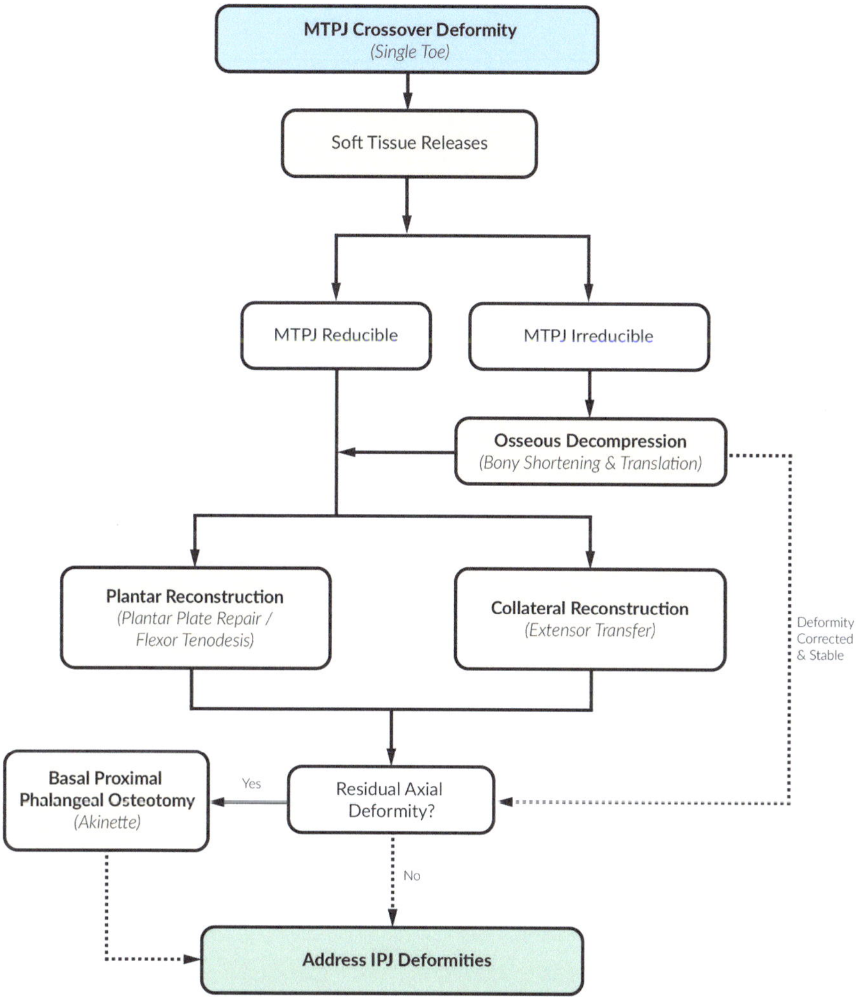

Fig. 2.3 Surgical algorithm for the management of combined sagittal and axial plane deformities of the MTPJ. The proposed algorithm is for a single toe, although other concurrent deformities in the hallux or other toes should also be addressed. *Modified with permissions from Malhotra et al.* [9] *Creative Commons Licence 4.0 (CC BY-NC).* https://creativecommons.org/licenses/by-nc/4.0/

is performed next, and this too can be performed safely percutaneously [20, 21]. This is often sufficient to correct mild, reducible deformities. In more severe cases, or in the case of a crossover toe, a tight collateral ligament may also need to be released. For a crossover toe the collateral which requires releasing is on the side the toe is deviated toward (i.e. the concave side of the deformity).

Osseous Decompression

In some cases, releases are insufficient to allow correction of the MTPJ deformity, often due to severe soft tissue contraction. In these cases, it may become necessary to shorten the bones (**osseous decompression**) to de-tension the soft tissues and allow the joint to reduce [18]. In the absence of severe contracture, bony shortening may still be desirable if the relative length of the metatarsal is too long (abnormal parabola). In these cases, the abnormal forces resulting from the relatively long metatarsal may have played a role in the initial pathology, and shortening the bone serves the added purpose of reducing forefoot overload [5, 22]. Osseous decompression is a powerful corrective technique, which can reduce the need for soft tissue releases and stabilisation in some cases.

Proximal Hemi-Phalangectomy (Stainsby Procedure)

Osseous decompression may be performed at metatarsal or the proximal phalanx. When done at the proximal phalanx, a hemi-phalangectomy may be performed as described by Briggs and Stainsby **(Stainsby Procedure)** [23]. In this procedure the plantar plate is detached from the proximal phalanx, and freed from the metatarsal, and the plantar fat pad is relocated. The EDL tendon is divided proximally, and its attachment distally is preserved. The extensor is concertinaed and tied down to the plantar plate or the flexor tendon. This is then held in place with a wire which passes into the metatarsal head. The results of this procedure in a single toe are not as good as when done in multiple toes (such as in patients with inflammatory arthritis), and therefore this procedure is considered a salvage option [23–25].

Open Distal Oblique Metatarsal Osteotomy (Weil's Osteotomy)

More commonly performed is a shortening lesser metatarsal osteotomy. Although there are many described techniques, two of the most common are the open oblique osteotomy popularised by Weil **(Weil's osteotomy)**, and the percutaneous distal metatarsal metaphyseal osteotomy **(DMMO)**. A Weil's osteotomy can be performed through a longitudinal incision. When multiple osteotomies are being performed the incision can be placed in the web spaces. Care is taken to preserve the extensor tendons and identify the MTPJ. The plantar plate is freed from the undersurface of the metatarsal head and then the osteotomy is performed. The direction of the osteotomy should begin just dorsal to the articular surface and aim to be parallel to the sole of the foot (this can be approximated by aiming towards the inferior aspect of the calcaneus). The metatarsal is then shortened by a few millimetres which can be judged by soft tissue tension and the appearance of the parabola on fluoroscopy. The position can be provisionally held with a 1.0 mm wire prior to fixing with a twist-off screw [26]. Care should be taken to ensure the shortening does not result in an imbalanced forefoot parabola, and the procedure may need to be performed on adjacent toes to recreate a balanced foot [5]. Excellent medium-to-long term results have been reported with this procedure [27]. The Weil's osteotomy is versatile as it can be used in the setting of a crossover toe by translating the metatarsal head medially or laterally prior to fixation—the translation needs to be *towards* the direction of toe angulation as this will reduce the tension on the collateral on the concave side of the deformity and tighten the collateral on the convex side [28]. The key complications of the Weil's osteotomy are stiffness and a 'floating toe' [29]. A floating toe may occur due to loss of tension of the plantar fascia due to shortening, which stops it functioning effectively during gait. At the same time there is concomitant depression of the metatarsal head that accompanies the shortening, which may cause the centre of rotation of the MTPJ to lie below the intrinsic muscles line of pull—this effectively defunctions the intrinsic muscle's ability to plantarflex the MTPJ [26, 30, 31].

Distal Metatarsal Metaphyseal Osteotomy (DMMO)

Minimally invasive surgery is gaining increasing popularity in the management of foot and ankle conditions and the lesser toes are no exception. Minimally invasive techniques are discussed in the relevant chapter, but in brief, DMMOs are performed through a single stab incision using a 2 mm burr angled at 45 degrees to the shaft of the metatarsal at the metatarsal neck [19]. The burr runs at low-velocity and high-torque and can be additionally angled to allow medial or lateral translation of the osteotomy. The osteotomy does not require fixation and early weightbearing allows the toes to 'find' their optimal position according to the forces applied and soft tissue tension. Swelling is common postoperatively although this usually settles by 3 months [32, 33]. Malhotra et al. reported on over 100 cases of DMMOs with 99% union rates, a mean shortening of 3-4 mm, and excellent clinical results in the short-to-medium term [34]. DMMOs can be used instead of open osteotomies in the vast majority of cases, are equally as effective, and may have a lower incidence of floating toes [35]. DMMOs and Weil osteotomies have also been successfully used as an isolated procedure in the correction of crossover toes, with no further stabilisation required [36]. However, in the authors' experience, more severe cases of crossover toe require additional soft tissue stabilisation.

Soft Tissue Stabilisation

There are many different techniques described for soft tissue stabilisation of the MTPJ. Reconstruction of the plantar plate controls movement in the sagittal and axial planes, whilst reconstruction of the collaterals predominantly controls movement in the axial plane. However, the plantar plate may often be degenerate, and therefore repair or reconstruction may not be possible. In these cases, the FDL tendon can be used to recreate the function of the plantar plate and plantar fascia, allowing the toes to dynamically plantarflex at the MTPJ.

Flexor to Extensor Transfer

The **flexor to extensor transfer** serves a dual purpose of flexing the MTPJ in cases of mild dorsal subluxation, as well as addressing a flexible PIPJ flexion deformity / hammer toe. The procedure is performed by first accessing the FDL through a longitudinal plantar incision under the proximal phalanx. The FDL is detached from the distal phalanx and split into two slips. These are tunnelled dorsally on either side of the phalanx and retrieved through a separate dorsal incision over the proximal phalanx. The two slips are then either sutured together or sutured to the extensor tendons. As the FDL no longer spans the IPJs, its pull then acts to plantarflex the MTPJ. At the same time the attachment to the extensor enables it to act like the intrinsic muscles and extend the PIPJ. This procedure is effective in milder deformity and may be coupled with a plantar plate repair for more severe deformities [37]. However, for a more severe deformity it is not sufficient and should be combined with osseous decompression [38]. This procedure is not commonly used by the authors.

Extensor Transfer

For the correction of less severe cross over toes, the collateral ligaments can be reconstructed using a slip of EDB [39, 40]. The authors' preferred technique is similar to that described by Hobizal et al. [41]. Through a longitudinal approach the EDB is identified and resected as proximally as possible, leaving sufficient length to weave through the proximal phalanx and metatarsal. The distal attachment is left intact. Tunnels are drilled perpendicular to the joint surface at about the level of the original collateral. The collateral is weaved through the drill holes of the proximal phalanx from either medial to lateral or lateral to medial (depending on which side the collateral reconstruction is required on). The EBD is then routed under the deep transverse metatarsal ligament and through the metatarsal drill holes. It is secured in place with an interference screw. The advantage of this technique is that it allows a shorter, more anatomic working length for the tendon. Going under the deep transverse metatarsal ligament allows it to exert some sagittal control and this can be adjusted by placing the tunnels more plantar if required. Although this technique works well for mild deformity, it is not sufficient in more severe deformity and the authors only use this technique for predominantly axial plane deformity [42–44].

Plantar Plate Repair

As discussed previously, the plantar plate plays an essential role in transmitting the forces of the plantar fascia to the proximal phalanx, and therefore exerts control of the MTPJ in the sagittal and (to some extent) the axial planes. Significant sagittal deformity (subluxation/dislocation) can therefore only occur when the plantar plate is disrupted. A **plantar plate repair** is therefore effective at restoring stability of the

MTPJ [45, 46]. A plantar plate repair can be performed through a dorsal or plantar approach. The plantar approach has an advantage of not requiring a metatarsal osteotomy for access to the plantar plate and can also allow a direct repair, at the cost of a scar on the weight bearing portion of the forefoot [37]. Through a dorsal approach a shortening osteotomy such as a Weil's osteotomy is required to gain access to the plantar plate—however, as osseous decompression is often required in any case, this is not a significant drawback. Previous authors have explored the potential of a dorsal approach without an metatarsal osteotomy on cadaveric models, but this requires extensive soft tissue dissection which may be better avoided in an already unstable toe [47]. The standard technique of a dorsal plantar plate repair involves a longitudinal incision and a Weil's osteotomy. Before the osteotomy is fixed, the head is retracted posteriorly to visualise the plantar plate. The plantar plate is freed from the metatarsal head, and any remnants detached from the proximal phalanx. Sutures are then placed through the plantar plate (a size 1 absorbable, braided suture may be used) and two drill holes are made in the proximal phalanx about 5 mm from the joint surface (these can be made with a 1.6 mm wire). The sutures from the plantar plate are then passed through these drill holes, from plantar to dorsal, the Weil's osteotomy is fixed, and the sutures are finally tensioned with the toe in slight plantarflexion. Commercially available jigs are available which may be used to aid in the passing of sutures through the plantar plate. The main drawback of this procedure is that it may be associated with stiffness of the toe, [38] and the plantar plate may be too degenerate to gain a proper purchase with sutures.

Flexor Tenodesis

Where the plantar plate is not of sufficient quality for reconstruction, the FDL tendon may be used in its place. The principle behind this **flexor tenodesis** is similar to that of the flexor to extensor transfer, but it is simpler to perform. The procedure starts off similarly to the plantar plate repair, but after the Weil's osteotomy, the plantar plate is divided and retracted so that the FDL tendon can be seen. The FDL is then pulled superiorly and distally using a tendon hook and a size 1 absorbable braided suture is passed from medial to lateral to gain purchase as proximally in the tendon as possible. The suture is then grasped and used to pull the tendon more distally and the suture is passed through the tendon as proximally as possible another couple of times. The rest of the procedure can be carried as with the plantar plate, but this provides a dynamic as well as static restraint to MTPJ subluxation. In cases of a cross over toe, this can be modified with only 1 hole drilled in the proximal phalanx and only one suture end passed through the proximal phalanx. If the plantar aspect of this drill hole is directed toward the convex side of the deformity, on tensioning the suture the FDL will pull the proximal phalanx into plantarflexion and medially/laterally—therefore acting as a plantar plate and collateral (Fig. 2.4).

The flexor tenodesis can also be done more distally without a Weil's osteotomy if performing a PIPJ fusion. In this case after preparing the PIPJ fusion, the flexor

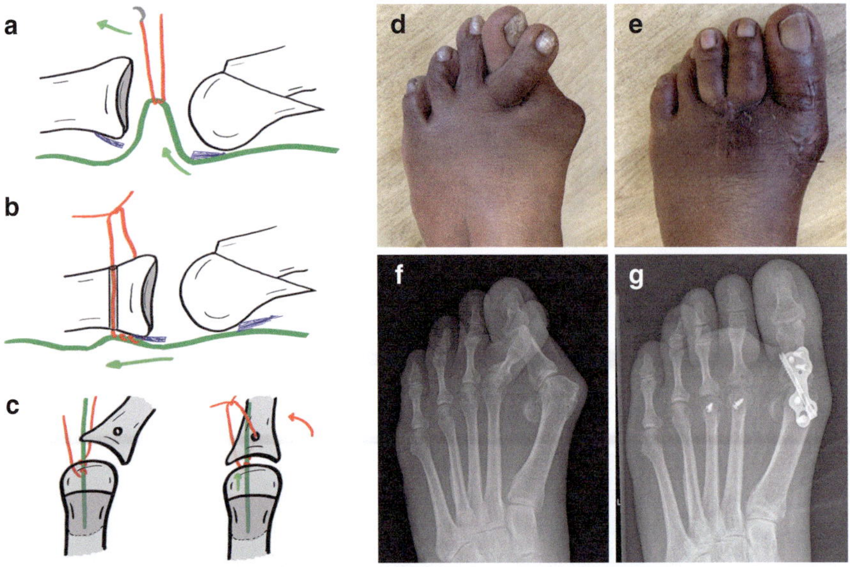

Fig. 2.4 Key steps for a flexor tenodesis used to correct a crossover toe deformity. After performing a Weil's osteotomy and dividing the plantar plate (blue), the FDL tendon (green) is retrieved, and a suture is passed through it three times (**a**). The suture is then passed through a drill hole in the proximal phalanx and tensioned with a toe in slight plantarflexion (after fixation of the osteotomy) (**b**). For a severe crossover toe, a single hole may be used with the plantar exit closer to the convex side of the deformity (lateral in this example). The other strand of suture is passed on the convex side of the deformity as well and the toe held in position whilst the suture is tensioned and tied—this allows the FDL to act as the plantar plate and a collateral (**c**). (**d** and **e**) show the pre- and post-operative clinical results of this technique being used to treat a severe crossover toe. (**f** and **g**) show the pre- and post-operative radiographic results in the same patient—an MTPJ fusion was used to correct the severe hallux valgus and a balancing Weil's osteotomy was used for the third metatarsal. Only a single drill hole was used, and this can be seen in the second proximal phalanx (**g**)

tendon can be found inferior to the phalanges and brought out and secured with sutures in the manner described above. The 2 ends of the suture can be brought up the side of the proximal phalanx and sutured together or to the extensor after the PIPJ is fixed (Fig. 2.5). This is similar to but simpler than a flexor to extensor transfer. The flexor tenodesis is the author's preferred method of soft tissue stabilisation. There are also commercially available implants which further simplify this procedure.

Basal Proximal Phalangeal Osteotomy (Akinette)

In cases of residual deformity either at the MTPJ or within the proximal phalanx, an Akinette procedure can be performed—this results in a straight, functional toe even if the MTPJ is not perfectly reduced [48, 49]. This can either be performed open,

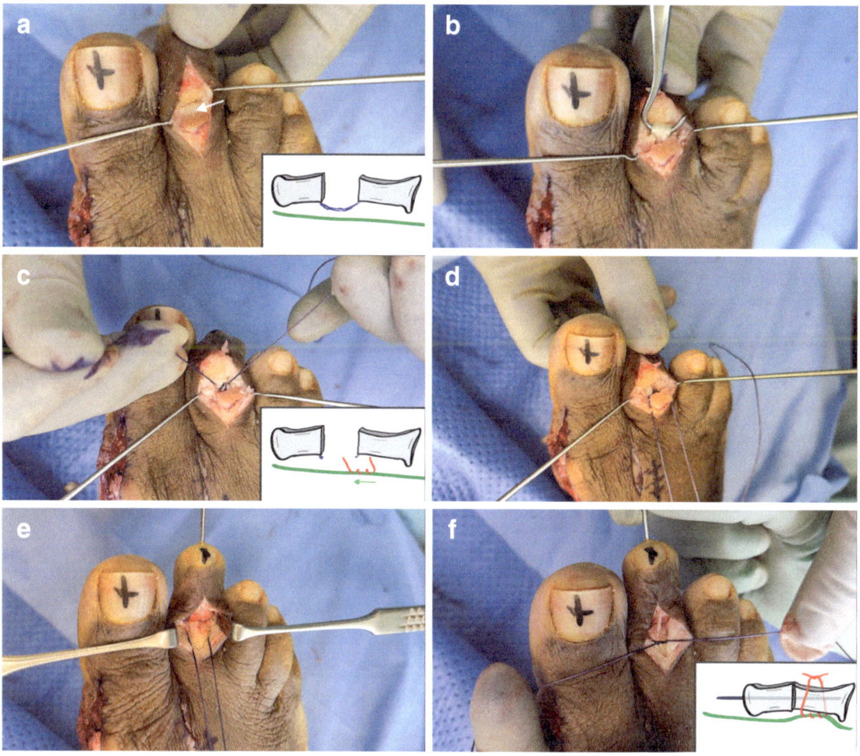

Fig. 2.5 Key steps for the flexor tenodesis being performed through a PIPJ fusion. After resection of the PIPJ the plantar capsule can be seen (white arrow) (**a**). This needs to be divided and then the FDL tendon can be retrieved using a small tendon hook (**b**). A suture is passed through the tendon and three loops passed through to improve hold on the tendon—these should be as proximal as possible (**c**). The slips of suture are passed on either side of the proximal phalanx (**d**) which is then fused in the preferred method, with a wire in this example (**e**). Finally, with the toe slightly plantarflexed, the suture is tensioned over the proximal phalanx (**f**)

and secured with a wire, or it can be performed percutaneously [19, 50]. When performed percutaneously a 2 mm × 8 mm short burr is used to perform an osteotomy of half of the width of the phalanx, within the proximal metaphysis. The plantar aspect of the cut is often taken all the way across, leaving only a dorsolateral or dorsomedial hinge. The toe can then be manipulated into position and is usually stable. Fixation is therefore not required, although dressings to hold it in place are applied for 2 weeks [50].

Addressing the PIPJ

After the MTPJ is stabilised and deformities corrected, the PIPJ should be addressed next. Our suggested algorithm for managing PIPJ deformities is illustrated in Fig. 2.6.

For flexible deformities, numerous soft tissue options are available. An FDB tenotomy can be performed and this can be done open or percutaneously [18, 51]. However, this technique does not afford much control of toe position and therefore a flexor to extensor transfer (described in previous sections) is preferred, although this can result in a stiff toe and loss of prehensile function [52–54]. Satisfaction rates with a flexor to extensor transfer have been reported to be between 80–90% [55–57].

Management of Fixed Deformities

Fixed deformities require osseous decompression with excision of the PIPJ to allow reduction. Following joint excision, the proximal and middle phalanx are often fused (PIPJ fusion). This can be done through a transverse or longitudinal incision over the PIPJ. The collaterals are released, and the proximal phalangeal bone is excised at the levels of the condyles. The middle phalanx articular surface is also prepared, and the joint surfaces apposed. Fixation with a wire or implant is used to hold the joints together.

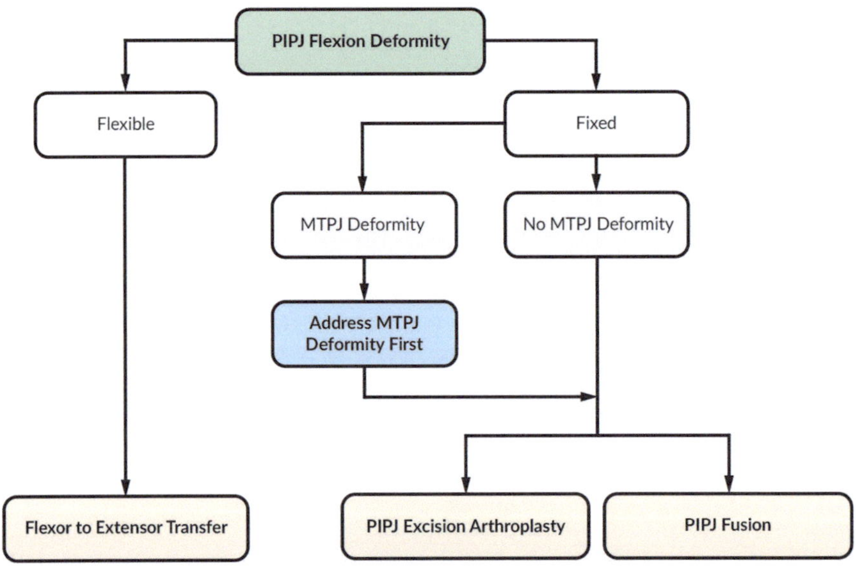

Fig. 2.6 Surgical algorithm for the management of PIPJ deformities. Concurrent deformities in the hallux or other toes should also be addressed. *Modified with permissions from Malhotra et al.* [9] *Creative Commons Licence 4.0 (CC BY-NC).* https://creativecommons.org/licenses/by-nc/4.0/

Although fusion has long been the gold standard, about 20% of patients may only ever develop a fibrous union, although this does not appear to adversely affect outcome [13]. Schrier et al. conducted a randomised controlled trial to compare PIPJ excision versus fusion. In both groups they passed a wire through the tip of the toe, into the proximal phalanx and then into the metatarsal head. The main difference between groups was that in the excision group they resected more bone and did not attempt to compress the joint surfaces. They report equivalent results in both groups [58]. Other authors have raised concerns that PIPJ excision may result in mal-alignment [16]. The authors prefer a PIPJ fusion as this allows other procedures to be carried out (such as a flexor tenodesis) where required. Patients are however counselled that they may have a fibrous rather than bony union, although failure to unite is unlikely to affect their outcome.

Wire Versus Intramedullary Implant

The traditional method of PIPJ fusion is with a 1.6 mm wire which remains in situ for up to 6 weeks. This is cheap, versatile and has the advantage of not leaving any metalwork in-situ. This is particularly advantageous in revision surgery, if the DIPJ becomes symptomatic, or in severe deformities (such as with neurological foot deformity) where there is abnormal anatomy and a 'zigzag' alignment of the phalanges is acceptable providing it results in a functional toe.

However, many patients find a wire sticking out of their toe for 6 weeks inconvenient. Therefore, several intramedullary implants are now available which can avoid the use of a wire and allow patients to return to their normal footwear earlier. Implants can also (theoretically) provide more control of position in the long term. Implants range from memory metal (Nitinol) and bio-composite materials to allografts, and there is little evidence to support the use of one over the other. The literature would suggest that although implants have good short to medium term results, these are not substantially better than wires, and certainly not as cost-effective [59–67].

Addressing the DIPJ

Our algorithm for treatment of DIPJ deformities is illustrated in Fig. 2.7. For flexible mallet toe deformities, a flexor tenotomy is often sufficient. This can be done through an open procedure, but a percutaneous tenotomy of the FDL at the level of the middle phalanx has good outcomes [25, 68].

For fixed deformities, as with PIPJ deformities, excision of the DIPJ is required. As with the PIPJ, this is often followed by a fusion with a wire. In 30% of cases only a fibrous union will result, but as with PIPJ fusions, this does not appear to adversely affect outcome [69]. The procedure is similar to the PIPJ fusion (described in the

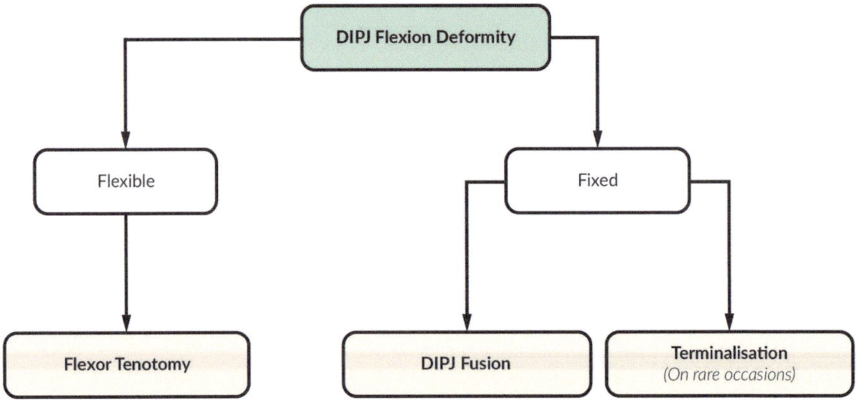

Fig. 2.7 Surgical algorithm for the management of DIPJ deformities. Concurrent deformities in the other toes and at the PIPJ should also be addressed. *Modified with permissions from Malhotra et al.* [9] *Creative Commons Licence 4.0 (CC BY-NC).* https://creativecommons.org/licenses/by-nc/4.0/

previous section), and once again intramedullary implants are available [70]. For low demand patients, at high risk of morbidity, amputation of the tip of the toe (terminalisation) is a salvage option which may be considered.

Complications

Complications are not infrequent after lesser toe surgery and may include malalignment, infection, wound complications, persistent swelling, chronic pain, recurrence, floating toes, stiffness, symptomatic metalwork, and ischaemia [71, 72]. Patients should be adequately counselled with regards to these risks prior to surgery.

Morton's Neuroma

Morton's neuroma, or interdigital neuroma, is a benign lesion most commonly occurring within the second or third intermetatarsal space. It is not a nerve tumour or neuroma, but rather a compressive neuropathy with perineural fibrosis secondary to entrapment of the interdigital nerve under the deep transverse intermetatarsal ligament (**DTIML**). It is once again important to perform a thorough history and examination and to confirm the diagnosis as many patients may have alternate pathologies such as metatarsalgia, capsulitis or **intermetatarsal bursitis** which are associated conditions [73, 74].

Operative Management

Once again, most patients can be managed successfully with nonoperative measures. Surgical treatment is indicated when conservative treatment has failed. It is imperative to ensure that the correct diagnosis is obtained prior to surgery, and that any associated pathologies are treated simultaneously. Numerous techniques are described which include excision of the lesion, neurolysis of the nerve, transposition of the nerve, or decompression of the intermetatarsal space.

Both neurolysis and neurectomy have been shown to be more effective in treating pain than injection therapy [75]. The results of **neurectomy** have been reported as 'excellent' in up to 80% of patients, although only two-thirds of patients are pain free, and numbness is a common complication [76, 77]. However, there is insufficient evidence to determine whether any alternative treatments are superior to neurectomy. **Neurolysis** has been shown to have similar efficacy as neurectomy although the results can be improved by **transposing the nerve** dorsally [78–80]. In this setting over 90% of patients can experience a symptomatic improvement, without the risk of numbness or neuroma, and a future neurectomy remains an option in case of recurrence [78, 80].

Minimally invasive decompression has been described although the results are variable and reoperation rate high. Other adjunctive procedures include gastrocnemius recession and shortening metatarsal osteotomies to treat associated pathology, although there is little high quality evidence to support their routine use, and therefore these are best reserved for cases where there is clear cut concomitant pathology [78, 81].

Neurectomy

This procedure can be approached from either dorsal or plantar. The dorsal approach is preferred by many surgeons due to fewer postoperative complications and a faster recovery.

For the dorsal approach, a 3–4 cm longitudinal incision is made over the appropriate webspace on the dorsum of the foot. The extensor tendons are retracted, and the superficial sling of intermetatarsal tissue is divided. The DTIML is identified and divided whilst protecting the neurovascular bundles. The neuroma is normally visible beneath this—use of a lamina spreader between the metatarsals may facilitate neuroma identification and excision. The distal digital branches are the identified and transected and the remaining nerve carefully dissected and then divided proximal to the neuroma to ensure complete removal. Gentle traction on the nerve to ensure as proximal a resection as possible is advisable as this allows the stump to retract into the soft tissues. The excised nerve will often have the classic 'Y' shape with the two distal limbs and the single proximal limb.

Neurolysis and Nerve Transposition

This procedure is similar to the neurectomy, but care is taken to preserve the dorsal transverse tissue during division. After division of the DTIML, the nerve is similarly identified, but instead of resecting it, the nerve is gently freed from the surrounding tissues and any bursitis excised. The nerve is then transposed dorsal to the dorsal transverse tissue, which is repaired. The nerve then lies on a sling of tissue in a dorsal location.

Complications

Complications from surgical intervention include wound infection, recurrence, stump neuroma formation (after neurectomy), persistent pain and nerve damage. Stump neuroma formation can be minimised by ensuring complete neuroma excision, excising the neuroma with a margin of healthy tissue and burying the nerve stump into surrounding soft tissues/muscle. It is advisable to avoid simultaneous surgery on neuromas in neighbouring intermetatarsal spaces to avoid the risk of compromising the neurovascular supply to a toe. Comprehensive patient counselling on realistic expectations and potential recurrence, ongoing pain and nerve damage is crucial for optimal management.

Conclusion

Lesser toe deformities are complex and can occur at multiple levels. It is important to understand the underlying pathology of the deformity and to carefully assess each aspect of the deformity. A stepwise approach aimed at stabilising the MTPJ and then addressing any associated IPJ deformities is required.

References

1. Saro C, Bengtsson AS, Lindgren U, Adami J, Blomqvist P, Fellander-Tsai L. Surgical treatment of hallux valgus and forefoot deformities in Sweden: a population-based study. Foot Ankle Int. 2008;29(3):298–304.
2. Hughes J, Clark P, Klenerman L. The importance of the toes in walking. J Bone Joint Surg Br. 1990;72(2):245–51.
3. Klenerman LBW. The human foot: a companion to clinical studies. Springer; 2006.
4. Hicks JH. The mechanics of the foot. II. The plantar aponeurosis and the arch. J Anat. 1954;88(1):25–30.
5. Maestro M, Besse JL, Ragusa M, Berthonnaud E. Forefoot morphotype study and planning method for forefoot osteotomy. Foot Ankle Clin. 2003;8(4):695–710.

6. Dominguez G, Munuera PV, Lafuente G. Relative metatarsal protrusion in the adult: a preliminary study. J Am Podiatr Med Assoc. 2006;96(3):238–44.
7. Morton DJ. Metatarsus Atavicus: the identification of a distinctive type of foot disorder. J Bone Joint Surg Am. 1927;9(3):531–44.
8. Harris RI, Beath T. The short first metatarsal; its incidence and clinical significance. J Bone Joint Surg Am. 1949;31A(3):553–65.
9. Malhotra K, Davda K, Singh D. The pathology and management of lesser toe deformities. EFORT Open Rev. 2016;1(11):409–19.
10. Coughlin MJ. Crossover second toe deformity. Foot Ankle. 1987;8(1):29–39.
11. Coughlin MJ. Subluxation and dislocation of the second metatarsophalangeal joint. Orthop Clin North Am. 1989;20(4):535–51.
12. Coughlin MJ. Second metatarsophalangeal joint instability in the athlete. Foot Ankle. 1993;14(6):309–19.
13. Coughlin MJ, Dorris J, Polk E. Operative repair of the fixed hammertoe deformity. Foot Ankle Int. 2000;21(2):94–104.
14. Stainsby GD. Pathological anatomy and dynamic effect of the displaced plantar plate and the importance of the integrity of the plantar plate-deep transverse metatarsal ligament tie-bar. Ann R Coll Surg Engl. 1997;79(1):58–68.
15. Darcel V, Piclet-Legre B. Lesser-toe deformity. Orthop Traumatol Surg Res. 2023;109(1S):103464.
16. Dhukaram V, Hossain S, Sampath J, Barrie JL. Correction of hammer toe with an extended release of the metatarsophalangeal joint. J Bone Joint Surg Br. 2002;84(7):986–90.
17. Dhukaram V, Chapman AP, Upadhyay PK. Minimally invasive forefoot surgery: a cadaveric study. Foot Ankle Int. 2012;33(12):1139–44.
18. Myerson MS, Shereff MJ. The pathological anatomy of claw and hammer toes. J Bone Joint Surg Am. 1989;71(1):45–9.
19. Redfern DJ, Vernois J. Percutaneous surgery for metatarsalgia and the lesser toes. Foot Ankle Clin. 2016;21(3):527–50.
20. Gilheany M, Baarini O, Samaras D. Minimally invasive surgery for pedal digital deformity: an audit of complications using national benchmark indicators. J Foot Ankle Res. 2015;8:17.
21. Debarge R, Philippot R, Viola J, Besse JL. Clinical outcome after percutaneous flexor tenotomy in forefoot surgery. Int Orthop. 2009;33(5):1279–82.
22. Vandeputte G, Dereymaeker G, Steenwerckx A, Peeraer L. The Weil osteotomy of the lesser metatarsals: a clinical and pedobarographic follow-up study. Foot Ankle Int. 2000;21(5):370–4.
23. Briggs PJ, Stainsby GD. Metatarsal head preservation in forefoot arthroplasty and the correction of severe claw toe deformity. Foot Ankle Surg. 2001;7(2):93–101.
24. Conklin MJ, Smith RW. Treatment of the atypical lesser toe deformity with basal hemiphalangectomy. Foot Ankle Int. 1994;15(11):585–94.
25. Coughlin MJ. Lesser toe deformities. In: Coughlin MJSC, Anderson RB, editors. Mann's surgery of the foot and ankle. 9th ed. Elsevier; 2014. p. 322–424.
26. Garcia-Fernandez D, Gil-Garay E, Lora-Pablos D, De-la-Cruz-Bertolo J, Llanos-Alcazar LF. Comparative study of the Weil osteotomy with and without fixation. Foot Ankle Surg. 2011;17(3):103–7.
27. Hofstaetter SG, Hofstaetter JG, Petroutsas JA, Gruber F, Ritschl P, Trnka HJ. The Weil osteotomy: a seven-year follow-up. J Bone Joint Surg Br. 2005;87(11):1507–11.
28. Devos Bevernage B, Deleu PA, Leemrijse T. The translating Weil osteotomy in the treatment of an overriding second toe: a report of 25 cases. Foot Ankle Surg. 2010;16(4):153–8.
29. Klinge SA, McClure P, Fellars T, DiGiovanni CW. Modification of the Weil/Maceira metatarsal osteotomy for coronal plane malalignment during crossover toe correction: case series. Foot Ankle Int. 2014;35(6):584–91.
30. Migues A, Slullitel G, Bilbao F, Carrasco M, Solari G. Floating-toe deformity as a complication of the Weil osteotomy. Foot Ankle Int. 2004;25(9):609–13.

31. Garg R, Thordarson DB, Schrumpf M, Castaneda D. Sliding oblique versus segmental resection osteotomies for lesser metatarsophalangeal joint pathology. Foot Ankle Int. 2008;29(10):1009–14.
32. Haque S, Kakwani R, Chadwick C, Davies MB, Blundell CM. Outcome of minimally invasive Distal Metatarsal Metaphyseal Osteotomy (DMMO) for lesser toe Metatarsalgia. Foot Ankle Int. 2016;37(1):58–63.
33. Henry J, Besse JL, Fessy MH, AFCP. Distal osteotomy of the lateral metatarsals: a series of 72 cases comparing the Weil osteotomy and the DMMO percutaneous osteotomy. Orthop Traumatol Surg Res. 2011;97(6 Suppl):S57–65.
34. Malhotra K, Joji N, Mordecai S, Rudge B. Minimally invasive distal metaphyseal metatarsal osteotomy (DMMO) for symptomatic forefoot pathology—short to medium term outcomes from a retrospective case series. Foot. 2018;38:43–9.
35. Yeo NE, Loh B, Chen JY, Yew AK, Ng SY. Comparison of early outcome of Weil osteotomy and distal metatarsal mini-invasive osteotomy for lesser toe metatarsalgia. J Orthop Surg. 2016;24(3):350–3.
36. Sallent A, Methol G, Altayo M, Soza D, Duarri G, Maled I, et al. From second webspace syndrome to second cross over toe: clinical and radiological findings following Weil osteotomy with no soft tissue procedure. Foot Ankle Surg. 2023;29(2):171–6.
37. Bouche RT, Heit EJ. Combined plantar plate and hammertoe repair with flexor digitorum longus tendon transfer for chronic, severe sagittal plane instability of the lesser metatarsophalangeal joints: preliminary observations. J Foot Ankle Surg. 2008;47(2):125–37.
38. Thompson FM, Deland JT. Flexor tendon transfer for metatarsophalangeal instability of the second toe. Foot Ankle. 1993;14(7):385–8.
39. Lui TH, Chan KB. Technique tip: modified extensor digitorum brevis tendon transfer for crossover second toe correction. Foot Ankle Int. 2007;28(4):521–3.
40. Myerson MS, Jung HG. The role of toe flexor-to-extensor transfer in correcting metatarsophalangeal joint instability of the second toe. Foot Ankle Int. 2005;26(9):675–9.
41. Hobizal KB, Wukich DK, Manway J. Extensor Digitorum brevis transfer technique to correct multiplanar deformity of the lesser digits. Foot Ankle Spec. 2016;9(3):252–7.
42. Fuhrmann RA. Subligamentous transfer of the extensor digitorum brevis tendon for medial malalignment of the lesser toes. Operative Orthopadie und Traumatologie. 2009;21(1):88–96.
43. Barca F, Acciaro AL. Surgical correction of crossover deformity of the second toe: a technique for tenodesis. Foot Ankle Int. 2004;25(9):620–4.
44. Haddad SL, Sabbagh RC, Resch S, Myerson B, Myerson MS. Results of flexor-to-extensor and extensor brevis tendon transfer for correction of the crossover second toe deformity. Foot Ankle Int. 1999;20(12):781–8.
45. Nery C, Coughlin MJ, Baumfeld D, Mann TS. Lesser metatarsophalangeal joint instability: prospective evaluation and repair of plantar plate and capsular insufficiency. Foot Ankle Int. 2012;33(4):301–11.
46. Fleischer AE, Klein EE, Ahmad M, Shah S, Catena F, Weil LS Sr, et al. Association of Abnormal Metatarsal Parabola with Second Metatarsophalangeal Joint Plantar Plate Pathology. Foot Ankle Int. 2017;38(3):289–97.
47. Jastifer JR, Coughlin MJ. Exposure via sequential release of the metatarsophalangeal joint for plantar plate repair through a dorsal approach without an intraarticular osteotomy. Foot Ankle Int. 2015;36(3):335–8.
48. Davis WH, Anderson RB, Thompson FM, Hamilton WG. Proximal phalanx basilar osteotomy for resistant angulation of the lesser toes. Foot Ankle Int. 1997;18(2):103–4.
49. Kilmartin TE, O'Kane C. Correction of valgus second toe by closing wedge osteotomy of the proximal phalanx. Foot Ankle Int. 2007;28(12):1260–4.
50. Ray R, Lewis TL, Robinson P, Dearden PMC, Goff TAJ, Watt C, et al. Valgus second toe deformity treated with a percutaneous extracapsular closing-wedge osteotomy of the proximal phalanx. Foot Ankle Int. 2022;43(9):1157–66.

51. Frey-Ollivier S, Catena F, Helix-Giordanino M, Piclet-Legre B. Treatment of flexible lesser toe deformities. Foot Ankle Clin. 2018;23(1):69–90.
52. Taylor RG. The treatment of claw toes by multiple transfers of flexor into extensor tendons. J Bone Joint Surg Br. 1951;33-B(4):539–42.
53. Myers SH, Schon LC. Forefoot tendon transfers. Foot Ankle Clin. 2011;16(3):471–88.
54. Veljkovic A, Lansang E, Lau J. Forefoot tendon transfers. Foot Ankle Clin. 2014;19(1):123–37.
55. Barbari SG, Brevig K. Correction of clawtoes by the Girdlestone-Taylor flexor-extensor transfer procedure. Foot Ankle. 1984;5(2):67–73.
56. Boyer ML, DeOrio JK. Transfer of the flexor digitorum longus for the correction of lesser-toe deformities. Foot Ankle Int. 2007;28(4):422–30.
57. Losa Iglesias ME, de Bengoa B, Vallejo R, Jules KT, Trepal MJ. Meta-analysis of flexor tendon transfer for the correction of lesser toe deformities. J Am Podiatr Med Assoc. 2012;102(5):359–68.
58. Schrier JC, Keijsers NL, Matricali GA, Louwerens JW, Verheyen CC. Lesser toe PIP joint resection versus PIP joint fusion: a randomized clinical trial. Foot Ankle Int. 2016;37(6):569–75.
59. Ellington JK, Anderson RB, Davis WH, Cohen BE, Jones CP. Radiographic analysis of proximal interphalangeal joint arthrodesis with an intramedullary fusion device for lesser toe deformities. Foot Ankle Int. 2010;31(5):372–6.
60. Fazal MA, James L, Williams RL. StayFuse for proximal interphalangeal joint fusion. Foot Ankle Int. 2013;34(9):1274–8.
61. Konkel KF, Menger AG, Retzlaff SA. Hammer toe correction using an absorbable intramedullary pin. Foot Ankle Int. 2007;28(8):916–20.
62. Roukis TS. A 1-piece shape-metal nitinol intramedullary internal fixation device for arthrodesis of the proximal interphalangeal joint in neuropathic patients with diabetes. Foot Ankle Spec. 2009;2(3):130–4.
63. Coillard JY, Petri GJ, van Damme G, Deprez P, Laffenetre O. Stabilization of proximal interphalangeal joint in lesser toe deformities with an angulated intramedullary implant. Foot Ankle Int. 2014;35(4):401–7.
64. Sung W, Weil L Jr, Weil LS Sr. Retrospective comparative study of operative repair of hammertoe deformity. Foot Ankle Spec. 2014;7(3):185–92.
65. Harmer JL, Wilkinson A, Maher AJ. A midterm review of lesser toe arthrodesis with an intramedullary implant. Foot Ankle Spec. 2017;10(5):458–64.
66. Hendrick SE, Kannegieter E. SmartToe, ToeGrip and buried k-wire versus percutaneous k-wire fixation for 2nd PIPJ arthrodesis: a comprehensive review of outcomes. Foot. 2020;45:101692.
67. Mirmiran R, Younger M. Lesser Digit Implants. Clin Podiatr Med Surg. 2019;36(4):651–61.
68. Louwerens JWSJ. Lesser toe deformities. In: Bentley G, editor. European surgical orthopaedics and traumatology: the EFORT textbook. 6: SpringerReference; 2014. p. 3407–973.
69. Coughlin MJ. Operative repair of the mallet toe deformity. Foot Ankle Int. 1995;16(3):109–16.
70. Khan F, Kimura S, Ahmad T, D'Souza D, D'Souza L. Use of Smart Toe((c)) implant for small toe arthrodesis: a smart concept? Foot Ankle Surg. 2015;21(2):108–12.
71. Phisitkul P. Managing complications of lesser toe and metatarsophalangeal joint surgery. Foot Ankle Clin. 2018;23(1):145–56.
72. Gray J, Singh D. Ischemic toe after surgery for lesser toe deformities: an algorithm. Foot. 2021;48:101817.
73. Larsen SB, Sogaard SB, Nielsen MB, Torp-Pedersen ST. Diagnostic considerations of intermetatarsal bursitis: a systematic review. Diagnostics (Basel). 2023;13(2)
74. Ganguly A, Warner J, Aniq H. Central metatarsalgia and walking on pebbles: beyond Morton neuroma. AJR Am J Roentgenol. 2018;210(4):821–33.
75. Lu VM, Puffer RC, Everson MC, Gilder HE, Burks SS, Spinner RJ. Treating Morton's neuroma by injection, neurolysis, or neurectomy: a systematic review and meta-analysis of pain and satisfaction outcomes. Acta Neurochir. 2021;163(2):531–43.
76. Coughlin MJ, Pinsonneault T. Operative treatment of interdigital neuroma. A long-term follow-up study. J Bone Joint Surg Am. 2001;83(9):1321–8.

77. Bucknall V, Rutherford D, MacDonald D, Shalaby H, McKinley J, Breusch SJ. Outcomes following excision of Morton's interdigital neuroma: a prospective study. Bone Joint J. 2016;98-B(10):1376–81.
78. Choi JY, Hong WH, Kim MJ, Chae SW, Suh JS. Operative treatment options for Morton's neuroma other than neurectomy—a systematic review. Foot Ankle Surg. 2022;28(4):450–9.
79. Koti M, Maffulli N, Al-Shoaibi M, Hughes M, McAllister J. Long-term results of dorsal neuroma/nerve transposition in the surgical management of Morton's neuroma and correlation with intraoperative anatomical variations. J Orthop Surg Res. 2022;17(1):22.
80. Song JH, Kang C, Hwang DS, Kang DH, Kim YH. Dorsal suspension for Morton's neuroma: a comparison with neurectomy. Foot Ankle Surg. 2019;25(6):748–54.
81. Gougoulias N, Lampridis V, Sakellariou A. Morton's interdigital neuroma: instructional review. EFORT Open Rev. 2019;4(1):14–24.

Chapter 3
Surgery for Arthritis of the Big Toe

Jasdeep Giddie and Maneesh Bhatia

Hallux Rigidus

Hallux rigidus, Latin for 'stiff toe' describes a painful metatarsophalangeal joint (MTPJ) of the great toe which is characterised by restricted motion and peri-articular bone formation. It is the most common form of arthritis affecting the foot, and the incidence increases with age [1]. The prevalence of symptomatic radiographic first MTPJ osteoarthritis in adults over 50 years in the United Kingdom is 8% [2]. There are a number of surgical treatment options available. The key to selecting the 'best option' requires a detailed assessment which should always include the history of the presenting complaint, examination of the limb and appropriate investigations. During this chapter we will discuss individual treatment options available, their supporting evidence and surgical tips and tricks.

J. Giddie
Frimley Park Hospital NHS Foundation Trust, London, UK

M. Bhatia (✉)
Consultant Orthopaedic Foot Ankle Surgeon, University Hospitals Leicester, Spire Hospital Leicester and Nuffield Health Leicester, Leicester, UK

Associate Professor, University of Leicester, Leicester, UK

Professor, DeMontfort University Leicester, Leicester, UK

M. Bhatia (ed.), *Surgical Techniques of the Foot and Ankle*,
https://doi.org/10.1007/978-3-031-93742-2_3

Pathophysiology

While arthritis can be caused by traumatic or iatrogenic injuries that directly cause damage to the articular cartilage of the MTPJ of the big toe, the most common aetiology of hallux rigidus is idiopathic [3]. Genetic factors appear to play a role with two thirds of patients having a positive family history and bilateral MTPJ involvement [4]. The classic location of the cartilage loss is on the dorsal half to two thirds of the metatarsal head [5]. Due to the on-going degenerative process proliferation of bony osteophytes on the dorsal and dorso-lateral aspect of the metatarsal head develop creating a bony ledge that causes an abutment of the proximal phalanx. Consequently the normal coupling of the centre of rotation of the proximal phalanx and metatarsal head is disrupted, leading to eccentric gliding of the proximal phalanx on the metatarsal head [6]. Biomechanical and structural factors, such as long first metatarsal, metatarsus elevatus, and metatarsus adductus can also lead to increased risk of hallux rigidus [7, 8]. Inflammatory conditions are a known risk factor and cause generalised joint destruction.

Signs and Symptoms

Patients will typically present with pain and stiffness that is worse with dorsiflexion activities e.g. running and climbing stairs. During ambulation pain can be exacerbated during the toe off and heel rise. Flexible and high heeled shoes can cause pain due to the restricted dorsiflexion whilst stiff soled shoes can help relieve some of the pain.

Salient examination points include:

1. Swelling around the MTPJ
2. Pain initially more localized to the dorsolateral aspect of the MTPJ
3. Pain whilst dorsiflexing the joint
4. Reduced range of motion of the joint
5. Pain on axial loading of the joint 'grind test'
6. Hyperextension of the interphalangeal joint (IPJ) to compensate for a stiff MTPJ.
7. Lateral foot overload in order to avoid the dorsiflexion of the MTPJ

Pain on dorsiflexion with a negative grinds test suggests grade 1 and 2 disease with less than 25% of the joint surface involvement. A positive grind test suggests more than 25% joint involvement—grade 3 and 4 disease [9] (Table 3.1). Examination of IPJ is key as an arthritic IP and MTPJ warrants a surgical plan where both joints are not fused to avoid an abnormal gait pattern.

Table 3.1 Coughlin and Shurnas clinical radiographic system for Grading Hallux Rigidus [9]

Grade	Dorsiflexion	Radiographic	Clinical Findings
0	40° to 60° and/or 10% to 20% loss compared with normal side	Normal	No pain; only stiffness and loss of motion on examination
1	30° to 40° and/or 20% to 50% loss compared with normal side	Dorsal osteophyte is main finding, minimal joint-space narrowing, minimal periarticular sclerosis, minimal flattening of metatarsal head	Mild or occasional pain and stiffness, pain at extremes of dorsiflexion and/or plantar flexion on examination
2	10° to 30° and/or 50% to 75% loss compared with normal side	Dorsal, lateral, and possibly medial osteophytes giving flattened appearance to metatarsal head, no more than ¼ if dorsal joint space involved on lateral radiograph, mild-to-moderate joint-space narrowing and sclerosis, sesamoids not usually involved	Moderate-to-severe pain and stiffness that may be constant; pain occurs just before maximum dorsiflexion and maximum plantar flexion on examination
3	≤10° and/or 75% to 100% loss compared with the normal side. There is notable loss of metatarsophalangeal plantar flexion as well (often ≤10° of plantar flexion)	Same as in grade 2 but with substantial narrowing, possibly periarticular cystic changes, more than ¼ of dorsal joint space involved on lateral radiograph, sesamoids enlarged and/or cystic and/or irregular	Nearly constant pain and substantial stiffness at extremes of range of motion but not at mid-range
4	Same as in grade 3	Same as in grade 3	Same criteria as grade 3 but there is definite pain at mid-range of passive motion

Radiographic Evaluation

Imaging should consist of weight bearing anteroposterior (AP), lateral and oblique views of the affected side. On the AP view, non-uniform joint space narrowing with flattening and widening of the metatarsal head with subchondral sclerosis and bony cysts may be visualised. On the lateral view, dorsal osteophytes over the base of the proximal phalanx and the metatarsal head can be seen. These osteophytes are more often on the lateral than medial side of the metatarsal head.

Classification

The gold standard accepted classification for hallux rigidus is one proposed by Coughlin and Shurnas [9]. It is based on both clinical and radiological findings.

Non-operative Treatment

Non-operative management can be effective in a proportion of patients and should always be explored prior to surgery.

(a) **Activity modification**

Non load bearing exercises such as swimming or biking rather than running.

(b) **Footwear modification**

Stiff soled shoes with a wider toe box to accommodate dorsal osteophytes can be useful. A rocker bottom sole can also be added to decrease dorsiflexion motion of the first MTP joint by rocking the foot from heel-strike to toe-off.

(c) **Medications**

Early disease characterized by synovial irritation can be managed with non-steroidal anti-inflammatories.

(d) **Orthotics**

Orthotics are designed to limit motion across the first MTP joint while providing cushioning and plantar pressure distribution. An insole with a Morton's extension under the first ray that reduces the MTPJ range of motion might help in early disease.

(e) **Intra-articular injections**

Intra-articular injections with steroid and local anaesthetic/hyaluronic acid have shown to provide temporary relief. Solan et al., noted approximately 6 months of benefit using a steroid, local anaesthetic and joint manipulation for mild to moderate arthritis [10]. There was limited benefit of these injections with more advanced degenerative changes.

Operative Treatment

There is no best single procedure for the treatment of hallux rigidus, the choice of a particular one depends on clinical examination, patient activity level, patient expectations, and radiological staging. Surgical treatment can broadly be divided into joint sparing and joint sacrificing procedures. The goals of surgery are to relieve pain, if possible maintain the MTP range of motion, provide stability and ultimately improve function and quality of life.

Set Up

Application of a thigh or ankle tourniquet with a sandbag under the buttock of the operated side. Ensure the patients feet are sat at the foot-end of the operating table.

Surgical Approach

A dorsal or medial approach is used to expose the first MTPJ. The extensor hallucis longus (EHL) is identified and protected. A full thickness capsular incision is made either medial or lateral to the extensor tendon. Capsular releases are performed on either side of the MTPJ.

Cheilectomy

The ideal patient for a cheilectomy has primarily dorsal symptoms from impingement, large dorsal osteophytes on radiographs with minimal to mild joint-space narrowing [3]. Preoperative pain at the midrange of MTP motion correlated with less predictable satisfactory results [11].

Surgical Technique

To aid exposure the proximal phalanx is plantar flexed. The dorsal 20–25% of the articular surface of the metatarsal head is resected along with any dorsal osteophytes from the metatarsal and proximal phalanx. This is done in an oblique fashion using an oscillating saw or a medium sized osteotome. The intra-operative range of motion is often greater than what the patients actually achieve. Easley et al., found intra-operative range of motion could be as high as 80–90° whereas clinical dorsiflexion ranged between 20° and 40° [12]. It is important to avoid resection greater than one-third of the dorsal metatarsal head, as this can lead to dorsal subluxation of the proximal phalanx [13].

Moberg Osteotomy

The Moberg osteotomy is a closing-wedge osteotomy (dorsiflexion osteotomy of the proximal phalanx).

In patients with early arthritic changes the degenerative cartilage is predominantly on the dorsal aspect of the metatarsal head. This osteotomy offloads contact pressure over the diseased cartilage and facilitates the third rocker of gait (heel raise). The centre of pressure on the first metatarsal head is now shifted in a plantar direction [14]. As a result, less forces act on the arthritic joint surface. The Moberg osteotomy can be combined with a cheilectomy. O'Malley et al. retrospectively examined 81 patients with grade III radiographic hallux rigidus and reported 85% satisfaction after cheilectomy with a Moberg osteotomy [15].

Surgical Technique

A similar approach as the cheilectomy is utilised. Care must be taken to protect the EHL during the approach and whilst performing the osteotomy. The osteotomy is performed using a size 10 oscillating saw. Ensure the integrity of the plantar cortex is maintained and therefore the flexor hallucis tendon (FHL) is not at risk. The osteotomy is then stabilised with internal fixation, most commonly a staple (Fig. 3.1). This is a stable osteotomy and full weight bearing and early range of movements is encouraged to achieve excellent dorsiflexion after this operation (Fig. 3.2).

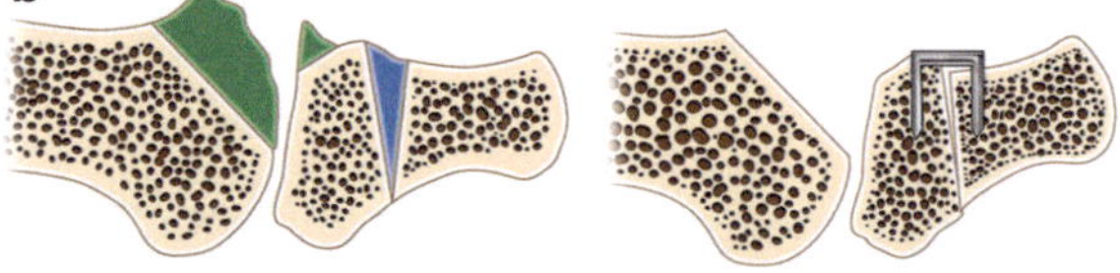

Fig. 3.1 (**a**, **b**) Moberg osteotomy

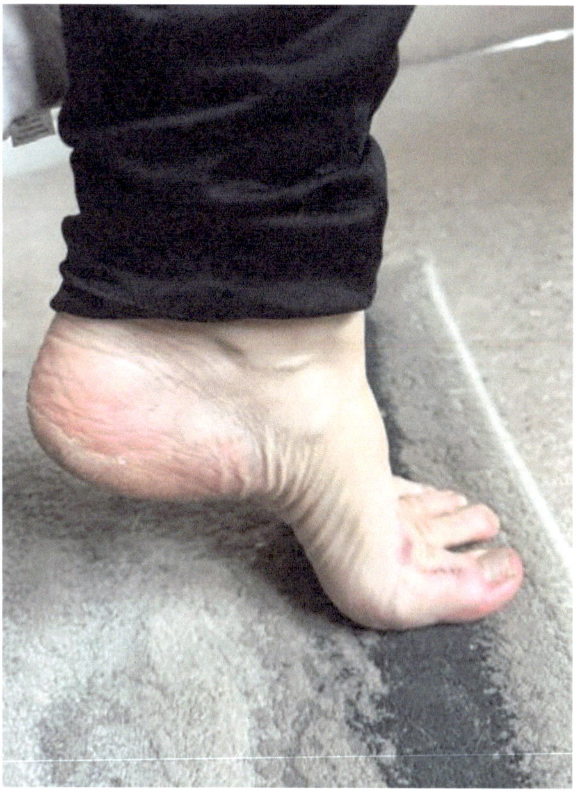

Fig. 3.2 Clinical photograph to demonstrate excellent dorsiflexion of first MTPJ following Moberg osteotomy 6 weeks post-surgery

Youngswick Osteotomy

The Youngswick osteotomy is effective in reducing symptoms and improving function in patients with mild to moderate hallux limitus or rigidus, provided appropriate patient selection and surgical technique is used. It is a modification of the Austin (Chevron) osteotomy of the first metatarsal, designed to provide dorsal decompression, shortening, and plantarflexion of the metatarsal head. The Youngswick osteotomy is typically indicated for:

1. **Hallux limitus/hallux rigidus:** Mild to moderate
2. **First metatarsal elevation:** Excessive dorsiflexion causing limited joint function
3. **Shortening of the first metatarsal:** Addressing metatarsalgia

Surgical Technique (as Described by Alessio Bernasconi)

The technique is performed using a medial/dorsomedial incision at the first MTPJ. As for all surgeries performed through this approach, care must be taken not to damage the dorsal medial cutaneous nerve of the hallux during subcutaneous dissection. After capsulotomy, the dorsal and medial osteophytes (classically found in this setting) can be removed using osteotomes, chisels or a 1-cm saw. The V-shaped osteotomy is performed through two cuts (dorsal and plantar) (Fig. 3.3). An additional second dorsal cut is made parallel to the first in order to remove a small bone segment. To the best of our knowledge, no agreement exists in literature regarding the thickness of this segment, which may range between 3 and 6 mm depending on the length of the first metatarsal and the desired decompression effect. The thicker the bone segment removed, the greater will be the relief at the joint with higher risk of transfer metatarsalgia. On the other side, the obliquity of the plantar cut will be planned based on the amount of desired plantarflexion, which is crucial especially in the setting of metatarsal elevation. The osteotomy is then traditionally stabilized using double-threaded cannulated screws (from 2 mm to 3.5 mm). Post surgery full weight bearing is permitted in a heel wedge shoe for 4 weeks. At 4 weeks after satisfactory X-rays weight bearing is permitted without the heel wedge shoe. Figures 3.4 and 3.5 demonstrate restoration of joint space and plantarisation of metatarsal head following this procedure (Figs. 3.4 and 3.5).

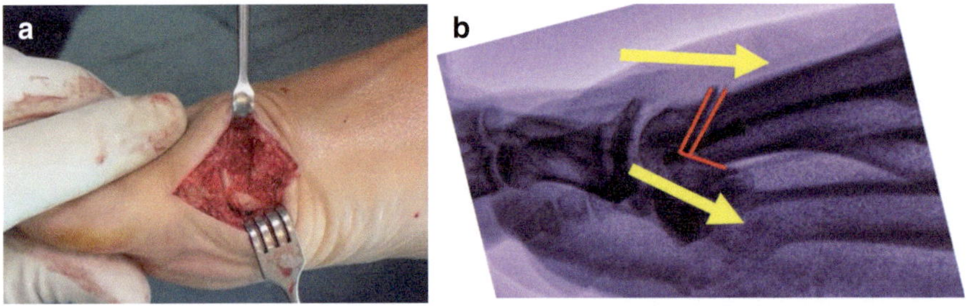

Fig. 3.3 (**a** and **b**) Clinical picture and Intra-operative images of a right first metatarsal following a V shaped osteotomy, removal of bone causing a decompression and plantarization of the first metatarsal head. (Figure courtesy of **Alessio Bernasconi**)

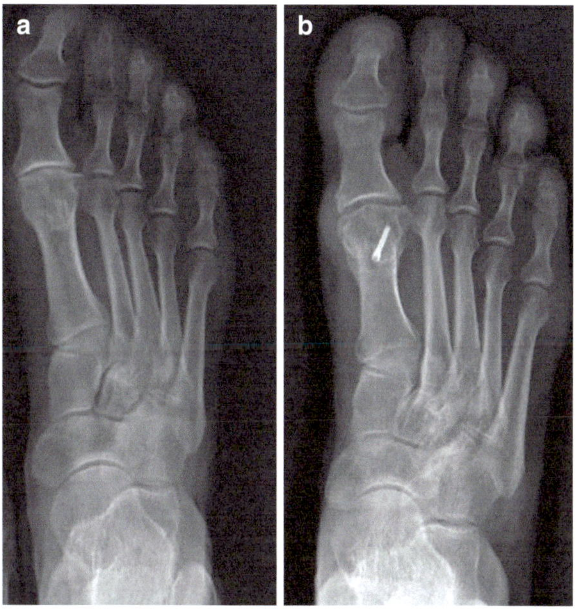

Fig. 3.4 (**a** and **b**) Pre and post operative AP radiographs of a right foot following a Youngswick osteotomy demonstrating longitudinal decompression and shortening of the first metatarsal. (Figure courtesy of **Alessio Bernasconi**)

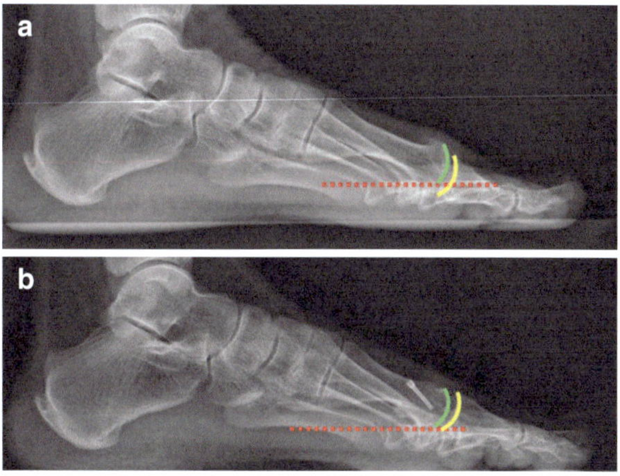

Fig. 3.5 (**a** and **b**) Pre and post operative lateral radiographs of right foot following a Youngswick osteotomy demonstrating plantarization of the first metatarsal head. (Figure courtesy of **Alessio Bernasconi**)

MTPJ Arthrodesis

For advanced arthritis MTPJ fusion remains the current gold standard of treatment with high satisfaction rates [16, 17]. Arthrodesis can also be used in patients with concomitant hallux valgus, hallux varus, rheumatoid arthritis and neuromuscular disorders. In patients with rheumatoid arthritis the soft tissue destruction and instability that ensues precludes joint sparing procedures. There are multiple joint preparation techniques and internal fixation devices for arthrodesis. In this next section we shall consider each individual step.

Surgical Approach

The first MTPJ can be exposed through medial or dorsal approaches. Medial approach (Fig. 3.6) is better in case of enlarged bunion and significant hallux valgus deformity. Another advantage of this approach is that the distal compression screw can be inserted through the same incision. Medial, lateral and a plantar capsular

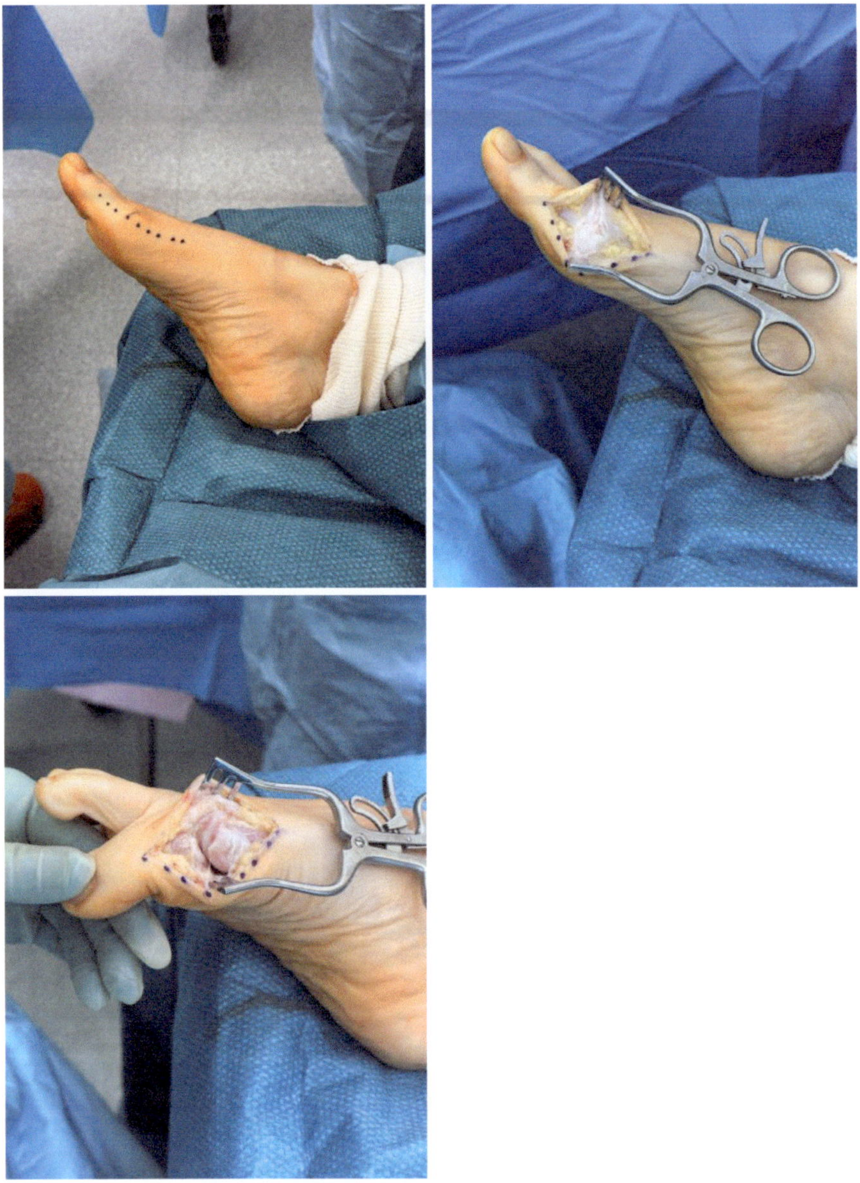

Fig. 3.6 Showing the medial approach—skin marking, medial capsule exposure and exposure of the joint following capsular release

release allows for disarticulation of the MTPJ. A curved periosteal elevator allows for a plantar capsule release and the authors recommend this release is performed between the metatarsal head and sesamoids and under the proximal phalanx.

Joint Preparation

The joint can be prepared by the following techniques:

1. Non-motorised—nibblers, osteotomes (Fig. 3.7) or rongeurs.
2. Motorised Saw, reamers or burr

Whilst flat cuts are easier to make, achieving optimal position of arthrodesis with congruous joint surfaces can be technically demanding [18]. Politi et al. on the other hand [19] found that flat cuts produced a more stable construct than conical reamers. Conical reamers permit for some change in angulation whilst maintaining bony contact (Fig. 3.8). In terms of union following joint fusion, the joint preparation method used makes no significant difference and either method can be adopted. In the case of soft bone it is better to avoid power instrumentation.

In patients with soft porotic bone e.g. rheumatoid arthritis, care must be taken whilst reaming as this can lead to iatrogenic fractures or undue shortening. We would recommend to use non-motorised instruments in preparing the joint surfaces in these cases . If using the reamer in these cases one must use it with caution at low torque/speed. The combination of high torque and firm pressure can be disastrous. Fenestration of the joint surface should be done following the reaming, where the subchondral surface is perforated using either a drill, or osteotomes (Fig. 3.9).

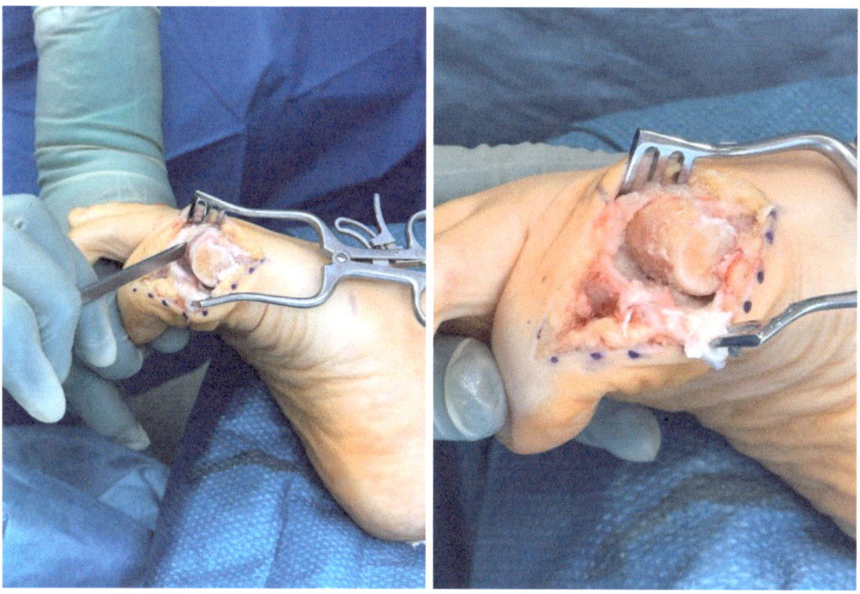

Fig. 3.7 Use of osteotome to prepare first metatarsal head

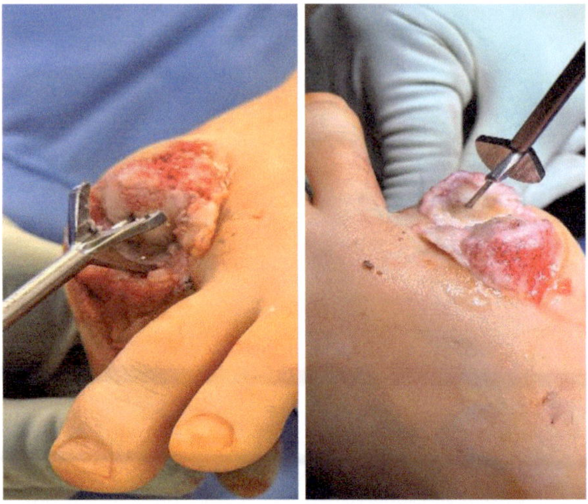

Fig. 3.8 (**a**) Cannulated reamers used to prepare metatarsal head (**b**) Preparation of the proximal phalanx

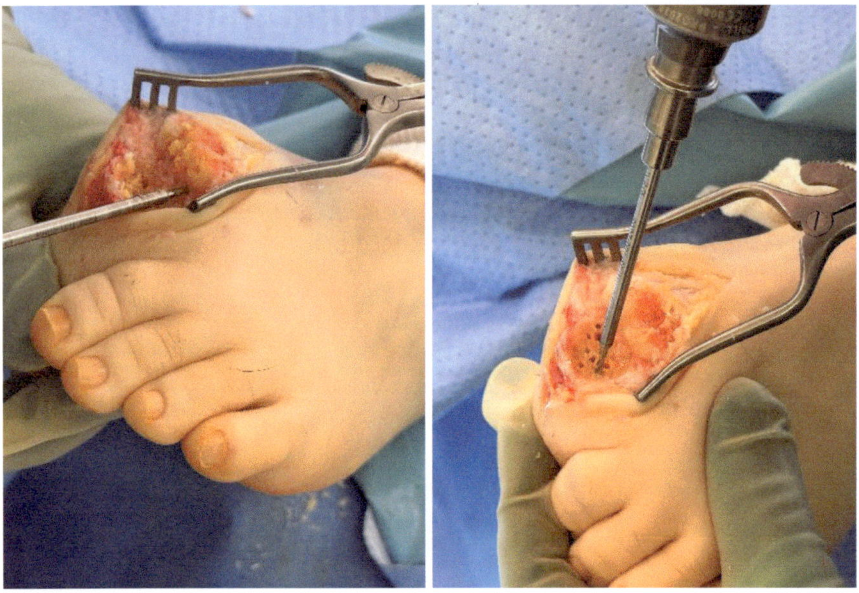

Fig. 3.9 (**a**) and (**b**): Fenestration of the proximal phalanx and metatarsal head.

Alignment of the Arthrodesis

Dorsiflexion is determined by simulated weight bearing. This should be assessed intra-operatively with the entire foot being placed on a foot plate (including the heel). The hallux should just make contact with the plate (Fig. 3.10). There should be flexibility of the IPJ to allow elevation and enable the surgeon to get a digit between the foot plate and the distal pulp. Rotational alignment is assessed from the

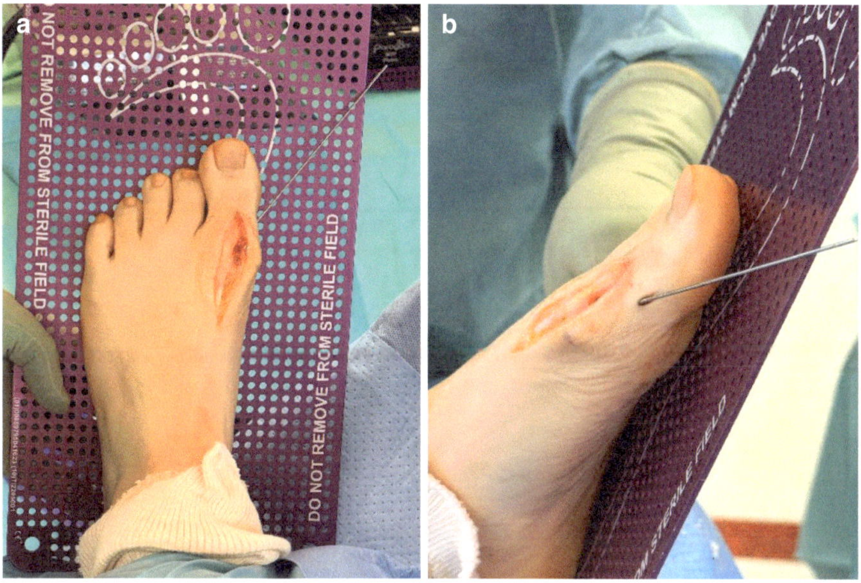

Fig. 3.10 (**a**) and (**b**): AP and Lateral View assessing simulated weight bearing of the great toe following insertion of the cannulated screw.

nail plate, which should be neutral. The optimal position of the first MTP joint is with neutral rotation and up to 10° of valgus and dorsiflexion.

Stabilisation

There are numerous devices that can be used to stabilise the MTPJ, which include crossed screws, a lag screw with a dorsal plate or staples. A recent systematic review of modes of fixation following MTPJ fusion which compared staples, screws and a dorsal plate with a lag screw technique found the highest rates of union were achieved using staples however better results across several outcome measures, including reduced complication incidence, stability, early ambulation, and good functional outcomes were found using a dorsal plate and lag screw technique [20]. The choice of implant depends on surgeon preference and cost. We would advocate the dorsal plate and lag screw technique for patients with soft porotic bone and or an associated hallux valgus.

Following joint preparation we would advise using a 1.6 mm k wire to stabilize the joint temporarily whilst assessing the position of the hallux (rotation, varus/valgus and sagittal plane). The insertion of the lag screw should follow. This can be placed from the medial border of the proximal phalanx across the joint and exiting lateral border of the metatarsal (Fig. 3.11a) or from medial border of the metatarsal across the joint and exiting the lateral border of the proximal phalanx (Fig. 3.11b). The former could lead to varus whereas the latter could cause valgus (Fig. 3.11a and b).

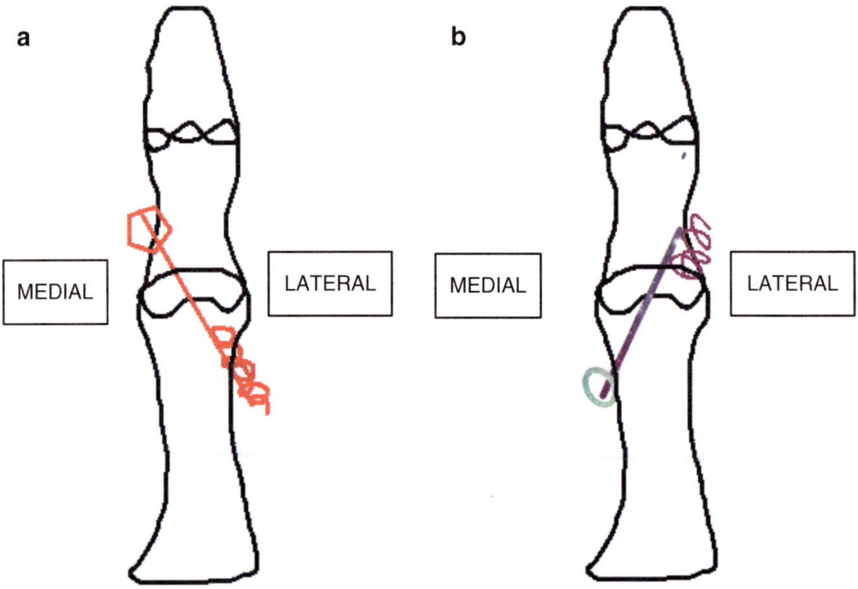

Fig. 3.11 (**a**) Lag screw insertion from proximal phalanx into metatarsal, compressing the medial side of the joint can alter the position into varus. (**b**) Lag screw insertion from metatarsal into proximal phalanx, compressing lateral side of the joint, can alter position into valgus

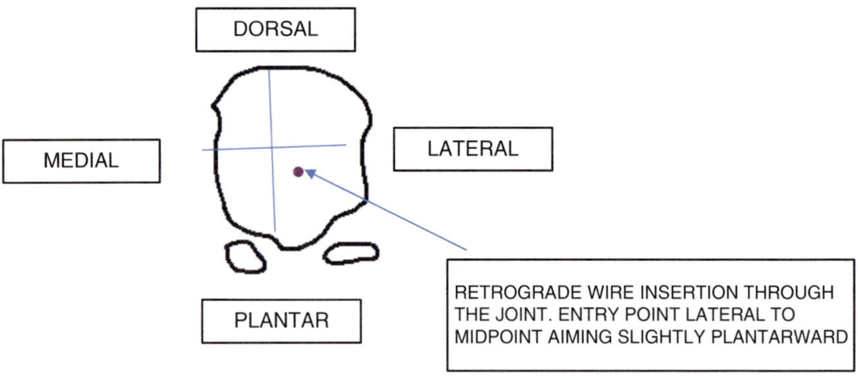

Fig. 3.12 En face view of Metatarsal head: Retrograde insertion of k wire through metatarsal head

A tip is to drive the guide wire for the cannulated lag screw well beyond the far cortex after measuring its depth. Although care should be taken whilst using the cannulated drill not to bend or break the guide wire, however, if the guide wire breaks it can be retrieved relatively easily if it is penetrated beyond the cortex. Another surgical tip is 'retrograde' wire insertion technique using a double ended k wire. The joint is exposed to enable the surgeon to view the metatarsal head en face (Fig. 3.12). The wire can then be inserted into the metatarsal head aiming in plantar direction and exiting the medial cortex of the metatarsal. The joint is then reduced and held in place whilst the wire is then advanced to traverse the joint and into the proximal phalanx on the lateral aspect.

The combination of one distal compression screw and a locking plate is the preferred fixation option of the authors for first MTPJ fusion surgery (Fig. 3.13). Once locking screws are used for the proximal phalanx, the use of non-locking screw in the oblong hole on the metatarsal side provides additional compression (Fig. 3.13c).

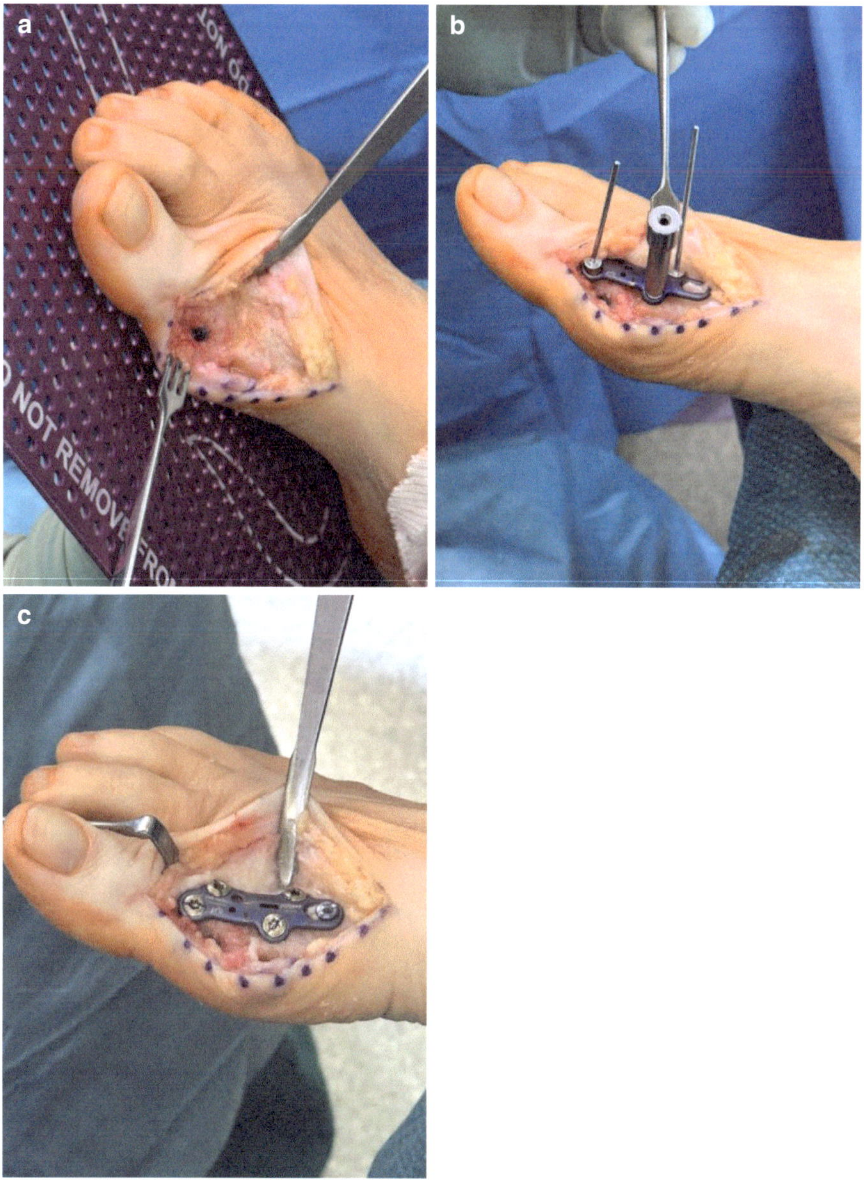

Fig. 3.13 (**a**) Use of the compression screw inserted from medial aspect of base of proximal phalanx into metatarsal head. (**b**) Temporary stabilisation of locking plate. (**c**) Final stabilisation of locking pate

MTPJ Arthroplasty

The main advantage of arthroplasty over arthrodesis is the preservation of movement without the risk of malunion or non-union. Both total joint arthroplasty and hemiarthroplasty of the proximal phalanx or metatarsal have been developed with various materials being used. Despite the potential benefit of maintaining joint motion while relieving pain, multiple complications have been documented for arthroplasty, including implant failure, soft tissue instability, aseptic loosening of components, pathological wear, limited soft tissue coverage and infection [21, 22]. To help categorize the history and the various implants available, Cook et al., categorized them into 4 generations: [23].

- First generation: material—silicone: design—hemiarthroplasty and total
- Second generation: material—improved silicone: design— hemiarthroplasty and total implants with grommets
- Third generation: material—metallic: design—hemiarthroplasty and total implants that are press fit
- Fourth generation: material—metallic: design—hemiarthroplasty and total implants that have a threaded stem

The success and benefit of implants documented in the literature should be scrutinized given the high degree of heterogeneity amongst the studies. In addition, there remain complications including revising implant failure which can be challenging due to bone loss.

Silastic MTPJ Replacement

The silastic implant is designed to act as a sloppy hinged dynamic spacer. It has no inbuilt ability to correct deformity or maintain correction. It is not directly attached to bone, allowing self- alignment in the axis of the joint [24]. Properties of silastic implants include:

1. Low modulus of elasticity reduces stress shielding and promotes bone loading.
2. Viscoelastic properties with high resistance to fatigue

The silastic implant has had a poor reputation when used in the past that can be attributed to two main causes: use of a single stemmed implant and poor patient selection (hallux valgus deformity). A retrospective review of 106 double stemmed silastic implants by Clough et al., found the survivorship of 97.2% at a mean of 5 years, with improvements in patient reported outcome measures (PROM) [24]. The main indications for use of Sialistic MTPJ replacement includes females over the age of 60 years, with end stage arthritis and a well aligned hallux.

Surgical Technique

The head of the first metatarsal is excised distal to the metaphyseal flare at the longest diameter of the metatarsal head. A size 10 oscillating saw is used to resect the portion of the head in 10° valgus. The base of the proximal phalanx is also resected. We recommend the use of a 2.5 mm drill for creating an entry point in the centre of the metatarsal head and proximal phalanx which can then be widened using the rasps. The rasps are numbered 0–7, 0 being the smallest with a sequential increase in diameter and length. The recommendation is to start with size 0 and work on the metatarsal followed by the proximal phalanx. Implant size is dependent upon the rasps used. The intramedullary canal is shaped in a rectangular fashion to accept the implant stem. The canals are washed out and cleared of any debris before implant insertion—a thin suction (Frazier) facilitates this. The (longer) stem of the implant is inserted in the intramedullary canal of the first metatarsal with the open portion of the hinge positioned dorsally. The toe is then flexed, and the distal (shorter) stem is inserted into the proximal phalanx. Prior to insertion, dip the implant in saline and use a non-toothed forceps to handle the implant. The grommets are not required [25].

Revision MTPJ Surgery

Revision surgery following MTPJ arthrodesis or replacement can be challenging due to bone loss. Excessive shortening can lead to transfer metatarsalgia and therefore metatarsal length needs to be preserved. Restoration of first ray length and alignment often cannot be achieved with in situ fusion and reconstruction techniques with bone graft are therefore required [26]. Revision surgery following an MTPJ fusion or arthroplasty may be required due to infection, aseptic non-union, mal union, synovitis, implant migration and osteolysis. Infection should be excluded through the baseline investigations including blood tests, appropriate imaging and swabs if appropriate. Deep tissue sampling off antibiotics should identify a causative organism. Local antibiotic elution can be achieved using bioabsorbable antibiotic carriers such as Stimulan [27] or Cerament [28], which provide the added advantage of preventing contracture of soft tissue. A staged revision can then be performed once infection clearance has been achieved. Our routine practice for deep infection with underlying osteomyelitis would be 6 weeks of antibiotics, followed by a 2-week holiday period (off antibiotics) with repeat inflammatory markers prior to definitive surgery.

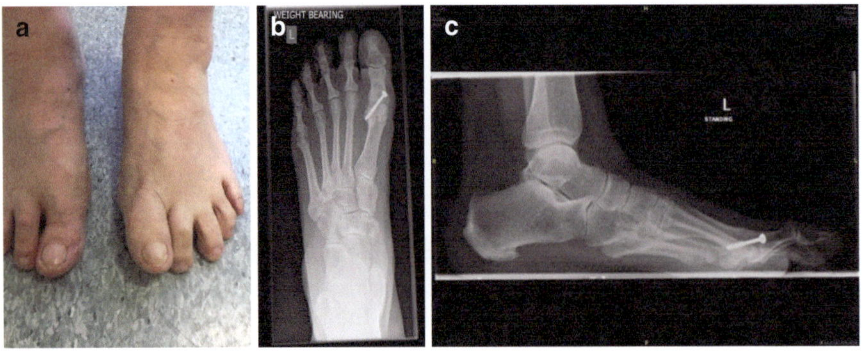

Fig. 3.14 (**a**) Clinical photograph dorsal mal union following left foot MTPJ fusion. (**b** and **c**) AP and lateral radiograph left foot hallux dorsal malunion

Metatarsophalangeal Joint Malunion

Malunion can occur in 3 planes:

1. Coronal plane—varus/valgus
2. Sagittal plane—dorsi/plantar flexion
3. Rotational

Malunion of the arthrodesis site is poorly tolerated. Excessive plantar flexion can lead to pressure at the plantar pulp of the hallux and excessive dorsiflexion can lead to pain at the tip of the toe due to compensatory flexion of the IPJ and transfer metatarsalgia (Fig. 3.14). A systematic review by Roukis et al. [29] reported a 6.1% incidence of malunion.

Metatarsophalangeal Joint Non-Union

As per Roukis et al. the overall incidence of nonunion following first MTPJ fusion is 5.4%. Only one thirds of radiological non unions are symptomatic [29]. Metal work removal alone could improve pain in about 50% of the symptomatic non unions. Revision fusion can be performed using more robust fixation and bone graft from calcaneus is usually sufficient if there is not too much bone loss or shortening (Figs. 3.15 and 3.16).

However, in cases with bone loss, restoration of length can be achieved through bone block arthrodesis which can be allograft or autograft. Luk et al., described

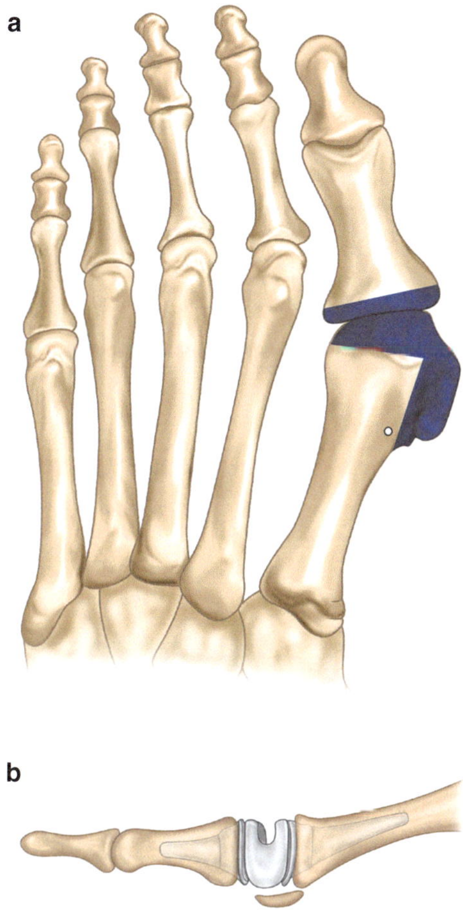

Fig. 3.15 (**a**, **b**) Picture demonstrating osteotomy of the head of the metatarsal and base of the proximal phalanx. Lateral view demonstrating implant positioning with hinge aligned dorsally

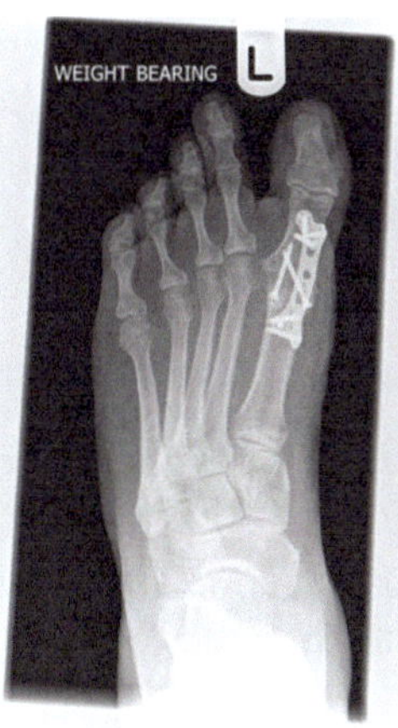

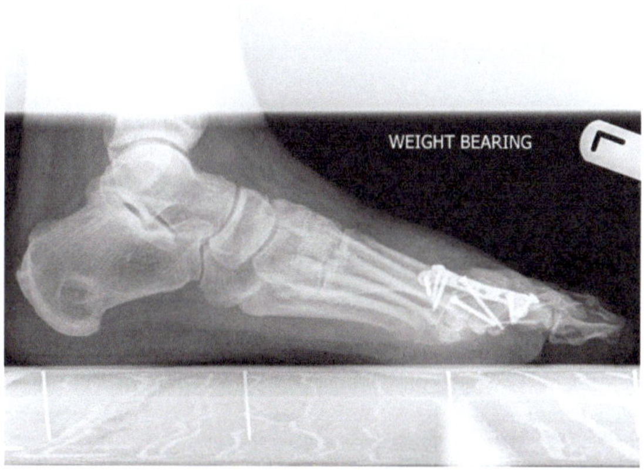

Fig. 3.16 Weight bearing AP and lateral view following revision MTPJ fusion for non-union with bone grafting from calcaneum

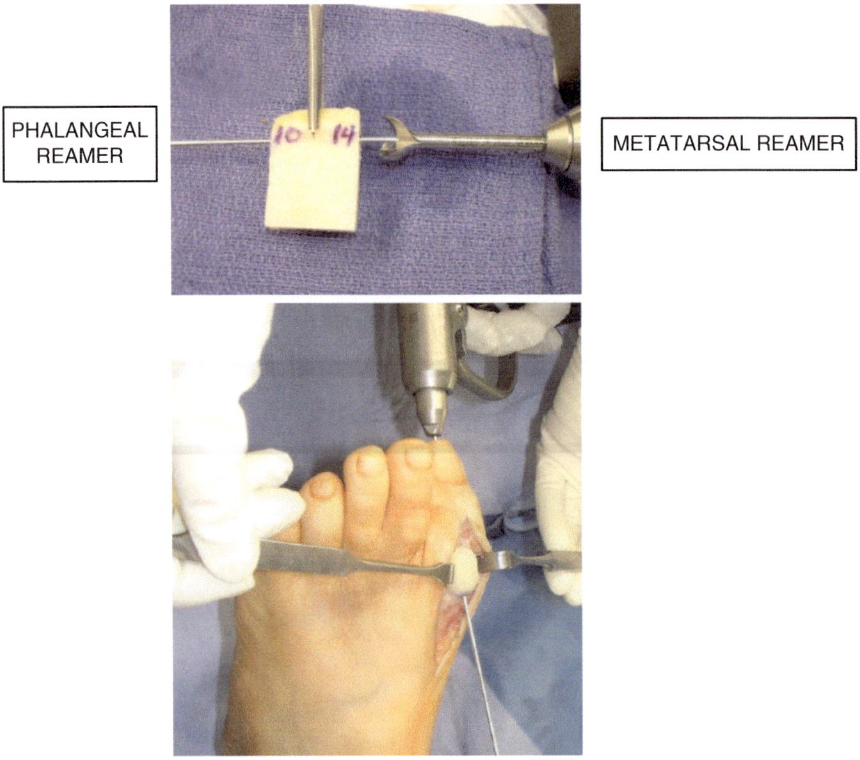

Fig. 3.17 (**a**) The allograft bone is prepared with reamers matching the sizes used for the metatarsal head and base of the phalanx. (**b**) The bone graft is placed in the defect and held with a K-wire before final fixation [30].

using interpositional bone block allograft in their patients [30]. They used a spherical reaming technique for preparation of the allograft. Their described technique can be used for both allograft and autograft (tricortical iliac crest) (Fig. 3.17).

Malagelada et al., described a technique of longitudinal (proximo-distal) bone dowel arthrodesis [26].

Surgical Technique (Dowel Technique) (Fig. 3.18)

A structural bi-cortical autograft measuring an additional 2 cm from the measured bone gap is harvested from the iliac crest and is then contoured in shape of a dowel. Cancellous bone graft is also harvested. The dowel is then inserted into the metatarsal cavity first followed by the proximal phalangeal cavity. The position of the toe is assessed against a flat surface to simulate the weight-bearing situation, as per a

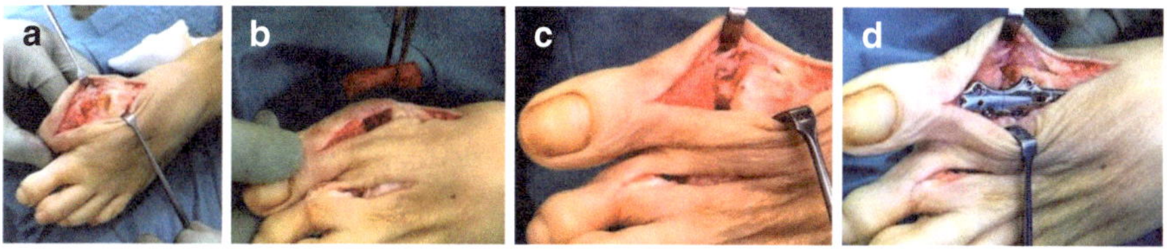

Fig. 3.18 (**a**) Preparation of the joint with intra-medullary holes in the base of the proximal phalanx and the metatarsal head. (**b**) Structural iliac crest bone graft prepared in a dowel shape of the required size and contoured to fit into the intramedullary holes (**c**) Dowel bone graft inserted in the MTPJ and evidence of the lengthening achieved. (**d**) Low-profile plate inserted for internal fixation and the remaining gap that is packed with cancellous bone graft [26]

standard arthrodesis. The correct position is held with the help of the dowel, which provides intrinsic stability while internal fixation is performed. Cancellous bone graft from the iliac crest is packed in around the dowel.

Advantages of the dowel-shaped bone graft include:

1. Inherently stable
2. Used for restoring length and large defects
3. The intramedullary position of the dowel graft is in direct contact with the endosteal blood supply.

Restoration of length can cause skin problems; therefore we would recommend downsizing the graft to ensure the soft tissues are not under tension.

First MTPJ Fusion for Deformity Correction

First MTPJ fusion can be performed for severe hallux valgus correction especially in elderly patients or as a revision procedure to correct iatrogenic deformity (Fig. 3.19). It can be technically difficult surgery and some technical tips are:

(a) Slight eccentric placement of guide wire for reaming: This can be useful for deformity correction
(b) Caution with the use of power instruments: The bone quality can be poor.
(c) Correction of supination in hallux valgus: The proximal phalanx in hallux valgus deformities, supinates. This additional deformity will need correction to ensure a mal union does not occur.
(d) Use of robust fixation and consideration of bone graft from calcaneus: Hallux valgus is a significant risk factor for non-union following first MTPJ fusion. A combination of compression screw, locking plate and bone graft is useful to prevent this complication.

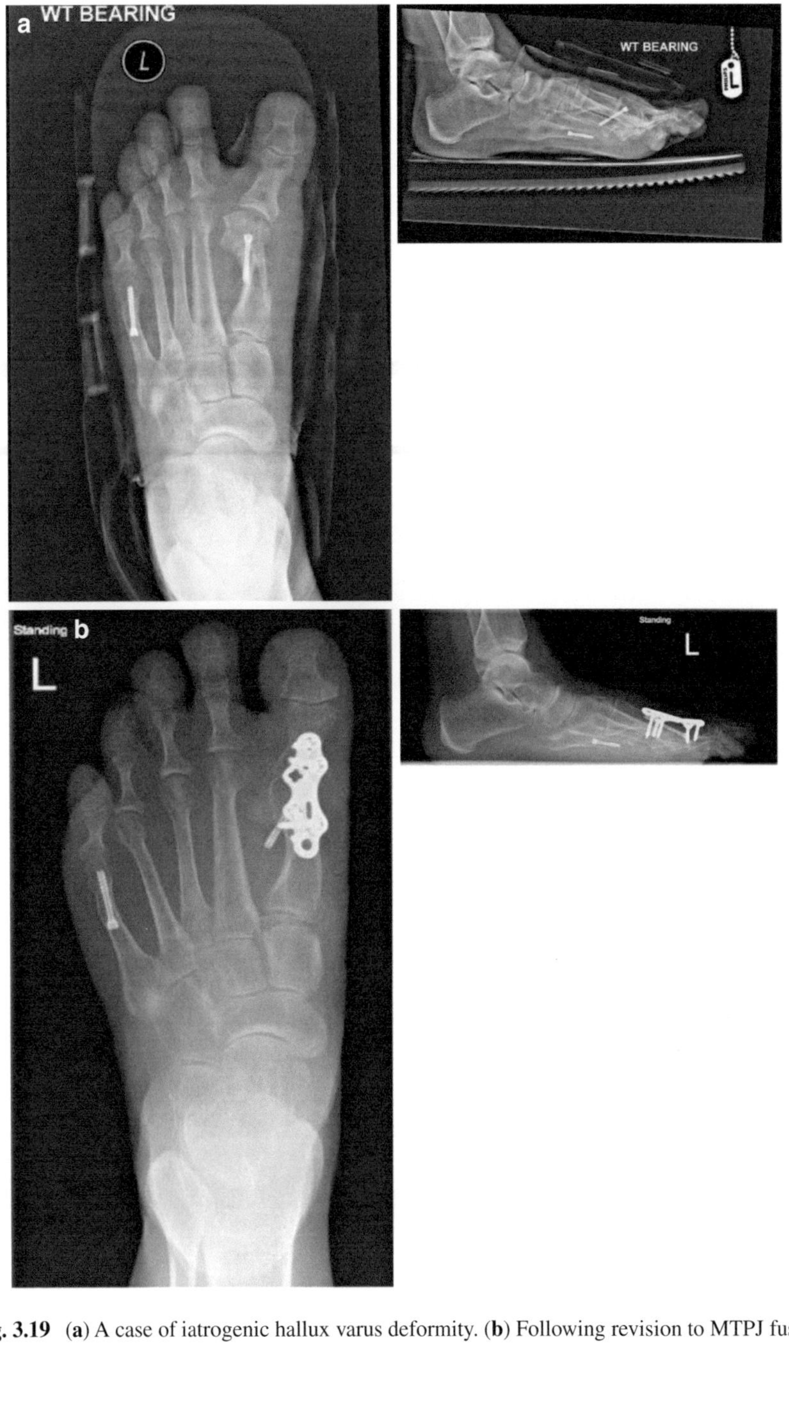

Fig. 3.19 (**a**) A case of iatrogenic hallux varus deformity. (**b**) Following revision to MTPJ fusion

Conclusions

Hallux rigidus is a common pathology that presents to foot and ankle clinics. Following an appropriate assessment, once a decision has been made to proceed with surgical intervention, there are several different operations that can be utilised. The choice is dependent upon the patient, radiographs, deformity, equipment available and surgical preference. Whichever procedure is chosen at final outcome ensures the toe is plantigrade and avoids shortening the hallux significantly as this can lead to metatarsalgia.

References

1. Bowen C, Gates L, McQueen P, Daniels M, Delmestri A, Drechsler W, Stephensen D, Doherty M, Arden N. Natural history of radiographic first metatarsophalangeal joint osteoarthritis: a nineteen-year population-based cohort study. Arthritis Care Res (Hoboken). 2020;72(9):1224–30.
2. Roddy E, Thomas MJ, Marshall M, Rathod T, Myers H, Menz HB, Thomas E, Peat G. The population prevalence of symptomatic radiographic foot osteoarthritis in community-dwelling older adults: cross-sectional findings from the clinical assessment study of the foot. Ann Rheum Dis. 2015;74(1):156–63.
3. Ho B, Baumhauer J. Hallux Rigidus. EFORT Open Rev. 2017;2(1):13–20. https://doi.org/10.1302/2058-5241.2.160031.
4. Coughlin MJ , , Shurnas PS . Hallux rigidus: demographics, etiology, and radiographic assessment. Foot Ankle Int 2003;24:731–743.
5. Moberg E. A Simple Operation for Hallux Rigidus. Clin Orthop Relat Res (1976–2007). 1979;142:55–6.
6. Shereff MJ , , Bejjani FJ , , Kummer FJ . Kinematics of the first metatarsophalangeal joint. J Bone Joint Surg Am 1986;68-A:392–398.
7. Migues A, Slullitel G. Joint-preserving procedure for moderate hallux rigidus. Foot Ankle Clin. 2012;17:459–71. https://doi.org/10.1016/j.fcl.2012.06.006.
8. Hamid KS, Parekh SG. Clinical presentation and Management of Hallux Rigidus. Foot Ankle Clin. 2015;20:391–9. https://doi.org/10.1016/j.fcl.2015.04.002.
9. Coughlin MJ, Shurnas PS, Hallux rigidus. Grading and long-term results of operative treatment. J Bone Joint Surg Am. 2003;85-A:2072–88.
10. Solan MC, Calder JD, Bendall SP. Manipulation and injection for hallux rigidus. Is it worthwhile? J Bone Joint Surg Br. 2001;83(5):706–808.
11. DuVries H. Surgery of the foot. St. Louis: Mosby Year Book; 1959. p. 392–9.
12. Easley ME, Davis WH, Anderson RB. Intermediate to long-term follow-up of medial-approach dorsal cheilectomy for hallux rigidus. Foot Ankle Int. 1999;20:147–52.
13. Nawoczenski DA, Ketz J, Baumhauer JF. Dynamic kinematic and plantar pressure changes following cheilectomy for hallux rigidus: a mid-term follow up. Foot Ankle Int. 2008;29:265–72.
14. Kim PH, Chen X, Hillstrom H, et al. Moberg osteotomy shifts contact pressure plantarly in the first metatarsophalangeal joint in a biomechanical model. Foot Ankle Int. 2016;37:96–101.
15. O'Malley MJ, Basran HS, Gu Y, Sayres S, Deland JT. Treatment of advanced stages of hallux rigidus with cheilectomy and phalangeal osteotomy. J Bone Joint Surg Am. 2013;95-A:606–10.
16. Flavin R, Stephens MM. Arthrodesis of the first metatarsophalangeal joint using a dorsal titanium contoured plate. Foot Ankle Int. 2004;25:783–7.
17. Coughlin MJ, Grebing BR, Jones CP. Arthrodesis of the first metatarsophalan geal joint for idiopathic hallux valgus: intermediate results. Foot Ankle Int. 2005;26:783–92.

18. Mahadevan D, Korim MT, Ghosh A, Allen PE, Bhatia M, Mangwani J. First metatarsophalangeal joint arthrodesis—do joint configuration and preparation technique matter? Foot Ankle Surg. 2015;21(2):103–7. https://doi.org/10.1016/j.fas.2014.10.002.
19. Politi J, John H, Njus G, Bennett GL, Kay DB. First metatarsal-phalangeal joint arthrodesis: a biomechanical assessment of stability. Foot Ankle Int. 2003;24:332–7.
20. Kang YS, Bridgen A. First metatarsophalangeal joint arthrodesis/fusion: a systematic review of modern fixation techniques. J Foot Ankle Res. 2022;15:30. https://doi.org/10.1186/s13047-022-00540-9.
21. Horisberger M, Haeni D, Henninger HB, Valderrabano V, Barg A. Total arthroplasty of the metatarsophalangeal joint of the Hallux. Foot Ankle Int. 2016;37:755–65. https://doi.org/10.1177/1071100716637901.
22. Nagy MT, Walker CR, Sirikonda SP. Second-generation ceramic first metatarsophalangeal joint replacement for Hallux Rigidus. Foot Ankle Int. 2014;35:690–8. https://doi.org/10.1177/1071100714536539.
23. Cook E, Cook J, Rosenblum B, Landsman A, Giurini J, Basile P. Meta-analysis of first metatarsophalangeal joint implant arthroplasty. J Foot Ankle Surg. 2009;48(2):180–90. https://doi.org/10.1053/j.jfas.2008.10.009.
24. Clough TM, Ring J. Silastic first metatarsophalangeal joint arthroplasty for the treatment of end-stage hallux rigidus. Bone Joint J. 2020;102-B(2):220–6. https://doi.org/10.1302/0301-620x.102b2.bjj-2019-0518.r2.
25. Operative Technique – Swanson Flexible Hinge Toe.pdf
26. Malagelada F, Welck MJ, Clark C. The dowel technique for first metatarso-phalangeal joint arthrodesis in revision surgery with bone loss. Foot Ankle Surg. 2018;24(3):224–8. https://doi.org/10.1016/j.fas.2017.02.009.
27. https://biocomposites.com/our-products/stimulan/
28. https://www.bonesupport.com/en-eu/products/cerament-bone-void-filler/
29. Roukis TS. Nonunion after arthrodesis of the first metatarsal-phalangeal joint: a systematic review. J Foot Ankle Surg. 2011;50(6):710–3. https://doi.org/10.1053/j.jfas.2011.06.012.
30. Luk PC, Johnson JE, McCormick JJ, Klein SE. First metatarsophalangeal joint arthrodesis technique with interposition allograft bone block. Foot Ankle Int. 2015;36(8):936–43. https://doi.org/10.1177/1071100715577953.

Chapter 4
Surgery for Arthritis of Midfoot

Manuel Monteagudo

Introduction

Midfoot arthritis is characterized by pain and swelling in the midfoot, which is worsened by standing and walking. Symptoms usually develop gradually over time, although faster after major midfoot trauma, such as a navicular fracture. Post traumatic midfoot arthritis is much more common than primary arthritis [1]. Other etiologies include inflammatory diseases and neuropathic conditions [2]. The tarsometatarsal joint is most involved when compared to other midtarsal joints [3]. Physical examination reveals generalized swelling and tenderness most commonly in the medial and dorsal aspects of the midfoot, with osteophytes often palpable because of the underlying arthritis. Clinical gait analysis commonly shows valgus collapse around the midfoot that is frequently combined with some degree of forefoot abduction [4]. Weight-bearing x-rays generally demonstrate loss of joint space in the midfoot joints and allow us to understand the type of deformity and location of the apex of collapse. Magnetic resonance imaging and computerized tomography are useful to quantify bone stock and address the extent of arthritis in surrounding joints. SPECT-CT may reveal subtle areas of arthritis that could otherwise go undiagnosed. Non-operative treatment consisting of the use of a stiff-soled comfort shoe, activity modification, and weight-loss, can be effective [5]. In the presence of deformity, insoles may play a role in the management of midfoot arthritis by redistributing weight and loads towards unaffected joints [6]. If non-operative treatment fails to alleviate pain and improve function, surgery is usually linked to a

M. Monteagudo (✉)
Foot and Ankle Unit—Trauma & Orthopaedics—Hospital Universitario Quironsalud, Madrid, Spain

Department of Medicine, Faculty of Medicine, Health and Sports, European University of Madrid, Madrid, Spain

M. Bhatia (ed.), *Surgical Techniques of the Foot and Ankle*,
https://doi.org/10.1007/978-3-031-93742-2_4

satisfactory outcome which most authors report to be in the range of 90% [7–9]. Arthrodesis is the most common procedure performed for midfoot arthritis but joint preserving surgery with osteotomies may be indicated in rare cases of asymmetric joint affection. In this chapter we will focus on surgical techniques available for arthritis of the midfoot and will try to provide the reader with some of the tips and tricks we have learned through years of success and failure.

Background and Pathogenesis

Trauma is the most common origin of midfoot arthritis. The triceps surae and plantar fascia act as a tension band usually generating dorsal compression of the affected joints which explains a frequent pattern of more dorsal than plantar wear in midfoot arthritis. Müller Weiss disease (MWD) is an example of asymmetrical arthritis where the talonavicular joint is affected laterally but not medially [10]. In the case of MWD, alteration of hindfoot mechanics leads to the development of a midfoot-driven hindfoot varus with subsequent loss of sagittal plane motion in the midtarsal joints.

Key Points in Examination

The combination of a thorough physical examination including visual gait analysis with the correct interpretation of weight bearing radiographs of both feet should allow us to make a diagnosis of most cases of midfoot arthritis and the associated deformities.

Clinical Examination—*Visual Gait Analysis and Deformity assessment*
We routinely ask the patient to walk barefoot in our clinic to start with visual gait analysis. In many patients it is evident that there is deformity and sometimes the apex of collapse is visible. Tarsometatarsal arthritis typically presents with valgus and abduction collapse. When deformity is in the Chopart joint, valgus is also more common than varus. In those cases, it is important to address whether the medial prominence corresponds to the talar head (true collapsing/flatfoot) or to the medial tuberosity of the navicular (*"paradoxical varus flat foot"in MWD).* In MWD, varus may be obvious or subtle. In subtle cases, grasping the patient's heel while asking the patient to do a bipodal toe-off may be of help. The "palpable" varus is maintained throughout the entire length of the toe-off and up to the plantigrade position of the foot, unlike valgus flatfoot in which (when the subtalar is mobile) the heel shifts from valgus to varus with the bipodal or monopodal heel rise [10]. Tenderness in midfoot arthritis is mostly dorsal but can also extend to the lateral and medial regions of the foot and ankle depending on how deformity behaves, altering the mechanical balance of the foot and ankle.

Imaging Studies—*Less Is More*
Weight bearing radiographs of both feet provides most of the information necessary to complete the diagnosis of midfoot arthritis and to know about the origin of deformity. Computerized tomography (CT) can help quantifying arthropathy, bone stock, and addressing osteoarthritis in the neighbouring joints. Magnetic resonance imaging (MRI) often reveals bone marrow oedema and associated soft-tissue injuries. Other tests such as SPECT-CT scintigraphy or weight-bearing CT can help to assess subtalar joint congruency and subtle associated lesions in the neighbouring joints [11].

Other Investigations
Posttraumatic cases may have suffered vascular damage that should be addressed preoperatively (revascularization prior to arthrodesis) as a well vascularized bone is paramount to obtain a solid fusion.

Management

Conservative treatment should be considered before surgery regardless of the type of arthritis or pain.

Non-operative Treatment

As with any mechanical pathology of the foot, conservative treatment should always precede any surgical indication [5]. In our experience, physical means of rehabilitation and anti-inflammatory medication generally have little effect in the treatment of midfoot arthritis. Mechanical foot problems need mechanical-based solutions. The use of insoles with a pronatory/supinatory wedge depending on type of deformity may work in most patients [11, 12]. Rocker bottom shoes are especially indicated in the presence of midfoot arthritis without deformity when insoles have a lower impact on rebalancing the foot [12].

Operative Treatment

Those patients who fail to respond to conservative treatment and suffer from limiting pain and dysfunction may be considered for surgery. Conventional surgical treatment for midfoot arthritis consists of performing arthrodesis of the painful arthritic segments [4].

There are some general considerations common to most surgical procedures when treating midfoot arthritis [7, 13]. Most techniques are performed with the patient in supine position under a tourniquet and fluoroscopy should be available. Soft-tissue stripping should be kept down to a minimum to expose the affected joint(s). Mini distractors and lamina spreaders are tools that favour joint exposure. Joints are prepared using a combination of curettes and osteotomes and then drilled with a fluted 2-mm drill bit to fenestrate all the surfaces to finally fish scale them with a 3-mm osteotome. Temporary percutaneous K-wires can be used to stabilize the joint into the desired position. Grafting largely depends on the host vascularity and graft bed. Under ideal conditions of a young healthy patient, harvesting may be from the distal tibia (medial malleolus) or the calcaneus where low volume of cancellous bone may be obtained by using an 8-mm core reamer or trephine (Fig. 4.1). When more volume of grafting is needed or host biology is poor with reduced vascularity, iliac crest is usually the location of choice. Visual and radiographic checks should be made after provisional fixation with K-wires and after final fixation with plates and screws. A good tip to avoid malpositioning is that the head of the talus, on any fluoroscopic projection/view, should be projected towards the head of the first metatarsal. If it points medially to the first metatarsal head, a valgus malalignment should be expected whereas varus will be the result of malposition of the talar head pointing anywhere lateral with respect to the head of the first metatarsal (Fig. 4.2). Fluoroscopy should also be used to confirm guide wire placement and length. Partially threaded cannulated titanium lag screws are placed crossing the joint. Following general principles of fixation in an arthrodesis, K-wires should be removed before advancing the screws to achieve compression. Fixation for most

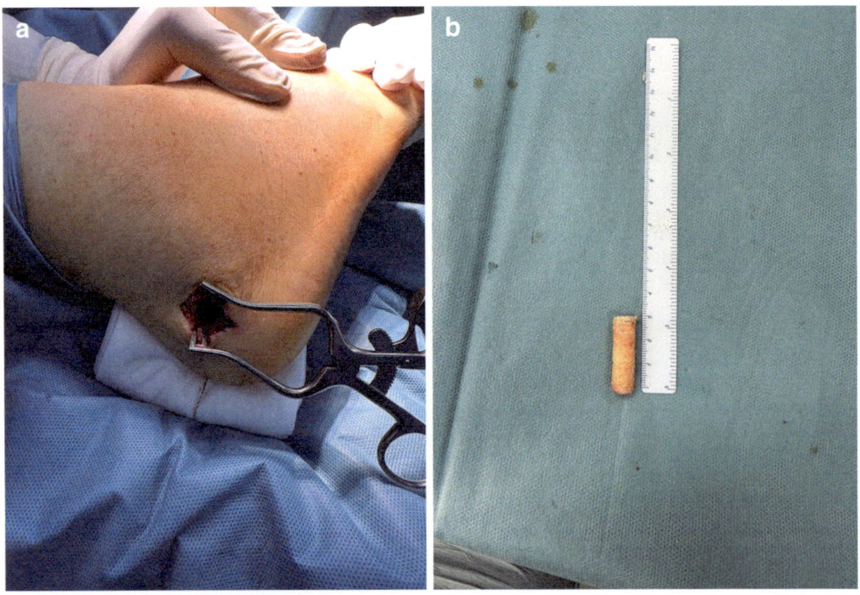

Fig. 4.1 Bone grafting is almost a necessity in most midfoot arthrodesis (**a**) Harvesting with trephine in the posterior tuberosity of the calcaneus. (**b**) Bone cylinder obtained after harvesting

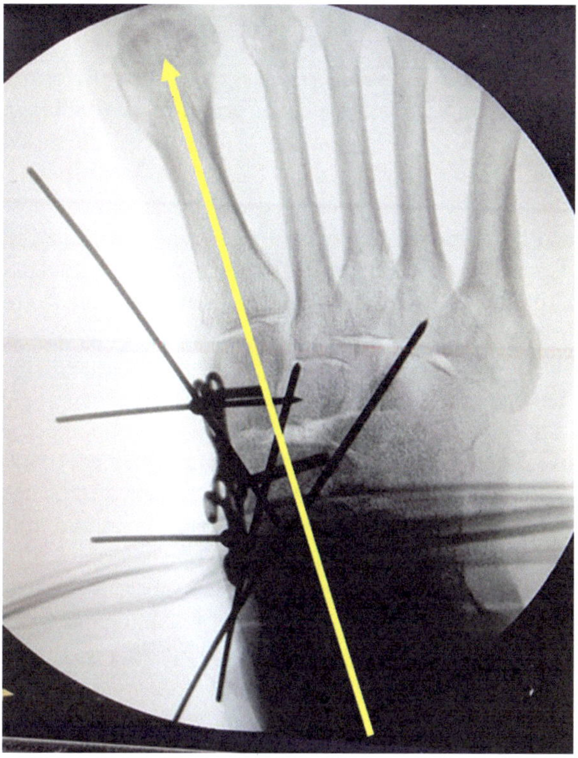

Fig. 4.2 Intraoperative fluoroscopic dorsoplantar view of the foot during midfoot arthrodesis surgery. The head of the talus should ideally point towards the head of the first metatarsal to ensure appropriate alignment is achieved after deformity correction

midfoot arthrodeses are typically carried out via a combination of cannulated partially threaded lag screws and a locking plate that spans either the dorsal, medial, lateral or medial plantar aspect of the joint. Plates in compression mode or with a ramp compression system are also used for midfoot fusions. Most plates are anatomical and need no bending or contouring [14]. To aid in the size selection, most sets of plates present with templates to select the one that best fits the patient, as they are a 1:1 match to plate size. Olive wires are useful in maintaining the plate in the desired position prior to the visualization of the foot under fluoroscopy. A slotted hole and distal placement of a K-wire allows for the distal segment to move proximally during compression. Final fluoroscopic images are obtained in multiple planes to confirm bone alignment and implant placement. The wound is closed in layers. Patients are placed in a splint for a week and then changed into a walker boot. Non-weight bearing period postoperatively varies depending on the type of procedure ranging from almost immediate-as-tolerated in joint preserving techniques to around 6 weeks for most arthrodesis. Realistic expectations include that any modification to the calcaneus-triceps loading axis or in midfoot joint motion requires a minimum of 6 months of "brain habituation" for the patient to reestablish a reliable gait.

Talonavicular Arthrodesis

Talonavicular arthrodesis (TN) is sometimes performed as an isolated procedure or in combination with subtalar arthrodesis (double fusion) and calcaneocuboid arthrodesis (triple fusion) [15]. Indications are varied from flatfoot deformity to posttraumatic arthritis [16]. TN arthrodesis has traditionally been regarded as technically difficult and associated with considerable rates of failure for both nonunion and malunion mainly because of the sclerosis found in the navicular in most cases of arthritis, especially in posttraumatic cases [15]. The geometry of the joint makes it difficult to work on it when it comes to debride the remaining cartilage. The optimal surgical approach for talonavicular arthrodesis is still uncertain with some authors showing the dorsal approach provides superior talonavicular joint preparation, especially the lateral ¼th of the talar head [17]. However, plate positioning may condition the approach. My favourite approach is through a medial incision over the joint that allows for an easier placement of implants and deformity correction (Fig. 4.3). A linear capsulotomy is followed using a mini distractor to open the joint. Subchondral drilling is especially important in the navicular side to promote subchondral bleeding. In cases of subtle deformity, it is important to be very conservative in cartilage resection to preserve anatomy and surface-contact for the arthrodesis. Arthroscopic approach may be an option in cases of in-situ fusions [18]. Cases with severe valgus deformity are (paradoxically) technically easier to manage intraoperatively as a medial-based wedge may create two flat and cancellous surfaces with a better mechanical and biological scenario to favour fusion. I then fix the navicular on the talus by using a dorsal to plantar screw and a locking plate (Fig. 4.4). Talonavicular arthrodesis is associated with a rate of non-union that ranges from 3% to 37%. Many implants are used for TN arthrodesis (K-wires, staples, screws, plates, plates with built-in compression screw, intraosseous fix systems) but there is still no gold standard when it comes to the superiority of one fixation method due to the lack of high-quality studies [19–21]. I routinely use calcaneal autograft to fill any defect after fixation.

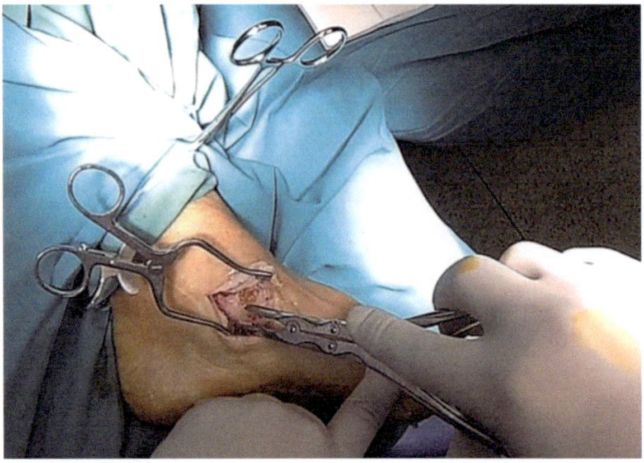

Fig. 4.3 Medial approach to the talonavicular is especially indicated when performing talonavicular arthrodesis for a severe flatfoot deformity. It allows optimal exposure of the talar head

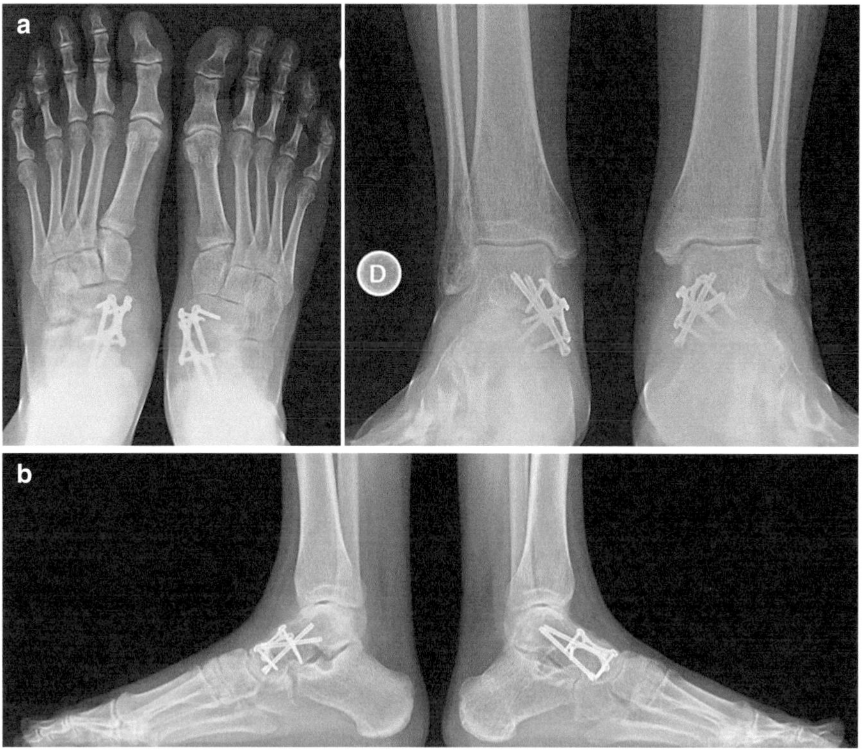

Fig. 4.4 Postoperative x-rays one year after bilateral isolated talonavicular arthrodesis in a rheumatoid case of bilateral talonavicular arthritis. Weight bearing radiographs in dorsoplantar view of both feet and anterolateral of both ankles (**a**) and lateral (**b**) views showing fixation with compression screw and locking plate

Tip: To effectively curette the remaining cartilage of both the talar head and the navicular, I prefer to start with the more-difficult-to-work-on navicular surface to be able to lean against the arthritic hard surface of the talar head. In the past, when I started curetting the talar head in the first place, I sometimes inadvertently crushed the subchondral surface and compressed the cancellous bone while working on the navicular thus creating an big iatrogenic defect that had to be filled before fixation.

Naviculocuneiform Arthrodesis

Naviculocuneiform (NC) arthrodesis has become a popular procedure for the management of collapsing flatfoot deformity when the apex of deformity is located at the NC joint [22]. With patient supine, an incision is made in the interval between the tibialis posterior and the tibialis anterior tendons, over the NC joint. Dissection is carried down to the medial cuneiform and the navicular to expose the medial surface of these bones and to reference talonavicular and cuneiform-metatarsal joints. Should the middle and lateral cuneiforms be included in the arthrodesis, an additional dorsal approach will allow working in the intercuneiform joints. Removal of cartilage or wedge-resection is performed using the general guidelines as explained previously. Temporary fixation may be achieved by placing a K-wire from dorsal distal to plantar proximal across the medial cuneiform after adequate joint positioning. A lag screw should ideally be placed across a plate or miss-the-plate fashion distally from the medial aspect of the medial cuneiform to the central region of the navicular. Should arthritis affect the middle and lateral cuneiforms, screws should also cross the intercuneiform joints (Fig. 4.5). When using a medial plate, an L-shaped end of a retractor can be placed around the tibialis anterior tendon to expose the distal holes on the plate and allow for an easier, secure fixation. Historically, NC fusion is apparently less reliable than surrounding arthrodesis, with reported nonunion rates ranging from 6.5% [23] to 25% [24], and only around 64% of patients rating their outcome as good or excellent [25]. NC arthrodesis may include just the medial cuneiform or extend to the rest of the cuneiforms depending on the degree of joint degeneration. Some authors regularly include the three cuneiforms which potentially adds better fixation possibilities to enhance primary stability in the pursuit of fusion [24]. In one study, overall nonunion rate for isolated naviculo-medial cuneiform fusion was 23% and fusing all three joints regardless of fixation constructs resulted in 18% nonunion [24]. Again, as with TN arthrodesis, there is still no gold standard when it comes to the superiority of one fixation method due to the lack of high-quality studies [23, 24, 26, 27].

Tip: Some patients present with a prominent navicular tuberosity and the template for a NC plate does not achieve an anatomic fit to the navicular. A portion of the navicular tuberosity may then be removed until correct fit of the template to bone is achieved. The removed bone can also be used as an autograft.

Tarsometatarsal Arthrodesis

Posttraumatic tarsometatarsal (TMT) arthritis commonly affects the medial part of the joint causing progressive arch collapse and foot abduction [28]. Almost invariably the first TMT joint is affected by degenerative changes and a medial approach is preferred. Should the second and third TMT joints be affected they should be included in the arthrodesis, with an additional dorsal approach to allow working in the intercuneiform and lesser TMT joints. Care is taken to avoid and protect the neurovascular structures, especially superficial sensory nerves that cross the dorsal aspect of the joint. TMT joint is exposed and assessed. Decortication of cartilage must be performed in a way to preserve as much subchondral bone as possible dorsally to avoid dorsiflexion of the lesser metatarsals. Passive dorsiflexion of the first metatarsophalangeal joint allows to place the first metatarsal in the adequate plantar flexion with respect to the cuneiform. First TMT joint is temporarily fixed with K-wires and followed by the second and third. Once the fusion sites are thoroughly prepared, bone graft is packed dorsally between the surfaces to be arthrodesed. In cases of long-standing deformities with arch collapse and abduction a medial and plantar based wedge of the affected joint may be excised to achieve anatomic

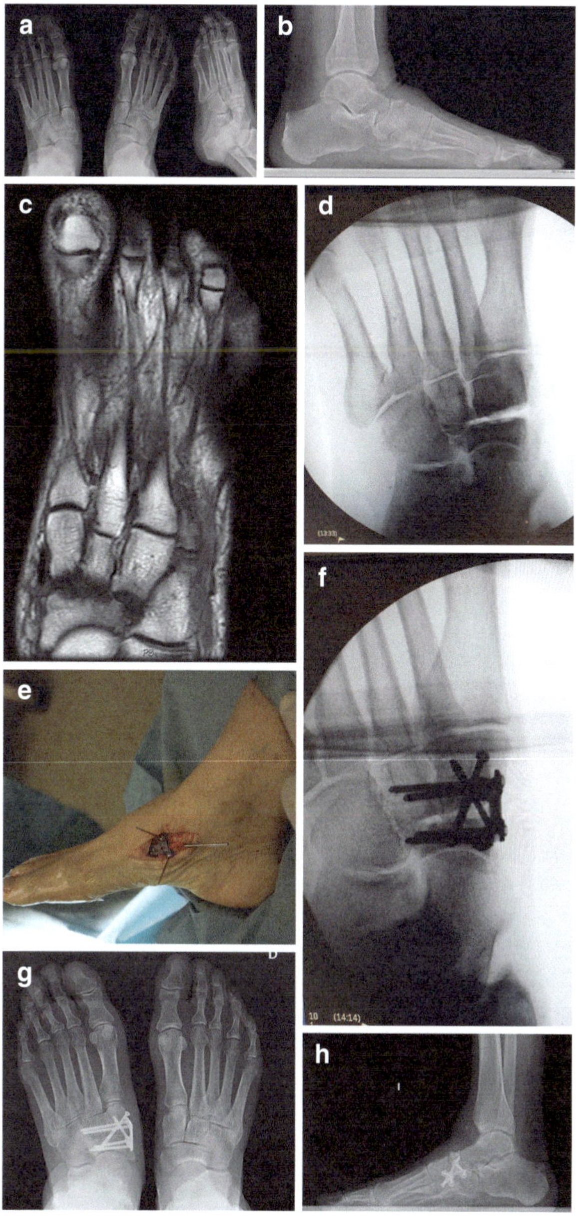

Fig. 4.5 Naviculocuneiform arthritis. (**a**) Dorsoplantar and oblique views of weightbearing x-rays showing abduction deformity and (**b**) lateral view with visible collapse with apex at the CN joint. (**c**) Magnetic resonance imaging confirming involvement of all cuneiforms. (**d**) Osteotomy with wedged resection of the affected joints to restore alignment. (**e**) Medial positioning of the plate after temporary fixation with K-wires. (**f**) Intraoperative fluoroscopy showing definitive fixation with compression screw and plate with ramp compression. (**g**) Dorsoplantar view of postoperative weightbearing x-rays 12 months after surgery. (**h**) Lateral view 12 months after surgery

correction before conventional fixation (Fig. 4.6). Again, as with the rest of midfoot arthrodesis, there is no optimal fixation strategy due to the lack of high-quality studies. Isolated plate fixation, smoking, and postoperative nonanatomic alignment seem to significantly increase the rate of nonunion but concomitant use of autogenous bone graft significantly decreased this risk [29]. Risk factors of nonunion were

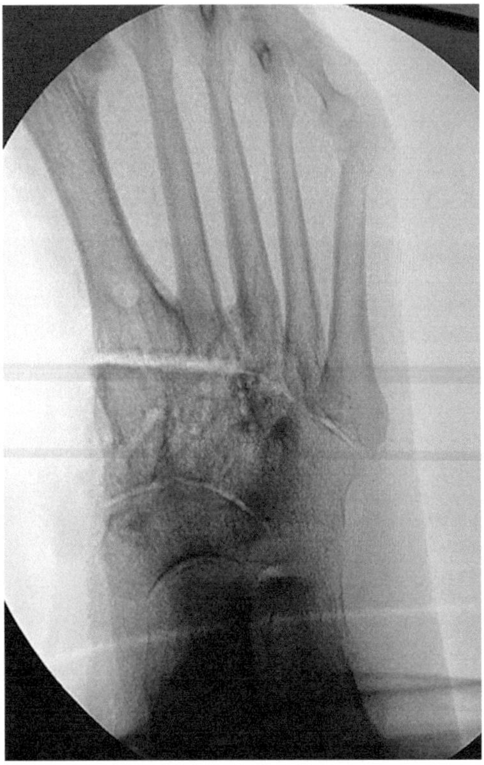

Fig. 4.6 Intraoperative fluoroscopic image showing resection-osteotomy through arthritic TMT 1–3 joints prior to arthrodesis

investigated revealing that diabetes mellitus, compression screw fixation alone, lack of adjuvant bone graft, and postoperative non anatomical alignment are independent predictors of nonunion following midfoot arthrodesis [30, 31]. The combination of a lag screw plus locking plate is apparently superior to crossed screw fixation [32], but new plating systems are continuously challenging biomechanical studies [33, 34]. My preferred method of fixation combines a lag screw plus plate with ramp compression (Fig. 4.7). TMT arthrodesis requires a longer non weight bearing period than other midfoot arthrodesis given the special mechanical requirements of the Lisfranc joint.

Tip: When a patient with TMT arthritis shows no signs of preoperative metatarsalgia and no gross deformity, "in situ" pinning TMT joints before preparing the articular surface may allow not to malposition (especially dorsiflexion) the TMT joint before definitive fixation.

Extended midfoot (Medial Column) Arthrodesis

Some posttraumatic cases develop arthritis in two or more adjacent joints, usually in the medial column. In cases where loss of bone stock after trauma alters the relationship between the medial and lateral columns, with relative shortening of the

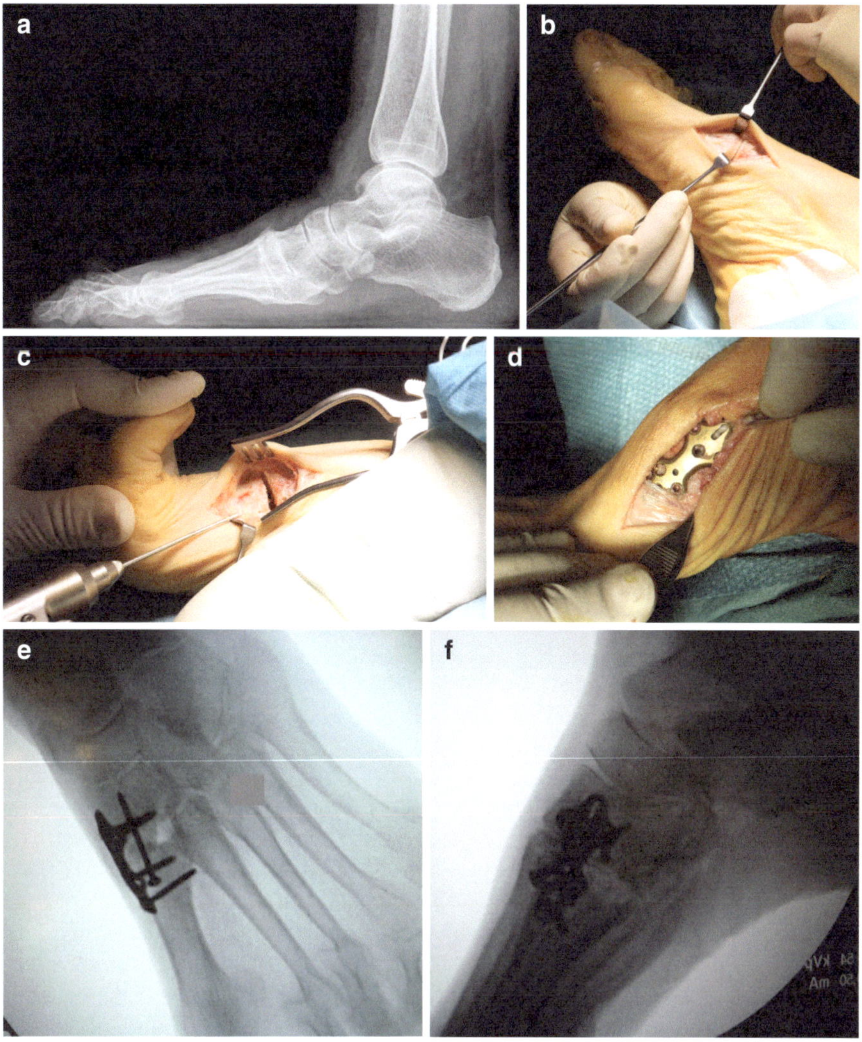

Fig. 4.7 First cuneiform-metatarsal arthritis sometimes presents with loss of medial arch height. (**a**) Lateral view weightbearing x-ray showing TMT1 arthritis and collapse. (**b**) Medial approach for TMT1 arthrodesis. (**c**) Positioning of TMT1 by dorsiflexion at the first metatarsophalangeal joint before temporary K-wire fixation. (**d**) Locking plate over the TMT1 joint. (**e**) Dorsoplantar fluoroscopic view of TMT1 arthrodesis with compression screw and locking plate. (**f**) Intraoperative fluoroscopic lateral view

medial column, bridging hardware and bone grafting will allow for the restoration of column length, shape, and foot alignment. Some indications for arthrodesis of the medial column (talus, navicular, medial cuneiform and first metatarsal) are Charcot arthropathy, posttraumatic reconstruction or severe rigid flatfoot deformity [35] (Fig. 4.8). Complication rate is still high and mainly resulting from inadequate

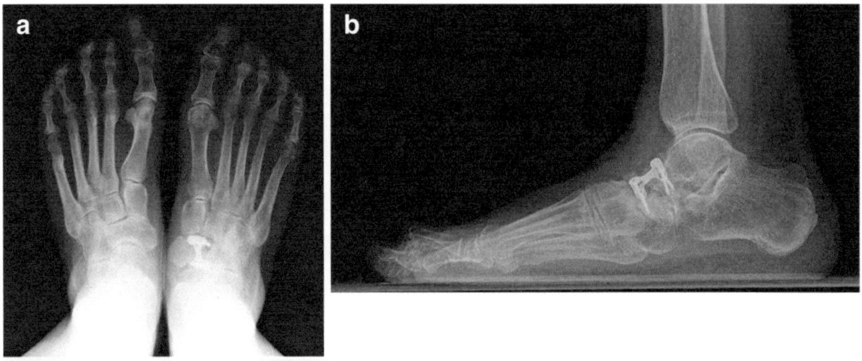

Fig. 4.8 Posttraumatic midfoot arthritis usually involves more than one joint. (**a**) Dorsoplantar view of weightbearing x-rays showing failed TN arthrodesis after navicular fracture. (**b**) Lateral view shows arthritic TN and NC joints with medial arch collapse

fixation [36] (Fig. 4.9). Special plates, designed for medial column arthrodesis, seem to offer more primary stability to reduce the complication rate [37]. There are specific plates to cover for almost any combination of arthrodesis of the medial column (Fig. 4.10).

Tip: When many joints have to be included in the arthrodesis, I prefer to harvest bone from the iliac crest so that I can pack every joint until the plate is flushed with the bones and grafting.

Joint preserving Surgery/Osteotomy

Some midfoot arthritis conditions present with asymmetrical cartilage wear and joint-preserving surgery may be a good alternative to an arthrodesis. Müller-Weiss disease (MWD) is a condition that involves a dysplastic navicular bone with asymmetric talonavicular arthritis and secondary hindfoot varus deformity [10]. Conventional talonavicular (or extended) arthrodesis does not address the underlying pathomechanics (varus hindfoot). An isolated valgus (Dwyer-type) osteotomy of the os calcis has shown to be effective in the shifting of the talar head medially to face healthy TN cartilage [38]. Fixation of the osteotomy is then performed with two 6.5- or 7.0-millimetre cannulated screws. The Dwyer-type calcaneal valgus osteotomy works for most cases. The osteotomy should be placed in the most anterior region of the calcaneus. The lateral based wedge of about 8–10 mm produces a greater valgus effect. The further away the osteotomy cut is placed with respect to the Achilles insertion, a longer lever arm will magnify the valgus effect. Adding a lateral displacement (reverse Koutsogiannis effect) to the Dwyer osteotomy permits to even gain more valgus (Fig. 4.11). In recent years, and in view of our results, this "super valgus"osteotomy—very anterior-lateral-closing-wedge plus lateral-sliding calcaneal osteotomy—has become our surgery of choice, regardless of the radiological stage at the time of surgery [39, 40] (Fig. 4.12). The only contraindication

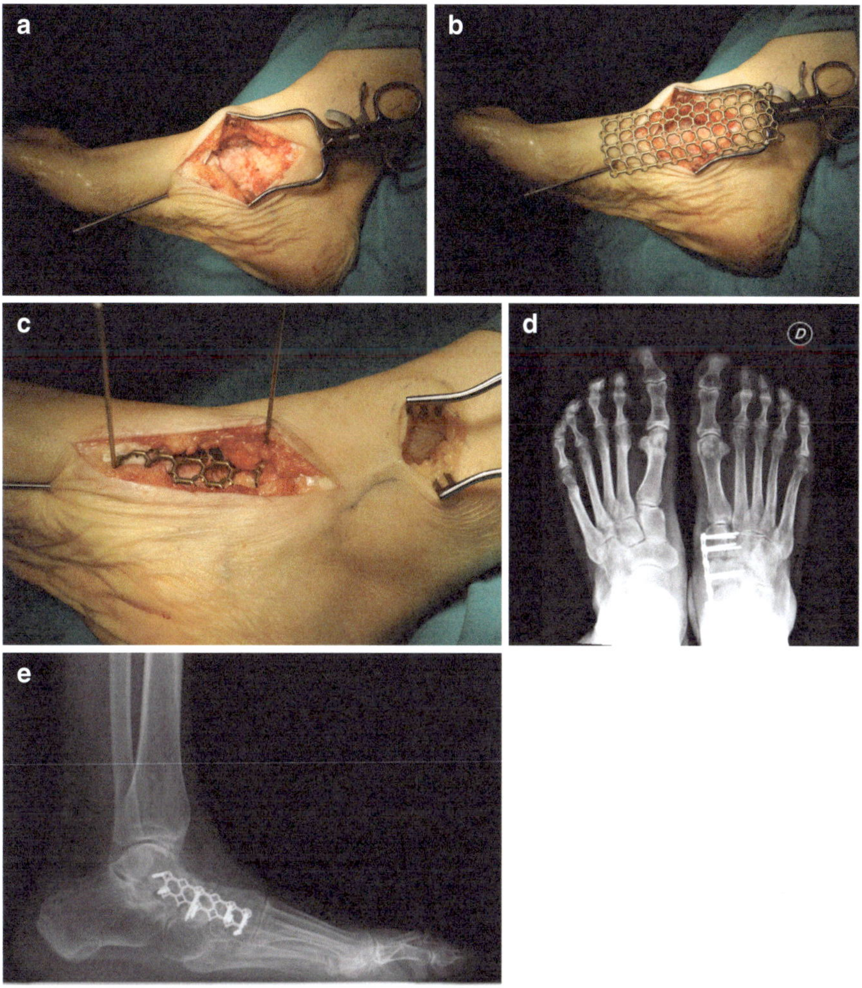

Fig. 4.9 Type of fixation may condition talonaviculocuneiform arthrodesis. (**a**) Temporary wire fixation after joint preparation through a medial approach. (**b**) Mesh plates were popular before specific platings were developed to cover medial column fusions. (**c**) Mesh plate adapted for a talonaviculocuneiform arthrodesis and approach over the medial malleolus for bone harvesting. (**d**) Dorsoplantar view of postoperative weightbearing x-rays 12 months after surgery. (**e**) Lateral view 12 months after surgery

for the super valgus osteotomy might be the presence of arthritis in the medial region of the talonavicular joint that would not allow medial migration of the talar head.

Tip: When attempting to shift the posterior region of the calcaneus laterally it is usually necessary to stretch/weaken the medial soft tissues by using a lamina spreader, to open and close the osteotomy several times, resulting in a controlled fractional elongation of the medial soft tissues including the plantar fascia. In my experience there is no need to section

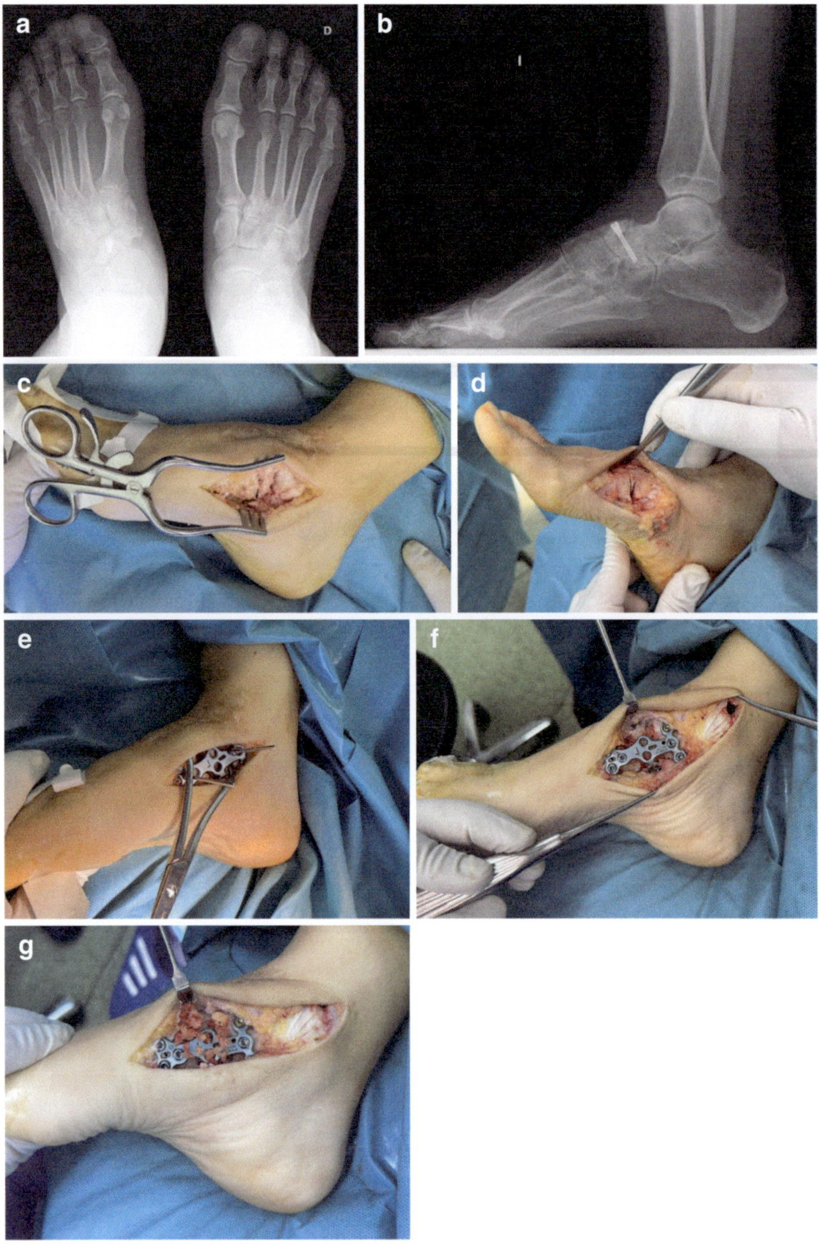

Fig. 4.10 Posttraumatic midfoot arthritis usually involves more than one joint. (**a**) Dorsoplantar view of weightbearing x-rays showing abduction deformity after failed surgery for comminute navicular fracture. (**b**) Lateral view showing dorsal migration and plantar compression of the navicular. (**c**) Intraoperative view after medial approach to the talonaviculocuneiform joints. (**d**) Joint preparation with dorsal wedge resection to restore medial column alignment. (**e**) Positioning of a specific anatomic talonaviculocuneiform fusion plate with olive wires. (**f**) Compression screw from dorsal to plantar and fixation of the plate with screws. Extensile approach allows for bone harvesting in the medial malleolus. (**g**) Bone graft is packed into the prepared joints to fill bone defects

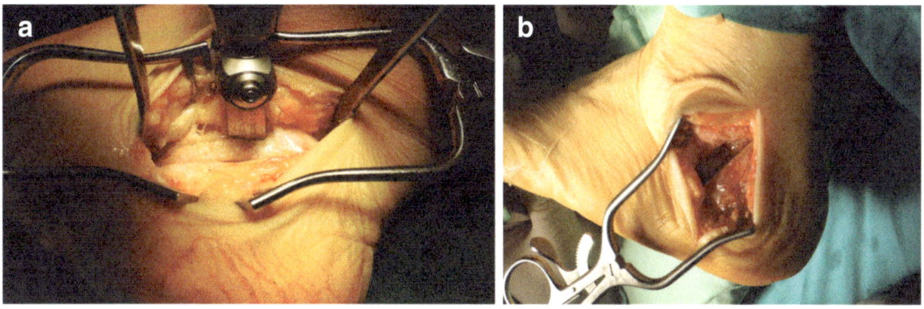

Fig. 4.11 An isolated supervalgus calcaneal osteotomy can change pathomechanics in MWD. (**a**) Dwyer osteotomy (8–10 mm of wedge) should be as far from the Achilles as possible to maximize valgus shifting. (**b**) Lateral displacement (8–10 mm-slide) of the osteotomy after medial soft tissue stretching

the plantar fascia to allow for a lateral slide, which might have unpredictable consequences, such as medial arch collapse and lateral column overload syndrome of the foot. When this effect is achieved, it is easy to add about 8 to 10 mm of lateral translation of the posterior calcaneal tuberosity.

Central Lisfranc arthritis affecting second and third TMT joints is frequently observed in patients with no history of previous trauma. The so-called “primary Lisfranc arthritis” does not affect the first ray. Some H-shaped plates have been developed for this specific uncommon type of arthritis. After years analysing central Lisfranc arthritis we believe it is a good example of asymmetrical arthritis with wear concentrating mainly in the dorsal aspect of the joint (with intact cartilage in the plantar half of the joint), possibly the result of an abnormal compression effect in patients with tight gastrocnemius and a short first metatarsal with respect to the second metatarsal (Fig. 4.13). Loads would then be distributed across the dorsal part of the second and third TMT joints causing slow progressive degeneration. Proximal gastrocnemius release apparently improves pain in patients with central TMT arthritis [41]. We usually combine proximal medial gastrocnemius release with shortening triple Weil osteotomies to decompress the dorsal aspect of the central region of the joint, and to transfer loads towards the first metatarsal.

Conclusions

Midfoot arthritis is an uncommon but challenging condition for the orthopaedic surgeon. With the rare exception of asymmetric arthritis in Müller Weiss disease and central Lisfranc, in which joint preserving surgery may be attempted, most arthritic midfoot joints will need an arthrodesis. Meticulous surgical technique is necessary to create the biological and mechanical environment for a successful fusion. Post traumatic degeneration presents with deformity, poor bone stock, within a geometry of bones that is not easy to fix with good primary stability. To enhance biology and

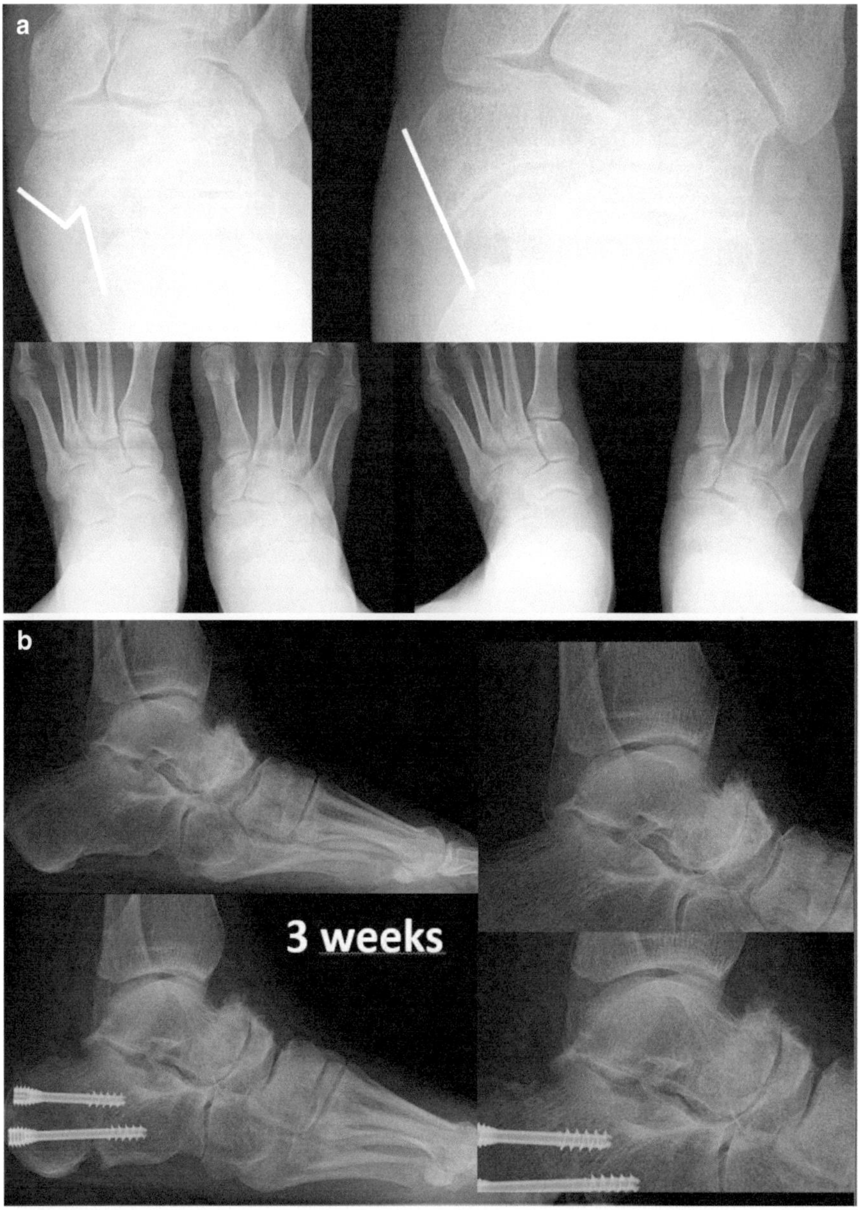

Fig. 4.12 Changes in alignment after osteotomy in MWD are visible around 3 weeks from surgery when the patient is allowed to weightbear. (**a**) Dosroplantar view of weightbearing x-rays preoperatively and postoperatively demonstrate medial displacement of the talar head to occupy the medial aspect of the TN joint. (**b**) Lateral views before and three weeks after surgery showing changes in the TN joint that is now "visible" because of the medial displacement of the talus

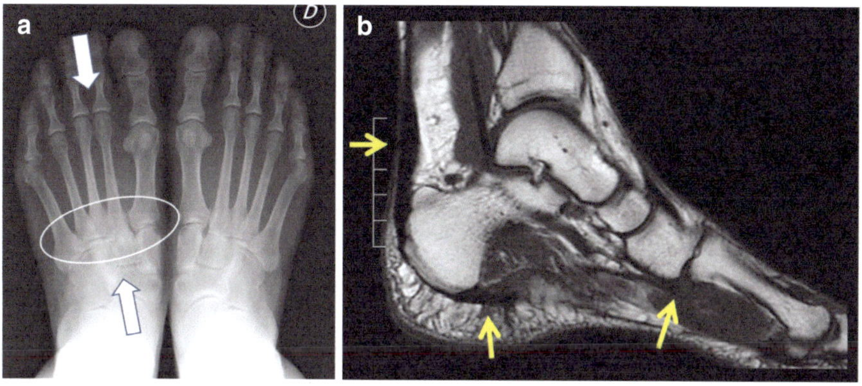

Fig. 4.13 The so-called "primary Lisfranc arthritis" typically involves the second and third TMT joints unlike the posttraumatic that almost invariably includes the first TMT joint. (**a**) Dorsoplantar view of weightbearing x-rays showing central TMT arthritis in a patient with index minus (short first metatarsal with respect to the second) and a tight gastrocnemius. Arrows show direction of abnormal loading transferred from the insufficient short first ray to the second and third (**b**) Magnetic resonance image of the same patient suggesting multiple disorders with the common aetiology of a tight gastrocnemius. Arrows show thickening of the Achilles tendon, the proximal plantar fascia, and asymmetric Lisfranc joint with dorsal compression and plantar widening

promote fusion in the midtarsal joints, bone grafting is routinely done with harvesting from the calcaneus for moderate defects or iliac crest when more bone is needed. The development of specific plating systems has helped in reducing the rate of nonunions to less than 10% in the most recent series. Malunion is mainly dependent on inadequate surgical (re)positioning of the bones, seldom reported, and possibly more common than nonunion.

Ethical Statement Not applicable for this article.

Conflict of Interest There are no conflicts for interest for the authors of this article.

Funding No financial support.

References

1. Kurup H, Vasukutty N. Midfoot arthritis—current concepts review. J Clin Orthop Trauma. 2020;11(3):399–405.
2. Patel A, Rao S, Nawoczenski D, Flemister AS, DiGiovanni B, Baumhauer JF. Midfoot arthritis. J Am Acad Orthop Surg. 2010;18(7):417–25.
3. Gougoulias N, Lampridis V. Midfoot arthrodesis. Foot Ankle Surg. 2016;22(1):17–25.
4. Verhoeven N, Vandeputte G. Midfoot arthritis: diagnosis and treatment. Foot Ankle Surg. 2012;18(4):255–62.
5. Lim PQX, Lithgow MJ, Kaminski MR, Landorf KB, Menz HB, Munteanu SE. Efficacy of non-surgical interventions for midfoot osteoarthritis: a systematic review. Rheumatol Int. 2023;43(8):1409–22.

6. Zhang H, Lin Lv M, Yang J, Niu W, Cheung JC, Sun W, Wong DW, Ni M. Computational modelling of foot orthosis for midfoot arthritis: a Taguchi approach for design optimization. Acta Bioeng Biomech. 2020;22(4):75–83.
7. Zonno AJ, Myerson MS. Surgical correction of midfoot arthritis with and without deformity. Foot Ankle Clin. 2011;16(1):35–47.
8. Bauer T. Percutaneous hindfoot and midfoot fusion. Foot Ankle Clin. 2016;21(3):629–40.
9. Nemec SA, Habbu RA, Anderson JG, Bohay DR. Outcomes following midfoot arthrodesis for primary arthritis. Foot Ankle Int. 2011;32(4):355–61.
10. Maceira E, Rochera R. Müller-Weiss disease: clinical and biomechanical features. Foot Ankle Clin. 2004;9(1):105–25.
11. Kim KC, Schmidt E, de Carvalho KAM, Lalevee M, Mansur N, Dibbern K, Auch E, Jasper R, Netto CC. Risk factors for midfoot arthritis associated with medical history by weight bearing computed tomography. J Foot Ankle Surg. 2024;63(5):532–6.
12. Orejana ÁM, Monteagudo M. Nonoperative treatment of Müller–Weiss disease. Foot Ankle Clin. 2024; in press
13. Den Hartog BD, Kay DB. Non-neuropathic midfoot multiplanar deformity: surgical strategies for reconstruction. Foot Ankle Clin. 2009;14(3):383–92.
14. Dang DY, Flint WW, Haytmanek CT, Ackerman KJ, Coughlin MJ, Hirose CB. Locked dorsal compression plate arthrodesis for degenerative arthritis of the midfoot. J Foot Ankle Surg. 2020;59(6):1171–6.
15. Barkatali BM, Sundar M. Isolated talonavicular arthrodesis for talonavicular arthritis: a follow-up study. J Foot Ankle Surg. 2014;53(1):8–11.
16. Ma S, Jin D. Isolated talonavicular arthrodesis. Foot Ankle Int. 2016;37(8):905–8.
17. Andrews NA, Patch DA, Torrez TW, Sutherland CR, Harrelson WM, Pitts C, Agarwal A, Shah A. Which surgical approach is optimal for joint preparation in talonavicular fusion—a cadaver study. Foot Ankle Surg. 2022;28(5):657–62.
18. Kumamoto W, Lui TH. Arthroscopic talonavicular arthrodesis for the management of talonavicular osteoarthritis. Arthrosc Tech. 2024;13(8):103006. https://doi.org/10.1016/j.eats.2024.103006. eCollection 2024 Aug
19. Lechler P, Graf S, Köck FX, Schaumburger J, Grifka J, Handel M. Arthrodesis of the talonavicular joint using angle-stable mini-plates: a prospective study. Int Orthop. 2012;36(12):2491–4.
20. Goh TS, Han JB, Lee SM, Kang SW, Shin WC, Woo SH. Screw only versus screw plus plate in isolated talonavicular arthrodesis. Foot Ankle Surg. 2022;28(7):1045–9.
21. Arumugam V, Ranjit S, Patel S, Welck M. What is the best fixation technique for isolated talonavicular arthrodesis?—a systematic review. Foot (Edinb). 2023 Mar;54:101966. https://doi.org/10.1016/j.foot.2023.101966. Epub 2023 Feb 10
22. Ajis A, Geary N. Surgical technique, fusion rates, and planovalgus foot deformity correction with naviculocuneiform fusion. Foot Ankle Int. 2014;35(3):232–7.
23. Chu AK, Wilson MD, Lee J, So E, Prissel MA, Hyer CF. The incidence of nonunion of the naviculocuneiform joint arthrodesis: a systematic review. J Foot Ankle Surg. 2019;58(3):545–9.
24. Kolyesnykov PO, Chong AC, Fischer NJ, Sweeter JM, McLister DA. Outcomes of naviculocuneiform arthrodesis with and without adjunct arthrodesis. J Foot Ankle Surg. 2024;S1067-2516(24):00279–5. https://doi.org/10.1053/j.jfas.2024.11.001.
25. Gougoulias N, Christidis P, Christidis G, Oshba H, Lampridis V. Naviculocuneiform joint arthrodesis in a cohort of 36 patients. Foot (Edinb). 2024;60:102115.
26. Kuestermann H, Ettinger S, Yao D, Schwarze M, Plaass C, Stukenborg-Colsman C, Claassen L. Biomechanical evaluation of naviculocuneiform fixation with lag screw and locking plates. Foot Ankle Surg. 2021;27(8):911–9.
27. Casciato D, Wynes J. The navicular cuneiform joint: updates on avoiding and managing a nonunion. Clin Podiatr Med Surg. 2023;40(4):613–21.
28. Panagakos P, Patel K, Gonzalez CN. Lisfranc arthrodesis. Clin Podiatr Med Surg. 2012;29(1):51–66.

29. Buda M, Hagemeijer NC, Kink S, Johnson AH, Guss D, DiGiovanni CW. Effect of fixation type and bone graft on tarsometatarsal fusion. Foot Ankle Int. 2018;39(12):1394–402.
30. Ahmad J, Lynch MK, Maltenfort M. Comparison of screws to plate-and-screw constructs for midfoot arthrodesis. Foot Ankle Int. 2018;39(8):922–9.
31. Lee W, Prat D, Wapner KL, Farber DC, Chao W. Comparison of 4 different fixation strategies for midfoot arthrodesis: a retrospective comparative study. Foot Ankle Spec. 2024;17(2):98–108.
32. Fraser TW, Miles DT, Huang N, Davis FB, Dunlap BD, Doty JF. Radiographic outcomes, union rates, and complications associated with plantar implant positioning for midfoot arthrodesis. Foot Ankle Orthop. 2021;6(3):24730114211027115. https://doi.org/10.1177/24730114211027115. eCollection 2021 Jul
33. Ettinger S, Altemeier A, Stukenborg-Colsman C, Yao D, Plaass C, Lerch M, Claassen L. Comparison of isolated screw to plate and screw fixation for tarsometatarsal arthrodesis including clinical outcome predictors. Foot Ankle Int. 2021;42(6):734–43.
34. Wininger AE, Klavas DM, Gardner SS, Ahuero JS, Harris JD, Varner KE. Plantar plating for medial naviculocuneiform arthrodesis in progressive collapsing foot deformity. Foot Ankle Orthop. 2022;7(1):24730114221088517. https://doi.org/10.1177/24730114221088517. eCollection 2022 Jan
35. Rammelt S, Murillo PAC. Lisfranc arthrodesis in posttraumatic chronic injuries. Foot Ankle Clin. 2022;27(4):745–67.
36. Nasser EM, LaPorta GA, Trott K. Medial column arthrodesis using an anatomic distal fibular locking plate. J Foot Ankle Surg. 2015;54(4):671–6.
37. Simons P, Sommerer T, Zderic I, Wahl D, Lenz M, Skulev H, Knobe M, Gueorguiev B, Richards RG, Klos K. Biomechanical investigation of two plating systems for medial column fusion in foot. PLoS One. 2017;12(2):e0172563. https://doi.org/10.1371/journal.pone.0172563. eCollection 2017
38. Monteagudo M, Maceira E. Management of Müller-Weiss disease. Foot Ankle Clin. 2019;24(1):89–105.
39. Li S, Myerson M, Monteagudo M, Maceira E. Efficacy of calcaneus osteotomy for treatment of symptomatic Müller-Weiss disease. Foot Ankle Int. 2016;38(3):261–9.
40. Buendía I, Gaviria ME, Monteagudo M, Maceira E, Martínez de Albornoz P. Enfermedad de Müller–Weiss, ¿cómo hemos cambiado? Rev Pie Tobillo. 2020;34(2):125–32.
41. Anselmo DS, Thatcher L, Erfle D. Gastrocnemius recession as an alternative to midfoot arthrodesis for painful midfoot arthritis. J Foot Ankle Surg. 2020;59(5):1106–8.

Chapter 5
Surgery for Arthritis of Hindfoot

Alessio Bernasconi

Introduction

'Osteoarthritis of the hindfoot' generally corresponds to an advanced cartilage degeneration at the subtalar, talonavicular and calcaneocuboid joints. Out of multiple possible causes, the two most common are certainly trauma and progressive collapsing foot deformity (PCFD, previously known as flatfoot). A mixture of mechanical (malalignment and joint incongruency) and biological (inflammatory environment) factors lead to alter the cartilage and subchondral layers with a subsequent reduction of the physiological joint space. In clinical terms, this generates pain and functional limitation at the hindfoot, which are the main reasons that bring the patient to seek medical attention. If the conservative measures fail to provide relief, surgery may be indicated. Historically, in this context arthrodesis of one, two (double fusion) or three (triple fusion) joints has always represented the gold standard, leading to symptom resolutions at the price of a definitive stiffness of the hindfoot. During the last decades, arthroscopic approaches have been described, which may be technically more demanding but that allow to reduce the stress on surrounding soft tissues. Even more recently, and with a similar intent, percutaneous techniques have been reported, which will probably gain further space in the future. As a reminder, in this context the Achilles tendon is often shortened, and its lengthening (which can be safely performed percutaneously) may be recommended. Last, we will not discuss here joint-preserving techniques, which may have a role in the setting of moderate articular degeneration and selected cases, being aimed to mechanically realign the hindfoot, indirectly re-balance the painful joint and provide relief without need to create iatrogenic stiffness (fusion).

A. Bernasconi (✉)
Department of Public Health, Orthopaedic and Trauma Unit,
University Federico II of Naples, Naples, Italy

M. Bhatia (ed.), *Surgical Techniques of the Foot and Ankle*,
https://doi.org/10.1007/978-3-031-93742-2_5

Key Points in Assessment

The main reason why arthritis of the hindfoot leads to surgery is pain! It is therefore essential to define if the degeneration process at the subtalar, talonavicular and calcaneocuboid joints is actually related to the symptoms which bring the patients to our attention. Due to the superficial position of joints in the foot, tenderness on palpation of each joint generally reflects an underlying inflammatory process related to impaired function of the same joint. Heel-raise test (single and double) and Jack's test (plantar fascia tightens while great toe is passively dorsiflexed) may be useful to verify the flexibility of the deformity. A standard radiographic approach through weight bearing anteroposterior and lateral radiographs of feet and ankles usually represents first-line imaging. However, if available, the use of three-dimensional measurements of weight-bearing computed tomography (WBCT) might provide a more accurate idea of the real degree of hindfoot malalignment. Obviously, magnetic resonance imaging (MRI) is the gold standard to assess soft tissues such as tendons (detecting either tenosynovitis or tendinosis or tendon tears) and ligaments. Once the diagnosis has been confirmed, fusion procedures may be considered and discussed with the patient, focusing on the fact that a well-aligned arthrodesis of one or multiple joints may help the patient get rid of the pain at the price of different degrees of stiffness of the hindfoot.

Subtalar Arthrodesis

Subtalar arthrodesis is the most common fusion procedure at the hindfoot.
Although the joint is made up of three different components (anterior facet, middle facet and posterior facet), most authors have reported preparing and fixing only the posterior facet with good clinical results. So far, evidence suggests that there is no formal need to prepare and fix also the middle and anterior facet [1].

Lateral Approach

The most common approach to the subtalar joint is lateral. The patient can be positioned in a lateral position or supine with a sandbag under the gluteus in order to internally rotate the lower limb and better visualize the lateral aspect of the hindfoot. A thigh tourniquet is positioned and inflated at 250–300 mmHg. The skin landmarks are the lateral malleolus, the base of the fifth metatarsal and, if possible, the base of the fourth metatarsal (which is more difficult to find but that can be imagined slightly dorsomedially to the base of the fifth). The 7- to 8-cm skin incision starts approximately 1 cm distal to the tip of the malleolus and is directed anteriorly towards the base of the fourth metatarsal. Some others recommend considering the sinus tarsi as the main landmark and incise posteriorly to it (Fig. 5.1). During the approach injuries to the sural nerve (which lies halfway between the tip of the lateral malleolus and the posterior skin of the heel) should be prevented by blunt dissection of the subcutaneous tissues at the posterior part of the joint. More deeply, peroneal tendons are identified and protected using a mini-hohmann elevator positioned posteriorly to the joint. Distally to the sinus tarsi, the extensors retinaculum and the underlying proximal insertion of the extensor digitorum brevis muscle belly are visualized and detached if needed. The calcaneofibular ligament is sectioned and a capsulotomy performed until the sinus tarsi, to approach the subtalar joint. In stiffer cases, attention must be paid since the joint may be not easily identifiable and using osteotomes or chisels may lead to false routes in the calcaneus bone. Positioning a Hintermann distractor in the talus and the calcaneus may help progressively jack the joint out (Fig. 5.1). Once a satisfactory view has been obtained, the joint can be prepared either in a traditional way with classical instruments (osteotomes, curettes, chisels) either with motorized tools (a 1-cm saw blade or a burr) in order to remove remnants of cartilage and sclerotic bone and get to fresh bleeding bone. The visualization on the medial aspect of the joint of the tendon of the flexor hallucis longus confirms that the whole width of the facet has been prepared (Fig. 5.2).

In the authors' experience, in cavovarus feet the preparation of the posterior facet alone does not allow to derotate the talus over the calcaneus thereby it is difficult to restore the talocalcaneal angle. Therefore, in these cases it may be useful to prepare

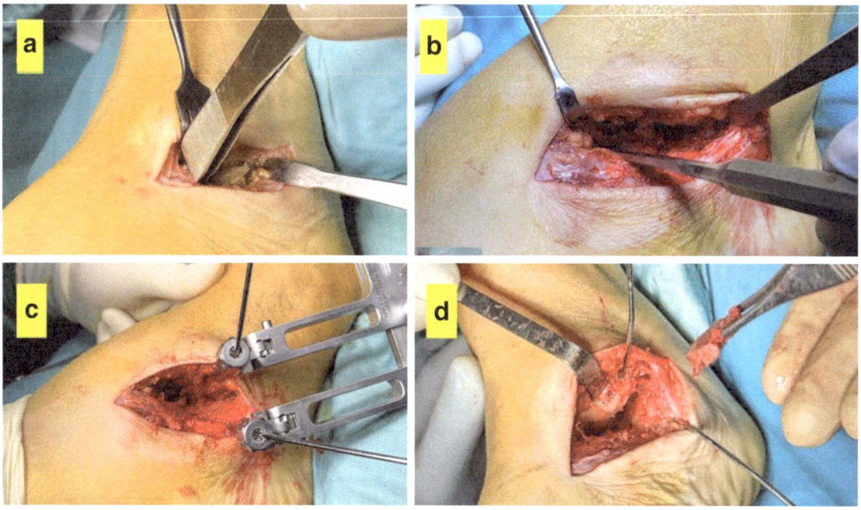

Fig. 5.1 Different phases of a subtalar fusion through a lateral incision. (**a**) Positioning a small forceps into the sinus tarsi may allow to identify the anterior border of the posterior facet of the subtalar joint, which is useful especially in particularly rigid and tight deformities. (**b**) The joint is exposed. (**c**) An Hintermann distractor is helpful to open the joint up and prepare it. (**d**) Tricortical bone graft may be placed in between the articular surfaces in order to increase the talocalcaneal height and add a biological support for fusion

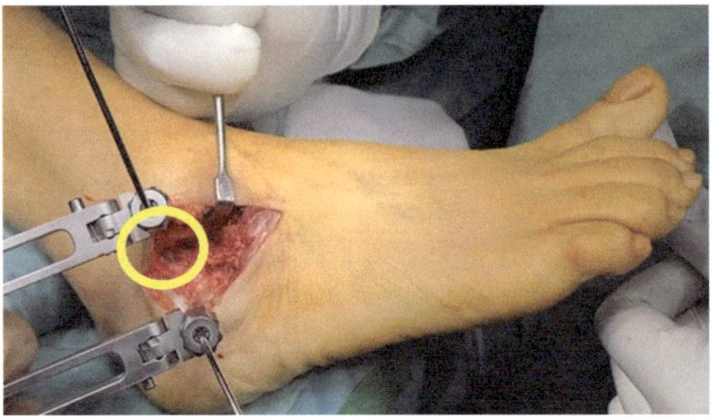

Fig. 5.2 Identifying the flexor digitorum longus tendon (moving the hallux is helpful to find it) allows to ensure that the whole width of the joint has been prepared

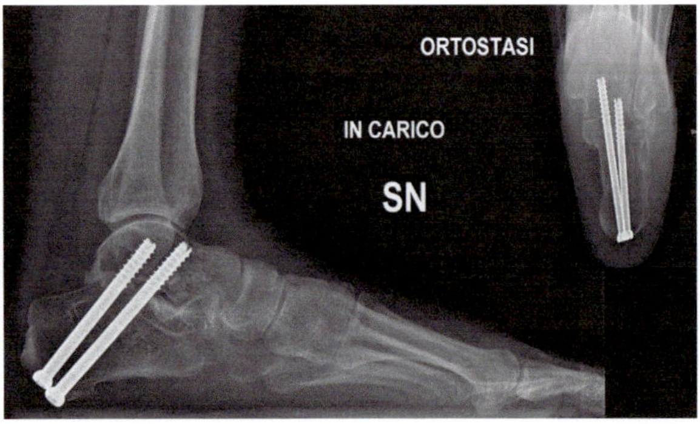

Fig. 5.3 Among different techniques to fix the subtalar joint, one of the most common is using two cannulated screws from the calcaneus into the talus

in addition the middle and the anterior facets which can be found just anteriorly to the sinus tarsi. A more generous detachment of the extensor digitorum brevis muscle belly will be necessary to expose the anterior part of the calcaneus.

Fixation of the joint can be achieved in multiple ways. Cannulated screws represent the most common method adopted and may vary in diameter (from 5.5 mm to 8 mm), in number (from 1 to 3) and in direction (only anterograde, only retrograde or combined) based on surgeon's preference (Fig. 5.3). While in some studies three screws have led to a lower risk of non-union [2, 3], the two-screw construct remains the most common worldwide. Fluoroscopy is essential to verify the position of the metalwork throughout the procedure. A correct procedure may allow to realign the hindfoot and restore a more physiologic foot tripod (Fig. 5.4).

Medial Approach

The medial approach to the subtalar fusion is less frequently used. The incision is generally placed around 1 cm below the medial malleolus (Fig. 5.5). After blunt dissection, the tibialis posterior tendon is identified and moved slight dorsally in order to visualize the medial border of the posterior subtalar facet; the flexor

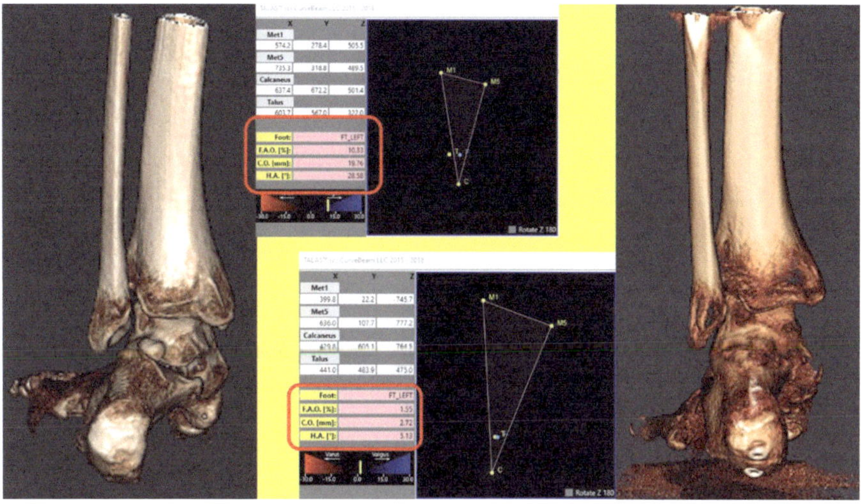

Fig. 5.4 Three-dimensional reconstructions from weight-bearing CT imaging which demonstrate the correction of the alignment of the hindfoot after subtalar arthrodesis. Dedicated software allows the calculation of the Foot and Ankle Offset (TALAS, CURVEBEAM AI) to quantify such correction

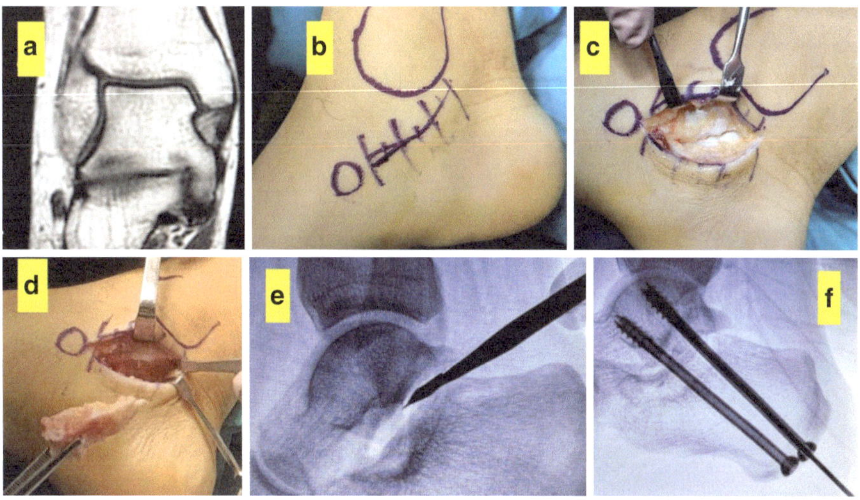

Fig. 5.5 Different steps of a coalition resection through a medial approach at the subtalar joint followed by fusion. In **a** the coalition is identified on the coronal plane. In **b** the incision is shown, placed over the skin projection of the tibialis posterior tendon. In **c** the tibialis posterior (above) and the flexor digitorum longus (below) tendons are identified. In **d** the coalition is resected, allowing (**e**) an access to the joint. In **f** final fixation with two cannulated screws

digitorum longus tendon will be retracted plantarly along with the flexor hallucis longus and the neurovascular bundle (Fig. 5.5). In some conditions, the medial approach may prove particularly useful:

- A rigid hindfoot due to a talocalcaneal coalition which usually is developed on the medial side of the subtalar joint; approaching medially may allow to easily visualize the coalition and resect it, then proceeding to prepare the subtalar joint for arthrodesis:
- Severely deformed valgus hindfoot, in which a medial incision heals without excessive tension as opposed to a lateral one which would be at high risk of dehiscence or breakage;
- Need to perform a double fusion and not ideal skin conditions which may bring the surgeon to opt for a single medial incision to approach both the subtalar and the talonavicular joint.

On the other side, it must be taken in mind that an excessive soft tissue resection of the medial aspect of the talus may lead to inadvertently detach the distal insertion of the deltoid ligament, which may generate a iatrogenic valgus collapse at the tibiotalar joint (especially after fusion of the subtalar joint which by definition overloads tibiotalar structures).

Talonavicular Arthrodesis

Talonavicular arthrodesis is usually indicated in case of joint degeneration and/or joint instability which may lead to an abnormal increase in the talonavicular uncoverage percentage and lateral (in progressive collapsing foot deformity) or medial (in cavovarus feet) subluxation or dislocation of the navicular over the talar head. It can be performed as isolated arthrodesis or in the context of a double or triple fusion.

Overall, three windows can be considered for approaching the joint, which could be called medial, dorsomedial and dorsolateral. Each one of them can be used as a single incision or they can be combined in order to allow the surgeon to maximize the amount of joint which can be appropriately prepared for fusion (Fig. 5.6).

The medial incision is placed slightly dorsally to the tibialis posterior tendon and medially to the tibialis anterior tendon, being represented by a horizontal line drawn from the anterior border of the medial malleolus to the medial tuberosity of the navicular. After subcutaneous dissection, the tibialis posterior is identified and either protected plantarly or split to get access to the joint capsule. The capsulotomy enables access to the joint. All the other steps to prepare the joint (positioning of a Hintermann distractor, use of non-motorized or motorized tools to remove the cartilage and the sclerotic bone and get to the bleeding bone) overlap those described for the subtalar joint.

The dorsomedial approach can be considered for those cases where the medial approach does not allow a satisfactory access to the central and lateral part of the joint, which is not infrequent due to the rounded shape of the talonavicular joint. In

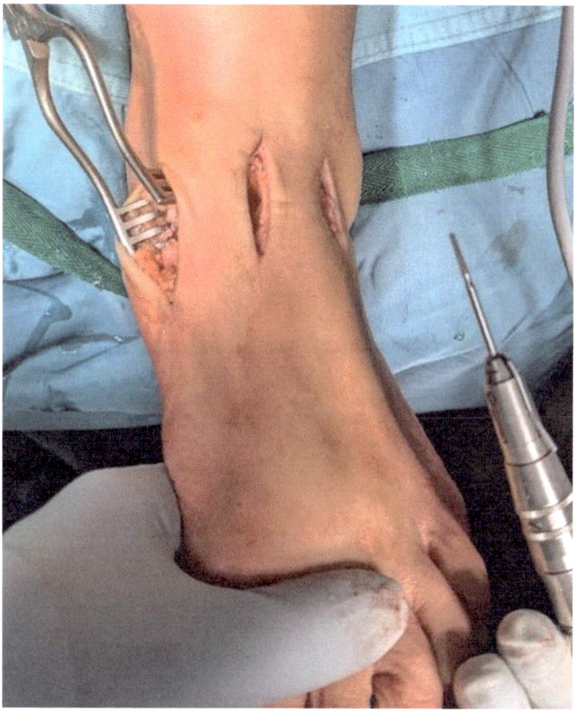

Fig. 5.6 Three portals to access the talonavicular joint. A high-speed burr may help to debride the cartilage and the sclerotic bone and prepare the surfaces for the arthrodesis

this case, the incision is placed vertically just lateral to the tibialis anterior tendon. After subcutaneous dissection, the extensor hallucis longus is protected laterally along with the tibialis anterior neurovascular bundle and the extensor digitorum longus tendon. The dorsal capsule is excised and the central part of the joint can be easily accessed. A mini-Hohman distractor positioned under the tibialis anterior tendon allows to join the spaces created with the medial and dorsomedial approach and to make sure that most of joint is adequately prepared.

The dorsolateral approach is more rarely used, but it is particularly useful for deformed navicular in which lateral osteophytes or fractured pieces of bone may generate pain and need to be removed. In this case the vertical incision is positioned over the projection of the navicular-lateral cuneiform joint. Since no obvious skin landmarks can be recommended for this approach, we recommend using a needle under fluoroscopy in order to center the incision in the right spot. Positioning the foot in order to get a slightly oblique dorsoplantar view (i.e. rotating internally the foot) may help better visualize this joint. As a rule of the thumb, the line of the incision will start approximately 1 cm anteriorly to the sinus tarsi and will be drawn toward the fourth toe. Considering that the superficial peroneal nerve lies anteriorly and laterally at the ankle, care should be recommended in subcutaneous dissection using the 'nick and spread' technique in order to identify it or push it away laterally with the soft tissues.

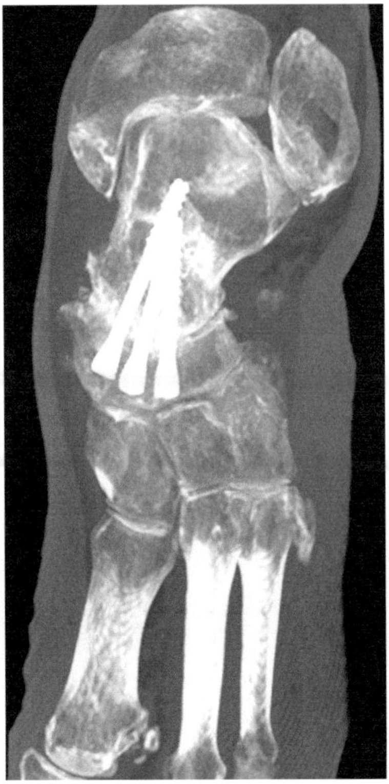

Fig. 5.7 Talonavicular fusion achieved using three cannulated screws (6-month CT imaging)

Fixation of the joint can be achieved using 4- or 5-mm compression screws (usually one to three positioned from distal to proximal) (Fig. 5.7). Care must be taken to ensure the head of the screws is sufficiently deep in the subchondral bone of the navicular in order to avoid soft tissue irritation in the dorsal midfoot.

Calcaneocuboid Arthrodesis

As for other procedures described above, the calcaneocuboid arthrodesis is indicated for treating symptomatic joint degeneration. Unlike the subtalar and talonavicular joints, the isolated arthrodesis of the calcaneocuboid joint is almost never performed since from a biomechanical standpoint the other two joints become rigid and potentially symptomatic, leading to a high risk of recommending a triple fusion in a short delay of time. From a surgical point of view, the incision to access the calcaneocuboid joint corresponds to the anterior extension of the same incision described for the subtalar joint. A needle may help to identify the calcaneocuboid joint. After elevation of the proximal insertion of the extensor digitorum brevis, the capsule is found plantarly. The joint is prepared as usual. Fixation is achieved either using one cannulated screw (in retrograde or antegrade direction), staples or (more rarely) plates.

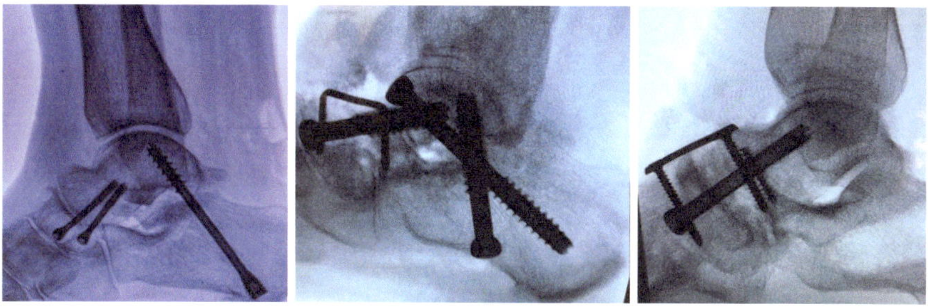

Fig. 5.8 Multiple ways to stabilize hindfoot joint using a combination of screws, plates and staples (on the left and at the center two double fusions; on the right a talonavicular fusion)

General Operative Considerations

Taking into account the three hindfoot joints, it is desirable to fuse only the painful degenerated joints (Fig. 5.8). This will allow as much as possible the hindfoot function as shock absorption and propulsion of the body.

Use of Graft

In general terms, two types of graft could be considered: (1) a structural one, such as a tricortical piece harvested from the iliac crest or an allograft, used to restore an appropriate height of the talocalcaneal complex and to add 'fresh' bone whenever sclerotic surfaces are identified even after the traditional joint preparation; (2) cancellous bone graft, which can be harvested from the tibia, the fibula or the calcaneus, which doesn't have structural properties but which helps boost biologically the process of fusion.

Bone Block Distraction Arthrodesis

With regard to the subtalar joint, it can be observed in some cases a loss of height of the calcaneus due to a previous thalamic fracture or to an advanced PCFD. In these cases:

- The Achilles tendon is usually short, so it may be worth considering a percutaneous triple hemisection of the tendon (Hoke procedure) to let the calcaneus tuberosity move down;
- A distraction arthrodesis is indicated in order to restore a more natural kinematics at the hindfoot and reduce the risk of anterior impingement at the tibiotalar joint; this generally requires a structural bone graft which is either harvested from the iliac crest or as allograft molded to fit the joint space (Figs. 5.9 and 5.10):

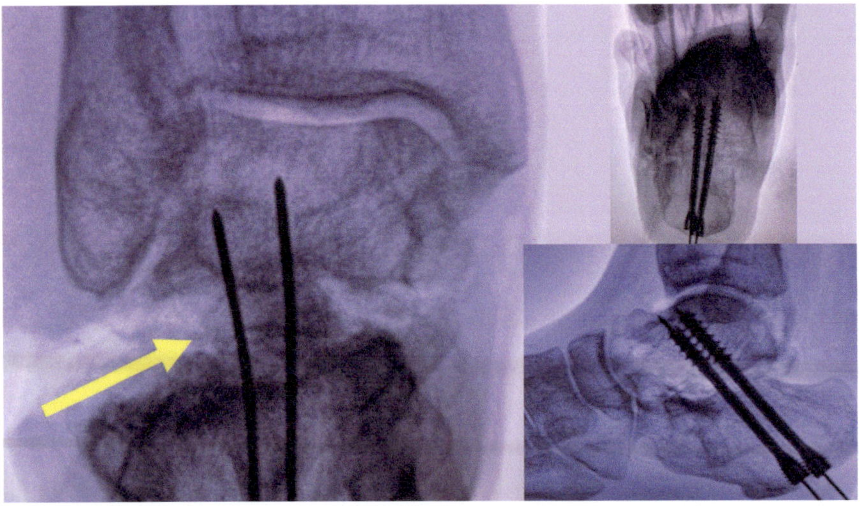

Fig. 5.9 The arrow indicated a structural tricortical graft used to perform a distraction subtalar arthrodesis

- A longitudinal (vertical) approach can be considered, incising the skin halfway between the posterior border to the lateral malleolus and the Achilles tendon, until the superior border of the posterior tuberosity of the calcaneus; a careful dissection of soft tissue is mandatory in order to avoid iatrogenic damage to the sural nerve. The biggest advantage of such approach will be an easier closure after the distraction of the subtalar joint since the incision will be parallel to the vector of lengthening. On the other side the posterior facet will be slightly harder to visualize and to prepare for fusion;
- A standard horizontal approach is still usable, but particular attention will be needed for closing soft-tissues since the risk of wound dehiscence due to excessive tension will be significant; in the end, the choice between a vertical and a horizontal approach will depend on the surgeon's experience and on the amount of distraction needed.

Triple Versus Double Arthrodesis

The triple and the double fusion (which differ by the involvement or not of the calcaneocuboid joint) are considered similar from a functional standpoint. A growing number of authors have been performing double arthrodesis in order to reduce the operative time, the damage on soft tissue and the risk of irritation from metalwork [4]. To date, there is no clear comparative study comparing the two techniques. However, in the authors 'experience, while in PCFD correction a double arthrodesis may allow to satisfactorily restore a good congruence at the Chopart joint with a

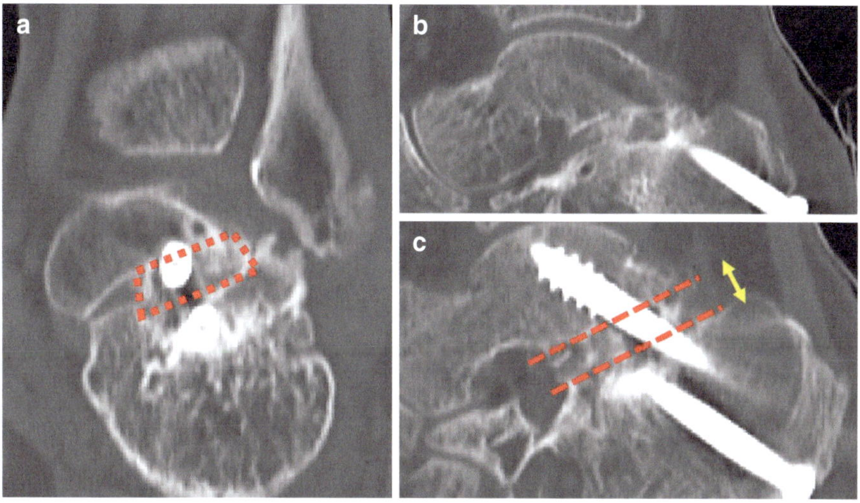

Fig. 5.10 On postoperative CT images the integration of the graft at the fusion site may be verified

distraction of the lateral column, in cavovarus feet it will be necessary to approach the calcaneocuboid joint in order to shorten the lateral column and re-align the foot.

Arthroscopic Techniques

General Concepts

Upon review of the literature, the complication rate after traditional subtalar arthrodesis has been reported up to 34% of cases [5], with wound dehiscence accounting for approximately 4% of them [6]. This is probably one of the main reasons why arthroscopic approaches to the subtalar joint have been found appealing from a number of foot and ankle surgeons, especially those with a previous training in small joints arthroscopy. Considering the anatomy of the subtalar joint (especially the posterior facet which is the main target for fusion procedures), two arthroscopic approaches are possible: the posterior approach and the anterolateral approach.

Posterior Arthroscopic Subtalar Arthrodesis (PASTA)

Surgery can be performed under regional or general anesthesia. A tourniquet is generally inflated at the upper thigh. The patient lies prone, with a support placed under the leg in order to allow some movement of the ankle. Distraction is usually not needed. A 4-mm 30-degrees arthroscope is used. Skin landmarks to place portals are the lateral malleolus, the medial and lateral borders of the Achilles tendon, and the sole of the foot. A line is drawn from the tip of the lateral malleolus to the Achilles tendon, parallel to the plantar aspect of the foot. The posterolateral and posteromedial portals are positioned just above this line, laterally and medially to the Achilles tendon. The posterolateral portal is commonly made first, using the 'nick and spread' technique. A mosquito clamp is directed anteriorly, pointing toward the first intermetatarsal space. Once bone is felt, a blunt obturator and the trocar are introduced following the same direction, in order not to cross the neurovascular bundle. Then, the posteromedial portal is made at the same level as the posterolateral one but on the medial side of the Achilles tendon. After the skin incision, a mosquito clamp is introduced and directed toward the trocar at a 90-degree angle, then is progressed anteriorly until both the trocar and the clamp touch the posterolateral aspect of the subtalar joint. The crural fascia is often penetrated in order to create a working area in the posterior aspect of the ankle. The subtalar joint capsule and fat tissues around are removed. The flexor hallucis longus (FHL) tendon remains the most important inner landmark during the procedure ensuring that all instruments are kept laterally to it, since on the other side (medially) the tibialis posterior neurovascular bundle lies. Classical 3.5-mm motorized instruments and nonmotorized tools (small chisels, osteotomes, graspers and scissors) are used to perform soft-tissue and bony debridement as needed. The subtalar joint has to be prepared as for all fusion procedures, by removing residual cartilage and superficial sclerotic bone until bleeding bone appears (Fig. 5.11). The joint is debrided from posterolateral to posteromedial and from anterolateral to anteromedial. The sinus tarsi represents the anterior limit of the posterior subtalar joint. An anterior third portal can be made at the sinus tarsi in order to ensure an adequate preparation of the anterior half of the posterior facet. Stabilization of the talocalcaneal block can be achieved using anterograde or retrograde cannulated screws (using from one to three screws with a diameter ranging from 5.5 to 8 mm) (Fig. 5.12). The postoperative protocol follows the same rules as for open subtalar arthrodesis.

Anterolateral Arthroscopic Subtalar Arthrodesis (ALAPSTA)

The patient is placed in the lateral position on the operating table under general or regional anesthesia and a well-padded high-thigh tourniquet is inflated. The position may also be supine with a pad positioned under the homolateral gluteus maximus muscle to obtain lower limb internal rotation. Main skin landmarks are identified as the lateral malleolus, the base of the fifth metatarsal bone and the anterior process of calcaneus corresponding to the floor of the sinus tarsi. The calcaneocuboid joint and the sural nerve trajectory can be considered additional landmarks (Fig. 5.13). A 'soft point' (sinus tarsi lateral projection) and the superficial peroneal nerve trajectory (if seen through the skin) are also marked. By introducing a posteriorly-oriented needle in the sinus tarsi, 10 to 15 cc of a 0.9% saline solution are injected. The consequent slight forefoot dorsiflexion and adduction confirm the correct position

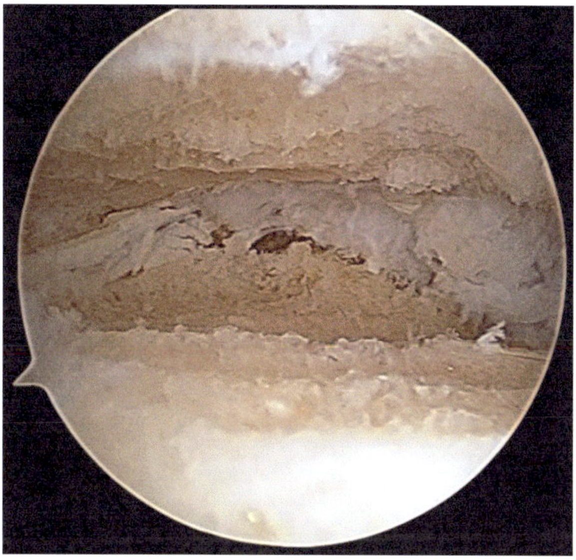

Fig. 5.11 Visualisation of bony surfaces after joint preparation. (Courtesy of Dr. Jesus Vila Y Rico)

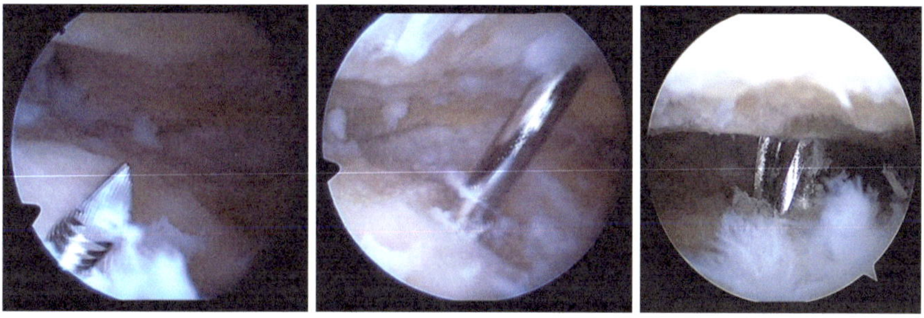

Fig. 5.12 Temporary placement of K-wires before positioning of screws. (Courtesy of Dr. Jesus Vila Y Rico)

of the needle. First, the posterior (or middle) portal is placed 1 to 5 mm distal to the malleolar tip, the posterior limit of the 4–5 mm horizontal incision corresponding to the vertical projection of the malleolar tip along the axis of the fibula (Fig. 5.13).

This is followed by blunt dissection of the subcutaneous tissue and of the extensor retinaculum by using a Halstead mosquito clamp parallel to the main posterior subtalar joint axis and perpendicularly to tibia. An arthroscope sheath and a blunt obturator are then introduced and slightly moved back and forth to create an adequate working chamber. The obturator is then removed and a 4.0-mm 30° arthroscope is positioned (hydraulic pump at 50 mmHg pressure). The second more anterior portal is placed with the help of a guide needle under direct endoscopic vision (Fig. 5.14). The 5-mm incision is positioned in the sinus tarsi and parallel to the sole of the foot—on a line that we call « the equator » of the sinus tarsi. Subcutaneous tissues are tackled in the way previously described, and a 4.5-mm arthroscopic synovial resector is introduced to prepare the subtalar joint.

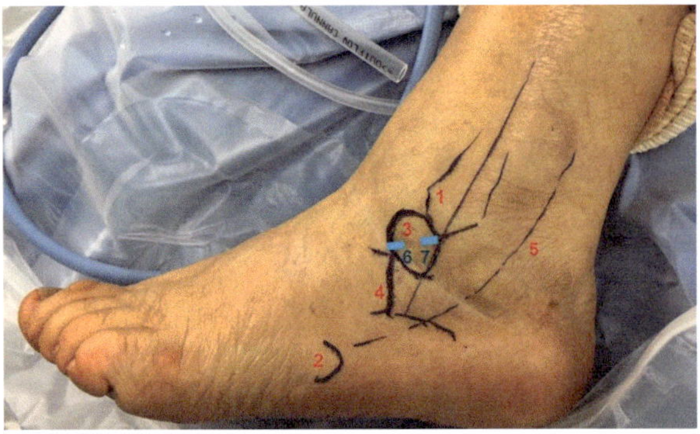

Fig. 5.13 External anatomy of portal placement during arthroscopic right posterior subtalar arthrodesis. Main landmarks are identified as the lateral malleolus (1), the base of the fifth metatarsal bone (2), the sinus tarsi (3), the calcaneocuboid joint (4) and the sural nerve skin projection (5). The anatomic location of the subtalar arthroscopy portals is marked (6 and 7)

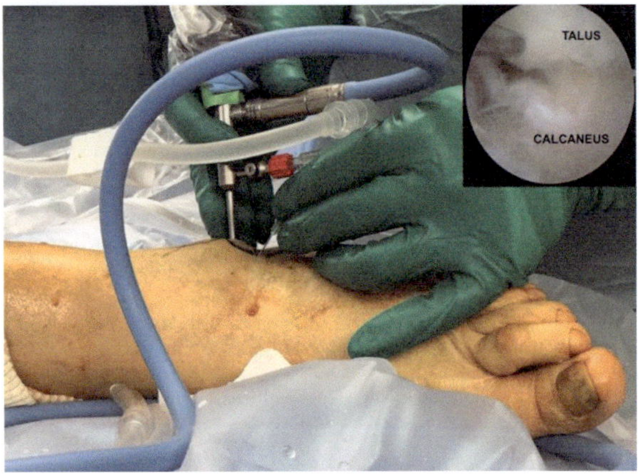

Fig. 5.14 Placement of the anterior portal to perform an ALAPSTA. After the introduction of an arthroscope in the first (more posterior) lateral portal, a needle is used to control the position of the second (more anterior) portal and to find out the correct orientation of the shaver that will replace the needle. In the right little box, the arthroscopic check of the needle is placed in the lateral space defined by the talus (superiorly) and the calcaneus (inferiorly)

After a careful synovectomy and debridement of the fibrous scar tissue, the anterior aspect of posterior subtalar joint, the talus superiorly, calcaneus inferiorly and sinus tarsi ligament antero-laterally may be visualised. Joint debridement is usually performed using a 4-mm arthroscopic burr, starting at the anterolateral angle and realising 180° rotation movements from lateral to medial. Thereafter, the burr is placed medially to remove cartilage from the half of the joint (movements from medial to lateral), and after again laterally to continue the resection along the lateral joint aspect up to the posterior area. The shaver shield protects the peroneal tendons and the calcaneo-fibular ligament. Due to the absence of external distraction and to the physiologic postero-medial joint surface curvature, we use a rigid curette (better if curved) to complete the debridement (Fig. 5.15). The flexor hallucis longus (FHL) tendon lies behind the talar postero-medial process, so it should be used as posterior limit in the resection to avoid damage to the latter and to the tibial nerve. Exchanging the portals allows to prepare the more medial joint aspect and to debride the residual cartilage, with no risk for the talar medial process. Following this procedure, the articular surfaces may be prepared almost completely. After this, the tourniquet is deflated to appreciate a consistent trabecular bone bleeding and to exclude vascular lesions. Bone grafting is never used in our experience, even if theoretically possible. While cartilage has to be removed as far as possible, the subchondral bone small

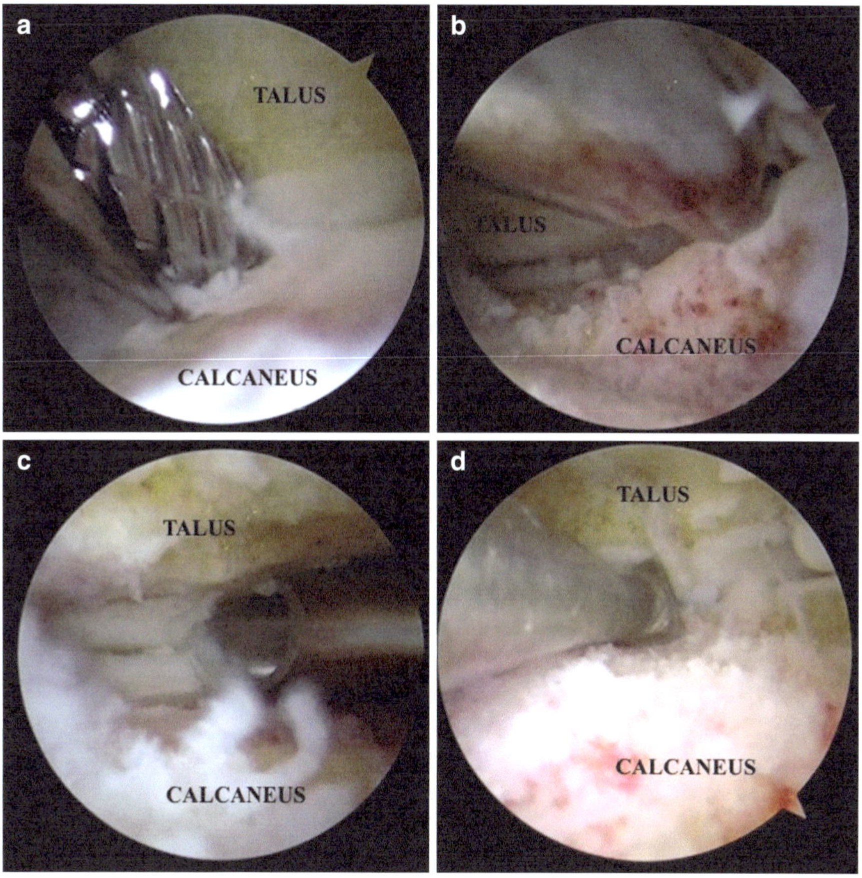

Fig. 5.15 ALAPSTA of left hindfoot in a patient with severe idiopathic subtalar arthritis. The patient is placed in the lateral position. In **a**, **b** and **d** visualization is performed through the posterior portal, while in **c** through the anterior one. The sequence shows different phases of the cartilage debridement in the posteromedial (**a**), posterior (**b**), and posterolateral area of the subtalar joint. A curette is generally used to remove the residual cartilage (**d**)

irregularities must be left in place as they contribute to augment the total contact surface, thus helping the healing process (Fig. 5.15). Skin portals are closed by two absorbable sutures. Fixation is generally performed as described above.

Percutaneous Techniques

Percutaneous techniques are gaining momentum to perform forefoot and hindfoot osteotomies. Already in 2016, percutaneous hindfoot and midfoot fusions were discussed in literature as a way to reduce the morbidity and speed up the recovery of patients [7]. The best indications were fusions for mild-to-moderate reducible hindfoot and midfoot deformities in fragile patients with general or local bad conditions. While not may papers have been published so far (so that a clear indication towards or against this technique cannot be formulated), the principles to perform fusion procedures are a mixture of percutaneous surgery and arthrodesis techniques: small portals are placed along the same incisions which would be used for open techniques; appropriate blunt dissection with rongeurs or mosquito clamps until the bone is reached should be performed in order to 'move away' neurovascular and tendinous structure: high-speed burrs, whose position is verified under fluoroscopy, are used to prepare the joint: an appropriate irrigation system must be used in order to reduce the temperature of the burr and the subsequent risk of thermal necrosis. On the other hand, the need to consider a learning curve has been described as the main limitation for these techniques.

Postoperative Management

Traditionally, after hindfoot arthrodesis the foot is immobilized in a non weight bearing plaster cast for 6 weeks, followed by full weight bearing (as tolerated) in a boot and gradual recovery of movement for further 6 weeks. It's clear that this timeframe must be adapted to each single patient, with shorter times of immobilisation in young motivated patients with no comorbidity and good bone quality vs longer immobilization times in elderly patients affected by other conditions and reduced bone density.

References

1. Izzo A, Manzi G, D'Agostino M, Mariconda M, Patel S, Bernasconi A. Combined anterior and posterior vs isolated posterior facet fixation for subtalar arthrodesis: a proportional meta-analysis and systematic review of the literature. Orthop Traumatol Surg Res. Published online. 2024; https://doi.org/10.1016/J.OTSR.2024.104027.

2. Wirth SH, Viehöfer A, Fritz Y, Zimmermann SM, Rigling D, Urbanschitz L. How many screws are necessary for subtalar fusion? A retrospective study. Foot Ankle Surg. 2020;26(6):699–702. https://doi.org/10.1016/J.FAS.2019.08.017.
3. Jones JM, Vacketta VG, Philp FH, Catanzariti AR. Radiographic outcomes of isolated subtalar joint arthrodesis with varying fixation technique. J Foot Ankle Surg. 2022;61(5):938–43. https://doi.org/10.1053/J.JFAS.2021.12.016.
4. Burns PR, Powers NS. Double versus triple arthrodesis for flatfoot deformity: when, why, and how? Clin Podiatr Med Surg. 2023;40(2):315–32. https://doi.org/10.1016/J.CPM.2022.11.009.
5. Saragaglia D, Giunta J, Gaillot J, Tourné Y, Rubens-Duval B. Subtalar arthrodesis using a single compression screw: a comparison of results between anterograde and retrograde screwing. Eur J Orthop Surg Traumatol. 2022;32(8):1583–9. https://doi.org/10.1007/S00590-021-03141-7.
6. Rungprai C, Phisitkul P, Femino JE, Martin KD, Saltzman CL, Amendola A. Outcomes and complications after open versus posterior arthroscopic subtalar arthrodesis in 121 patients. J Bone Joint Surg Am. 2016;98(8):636–46. https://doi.org/10.2106/JBJS.15.00702.
7. Bauer T. Percutaneous Hindfoot and Midfoot fusion. Foot Ankle Clin. 2016;21(3):629–40. https://doi.org/10.1016/J.FCL.2016.04.008.

Chapter 6
Ankle Fusion

Maneesh Bhatia, Christian Plaass, and Hytham Afifi

Introduction: Nature of the Problem

Ankle arthrodesis remains the gold standard for treating advanced, painful ankle osteoarthritis. More than three decades ago, this procedure was adapted to arthroscopic techniques, leading to numerous studies reporting excellent results with a low complication rate [1].

Arthroscopic ankle arthrodesis (AAA) is an effective surgical approach for managing degenerative ankle disease, even in cases of moderate tibiotalar coronal deformity. Research indicates that AAA results in good to excellent functional outcomes, with nearly three-quarters of patients achieving favourable results at a mean follow-up of 86 months postoperatively [2].

Recent evidence from Lorente et al. [3] further supports the efficacy of AAA, demonstrating that while both arthroscopic and open ankle arthrodesis achieve comparable fusion rates, the arthroscopic approach is associated with reduced hospital stay and lower overall complication rates. Specifically, their systematic review and meta-analysis found that while fusion rates remain similar, arthroscopic techniques provide a faster recovery profile, making it a preferable option in appropriately selected patients [3].

M. Bhatia (✉)
Consultant Orthopaedic Foot Ankle Surgeon, University Hospitals Leicester, Spire Hospital Leicester and Nuffield Health Leicester, Leicester, UK

Associate Professor, University of Leicester, Leicester, UK

Professor, DeMontfort University Leicester, Leicester, UK

H. Afifi
University Hospitals Leicester NHS Trust, Leicester, UK

C. Plaass
Hannover Medical School, Hannover, Germany

M. Bhatia (ed.), *Surgical Techniques of the Foot and Ankle*,
https://doi.org/10.1007/978-3-031-93742-2_6

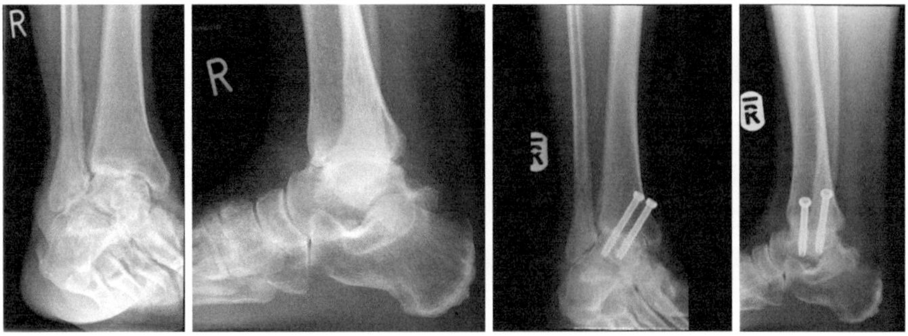

Fig. 6.1 Pre operative and post operative radiographs of a 72 years patient 5 months post-surgery (arthroscopic ankle arthrodesis) returning back to Martial arts and demonstrating excellent gait and range of movements

The main concerns against ankle fusion are in relation to affection of gait and loss of movements following ankle fusion surgery. However, the majority of patients undergoing arthroscopic ankle fusion make a good recovery including participation in sporting activities with a near normal gait and no significant restriction of range of movements as illustrated in Fig. 6.1.

Indications and Contraindications

The primary indications for AAA surgery include all causes of end-stage ankle arthritis, particularly cases where there is soft tissue compromise around the ankle joint. When evaluating the potential causes of ankle arthritis, soft tissue condition and management become significant considerations. Posttraumatic arthritis frequently develops in patients with severe ankle trauma, which may include open fractures or multiple surgical interventions leading to extensive scarring. AAA is also indicated for patients with inflammatory arthritis and elderly patients who may have compromised skin healing. The minimally invasive nature of AAA, with small arthroscopic portals and percutaneous screw fixation, makes it an ideal choice for these cases.

A common misconception is that deformity is a contraindication for AAA. However, literature suggests otherwise [4]. The critical factor in assessing deformity is whether the forefoot can be positioned flat on the ground. The surgeon must differentiate between deformity at the ankle joint, which can be corrected through joint preparation, and deformity below the ankle, which may require additional osteotomies to achieve proper alignment. Figure 6.2 illustrates an example where AAA has been performed in a patient with multiple medical comorbidities and poor soft tissue envelope with ankle arthritis and significant valgus deformity at the ankle joint.

Relative contraindications include:

- Poor skin quality: Previous surgical interventions or scars may necessitate modifications in screw placement to ensure healthy tissue coverage.
- Metalwork from prior surgeries: This may require adjustments in technique to accommodate existing implants.

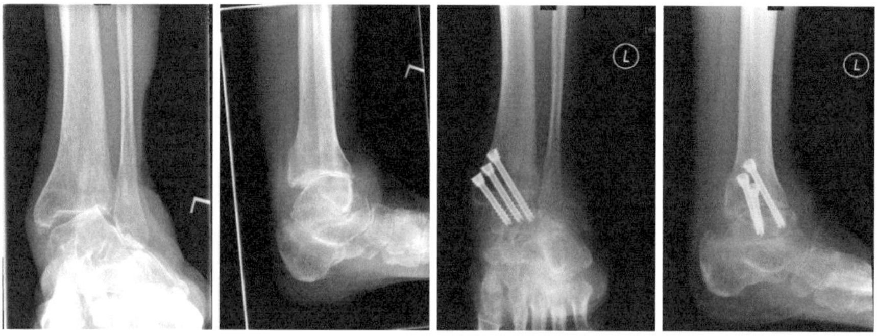

Fig. 6.2 Pre and post-surgery radiographs of a 76 years old patient with significant valgus deformity illustrating that a significant deformity can be addressed by arthroscopic ankle fusion

- Avascular necrosis of the talus: While sometimes considered a contraindication, it can be an indication for AAA if fusion is the goal.
- Poor vascularity: Should be carefully assessed for severity, as an arthroscopic approach minimizes the risk of wound healing complications.
- Smoking: Not an absolute contraindication but significantly increases the risk of nonunion. Patients should be counselled on cessation before surgery.
- Neuropathy: This increases the risk of nonunion, particularly in cases of early-stage active Charcot arthropathy.
- Active infection: This is an absolute contraindication to AAA and must be fully treated before considering arthrodesis [4].

Surgical Technique/Procedure (Anterior Ankle Arthroscopic Fusion)

Preoperative Planning

Before considering AAA, it is essential to confirm that the symptoms originate from the ankle. A thorough history and clinical examination remain the most effective methods for distinguishing ankle pathology from issues affecting adjacent joints. Standing anteroposterior and lateral radiographs and a CT scan serve as crucial diagnostic tools. Additionally, in presence of multiple joint arthritis, a targeted local anesthetic injection can help confirm whether the pain is localized to the ankle joint.

Preparation and Patient Positioning

Preoperative prophylactic intravenous antibiotics should be administered according to local protocols to minimize the risk of infection. The use of general or regional anaesthesia is recommended to ensure full limb relaxation during the procedure.

The patient is positioned supine on the operating table, with a sandbag placed under the ipsilateral buttock to maintain proper limb alignment. A thigh tourniquet may be inflated at the discretion of the surgeon, although it is possible to perform the entire procedure without a tourniquet. The leg is prepared up to the knee to allow adequate access for assessing limb alignment and to facilitate the placement of guidewires and screws for fixation. A knee support facilitates some flexion of the knee joint and this is helpful to apply traction (Fig. 6.3). Traction with a non-invasive device is useful in facilitating joint visualization and the senior author always uses it when performing AAA (Fig. 6.4).

Surgical Technique

The surgical technique involves the use of a standard 4.5-mm or 5.0-mm, 30-degree arthroscope ("knee scope"). To facilitate joint visualization, 20 mL of saline is injected into the joint to achieve distension (Fig. 6.5). A standard anteromedial portal (medial to the tibialis anterior tendon) is created for the insertion of the scope. This is performed following a skin incision and blunt dissection using a small clip. Under direct vision, an anterolateral portal (lateral to the extensor digitorum

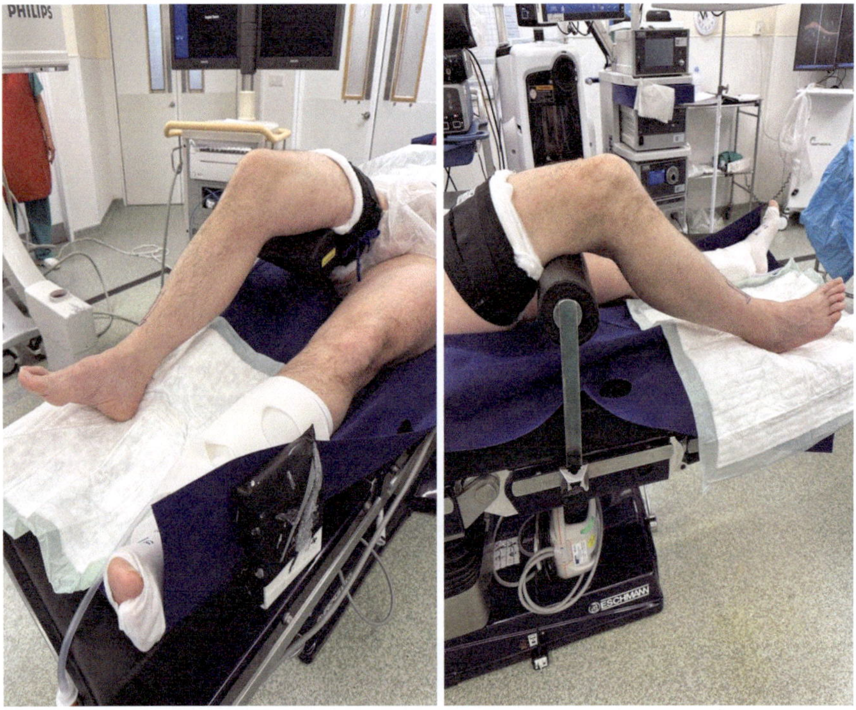

Fig. 6.3 Patient position

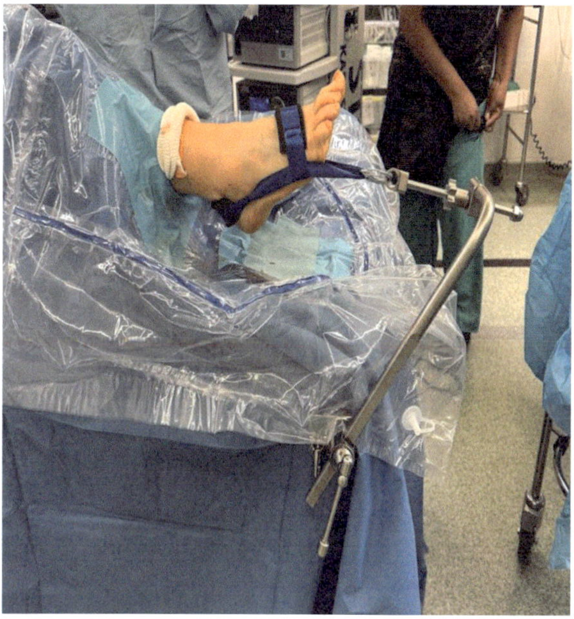

Fig. 6.4 Use of traction device in AAA surgery

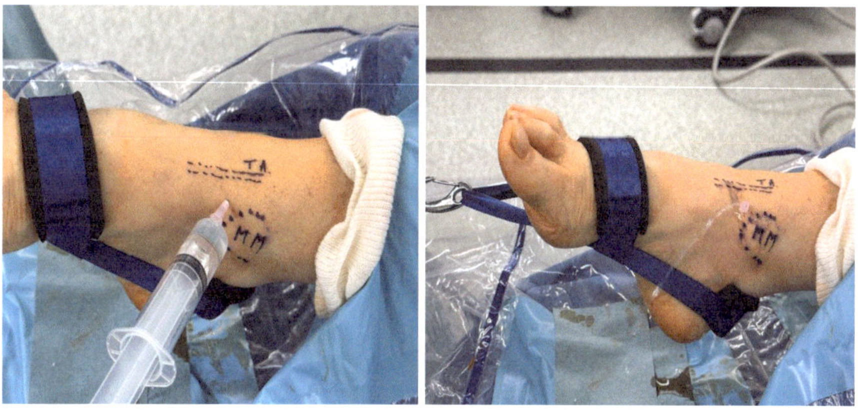

Fig. 6.5 Injection of saline through the anteromedial portal. A good flowback indicates intra-articular injection of fluid

communis) is established in the same manner (Fig. 6.6). Special care must be taken to avoid injury to the lateral superficial peroneal nerve, which is located subcutaneously.

For initial joint debridement, power instruments such as a 4.5-mm full-radius arthroscopic shavers are recommended, as they enhance visualization by clearing soft tissue and debris (Fig. 6.7). This is followed by the use of a motorized burr, preferably a barrel-shaped burr, is used to prepare the subchondral surfaces thoroughly (Fig. 6.8). To denude the cartilage from the posterior rim where burr can't reach, the use of a curette is beneficial (Fig. 6.9). Although preparation of medial and lateral gutters is not mandatory, a good clearance does aid healing and the senior author always prepares these. Figure 6.10 demonstrates satisfactory preparation of the joint surfaces prior to screw insertion.

For fixation, a cannulated compression screw system with a minimum diameter of 6.5 mm is used. Although anecdotal teaching and thinking is that in order to achieve compression, headed screws should be used, the senior author has used both headed and headless screws with equally good results. In most cases the use of two screws is sufficient. Both screws are placed medially (anterior and posterior). Figure 6.11 illustrates the setup of the image intensifier machine and placement of guide wires for cannulated screw insertion.

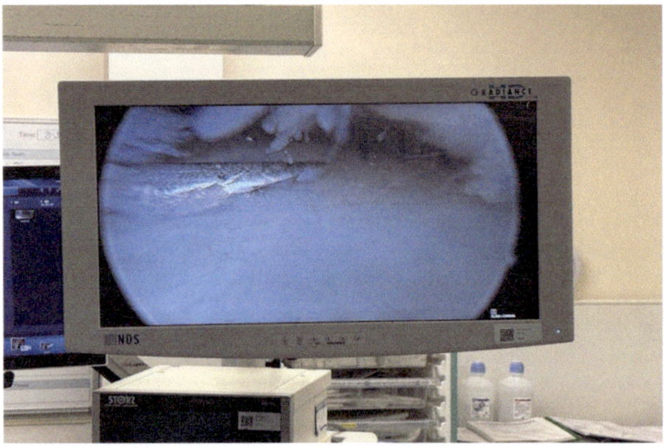

Fig. 6.6 Use of needle in the ankle joint to make the anterolateral portal under vision

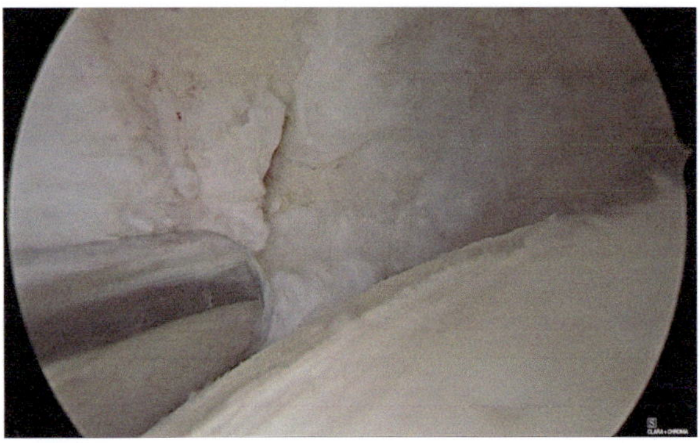

Fig. 6.7 Use of soft tissue shaver for early soft tissue debridement and synovectomy

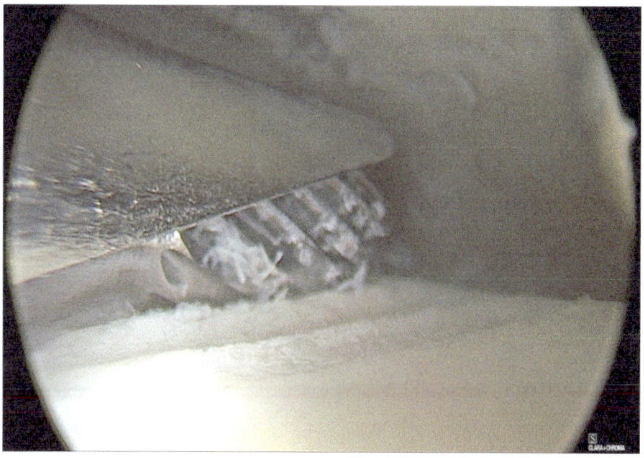

Fig. 6.8 Use of burr to denude cartilage

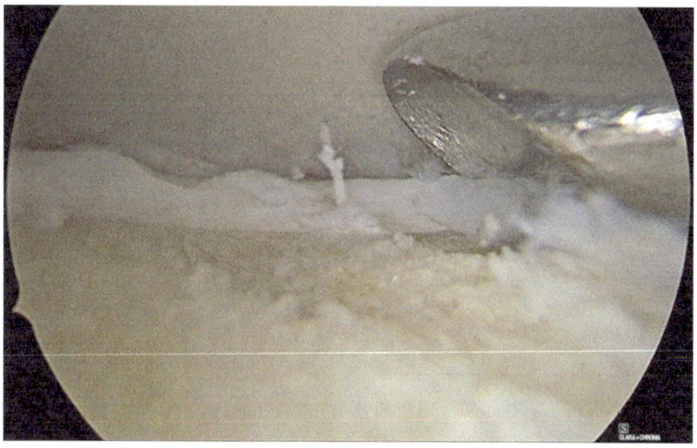

Fig. 6.9 Following use of burr to achieve subchondral preparation, a curette is used to reach the posterior rim where the burr can't reach

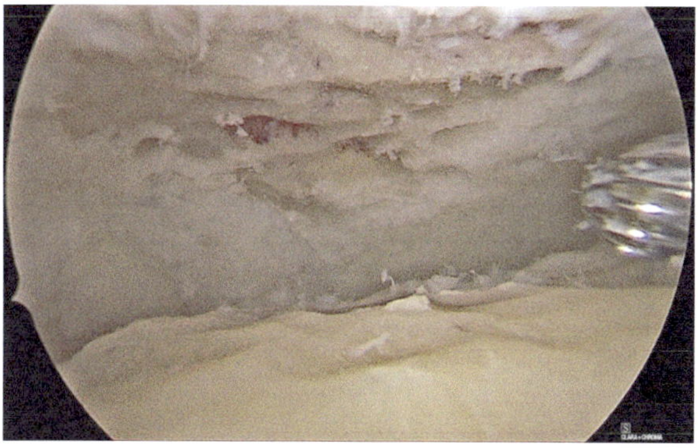

Fig. 6.10 Final preparation of the ankle joint during AAA to subchondral bleeding bone surfaces

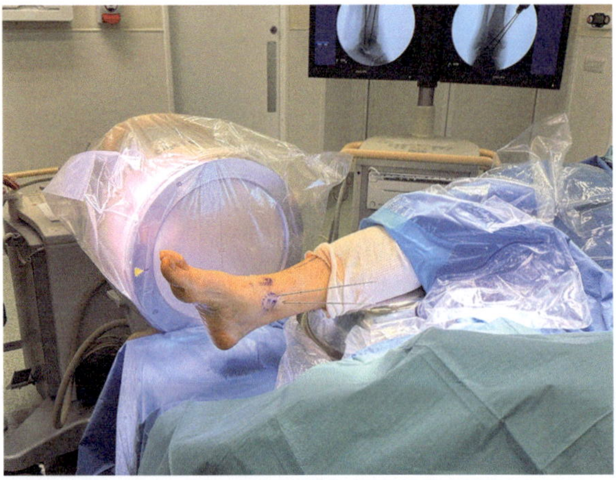

Fig. 6.11 Placement of two parallel medial guide wires for optimal cannulated screw placement in AAA surgery

Postoperative Care

- Immediately after surgery, sterile wound dressings are applied, and the limb is immobilized in a below-knee splint on the operating table.
- The patient remains non-weight bearing for the first 2 weeks postoperatively.
- From weeks 2–6, weight-bearing is permitted while the patient remains in plaster cast.
- After 6 weeks if there is satisfactory progression of healing on X-rays, then plaster is replaced with a removable boot.
- X-rays are performed at 6 weeks and then periodically.
- Most patients achieve good union between 8–12 weeks when physiotherapy is started.

Posterior Ankle Arthroscopic Fusion

Arthroscopic ankle arthrodesis (AAA) is most commonly performed via the standard anterior approach, utilizing anteromedial and anterolateral portals. However, some studies suggest that a posterior approach may result in a higher union rate [5]. The posterior approach allows for over 95% of the joint to be debrided, making it particularly useful in cases where:

- The patient requires talocalcaneal fusion in addition to tibiotalar arthrodesis.
- Large anterior osteophytes obstruct access to the ankle joint through the anterior approach.

However, the posterior approach is only technically feasible when:

- Equinus deformity is not present.
- The patient does not have a malunited posterior malleolus.

Given that most patients undergoing arthrodesis have post traumatic ankle arthritis, the applicability of the arthroscopic posterior approach for fusion remains limited [5].

Open Ankle Arthrodesis (OAA)

Open ankle arthrodesis (OAA) is traditionally regarded as the most reliable technique for correcting significant deformity in ankle arthritis. This approach offers several advantages over other arthrodesis techniques, including:

- Enhanced visualization of the joint.
- Improved access for joint preparation.
- Greater feasibility for performing corrective osteotomies.
- Lateral Transfibular approach is an excellent source of bone graft.
- OAA can be performed via different surgical approaches, depending on the specific deformity, including: Anterior, Posterior or Lateral Transfibular approach [6].

Surgical Technique/Procedure

Open anterior approach.

The open anterior approach is used in patients with:

(a) excessive anterior osteophytes causing equinus deformity, making AAA difficult,
(b) severe bony deformity or defects (Fig. 6.12a–c), or
(c) conditions requiring additional plate application due to bone quality, patient compliance, or neurogenic pathologies.

The procedure is performed with the patient in a supine position and a tight tourniquet applied. A standard anterior approach is used. To protect the neurovascular bundle, the ankle joint is accessed between the extensor hallucis longus and tibialis anterior tendons. The joint is distracted using a K-wire spreader on the medial side. Any remaining cartilage is removed with chisels and curettes, and the subchondral bone is microfractured (Fig. 6.13).

Repositioning is achieved using a pull-roll-push technique. The position is initially secured with a K-wire from the medial side. After verifying the correct positioning under fluoroscopy, a screw is placed to compress the talus against the medial gutter. In cases of severe varus malalignment, even after bony corrections, an alternative lag screw from the lateral side can help maintain the corrected position (Fig. 6.14).

In patients with increased risk of non-union a plate arthrodesis is recommended [7, 8]. The plate is fixed to the talar neck first. Typically, a compression hole in the

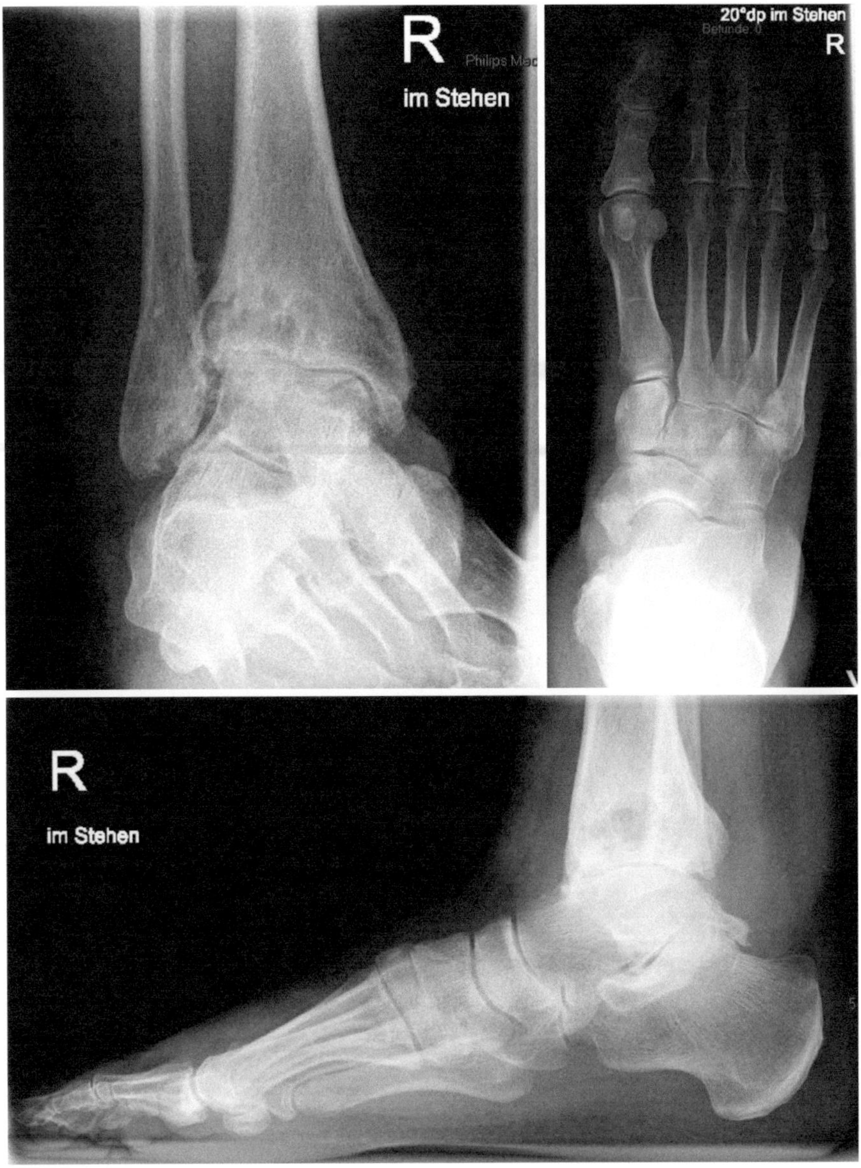

Fig. 6.12 (**a–c**) Ankle arthrosis with a defect in the distal lateral tibia

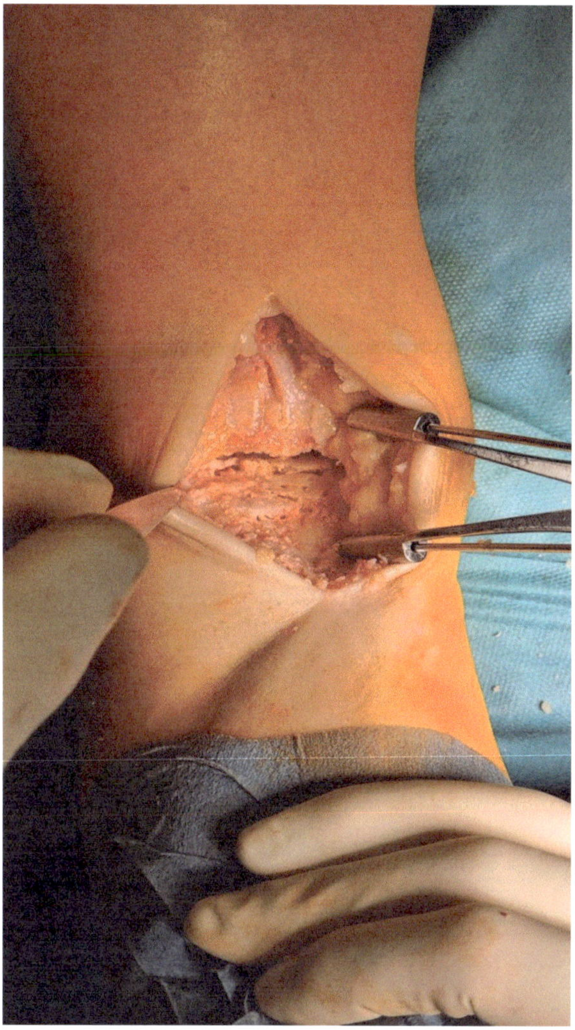

Fig. 6.13 A standard anterior ankle approach is used. A K-wire spreader is used to distract the joint. Any remaining cartilage is removed, cysts debrided and bone grafted

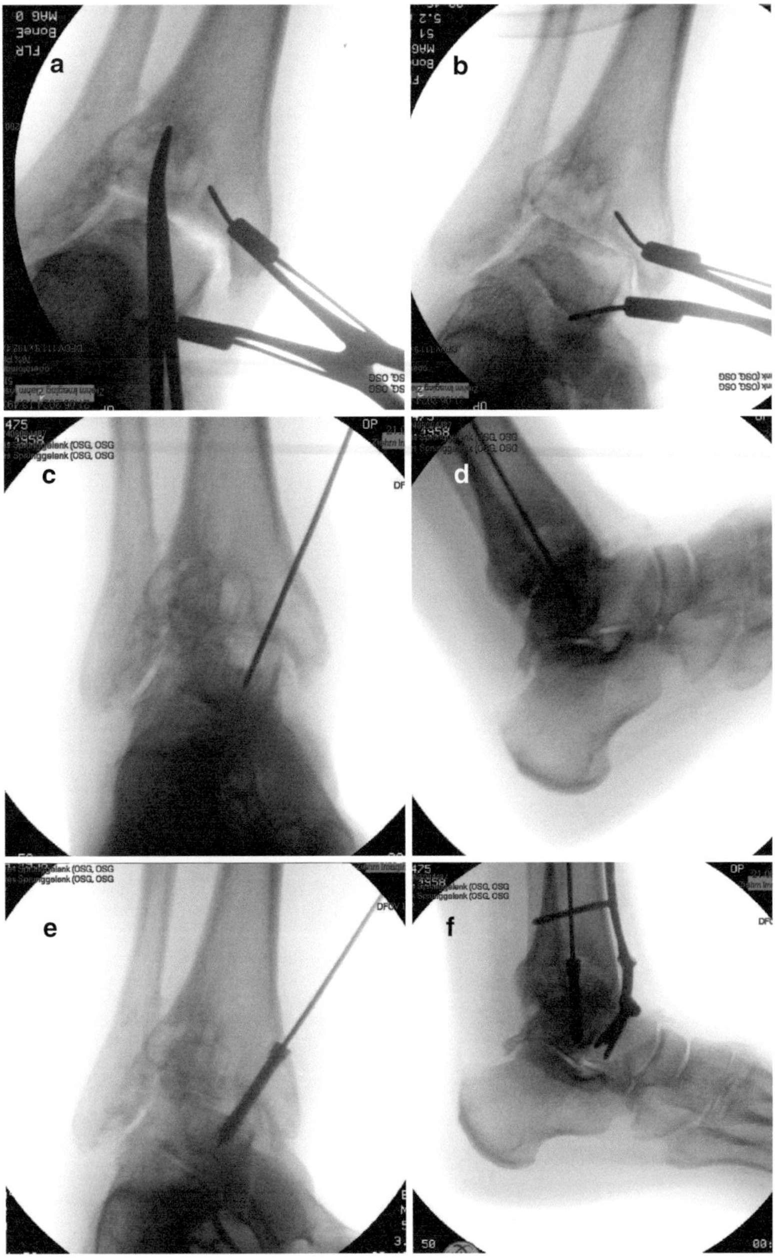

Fig. 6.14 The joint is debrided and distracted with a K-wire spreader. The bony defect is analysed (**a**). The bony defect is filled with auto- and allograft bone (**b**), the ankle reduced and temporarily fixed with a K-wire. The position of the reduction and position of the screw K-wire is checked fluoroscopically (**c**, **d**). A lag screw is then used to compress the talus against the tibia and the medial malleolus (**e**). The plate is then fixed to the talar neck and further compression applied using the compression hole of the plate and the position again checked fluoroscopically (**f**, **g**). Then the remaining screws are inserted and the position checked finally (**h**, **i**)

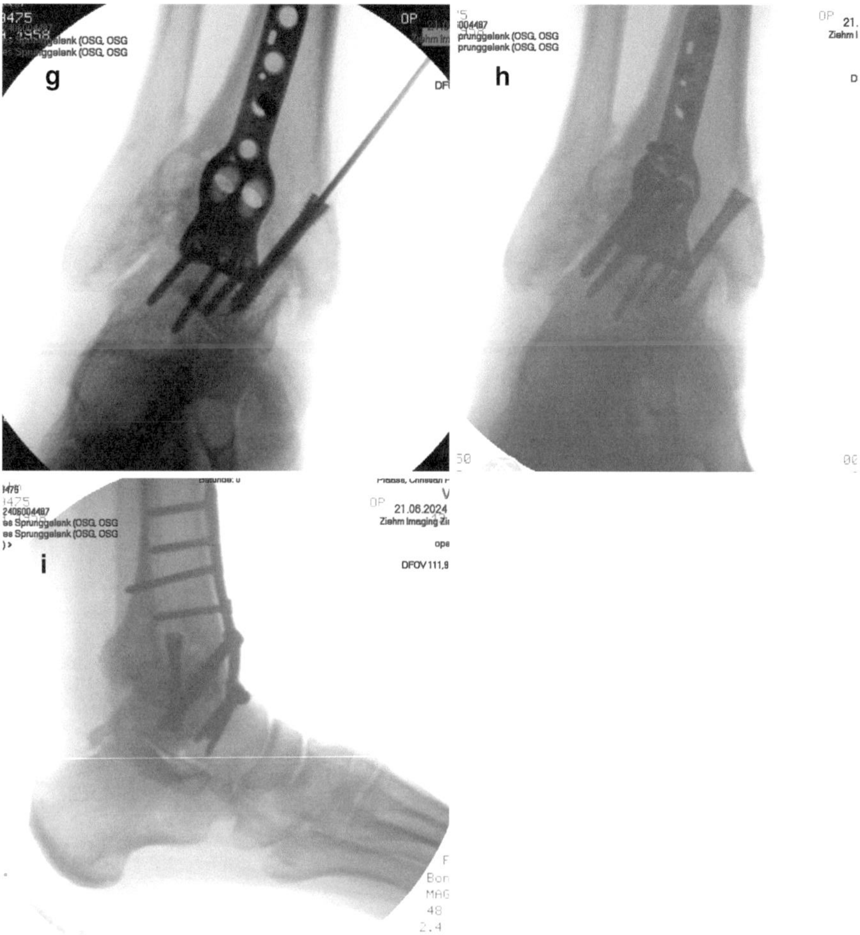

Fig. 6.14 (continued)

tibial part of the plate allows further compression (Fig. 6.15). The position is checked again fluoroscopically before securing the remaining plate screws. In patients with good bone quality, a standard 3- to 4-screw technique can alternatively be used.

Postoperative care includes non-weight bearing in a long walker until wound healing, followed by partial weight bearing depending on the patient's bone quality, for 6 weeks postoperatively. After an x-ray control, gradual weight bearing is then introduced, and once pain-free full weight bearing is achieved, a normal shoe with a slight rocker-bottom sole can be used after about 3 months (Fig. 6.16).

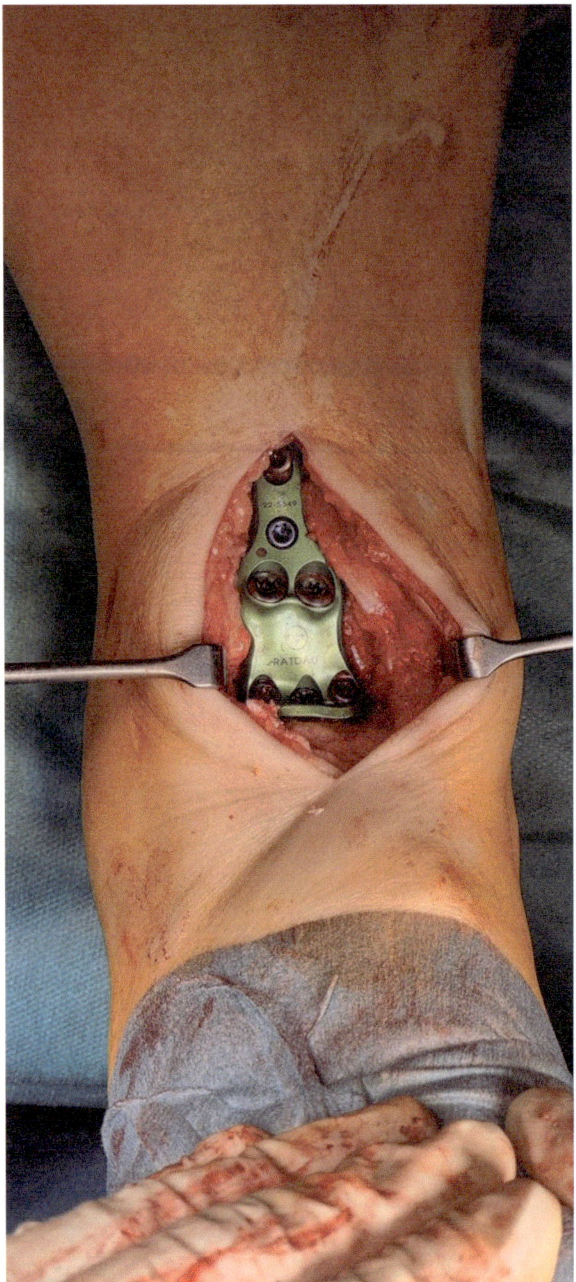

Fig. 6.15 An anterior ankle arthrodesis plate is used to improve stability in patients with bony insufficiencies

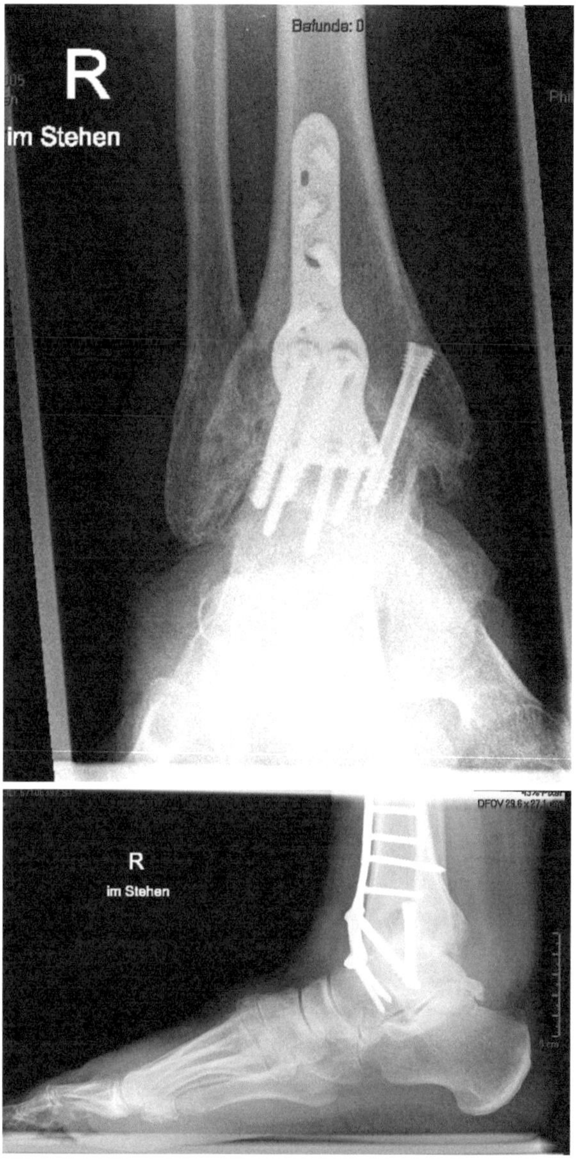

Fig. 6.16 Postoperative x-rays in a.p. (**a**) and lateral view (**b**) 3 months after operation, showing bony healing in a good position

Open Lateral Transfibular Approach

The lateral approach to the ankle provides an extensile exposure, offering excellent access to the tibiotalar joint and, when indicated, the distal subtalar joint. Fibula is divided in the middle to ease resection of fibula (Fig. 6.17).

Once the fibula is removed, the lateral aspect of the tibiotalar joint is visualised. Peroneal tendons should be protected (Fig. 6.18).

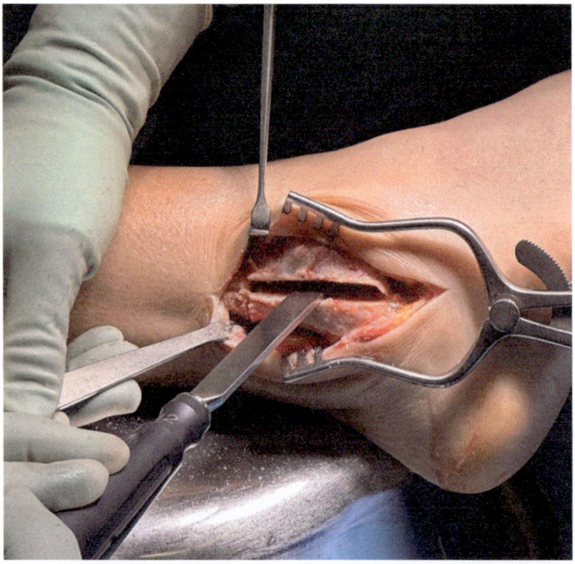

Fig. 6.17 Lateral Transfibular approach showing osteotomy of fibula

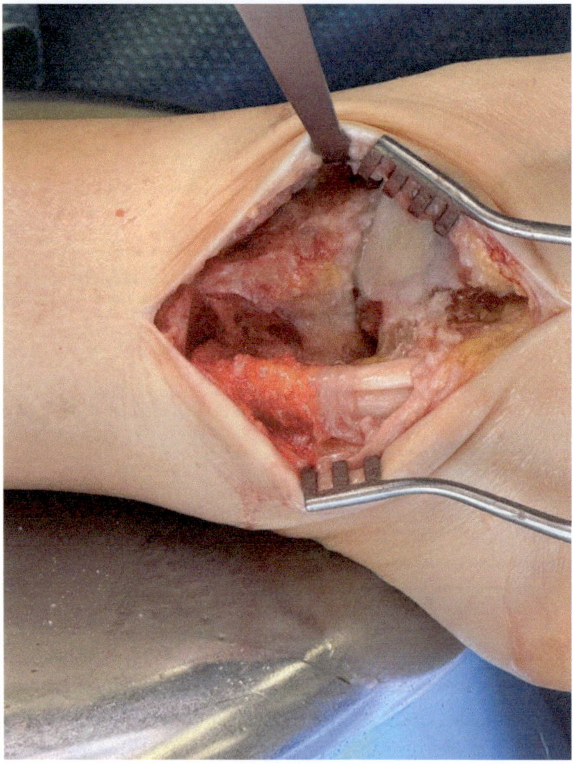

Fig. 6.18 Exposure of lateral ankle following resection of distal fibula

The next step is use of a distractor to enhance access to the ankle joint (Fig. 6.19).

The ankle joint is then prepared using a combination of osteotomes and rongeurs. A burr can be useful to prepare the medial gutter (Fig. 6.20a, b).

Figures 6.21, 6.22 and 6.23 illustrate fixation technique for Transfibular approach. Restoration of hindfoot alignment is the key step and should be confirmed clinically (Fig. 6.21a) and on radiographs (Fig. 6.21b). The reduction is held in satisfactory position with a 2 or 2.5 mm Kirschner wire (Fig. 6.21b).

This is followed by use of a compression lag screw (Fig. 6.22). Subsequently a lateral locking plate is used to provide rigid fixation (Fig. 6.23). Alternatively the fibula can be used as a bio-graft on the lateral side.

Post operative protocol is similar as described earlier following AAA. Total duration of plaster or boot is usually up to 12 weeks and full weight bearing is permitted throughout the use of plaster or boot. Figures 6.24 and 6.25 illustrate a case with significant deformity achieving good correction and union in less than 12 weeks.

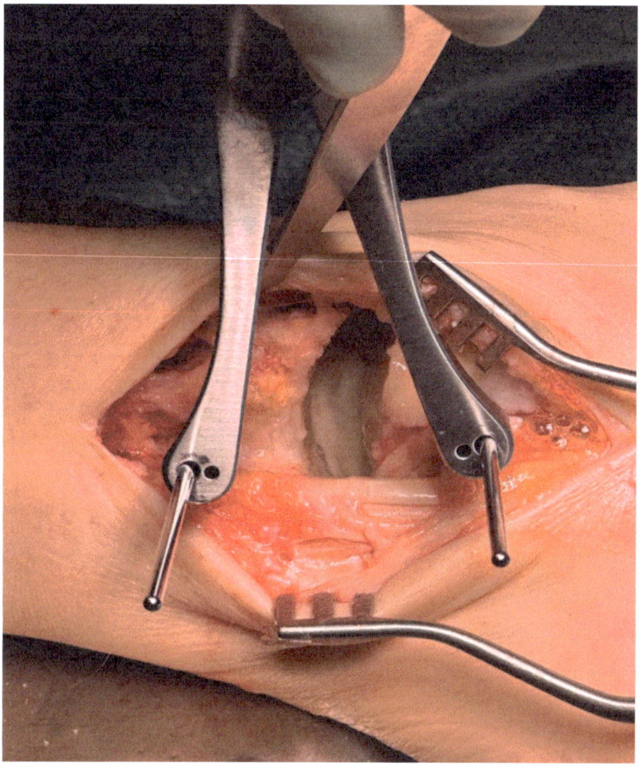

Fig. 6.19 Use of distractor demonstrating excellent view of ankle joint

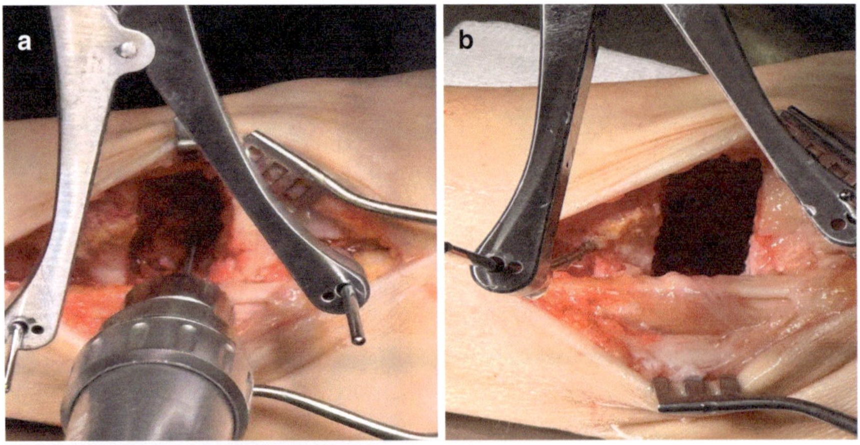

Fig. 6.20 (**a**) Use of burr to prepare medial gutter. (**b**) Final preparation

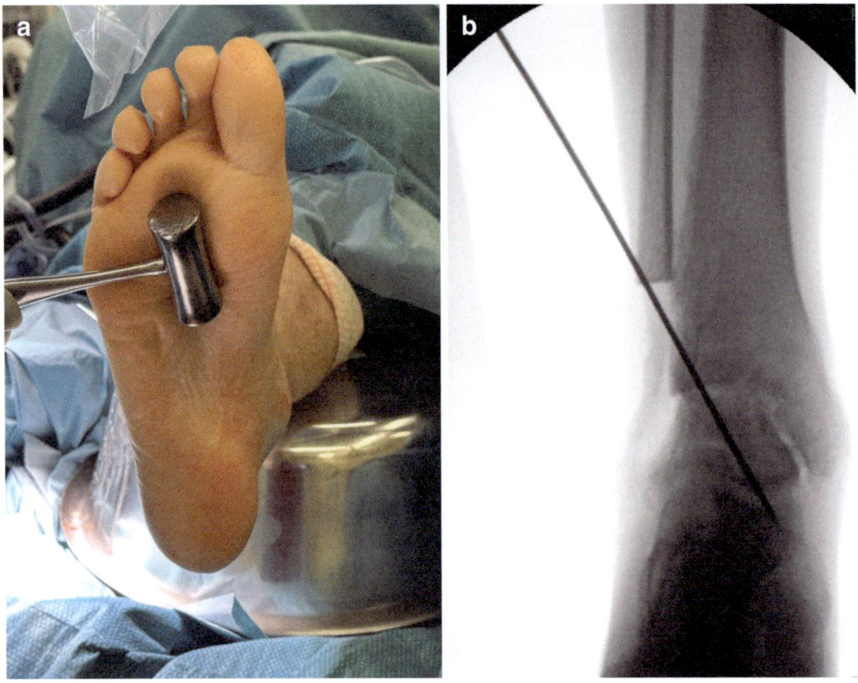

Fig. 6.21 (**a**) Illustration of deformity correction. (**b**) Satisfactory alignment maintained by a thick Kirschner wire

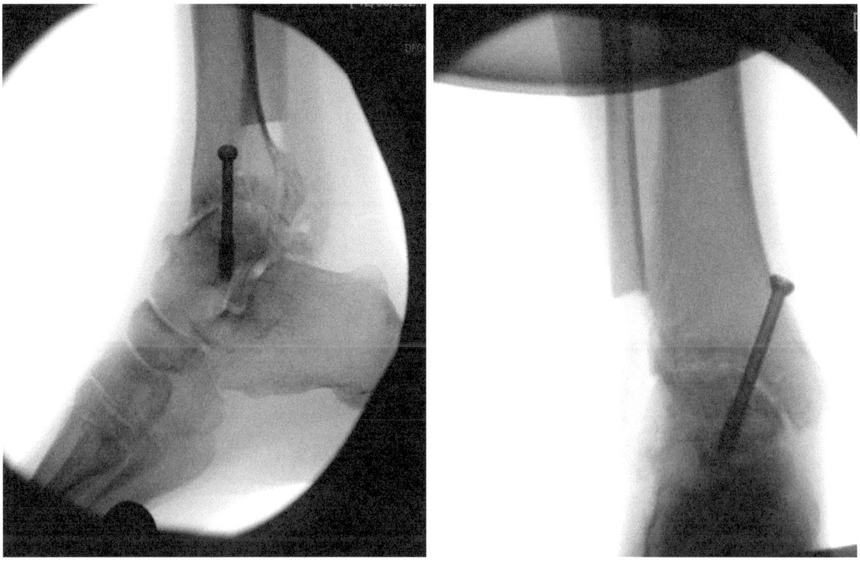

Fig. 6.22 AP & Lateral intraoperative images showing insertion of medial compression screw

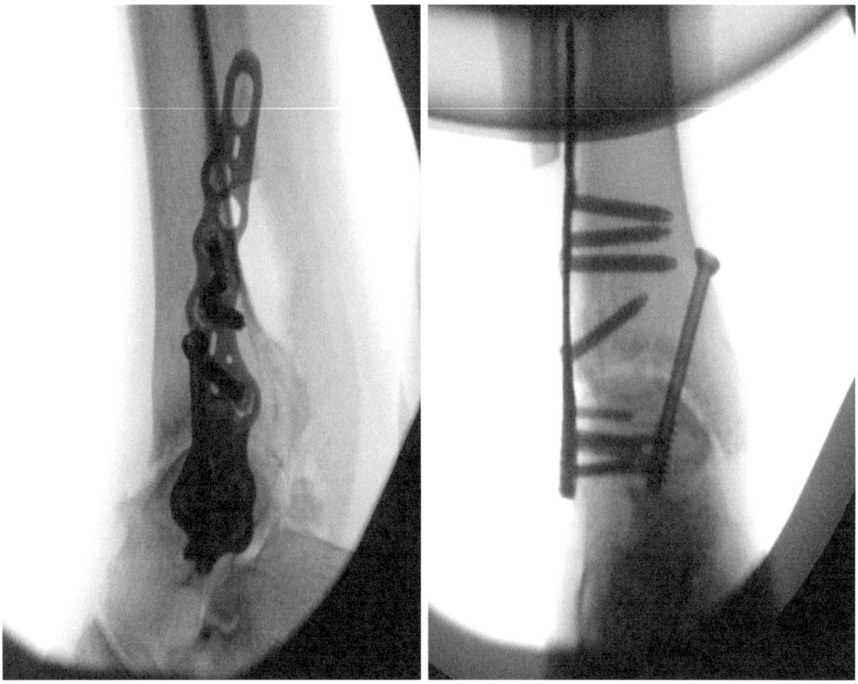

Fig. 6.23 Application of locking plate: AP and lateral intraoperative images

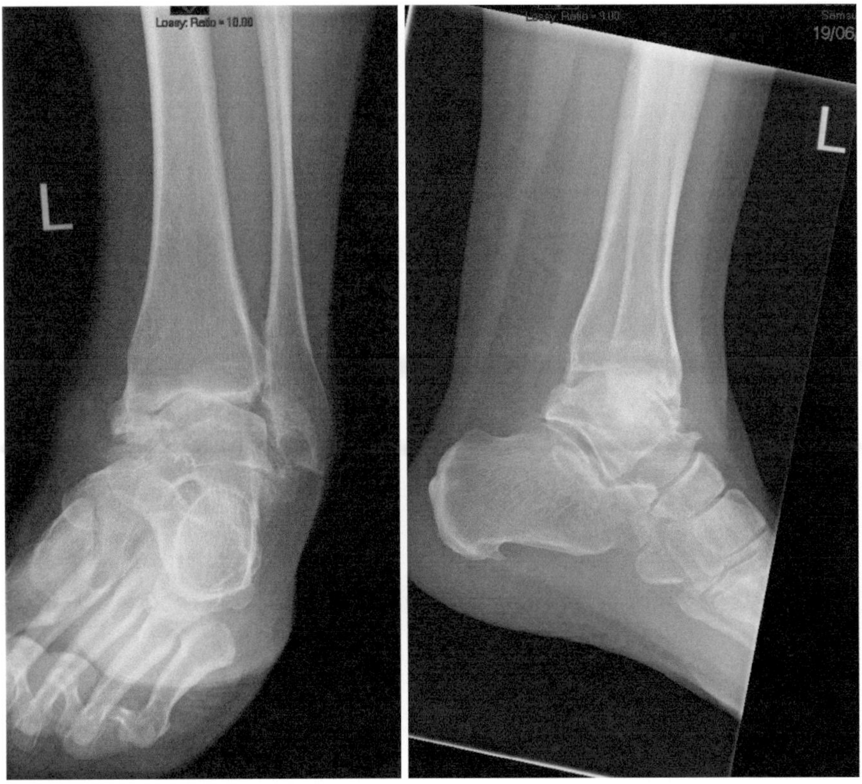

Fig. 6.24 AP and lateral radiographs of a young patient with severe fixed varus deformity with ankle arthritis

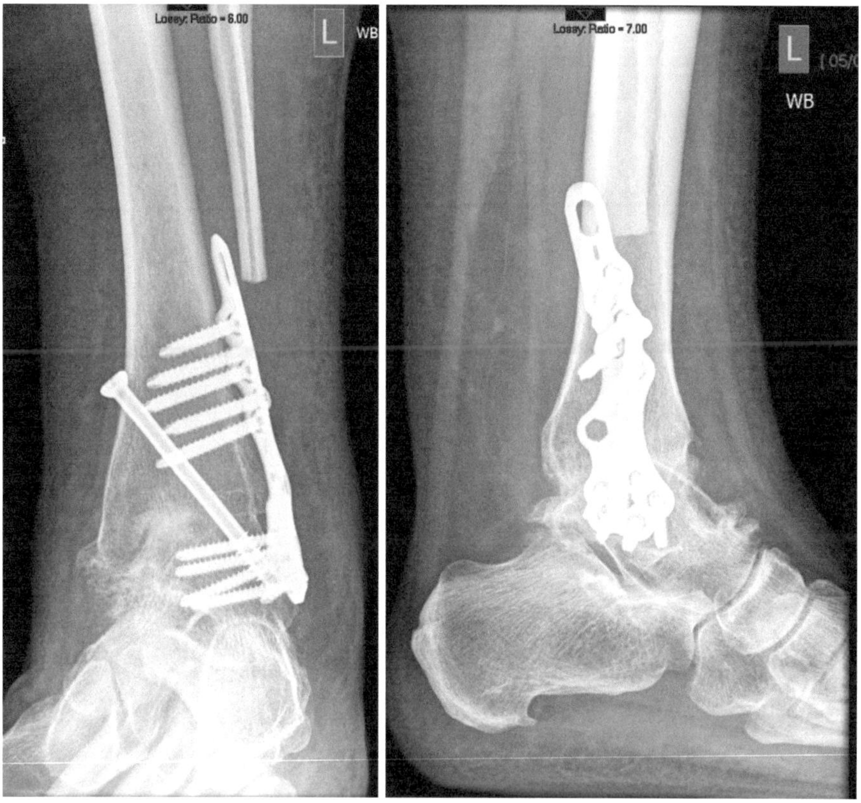

Fig. 6.25 AP and lateral radiographs of the same patient 11 weeks post open ankle fusion using Transfibular approach showing excellent correction of deformity and union

Open Posterior Approach for Tibiotalar Arthrodesis

The open posterior ankle approach is particularly indicated for patients who have sustained nonunion or malunion following a posterior malleolar fracture. It can also be considered primarily as a salvage procedure in cases where the anterior, medial, or lateral soft tissue envelope is compromised due to previous injury or surgical intervention. However, the posterior approach should be avoided in patients with poor vascular supply to the limb or the need for anterior incisions or simultaneous foot surgery, which may compromise healing. An example of posterior ankle fusion following secondary post traumatic arthritis of the ankle and nonunion of posterior malleolar fracture resulting in big bone defect on the posterior aspect of tibia is illustrated in Figs. 6.26, 6.27 and 6.28.

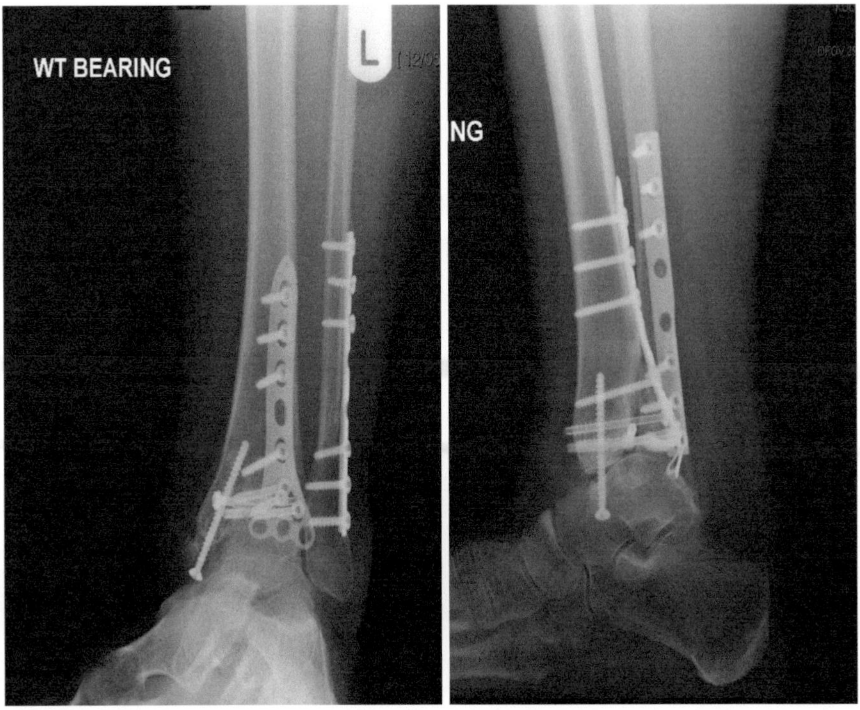

Fig. 6.26 Secondary post traumatic arthritis of ankle and non union of medial and posterior malleoli resulting in big bone defect on the posterior aspect of tibia

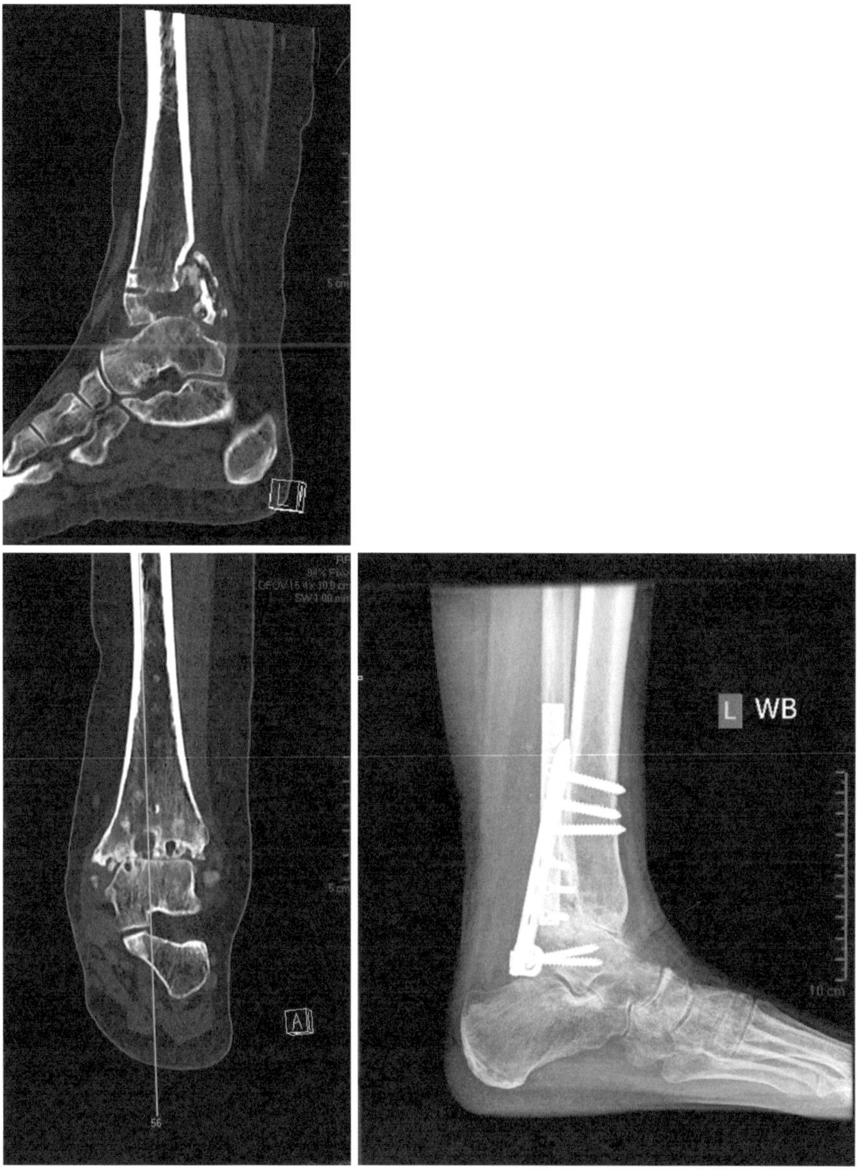

Fig. 6.27 CT scan images before fusion showing posterior malleolus non-union and OA

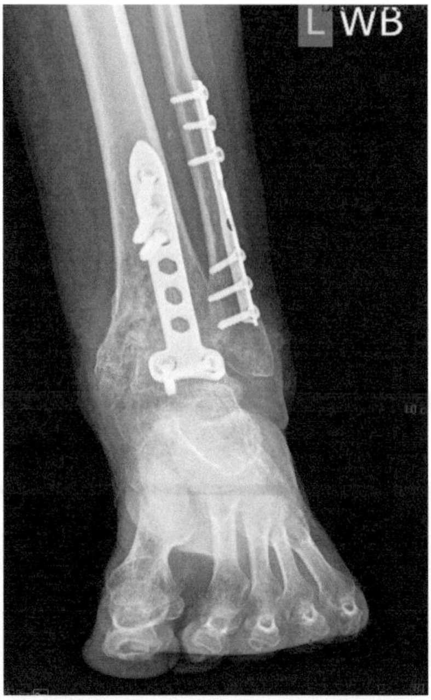

Fig. 6.28 Use of Posterior ankle fusion plate and bone graft resulting in excellent healing of the ankle fusion

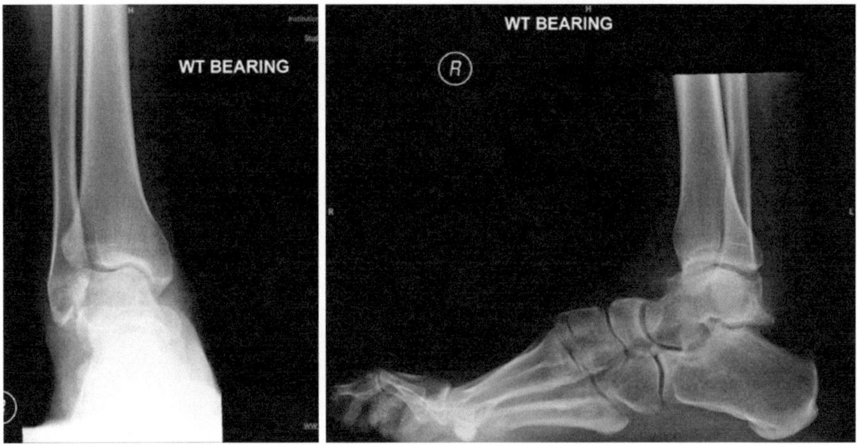

Fig. 6.29 Preoperative radiographs of a case with cavovarus deformity and ankle arthritis

Intramedullary Nail

In certain deformities or clinical conditions, tibiotalocalcaneal (TTC) arthrodesis may be preferred over isolated tibiotalar arthrodesis. In these cases, a retrograde intramedullary nail can be an excellent option due to its load-sharing capabilities, which provide superior biomechanical stability. However, this technique is only appropriate if the surgeon determines that sacrificing the subtalar joint is necessary [9]. An example of such a case is illustrated in Figs. 6.29 and 6.30.

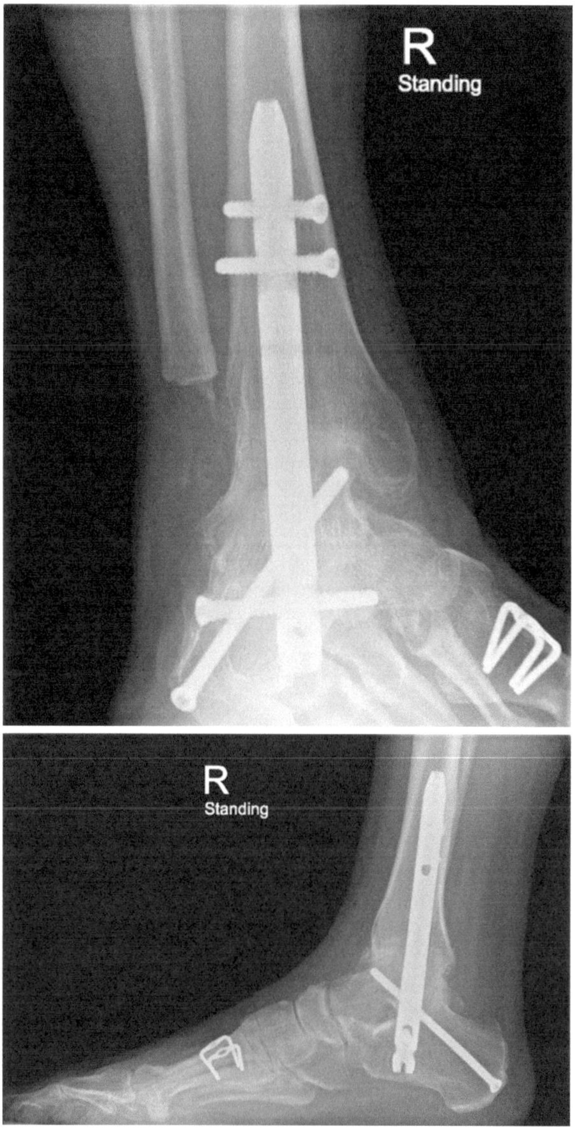

Fig. 6.30 Post operative radiographs of a case with cavovarus deformity and ankle arthritis showing excellent correction of deformity with the use of hindfoot nail and first metatarsal dorsiflexion osteotomy

Conclusion

Ankle arthrodesis remains a reliable treatment for ankle arthritis, particularly in cases with deformity. Arthroscopic ankle arthrodesis can address mild to moderate deformity. However, open technique of fusion is required in severe, fixed deformity. Tibio-talocalcaneal arthrodesis might be considered in cavovarus deformity, charcot joint or significant arthritis of the subtalar joint. Most patients are able to return to good function following successful ankle fusion surgery.

References

1. Bernasconi A. Arthroscopic ankle arthrodesis: a gold standard treatment for advanced painful ankle osteoarthritis. J Ankle Surg. 2017;
2. Jones CR, Wong E, Applegate GR, Ferkel RD. Arthroscopic ankle arthrodesis: a 2-15 year follow-up study. Arthroscopy. 2018;34(5):1641–9.
3. Lorente et al. This systematic review and meta-analysis compared arthroscopic versus open-ankle arthrodesis in patients with ankle osteoarthritis, analyzing fusion rates, operation time, hospital stay length, and overall complications. 2023;
4. Elmlund AO. Indications and contraindications for arthroscopic ankle arthrodesis. Orthop Rev. 2015;2015
5. Adukia V. Posterior ankle arthroscopic fusion: techniques and outcomes. Foot Ankle Surg. 2021;2021
6. van den Heuvel SBM, Doorgakant A, Birnie MFN, Blundell CM, Schepers T. Open ankle arthrodesis: a systematic review of approaches and fixation methods. Foot Ankle Surg. 2021;27(3):339–47. https://doi.org/10.1016/j.fas.2020.12.011.
7. Steginsky BD, Suhling ML, Vora AM. Ankle arthrodesis with anterior plate fixation in patients at high risk for nonunion. Foot Ankle Spec. 2020;13(3):211–8. https://doi.org/10.1177/1938640019846968.
8. Plaass C, Knupp M, Barg A, Hintermann B. Anterior double plating for rigid fixation of isolated tibiotalar arthrodesis. Foot Ankle Int. 2009;30(7):631–9. https://doi.org/10.3113/FAI.2009.0631.
9. Vier D. Fixation strategies and grafting in ankle arthrodesis. J Orthop Tech. 2021;2021

Chapter 7
Ankle Replacement Surgery

T. M. Clough, I. Abdelrahman, and J. Ring

Introduction

Ankle arthritis is a painful musculoskeletal condition, which significantly impacts on mobility and quality of life. Although its incidence is far less common than that of hip and knee arthritis, it is estimated at 30–47 cases per 100,000 population [1, 2]. Patients present with varying degrees of pain, swelling, stiffness, restriction of activity and, occasionally, deformity. Ankle arthritis can be classified based on aetiology: post traumatic, inflammatory or idiopathic [3]. There are a range of non-surgical treatments for ankle arthritis including lifestyle modification, analgesia, orthotics/braces and injections. When these have failed, surgical options include debridement and cheilectomy, osteotomy, arthrodiastasis and, in end stage disease, ankle fusion or ankle replacement. In this chapter we concentrate on ankle replacement surgery.

Fusion Versus Replacement

Ankle fusion has been considered for decades the gold standard treatment for end stage ankle arthritis. It can provide a stable pain free plantigrade hindfoot. The disadvantage of fusion is the loss of all ankle joint movement and the potential overload, particularly long-term, of surrounding joints.

Ankle replacement has the potential advantage over fusion of earlier post operative weight bearing and retaining range of motion, with theoretically better restoration of native ankle biomechanics and gait [4], thereby potentially "protecting"

T. M. Clough (✉) · I. Abdelrahman · J. Ring
Department of Foot & Ankle Surgery, Wrightington Hospital, Wrightington, Lancashire, UK
e-mail: tim.clough@doctors.org.uk; timothy.clough@wwl.nhs.uk; i.abdelrahman@nhs.net; joseph.ring@wwl.nhs.uk

M. Bhatia (ed.), *Surgical Techniques of the Foot and Ankle*,
https://doi.org/10.1007/978-3-031-93742-2_7

surrounding joints from arthrosis by allowing more natural hindfoot movement. This is of particular interest in those patients who have other hindfoot pathology or those having preexisting arthrodesis procedures e.g. subtalar joint fusions. The disadvantage of ankle replacements, as with any artificial joint, is the risk of ongoing pain, failure, wear, loosening and the need for revision [5, 6].

Ankle Anatomy and Biomechanics

The ankle is a diarthrodial capsular synovial joint formed superiorly by tibia/malleoli and inferiorly by talar dome. The stability is provided by three ligamentous complexes. The syndesmosis limits excessive motion between lower ends of tibia and fibula. Medial stability resisting valgus stress is provided by the deltoid ligaments with its superficial and primarily deep components. The lateral stability is provided by the anterior talofibular and calcaneofibular ligaments, which also combine to prevent excessive translation of the talus under the tibia [7].

The key motions of the ankle joint are plantar/dorsiflexion occurring in the sagittal plane, inversion/eversion through the coronal plane and minimal adduction/abduction occurring through the transverse plane. The combination of these motions upon ambulation through the tibiotalar and subtalar joints forms supination/pronation movements. The ankle joint has long been thought to be a simple hinged joint. However, it has a multi axial plane of movement with internal rotation occurring during dorsiflexion and external rotation occurring in plantar flexion. The axis of rotation of the ankle in the coronal plane is a vertical line passing through a central point between malleoli along the long axis of the tibia. In the sagittal plane, the axis of rotation in the sagittal plane is a vertical line along the long axis of the tibia intersecting the midline of the foot [7].

History of Total Ankle Replacement

Over the years, the total ankle replacement has undergone sequential evolution through several generations [8].

The initial designs in the 1970s failed to recreate the biomechanics of the ankle. They relied on large bone resections, cement fixation and poor bearing material. There were problems with alignment, biomechanics, bone stock and bearing failure all combined with poor management of soft tissues and inaccurate surgical placement. Failure rates were high, and outcomes were poor. Despite the poor outcomes of the initial designs, innovations continued, trying to reproduce the success seen in hip and knee arthroplasty.

In the 1980s, there were further attempts to create a durable ankle replacement. Second-generation designs were more successful due to a better understanding of the biomechanics and improvements in biomaterials. These implants fell into two main groups; fixed or mobile bearing. Second-generation designs. Include, but are not limited to, the STAR (Stryker, USA), the Agility (De-Puy, USA) and the Buechel-Pappas (De-Puy, USA).

Innovation in ankle arthroplasty design continued in the 1990s and 2000s with third-generation implants, particularly due to further understanding modes of failure and surgical techniques. This innovation enhanced the success of these third generation designs, which included the Salto (Tornier, France), Hintegra (Integra, France), Ankle Evolution System (AES) (Biomet, Belgium), Bologna-Oxford (BOX) (Finsbury, UK/France) and Mobility (Depuy, UK) and Zenith (Corin, UK). Due to failures, company policy and other factors many of the earlier designs of ankle replacement have been discontinued.

With the introduction of fourth generation designs such as the Infinity (Stryker, USA), which offer jigged, X-ray guided implantation with improved accuracy and reproducibility of implantation [9], outcomes have again improved [10]. There are also now reliable options for revision surgery (Inbone/Invision Stryker, USA) and for patient specific instrumentation (Prophesy Stryker, USA). The success of the modern generation of ankle replacement offers a reliable and reproducible alternative to ankle fusion. There is constant evolution in the world of orthopaedics with ongoing changes to implant design and manufacturing processes, increasing use of standing CT, custom made 3D printed implant and the increasing use of robotic assisted surgery and navigation in other areas of arthroplasty which may play a role in ankle replacement surgery in the future [11].

Patient Selection

As with any surgical procedure, careful patient selection and counselling are key. This is especially true of ankle replacements, where we aim to produce a well-functioning, long lasting implant via a technically demanding operation, which has a narrow margin of error [12].

Careful clinical appraisal of each patient is paramount, including review of their co-morbidities and level of function. Evaluation is made of the entire lower limb axis and presence of other joint pathology e.g. knee arthritis, tibial deformity etc. Alignment and balance of the forefoot, midfoot and hindfoot are reviewed, together with the presence of any other pathology e.g. flatfoot, cavus, Achilles tendinopathy, hindfoot/midfoot arthritis, or other previous joint fusions. Assessment is made of any deformity around the ankle, and its location, severity and correctability. Tightness/laxity of the medial and lateral ankle structures, as well as an assessment of the posterior structures is reviewed. Finally, a careful skin and soft tissue evaluation is key, paying particular attention to any scars, lymphoedema, or changes of chronic venous hypertension.

Indications and Contraindications

The ideal indication for total ankle arthroplasty is end stage ankle arthritis with a reasonable arc of preserved motion, neutral alignment, stable ligaments, good bone stock and a good soft tissue envelope. The indications can be extended to include revision for failed primaries and painful ankle nonunion/malunion.

Absolute contraindications include the presence of active infection, significant talar body avascular necrosis, grossly deformed or unstable ankle which cannot be corrected intra operatively, severe osteoporosis and neuropathic/neuromuscular or poorly vascularized lower limbs [13].

Assessment and Imaging

Preoperative radiological planning is an important step to assess suitability for total ankle replacement, anticipate difficulties and prepare accordingly. Weight bearing plain radiographs are usually the first imaging modality to be ordered to assess for degree of joint and surrounding joint arthritic involvement, bony stock status and alignment. Long leg views can be in use to assess the degree of any femoral or tibial deformities or any malalignment above the ankle. CT and MRI are increasingly used for more information regarding bone quality, cyst assessments, adjacent joint arthritic status and when additional combined soft tissue procedures are planned [14].

Assessment of more complex cases may be aided by using a patient specific instrumentation (PSI), with preoperative CT scanning, which allows templating of the implant for more accurate pre-operative planning [11, 15].

Implant Selection

There are currently 17 ankle replacement implant types historically listed in the UK National Joint Registry (NJR), which has been collecting data on ankle replacements since 2010 [10]. Several of these implants have now been discontinued for a variety of reasons. The choice of implant will depend on many factors, and each may exhibit its own advantages and disadvantages in terms of implantation, function and survival. It is beyond the scope of this chapter to discuss the merits and specifics of individual ankle replacements. Instead we aim to give an overview of the principles of ankle replacement surgery. When selecting any arthroplasty implant we need to look both at NJR data and the general literature, especially results from large, independent non-designer centre series.

Fixed Versus Mobile Bearing

The earlier generations of total ankle replacements were fixed bearing. From around 1996, in the UK and Europe, most designs then moved to mobile bearing systems, in the belief that improving bearing conformity would reduce polyethylene wear, aseptic loosening and thus improve survivorship. However, this did not prove to be the case, and since the introduction of the latest fixed bearing system (Infinity, Stryker) in the UK in 2014, this design now accounts for around 75% of primary TAR implantation in the UK [10].

Intra and Post-operative Care

Ankle replacement surgery is usually performed under a general or spinal/epidural anaesthetic. This can be supplemented with a regional anaesthetic block. Surgery can be performed as a day case in suitable patients [16, 17]. The patient is positioned supine, a pneumatic thigh tourniquet is usually used, and a sandbag is placed under the ipsilateral buttock to keep the front of the ankle facing the ceiling. Supported equipment - diathermy, suction, image intensifier must be carefully positioned within theatre. Surgery is performed in laminar flow, ultra clean orthopaedic theatres. It is the authors practice to use Toga gowns (Stryker) as a standard, and patients receive double skin preparations, with initial skin preparation in the anaesthetic room, and one further preparation in the operating room (Fig. 7.1). It is the authors practice to have X-ray coming in from the same side as the operated limb (Fig. 7.2).

Intravenous antibiotics are given at the start of the procedure, and further doses may be given postoperatively depending on local antibiotic prophylaxis policies. Suitable intra and postoperative thromboprophylaxis should be used again according to local policies this may include compression stockings, intermittent pneumatic compression and oral (eg aspirin, apixaban) or subcutaneous anticoagulants (eg dalteparin, enoxaparin). The choice of this will depend on patient risk factors, surgeon choice, local policies and licensing regulations.

Whichever implant is chosen, and once appropriate joint exposure has been performed, the specific jigs are used to aid alignment and precise cutting and fashioning of the bony cut surface (Figs. 7.3, 7.4, 7.5 and 7.6).

Postoperatively, once the patients' wounds are dressed some surgeons may place the patients into a below knee back slab, whilst others may place them into a walking boot. Depending on surgeons' preference the patient maybe non-weight bearing initially, or allowing to immediately partial or fully weight bear as tolerated. The wounds are usually inspected at 14–21 days, which will vary by surgeon. Once the wounds are healed the patient can begin weight bearing as tolerated in a removable boot and start gentle range of motion including early initial physiotherapy.

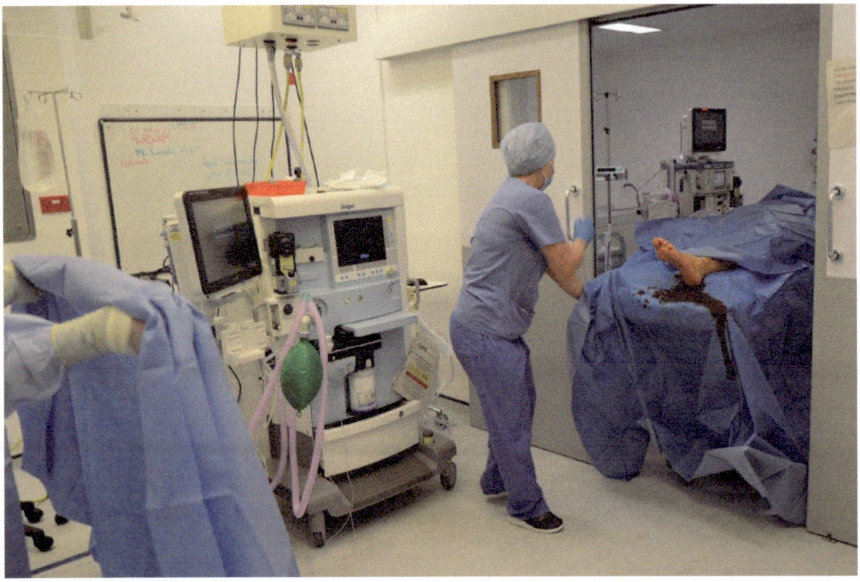

Fig. 7.1 Patient being brought into theatre from the anaesthetic room, pre-positioned and having had initial first sterile skin preparation in the anaesthetic room

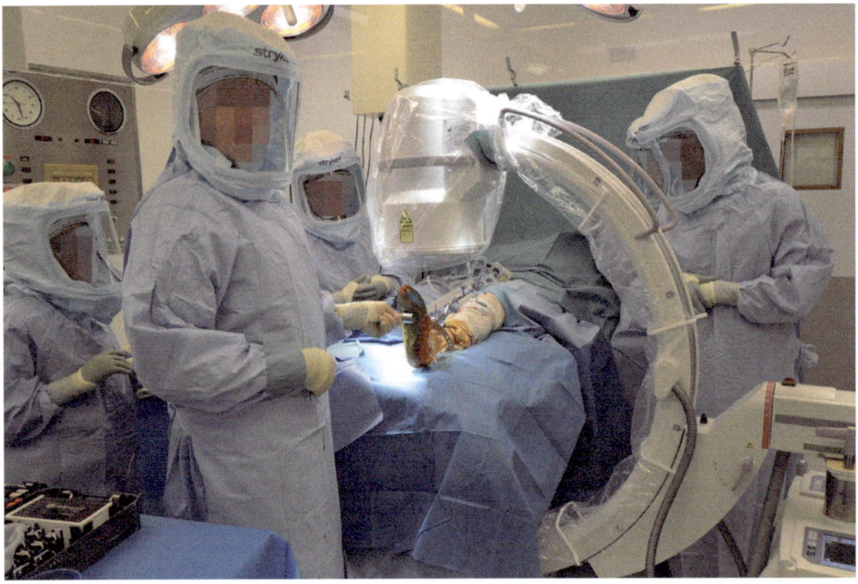

Fig. 7.2 Patient limb exposed. X-ray coming in from the same side as the operated limb. Instruments at the end of the table and on the unoperated side

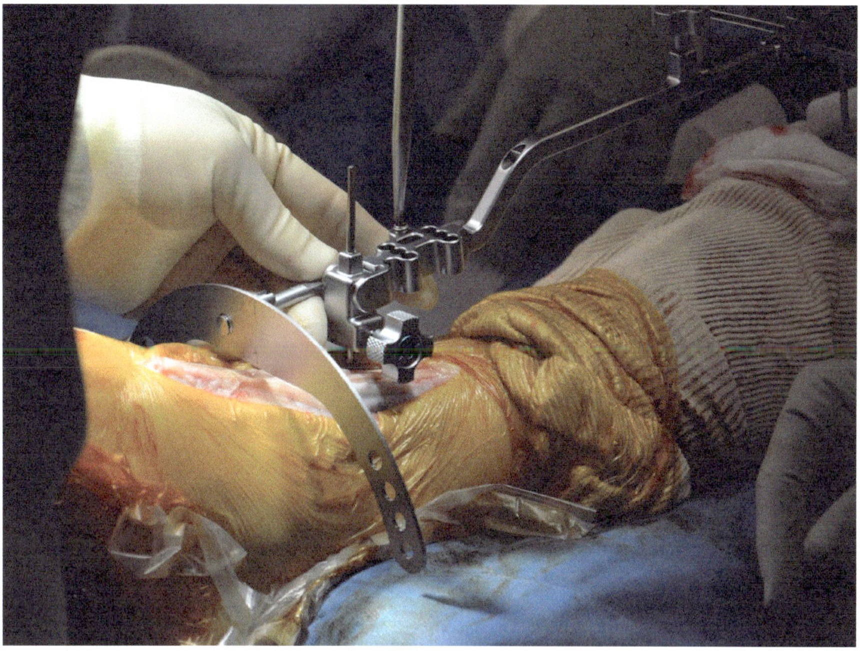

Fig. 7.3 Anterior alignment guide; positioned and checked with X-ray

Most patients will be reviewed regularly, usually seen at 6 weeks when they can start to wean from the boot. Further follow up will vary, but patients are usually seen at 3–6 months and at 12 months. Long term follow-up is recommended, either surgeon led, allied healthcare professional led, or patient led using a patient reported outcomes system. Most patients will be out of a boot by around 6 weeks and can return to light exercise, light work and driving at around this time. Most will start to see a slow early effect but by 6 months they should be feeling the benefits of the procedure.

Approaches

Anterior

The usual approach for ankle replacements is the anterior approach, as it provides excellent visualisation of the whole ankle joint.

A longitudinal skin incision is made over the centre of the ankle in line with the tibial crest and curved slightly medial beyond the ankle crease to avoid iatrogenic injury to the main trunk of the superficial peroneal nerve, which is identified and retracted. Deep fascia is sharply dissected lateral to tibialis anterior tendon, whose

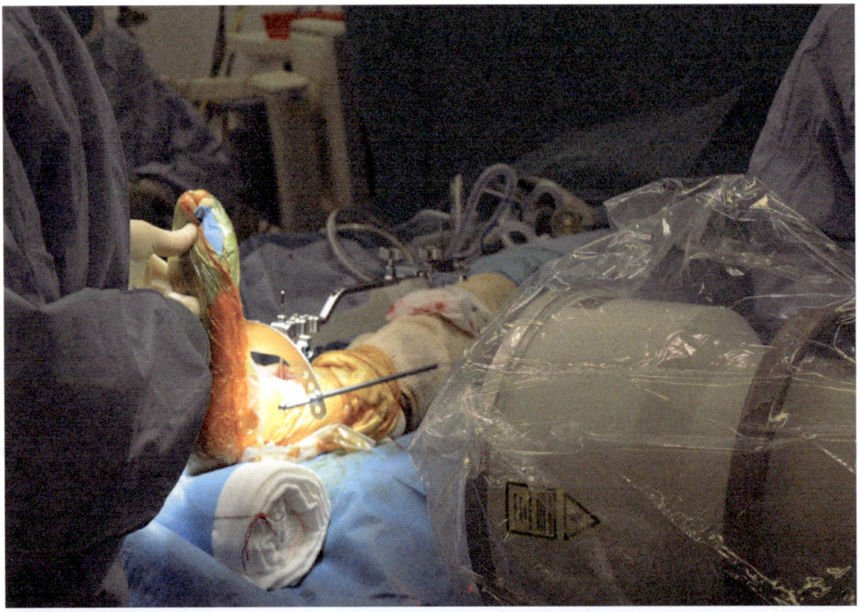

Fig. 7.4 Lateral alignment guide; positioned and checked with X-ray

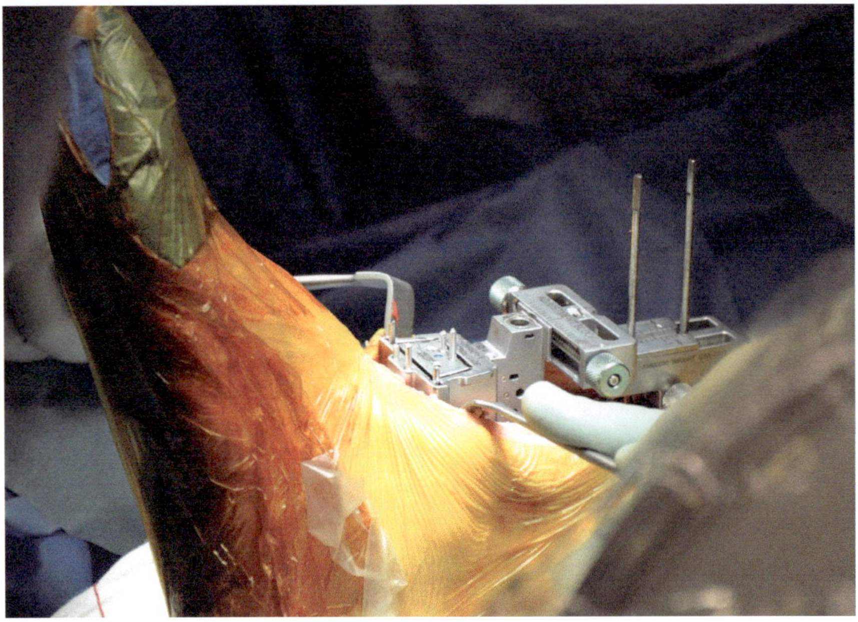

Fig. 7.5 Cutting guide

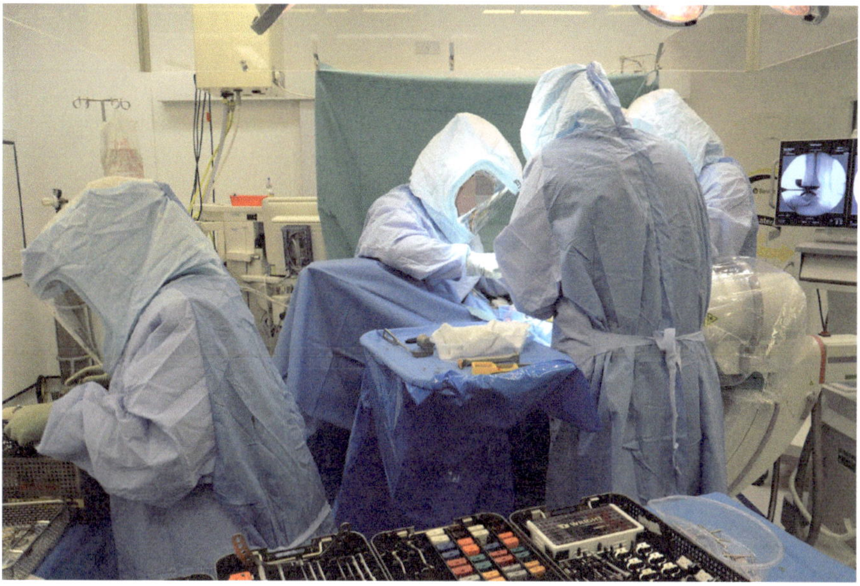

Fig. 7.6 Implant inserted

sheath is kept intact. Extensor hallucis longus tendon is identified for the EHL bed approach. Tibialis anterior tendon is retracted medially and EHL tendon is retracted laterally along with the anterior compartment neurovascular bundle. Crossing venous tributaries overlying the distal tibia periosteum and ankle joint capsule are coagulated using a diathermy. Two Hohmann retractors are placed around both malleoli. The distal tibia periosteum and joint capsule are sharply incised along the skin incision and the joint is visualized. Care must be taken to avoid iatrogenic nerve or tendon injury particularly during distal dissection [18].

Depending on surgeons training, experience implant used and preference the length and exact placement of this approach will vary. The approach needs to allow access to the entire ankle and allow visualisation of both the medial and lateral gutters. Failure to adequately visualise both gutters increases the risk of intraoperative malleolar fracture. The approach should also allow one to see the talonavicular joint at the distal end of the approach. The proximal extension will vary depending on the surgeon's preferences and implant used.

It is important to carefully incise and protect the extensor retinaculum to allow for repair at the end of the procedure, to prevent tendon bowstringing and risk of wound breakdown. Surgeons will vary the exact placement of the retinacular incision around the various tendons to either protect the neurovascular bundle or to keep the major tendons in situ for further wound security.

Lateral Transfibular

For completeness there is the option of a lateral approach for ankle arthroplasty which utilises a standard lateral approach and a fibular osteotomy to access the lateral ankle. This is specific for the Zimmer TM implant (Zimmer, USA) and requires fixation of the fibula upon completion of the arthroplasty using a standard plate and screws osteosynthesis technique.

Balancing the Ankle

The aim of an ankle replacement is to create a pain free, mobile, stable joint with a long lasting well-functioning implant. In order to achieve this the ankle implant must be well aligned to the coronal, sagittal and rotational limb axis, correctly sized, well balanced with stable fixation/integration to the bony interfaces. Additional procedures may need to be performed to achieve this goal.

Additional Procedures

A combined additional procedure with ankle arthroplasty might be needed to address concomitant deformities [19]. Sliding calcaneal osteotomy (open or minimally invasive) can be used to address residual varus or valgus deformity following implantation. Forefoot de-rotation or medial malleolus lengthening osteotomy can be also considered [20]. Additional posterior structures tightness can be addressed with posterior capsular release and Achilles lengthening. Lateral ligament stabilization is indicated for residual gross lateral instability. It is essential, at the end of the surgical procedure, to achieve a well-balanced, functioning prosthetic ankle in order to avoid early failure [21]. The frequency of additional procedures varies between the UK and North America with a large, prospective multicentre UK study reporting an additional procedure rate of 33% [22], whilst North American studies report rates of 70–79% [23, 24].

Surrounding Joint Fusions

If there is coexisting mild-moderate subtalar or talonavicular joint arthritis, this can be a good indication for ankle arthroplasty to potentially protect these joints [25]. However, if there is moderate-severe adjacent joint arthritis, then a combined ankle replacement and neighbouring joint fusion may be indicated. This can be performed at the time of the TAR (in the case of a talonavicular fusion), or, in the case of a subtalar joint fusion, can be performed either sequentially, or at the same time. Consideration must be made regarding approach to protect soft tissues and fixation techniques, to ensure there is no impingement on the implant or metal on metal contact [26].

Patient Specific Instrumentation

Many advances have been made in ankle arthroplasty and, as is the case for other joints, patient specific instrumentation (PSI) has been introduced, to be used in conjunction with certain implants. These involve creating a patient specific preoperative plan and jigs based on a CT scan of the patient ankle. This allows for more accurate planning, sizing and alignment with the potential added benefits of reducing operative steps, operative time and radiation exposure [11, 15]. This system is not available across all implants and companies. In a recent multicentre, prospective UK trial PSI accounted for 20% of the implants used [22]. Its use may increase in the ensuing years. However, currently there is no evidence to suggest it gives either significantly better PROMS postoperative scores, or better survivorship, as compared to non-PSI cases [22, 27].

Complications

As with any surgical procedure there are potential complications with ankle replacement surgery, and these must be discussed fully with the patient as part of an informed consent process. Complications can be minimised through meticulous surgical technique and careful patient selection [28–30]. They include wound healing problems, superficial or deep infection, malleolar fractures (often medial), periprosthetic fractures, aseptic loosening, polyethylene wear or fracture, medial gutter pain, stiffness, neurovascular injury, and thromboembolic complication [29].

Revision Surgery

A revision is defined as any operation where one or more components are added to, removed from, or modified in a joint replacement, or if a Debridement And Implant Retention (DAIR) with or without modular exchange is performed [10]. The indications for revision include aseptic loosening, infection, lysis, wear, malalignment, fracture, stiffness, pain, soft tissue impingement and component dislocation. This is a challenging surgical procedure best performed in a high-volume centre with an established MDT team experienced in both primary ankle replacements and in revision to fusion and arthroplasty.

The choice between revision to fusion or revision replacement would ideally be based through a MDT team discussion involving the patient at every stage, as part of a patient-centred, informed consent process. It depends upon the mode of failure, state of soft tissues, residual bone stock and concurrent deformity, and requires a balanced choice weighing up the surgical technicalities and the chances of long-term success with implant/fusion survival.

Revision to a fusion usually requires a void filler in the form of graft or a metallic cage, with appropriate fixation in the form of a hindfoot nail or fusion plate. Revision to arthroplasty usually requires the use of revision components which have additional stems/screws to stabilise the implant and an ability to accommodate any bone loss. Both surgical procedures are technically challenging, but the evidence supports both as viable options with good outcomes [31, 32].

The most devastating potential complication is that of deep infection. Generally, this is treated using the principles of infected arthroplasty treatment. These include careful multiple microbiology sampling to identify organisms, meticulous debridement after implant removal and usually a 2 staged procedure, with appropriate local and systemic antibiotic treatment between stages, guided by the microbiology results and clinical response [33, 34]. An infected ankle replacement can be revised to a fusion or to a revision arthroplasty depending on the specific clinical picture.

Due to the limited bone stock and thin, soft tissue envelope there is a risk of amputation when deep infection occurs after an ankle arthroplasty. This must be explained to the patient at primary listing and if this complication arises.

Major wound issues are a challenging issue beyond the scope of this chapter, and in some cases may require plastic surgery and, in the worst instances, amputation.

Tips and Tricks

Ankle replacement can be a challenging surgical procedure. In our opinion the key tips and tricks would be: careful patient selection and counselling, appropriate CPD, training in a unit performing a "suitable" volume of ankle replacements and MDT, and ideally centralisation of revision or complex primary procedures, as is best practice for other major joint arthroplasties. Efforts focused on reducing complications are key e.g. infection, tibial nerve injury, wound complication. Good knowledge and training of the operative technique for the implant used in your unit, supported by clear perioperative protocols and pathways when an issue arises after an ankle arthroplasty (eg malleolar fracture, VTE prophylaxis, day care arthroplasty, painful ankle replacements investigation) is vital.

Conclusion

Ankle replacements provide an excellent alternative to fusion in the treatment of end stage ankle arthritis. Like any arthroplasty procedure it requires careful patient selection, meticulous surgical technique and long term follow up. Patients should be counselled regarding the general and specific risks of ankle replacements as part of an informed consent process. We have outlined the need for careful patient selection, the setup and approach for ankle arthroplasty and some of the associated techniques and procedures which may be required to achieve a stable, balanced, mobile and long-lasting replacement.

References

1. Herrera-Perez M, Valderrabano V, Godoy-Santos AL, Netto C, González-Martín D, Tejero S. Ankle arthritis: comprehensive review and treatment algorithm proposal. EFORT Open Rev. 2022;7:448–59. https://doi.org/10.1530/EOR-21-0117.
2. Goldberg AJ, MacGregor A, Dawson J, et al. The demand incidence of symptomatic ankle osteoarthritis presenting to foot & ankle surgeons in the United Kingdom. Foot (Edinb). 2012;22(3):163–6. https://doi.org/10.1016/j.foot.2012.02.005.
3. Valderrabano V, Horisberger M, Russell I, Dougall H, Hintermann B. Etiology of ankle osteoarthritis. Clin Orthop Relat Res. 2009;467(7):1800–6. https://doi.org/10.1007/s11999-008-0543-6. PMID: 18830791; PMCID: PMC2690733.
4. Zygogiannis K, Thivaios GC, Kouramba A, Drakou A, et al. Comparison of post-operative gait parameters after total ankle arthroplasty and ankle fusion: a systematic review. Medicine (Baltimore). 2024;103(27) https://doi.org/10.1097/MD.0000000000038727.
5. Goldberg AJ, Chowdhury K, Bordea E, Blackstone J, Brooking D, Deane EL, Hauptmannova I, Cooke P, Cumbers M, Skene SS, Doré CJ. Total ankle replacement versus ankle arthrodesis for patients aged 50-85 years with end-stage ankle osteoarthritis: the TARVA RCT. Health Technol Assess. 2023;27(5):1–80. https://doi.org/10.3310/PTYJ1146. PMID: 37022932; PMCID: PMC10150410.
6. Li T, Zhao L, Liu Y, et al. Total ankle replacement versus ankle fusion for end-stage ankle arthritis: a meta-analysis. J Orthop Surg. 2024;32(1) https://doi.org/10.1177/10225536241244825.
7. Brockett CL, Chapman GJ. Biomechanics of the ankle. Orthop Trauma. 2016;30(3):232–8. https://doi.org/10.1016/j.mporth.2016.04.015. PMID: 27594929; PMCID: PMC4994968.
8. Gougoulias N, Maffulli N. History of total ankle replacement. Clin Podiatr Med Surg. 2013;30(1):1–20. https://doi.org/10.1016/j.cpm.2012.08.005. Epub 2012 Oct 6. PMID: 23164436.
9. King A, Bali N, Kassam A, Hughes A, Talbot N, Sharpe I. Early outcomes and radiographic alignment of the Infinity total ankle replacement with a minimum of two year follow-up data. Foot Ankle Surg. 2019 Dec;25(6):826–33. https://doi.org/10.1016/j.fas.2018.11.007.
10. No authors listed. UK NJR 21st Annual Report. October 2024. https://reports.njrcentre.org.uk/Portals/0/PDFdownloads/NJR%2021st%20Annual%20Report%202024_Ankles.pdf
11. Berlet GC, Penner MJ, Lancianese S, Stemniski PM, Obert RM. Total ankle arthroplasty accuracy and reproducibility using preoperative CT scan-derived, patient-specific guides. Foot Ankle Int. 2014;35(7):665–76. https://doi.org/10.1177/1071100714531232.
12. der Plaat V, Laurens W, Haverkamp D. Patient selection for total ankle arthroplasty. Orthop Res Rev. 2017:63–73.

13. Barg A, Wimmer MD, Wiewiorski M, Wirtz DC, Pagenstert GI, Valderrabano V. Total ankle replacement. Dtsch Arztebl Int. 2015;112(11):177–84. https://doi.org/10.3238/arztebl.2015.0177. PMID: 25837859; PMCID: PMC4390826.
14. Choi WJ, Kim BS, Lee JW. Preoperative planning and surgical technique: how do I balance my ankle? Foot Ankle Int. 2012;33(3):244–9. https://doi.org/10.3113/FAI.2012.0244.
15. April PM, Locke E, Meulenkamp B. Accuracy of a patient-specific total ankle arthroplasty instrumentation. Foot Ankle Int. 2023;44(11):1150–7.
16. Jain K, Murphy P, Karim T, Karski M, Clough TM. Results of enhanced recovery after primary ankle replacements. Foot (Edinb). 2017;31:13–5. https://doi.org/10.1016/j.foot.2017.01.001.
17. Elbashir M, Uzoigwe C, Kurup H. Day case ankle arthroplasty: are they safe and cost effective? A single-centre case-control study. J Clin Orthop Trauma. 2022;30:101919. https://doi.org/10.1016/j.jcot.2022.101919.
18. Lindsey BB, Hundal R, Bakshi NK, Holmes JR, Talusan PG, Walton DM. Ankle arthrodesis through an anterior approach. J Orthop Trauma. 2020;34(Suppl 2):S42–3. https://doi.org/10.1097/BOT.0000000000001838.
19. Franz AC, Krahenbuhl N, Ruiz R, Susdorf R, Horn-Lang T, Barg A, Hintermann B. Hindfoot balancing in total ankle replacement: the role of supramalleolar osteotomies. Int Orthop. 2020;44(9):1859–67. https://doi.org/10.1007/s00264-020-04681-z.
20. Doets HC, van der Plaat LW, Klein J-P. Medial malleolar osteotomy for the correction of Varus deformity during Total ankle arthroplasty: results in 15 ankles. Foot Ankle Int. 2008;29(2):171–7. https://doi.org/10.3113/FAI.2008.0171.
21. Ryssman DB, Myerson MS. Total ankle arthroplasty: management of Varus deformity at the Ankle. Foot Ankle Int. 2012;33(4):347–54. https://doi.org/10.3113/FAI.2012.0347.
22. Townshend DT, Bing A, Blundell C, Clough T, Davenport J, et al. Two to five-year outcomes of total ankle arthroplasty with the infinity fixed bearing implant a concise follow-up of a previous report. J Bone Joint Surg Am. 2023;105(23):1846–56. https://doi.org/10.2106/JBJS.22.01294.
23. Penner M, Hodges Davis W, Wing K, Bermenderfer T, Waly F, Anderson RB. The infinity Total ankle system: early clinical results with 2- to 4-year follow-up. Foot Ankle Spec. 2018;12(2):159–66. https://doi.org/10.1177/1938640018777601.
24. Nunley JA, Adams SB, Easley ME, DeOrio JK. Prospective randomized trial comparing Mobile-bearing and fixed-bearing total ankle replacement. Foot Ankle Int. 2019;40(11):1239–48. https://doi.org/10.1177/1071100719879680.
25. Dekker TJ, Hamid KS, Easley ME, DeOrio JK, Nunley JA, Adams SB. Ratio of range of motion of the ankle and surrounding joints after total ankle replacement: a radiographic cohort study. J Bone Joint Surg Am. 2017;99(7):576–82. https://doi.org/10.2106/JBJS.16.00606.
26. Kim BS, Knupp M, Zwicky L, Lee JW, Hintermann B. Total ankle replacement in association with hindfoot fusion. J Bone Joint Surg Br. 2010;92-B(11):1540–7. https://doi.org/10.1302/0301-620X.92B11.24452.
27. Yau J, Emmerson B, Kakwani R, Murty AN, Townshend DN. Patient-reported outcomes in total ankle arthroplasty: patient specific versus standard instrumentation. Foot Ankle Spec. 2024;17(1_suppl):30S–7S. https://doi.org/10.1177/19386400231179124.
28. Vale C, Almeida JF, Pereira B, Andrade R, et al. Complications after total ankle arthroplasty – a systematic review. Foot Ankle Surg. 2023;29(1):32–8. https://doi.org/10.1016/j.fas.2022.09.010.
29. Clough TM, Alvi F, Majeed H. Total ankle arthroplasty: what are the risks? Bone Joint J. 2018;100-B(10):1352–8. https://doi.org/10.1302/0301-620X.100B10.BJJ-2018-0180.R1.
30. Clough TM, Ring J. Total ankle arthroplasty. Bone Joint J. 2021;103-B(4):696–703. https://doi.org/10.1302/0301-620X.103B4.BJJ-2020-0758.R1.
31. Jennison T, Sharpe IT, Goldberg AJ. Outcome of conversion to fusion for a failed ankle replacement: a data linkage study using the National Joint Registry and NHS Digital. Foot Ankle Orthop. 2022:7(4). https://doi.org/10.1177/2473011421S00708.

32. Jennison T, Spolton-Dean C, Rottenburg H, Ukoumunne O, Sharpe I, Goldberg A. The outcomes of revision surgery for a failed ankle arthroplasty: a systematic review and meta-analysis. Bone Joint Open. 2022;3(7):596–606. https://doi.org/10.1302/2633-1462.37.BJO-2022-0038.R1.
33. Miner SA, Martucci JA, Brigido SA, DiDomenico L. Time to revision after periprosthetic joint infection in total ankle arthroplasty: a systematic review. J Foot Ankle Surg. 2023;62(1):186–90.
34. McNally M, Sousa R, Wouthuyzen-Bakker M, Chen AF, Soriano A, Vogely HC, Clauss M, Higuera CA, Trebše R. The EBJIS definition of periprosthetic joint infection. Bone Joint J. 2021;103-B(1):18–25. https://doi.org/10.1302/0301-620X.103B1.BJJ-2020-1381.R1.

Chapter 8
Joint Preserving Surgery in the Treatment of Ankle Osteoarthritis

Norman Espinosa and Stephan H. Wirth

Introduction

Osteoarthritis of the ankle joint can cause considerable discomfort for patients and restrict their daily and recreational activities. The aim of conservative and surgical treatments is to reduce or—in the best case—to fully eliminate pain while maintaining or restoring normal function of the ankle joint. In order to understand the therapeutic strategies correctly, it is necessary to briefly illustrate the etiological aspects and pathomechanisms that allow osteoarthritis to be divided into specific categories.

Etiologies

While knee and hip arthrosis is mainly caused by primary arthrosis, trauma-related causes play a major role in the development of ankle arthrosis. In the literature (considering both global and asymmetric osteoarthritis of the ankle joint), up to 70% of all ankle osteoarthritis cases are attributed to trauma [1, 2]. Statistically, 179/100,00 patients can be classified for the fractures [3] and in chronic instabilities 3.3/100,000 patients are identified who will then suffer from ankle osteoarthritis. [4]. For these reasons, osteoarthritis of the upper ankle joint becomes symptomatic 12–15 years earlier than osteoarthritis of the hip or knee joints.

N. Espinosa (✉)
FussInstitut Zurich AG, Institute for Foot and Ankle Reconstruction Zurich, Zurich, Switzerland
e-mail: espinosa@hin.ch

S. H. Wirth
Department of Orthopaedics, Uniklinik Balgrist, University of Zurich, Zurich, Switzerland
e-mail: stephan.wirth@balgrist.ch

M. Bhatia (ed.), *Surgical Techniques of the Foot and Ankle*,
https://doi.org/10.1007/978-3-031-93742-2_8

Pathomechanisms

The exact mechanisms of why trauma leads to ankle osteoarthritis are not yet fully understood. For high-energy trauma this is most easily explained: In addition to osseous destruction, the impact of the force also has a fatal effect on the cartilage tissue structure [5].

In contrast, the development of ankle osteoarthritis in low-energy trauma is more difficult to define. Nevertheless, residual malalignment, inadequate reduction of fractures or untreated or incorrectly treated ligamentous injuries, lead to altered force distributions within the ankle joint and thus to abnormal overloading of the articular cartilage, which in turn results in premature wear [6]. In this context, it should also be noted that local, persistent inflammatory processes in the ankle joint may play a role in maintaining or even accelerating these processes [7].

For this chapter, it is important to understand that it should be differentiated between global and asymmetric ankle osteoarthritis. While for global osteoarthritis, i.e. degeneration affecting the entire ankle joint, only arthrodesis or total ankle arthroplasty could be considered as therapeutic options, a completely new, joint-preserving treatment field opens up for so-called asymmetric ankle osteoarthritis.

Approximately two-thirds of patients with ankle osteoarthritis display an asymmetrical wear pattern [8]. However, as part of the kinematic chain, the transfer of forces through the hindfoot is not solely influenced by the ankle joint, but is also modulated by the functions of the adjacent joints (subtalar joint, tarsus) as well as muscles, tendons and ligaments.

The primary aim of joint-preserving surgery on the ankle joint is to preserve joint structure and function in the mid- to long term by surgically induced redirection of forces across the tibiotalar joint. In other words, the arthritic part of the joint will be relieved and the remaining, healthy zone in the joint becomes more loaded.

This chapter deals with the topic of joint-preserving surgery in the context of asymmetric ankle osteoarthritis and provides a step-by-step algorithm on how to manage those patients.

Types of Asymmetric Osteoarthritis

For the typification of asymmetric ankle arthrosis, it is advisable to think in all three dimensions. This results in the following patterns:

1. Misalignment of the ankle joint in the frontal plane [9, 10]

   Varus and valgus deformities

   (a) Local osteoarthritis of the medial talus dome and/or distal tibial plafond
   (b) Local arthritis on the lateral talus dome and/or distal tibial plafond

2. Misalignment of the tibia in the sagittal plane [11, 12]

   Extension: Subluxation of the talus ventrally, severe damage
   Flexion: Anterior

(a) Local osteoarthritis of the posterior talus and/or distal tibial plafond
(b) Localized osteoarthritis of the anterior talus and/or distal tibial plafond

3. Misalignments in the transverse plane: [13]

   External and internal rotation malpositions

   (a) Local osteoarthritis diagonal anteromedial—posterolateral
   (b) Local arthrosis diagonal anterolateral—posteromedial

4. Misalignments in two or all three planes.

Note: It is advisable to differentiate between congruent and incongruent deformities, as these forms might be addressed by either a dome or wedge osteotomy (Figs. 8.1a and 8.1b).

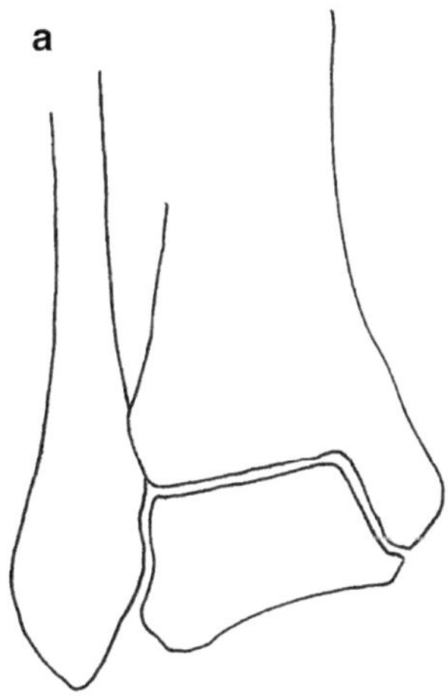

Fig. 8.1a Illustrated is a congruent varus ankle deformity

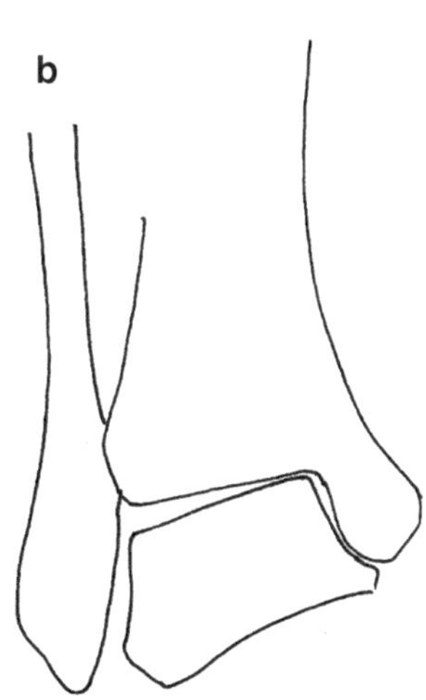

Fig. 8.1b Illustrated is an incongruent varus ankle deformity. Please note the tilting of the talus

General Indications and Contraindications

Indications:

Asymmetric valgus or varus arthrosis of the ankle joint
At least 50% of the joint surfaces remain intact.

Relative contraindications:

Age more than 70 years (individual, biological factors)
Hindfoot instabilities (can stabilization be achieved?)

Absolute contraindications

Severe instability of the hindfoot that can no longer be improved surgically
Severe vascular impairment
Severe neurological impairment
Inflammatory diseases
Infections
Neuroarthropathy

Imaging Required for Planning

The following images are required for correct planning of a correction:

1. Conventional radiographs: [14]
   (a) Anterior-posterior view of the ankle joint (ap)

       Medial, distal tibial articular surface angle (⟨)
       Medial distal tibio-talar angle (®)
       Incongruence: ®-⟨ >4° [8]

   (b) Hindfoot view (hindfoot alignment view or long-axial view) [15–17]

       Varus or valgus malalignment
       Long-axial view is more reliable, i.e. less susceptible, to rotation errors

   (c) Foot in 3 perspectives: dorsoplantar (dp), lateral, oblique [18]

       Subluxations of the talus in relation to the tibia
       Malpositions of the distal tibia

2. Full leg radiographs
   Determination of the anatomical and mechanical axes on the leg. Analysis of the hip and knee joint configurations with regard to hindfoot situation.

   These images are used to determine the so-called "Center of Rotation of Angulation" (CORA) [19, 20]. This corresponds to the apex of the deformity, if there is one. The CORA serves as a target for correction. The images also provide information on the extent of the osteoarthritis and any instabilities present.

3. CT and MR images:
   The CT and MR images are sensitive in detecting osteochondral lesions, as well as determining the ligamentous conditions.
   In recent years, weight-bearing CT scans of the hindfoot have emerged to help better understand the deformity in three dimensions [21]. Especially when it comes to the assessment of inframalleolar deformities and their correction [22–24].
   Fine-slice CT scans are used for condensed data collection of the hindfoot conditions, e.g. when virtual planning of corrective osteotomies is being considered.
4. SPECT-CT images:
   This method combines the high resolution of spiral CT with the high sensitivity of bone scintigraphy and helps to detect mechanically overloaded joint areas [25, 26].

Considerations on Osteotomy Techniques

Effects of the Types

In most cases, the CORA is found very close to or even at the level of the ankle joint (Fig. 8.1c). If a proximal wedge osteotomy (especially in cases with tilt of the talus, i.e. incongruent variant) is considered, this leads to translation of the distal fragment medially (valgus deformity) or laterally (varus deformity) (Figs. 8.1d and 8.1e). This means that a lateral overload would persist in the valgus case and a medial overload in the varus case. For this reason, a corrective translation to the lateral (in valgus deformity) or medial (in varus deformity) should be considered [11].

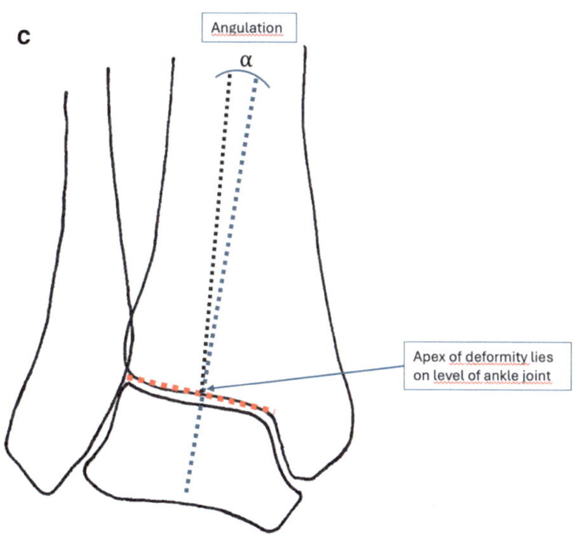

Fig. 8.1c The figure shows a valgus ankle deformity. The apex of the deformity falls onto the joint line. The angulation depicted is given by the intersection of the anatomical tibia axis and the perpendicular line through the center of the talar dome

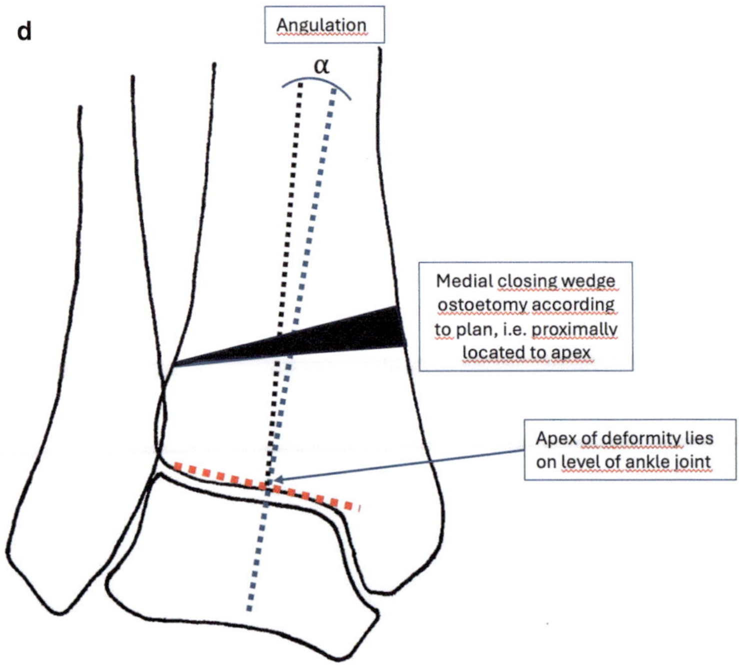

Fig. 8.1d The figure represents a medial closing wedge osteotomy performed proximal to the apex (which is located at level of the joint line). The black wedge will be removed

Fig. 8.1e The image shows the result of the osteotomy as shown in Fig. 8.1d. Because the osteotomy has been chosen proximal to the joint line the center of the talus is moved medially. In such a case either a lateral translation could be an option or better—a dome osteotomy

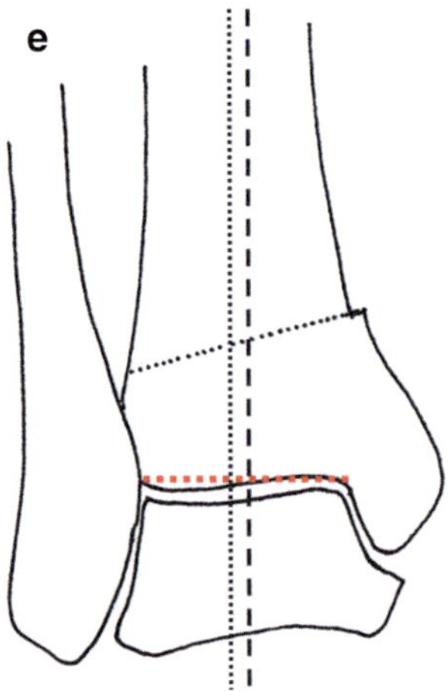

In patients with a CORA at the joint level itself and with a congruent deformity a spherical or dome-osteotomy is indicated (Figs. 8.2a and 8.2b).

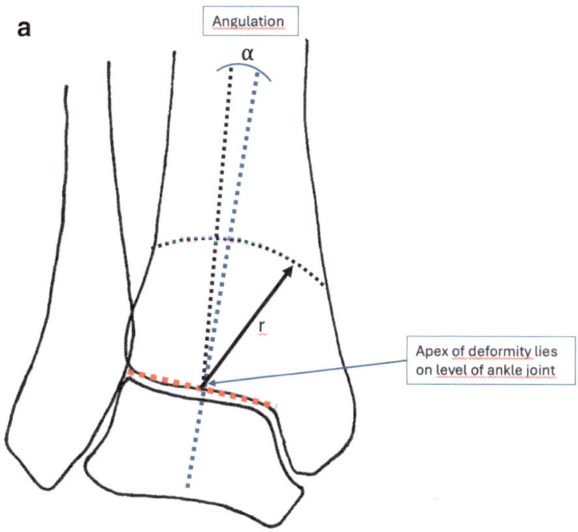

Fig. 8.2a In congruent deformities +/− apex of deformity located at level of joint level a dome osteotomy is preferred

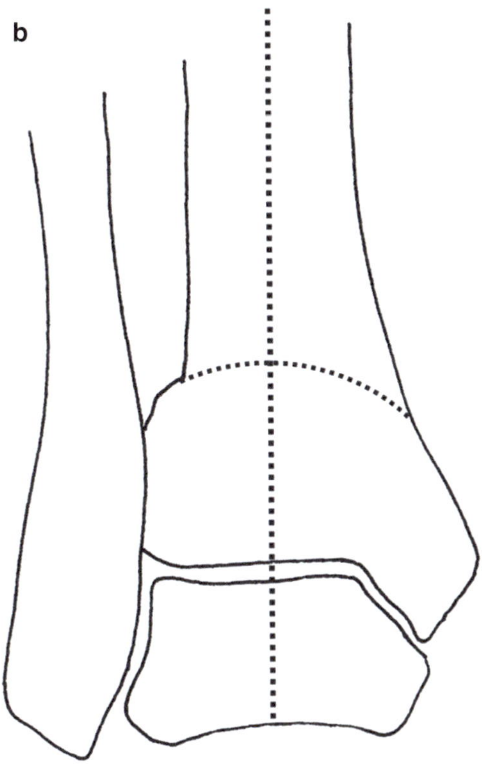

Fig. 8.2b The result after a dome osteotomy. The center of the talus runs directly through the anatomical axis of the tibia

The Role of the Fibula

The influence of the fibula is central and must always be taken into account in corrective osteotomies. A simple rule states: "The talus always follows the fibula".

If the correction has not yet been fully achieved with a medial-opening wedge osteotomy of the distal tibia, a shortening fibula osteotomy could be considered.

If the correction is not yet complete after a medial-closing wedge osteotomy of the distal tibia, a lengthening fibula osteotomy might be considered.

Although there still exists a controversy about additional fibular osteotomies [27] the authors reveal a liberal use of them during supramalleolar osteotomies. The aim is always to adjust the joint congruently in order to achieve reliable changes in intra-articular force transmission in the upper ankle joint [28].

Planning the Extent the Correction

Proper planning is essential in order to obtain the best correction. Surgeons should be aware of the geometric impact of their bony corrections. For this purpose a trigonometric approach can be helpful to calculate the needed amount of correction. Besides determination of the CORA it is also important to know how wide the base of the bony wedge will be.

The following formula can be used: [6].

$$H = \tan \langle\, ^{*}\, W$$

H = Base width of the bone wedge to be removed or inserted
$\langle$ = angle of the deformity + the amount of overcorrection desired
W = width of the tibia along the osteotomy line (in millimeters)

Note: Overcorrection means approx. +2° up to + 4°.

Figure 8.2c depicts the reference angles, which should at least serve as means to correct a deformity back to normal and Fig. 8.2d illustrates the analysis of how to proceed the planning.

Surgical Techniques

Malalignments above ankle joint (Fig. 8.3a)
Asymmetric varus ankle arthrosis

Medial-opening-wedge tibial osteotomy [29]
Indications:

- Incongruent varus malalignment, i.e. talar tilt in the ankle joint ($<10^\circ$ varus)

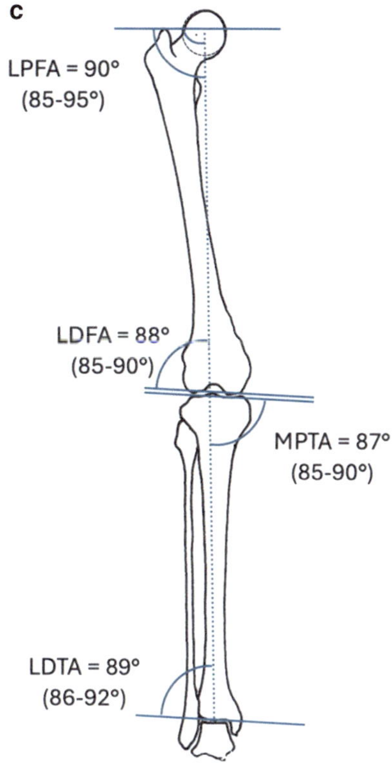

Fig. 8.2c The image shows the reference angles of the lower extremity: LPFA: Lateral proximal femoral angle; LDFA: Lateral distal femoral angle; MPTA: Medial proximal tibial angle; LDTA: Lateral distal tibial angle

Target:

- Slight overcorrection, i.e. 2° - 4° valgus of the tibial surface angle.
- After determining the CORA, the osteotomy is planned so that the anatomical tibial axis passes through the center of the upper ankle joint, or slightly lateral to it.

Advantages:

- Maintains lower-limb length
- Allows multiplanar corrections.

Disadvantages:

- Requires an allograft or autograft to fill the osteotomy
- Risk of nonunion
- Potential risk of neurovascular lesions

Note:

If the CORA falls on the joint line or very close to it, a dome osteotomy should rather be considered. If this is not possible or desired, the translation should be performed medially.

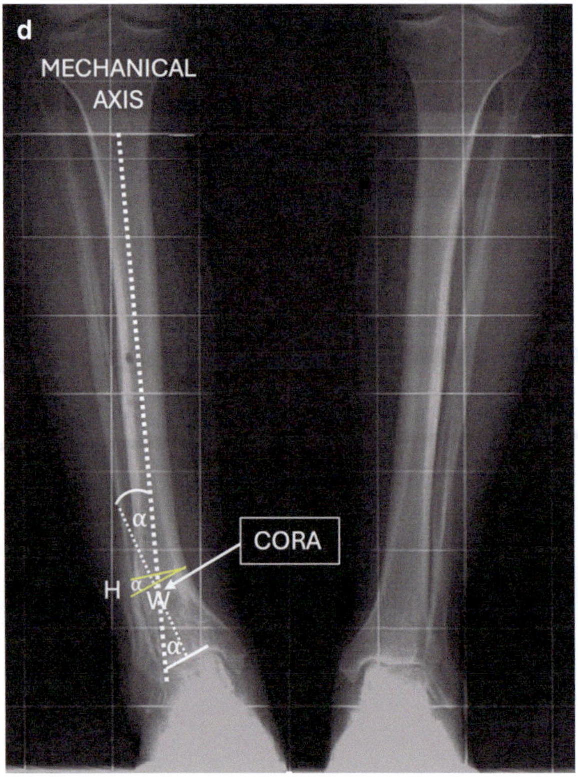

Fig. 8.2d The figure shows how the center of rotation of rotation of angulation (CORA) is defined. First the mechanical axis or the anatomical axis of the tibia (more or less the same in the tibia) is outlined. Second a perpendicular line is created running through the center of the tibial plafond. The intersection of both lines provides the CORA and the angle ⟨, which defines the amount of correction needed to adjust both lines. H: Height of base of wede; W: width of wedge along tibia at level of CORA (parallel to tibial plafond)

Tips and tricks:

In the case of an anterior subluxation of the talus, an anteromedial distraction can be applied during the medial opening tibial osteotomy. This allows the anatomical axis to be realigned with the center of rotation of the talus, thus achieving sagittal correction as well as frontal correction.

An additional fibula osteotomy should be considered for deformities over 10°.

Technique:

- The patient is positioned supine. The knee can be held slightly bent with the sandbag under the ipsilateral calf.
- The incision is made centrally over the medial malleolus
- The length of the incision averages approx. 7–10 cm
- This is followed by meticulous subcutaneous preparation and protection of the great saphenous vein and the saphenous nerve

Note: The two structures often run anterior to the incision (Fig. 8.3b)**.**

- Deep dissection until the periosteum of the medial tibia is reached
- Insertion of a Hohmann retractor anteriorly and posteriorly

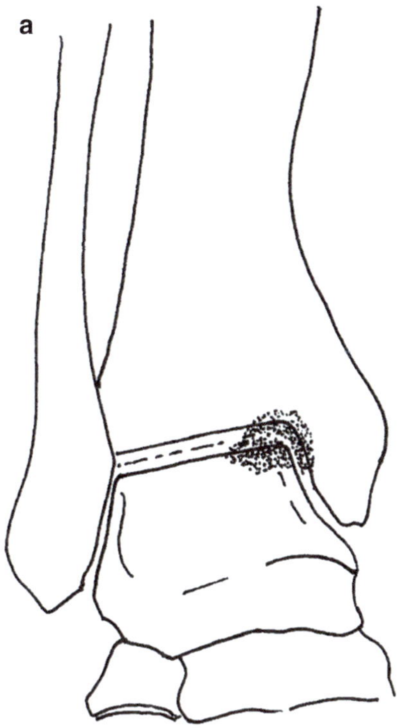

Fig. 8.3a Schematic drawing of an arthritic ankle joint. Please note: in this varus ankle the degenerative part of the joint is located medially

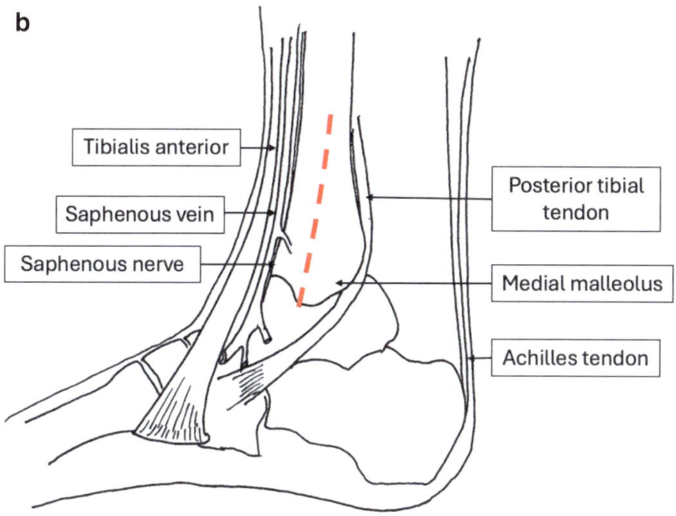

Fig. 8.3b Depicted are the anatomical relations between bones and soft-tissues. The red dotted line indicates the site of skin incision

- The proximal part of the posterior tibial tendon sheath must quite often be slightly incised so that the soft tissues can be folded posteriorly
- The authors now use an 8 mm Hohmann retractor anteriorly and a larger Hohmann-retractor posteriorly (wider hook, for better protection of the neurovascular, posteromedial bundle as well as the tendon structures)
- Once these steps have been completed, the tibia should be fully exposed
- A K-wire is placed under fluoroscopic control and inserted at the site of the osteotomy as preoperatively planned
- An oscillating saw is used to perform the osteotomy, which should remain incomplete (i.e. the lateral cortex of the tibia should not break)
- In addition to extensive irrigation, this always requires radiological control of the osteotomy depth
- You can manually check whether the osteotomy is moving or not
- A 15 mm osteotome is now inserted, which is carefully driven in from medial to lateral
- Two 10 mm osteotomes are inserted proximally and distally to the 15 mm osteotome, allowing the osteotomy to be opened in the gap
- Removal of the osteotomes and change to a laminar or—even better—Hintermann spreader
- The tibia is spread open until the calculated height of the wedge (reference at the medial cortex) is reached
- A prefabricated allogenic or autologous bone block is then inserted into the osteotomy
- The construct is fixed medially with a plate and thus secured (Fig. 8.3c).

At the end of this procedure, it must be checked whether the correction alone is sufficient or whether an additional fibular osteotomy is necessary.

Lateral Closing-Wedge Osteotomy [30]

Indications:

Incongruent varus malalignment, i.e. talar tilt in the ankle joint (>10° varus)

Target:

Slight overcorrection, i.e. 2° - 4° valgus of the tibial surface angle.

Advantages:

- Little influence on limb length
- Allows multiplanar corrections
- No bone graft necessary

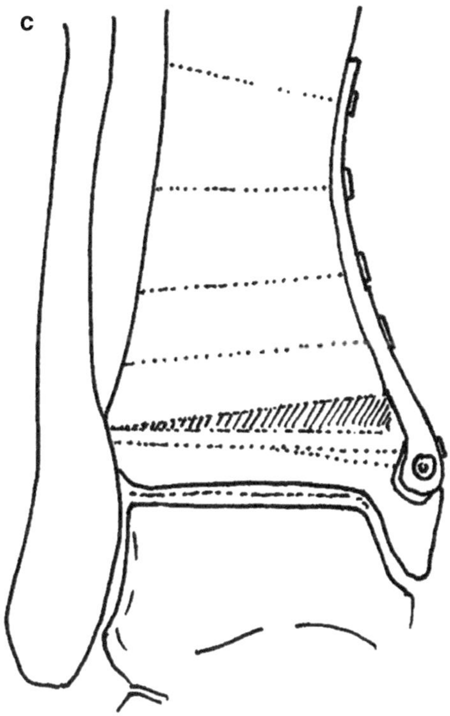

Fig. 8.3c The schematic drawing shows the result of the medial opening-wedge osteotomy. A plate has been put medially to secure the osteotomy. The gap, resulting from the osteotomy can be filled either be auto- or allograft

Disadvantages:

- Risk of medial cortex fracture is higher the larger the bony wedge is
- Preparation somewhat more complex than with medial-opening wedge osteotomy

Note:

If the CORA falls on the joint line or very close to it, a dome osteotomy should be used. If this is not possible or desirable, an additional medial translation should be performed.

Tips and tricks:

The superficial peroneal nerve perforates the intermuscular septum approx. 6–7 cm proximal to the tip of the fibula. This should always be taken into account when planning the approach

Technique:

- The patient is positioned in lateral decubitus with a tunnel cushion between the legs (Fig. 8.4a)
- The incision follows the dorsal edge of the fibula (Fig. 8.4b)
- The length of the incision averages approx. 10 cm
- This is followed by subcutaneous preparation

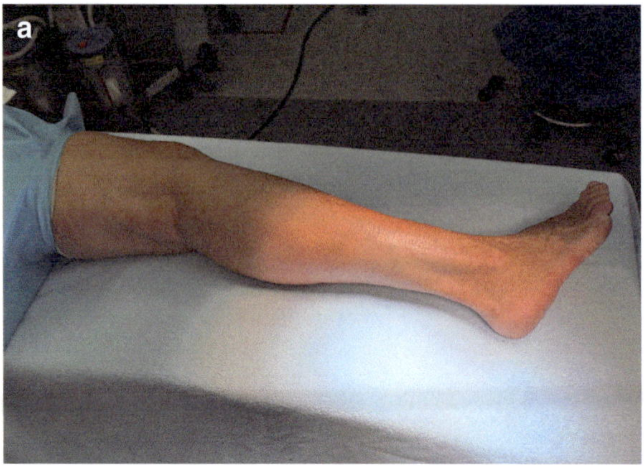

Fig. 8.4a The image depicts the positioning of the leg. The patient is placed on a lateral decubitus position

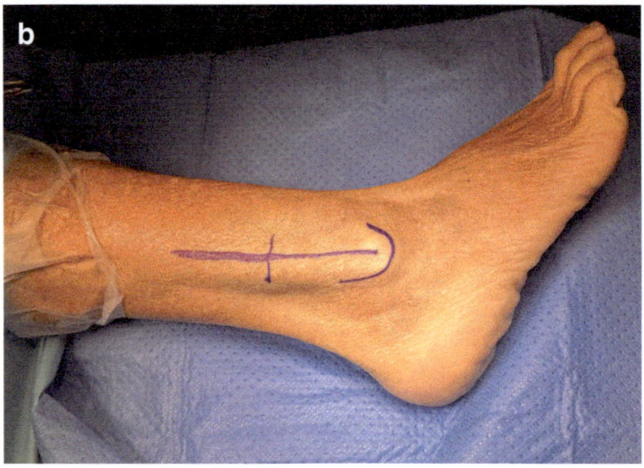

Fig. 8.4b The incision is marked on the lateral aspect of the fibula. The short line running perpendicular to the skin incision mark represents the level of the preoperatively planned osteotomy level

- Deep dissection is done until the periosteum of the fibula (*) is reached (Fig. 8.4c)
- The periosteum is spared
- The interosseous membrane is exposed ventrally with a raspatory
- The perforating vessels are spared during this process
- Next, the anterior soft tissues are lifted off the fibula (F) and a Hohmann retractor is inserted over the anterior part of the tibia (T) (Fig. 8.4d)
- Incision of the peroneal fascia along the posterolateral edge of the fibula
- The peroneal tendons and muscles are held away posteriorly with a Langenbeck hook
- The final detachment of the peroneal soft tissue is performed with a raspatory (Fig. 8.4e)
- The muscle belly of the flexor hallucis longus now becomes visible
- The fascia over the flexor hallucis longus is carefully split, which is done at the posterior edge of the fibula

Fig. 8.4c After the skin incision is done the fibula (asterix) is reached

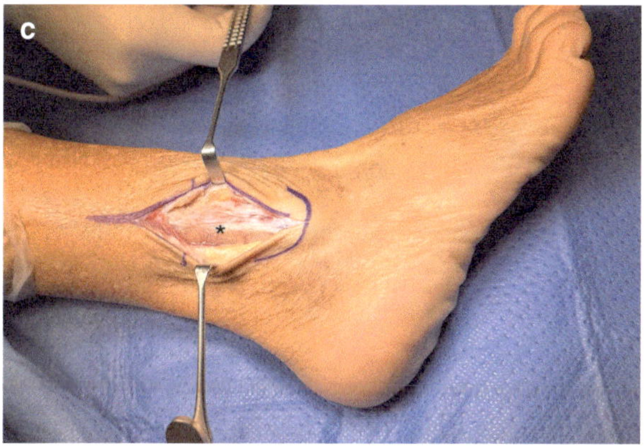

Fig. 8.4d Careful preparation is done. The soft-tissues are lift-off the fibula (F) and then - by help of a raspatory - the tibia (T). A small Hohmann-retractor is inserted anteriorly to the tibia to facilitate soft-tissue preparation

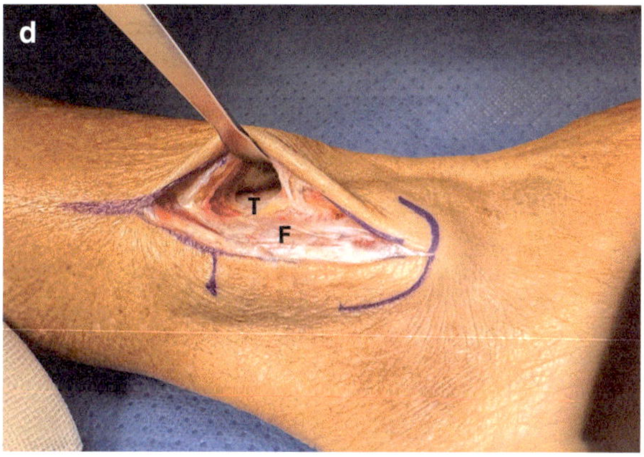

Fig. 8.4e On the posterior aspect a blunt raspatory is used to follow the back of the fibula and running over the dorsal aspect of the interosseus membrane until reaching the posterior wall of the tibia

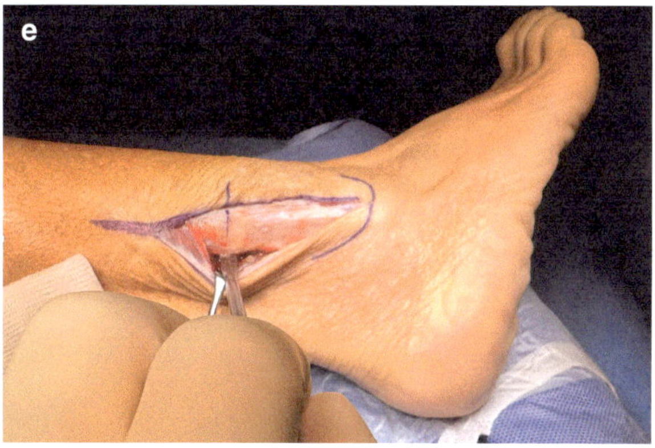

Note: The peroneal vessels should be left intact!

- The muscle fibers that originate from the fibula are sharply detached and then—by help of a an elevator—the soft tissues are bluntly elevated from the interosseous membrane and posterior tibia
- This creates a tunnel of approx. 2–3 cm in diameter
- A wide Hohmann retractor is placed into that tunnel so that it bypasses the entire posterior tibia and thus provides maximum protection for the soft tissue (Fig. 8.4f)
- A K-wire is now inserted approximately 3–5 cm proximal to the joint line (Fig. 8.4g)
- A second K-wire is inserted and the previously calculated width of the base at the fibula is marked with a monopolar cautery (Fig. 8.4h)
- The K-wires must be advanced to the medial side, without perforating the medial cortex (Fig. 8.4i)
- Both wires should cross or meet slightly lateral to the medial cortex
- The depth of the osteotomy is measured on the K-wire (Fig. 8.4j)

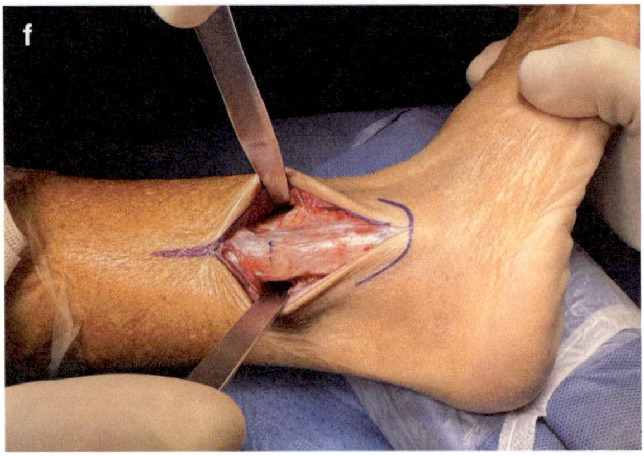

Fig. 8.4f Once the soft-tissues have been lift-off the anterior and posterior aspects of the fibula and tibia, a wide Hohmann retractor is inserted anteriorly and an Eva-hook posteriorly. Thus, the tibia and fibula become fully exposed while the neurovascular structures remain protected

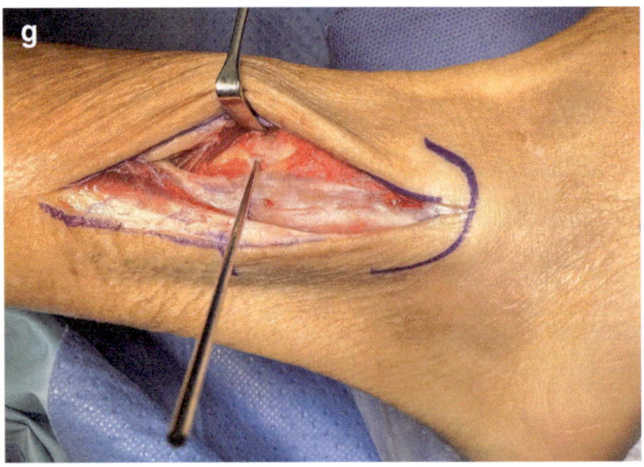

Fig. 8.4g A K-wire is inserted according to the preoperative planning and at the osteotomy-level. Fluoroscopy helps to check the level

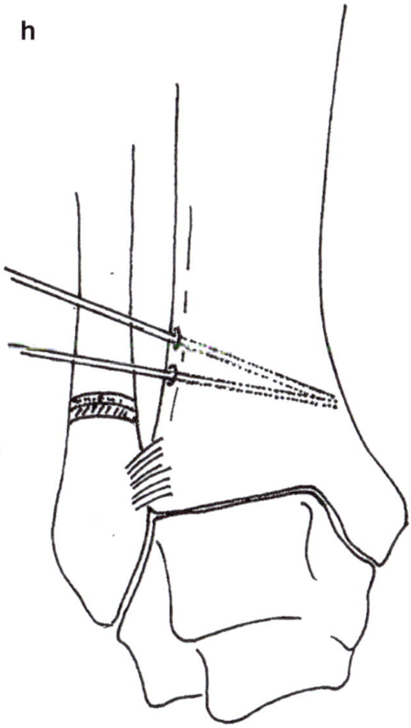

Fig. 8.4h The schematic drawing illustrates how both K-wires should be inserted. The authors enter both K-wires anterior to the fibula

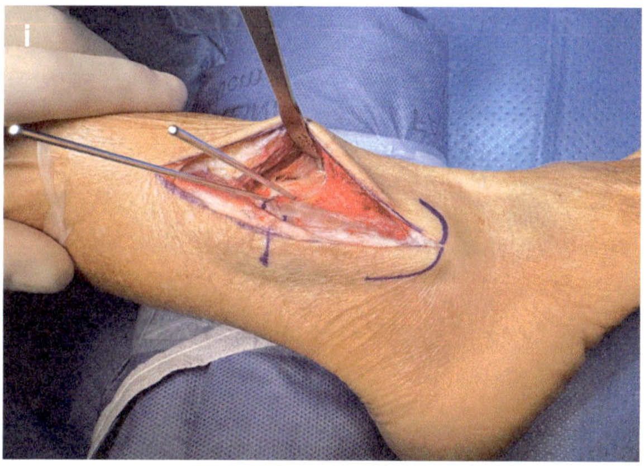

Fig. 8.4i The image shows how it looks like when both K-wires are inserted into the tibia

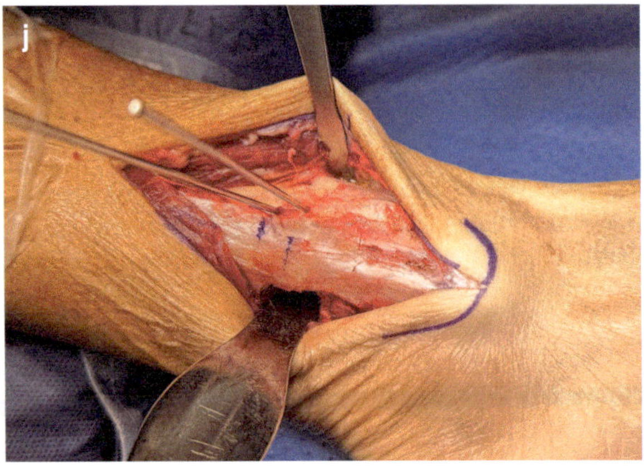

Fig. 8.4j After marking and checking the osteotomy lines an Eva-hook is inserted posteriorly and a Hohmann-hook is placed anteriorly

- The osteotomy is performed with an oscillating saw, which is then stopped approx. 5 mm in front of the medial cortex (in the ap-image) of the tibia
- Now follows the second osteotomy incision with the oscillating saw (Fig. 8.4k)
- The bone wedge can be removed
  Note: If the osteotomy is still too rigid, the medial cortex can be carefully weakened with an osteotome (Fig. 8.4l)
- The osteotomy can now be closed (Fig. 8.4m)
  Note: If the medial cortex breaks, a short plate must be placed medially, otherwise the osteotomy would gap at this point, the correction would be inadequate and the risk of nonunion is increased
- A 2-hole or modern anatomically-preshaped plate on the fibula (posterolateral) and a 3-hole plate or modern anatomically-pre shaped plate on the tibia (anterolateral) are often sufficient to secure the osteotomy adequately (Figs. 8.4n, 8.4o, 8.4p and 8.4q)

Asymmetric Valgus Arthrosis of the Upper Ankle Joint

Medial closing tibial osteotomy [31]

Indications:
Incongruent valgus malalignment, i.e. talar tilt in the ankle joint
Can be used for any valgus malposition
Target:
Slight overcorrection, i.e. 2° - 4° valgus of the tibial surface angle.
After determining the CORA, the osteotomy is planned so that the anatomical tibial axis passes through the center of the ankle joint, or slightly medial to it.
Advantages:

- Low risks regarding neurovascular integrity

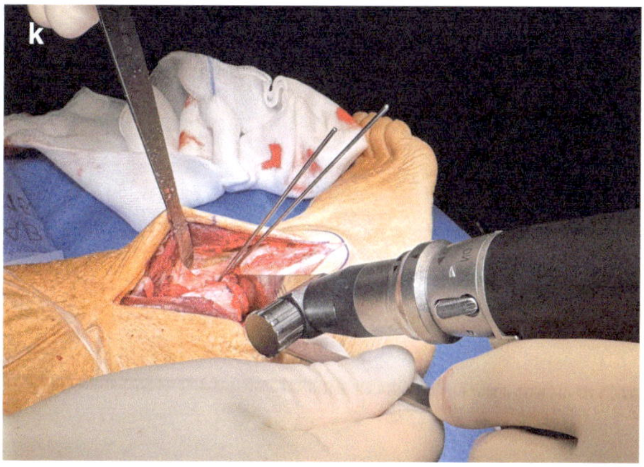

Fig. 8.4k The osteotomy is performed by means of an oscillating saw. Careful pumping actions help feel how the bones are cut. Do not saw too aggressive because otherwise the risk for medial tibial penetration rises

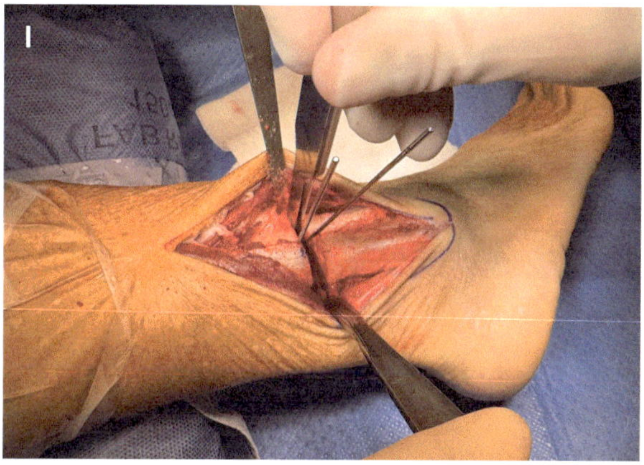

Fig. 8.4l Once the osteotomy is performed the bony wedge can be removed. Tipp: if the K-wires can be removed by hand the osteotomy lines have been cut perfectl

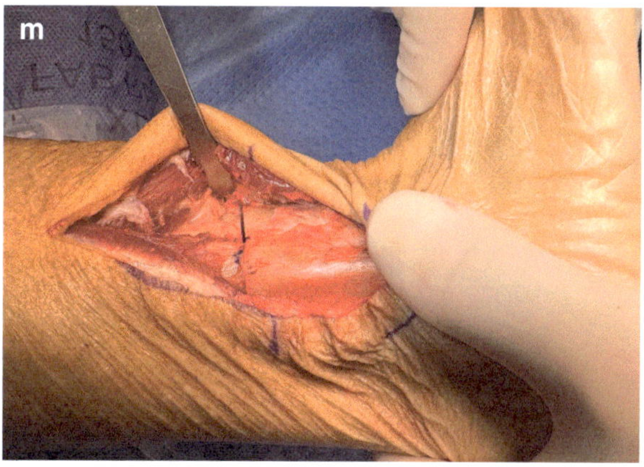

Fig. 8.4m The photograph illustrates the manual closure of the supramalleolar osteotomy

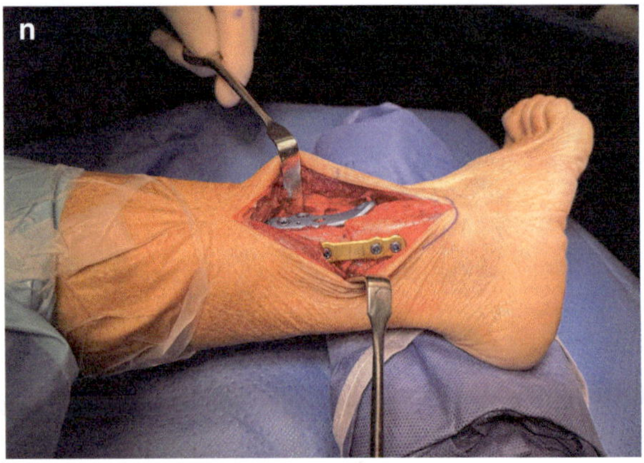

Fig. 8.4n The image shows the final fixation of the tibial and fibular osteotomy by means of plates

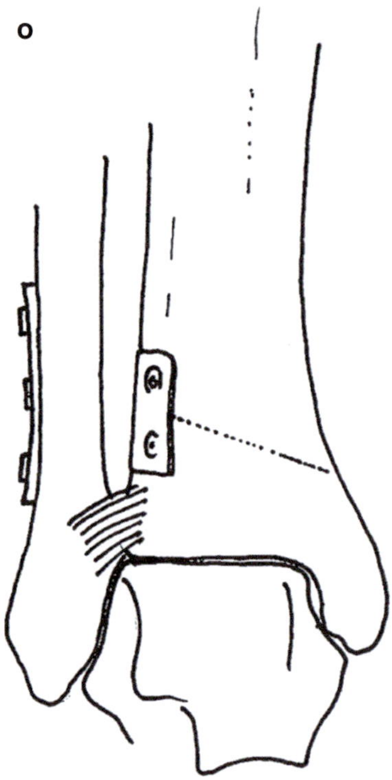

Fig. 8.4o Schematic drawing of the supramallelar lateral-closing-wedge osteotomy after plating

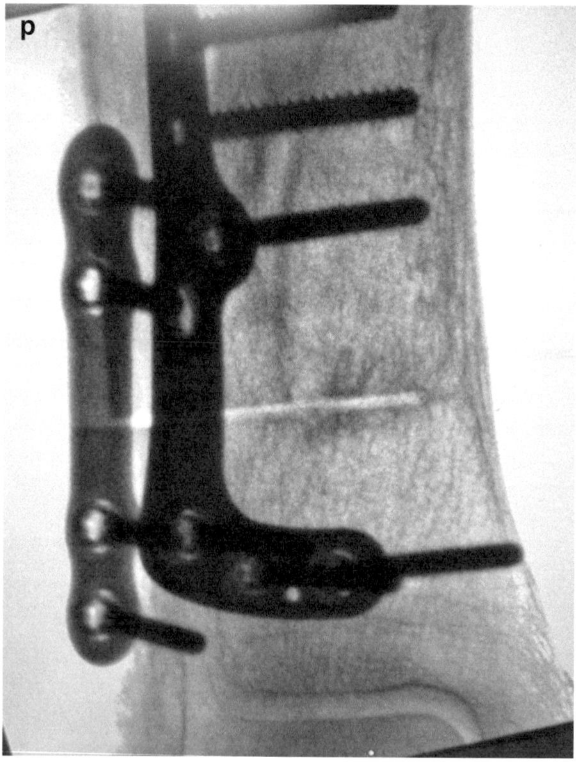

Fig. 8.4p Intraoperative fluoroscopy to check the ostoetomy and its fixation

- No bone block necessary
- Allows multi-planar corrections.

Disadvantage:

- Shortening of the leg length

Note:

If the CORA falls on the joint line or very close to it, a dome osteotomy should be used. If this is not possible or desired, the translation should be performed medially.

Tips and tricks:

For deformities that cannot be adequately corrected, an additional fibular lengthening osteotomy should be considered. To check the effect, the correction can be tested beforehand with a Hintermann spreader attached laterally (to the tibia and talus).

Technique (Figs. 8.1c, 8.1d and 8.1e):

- The patient is positioned supine. The knee can be held slightly bent with the sandbag under the ipsilateral calf.
- The incision is made centrally over the medial malleolus

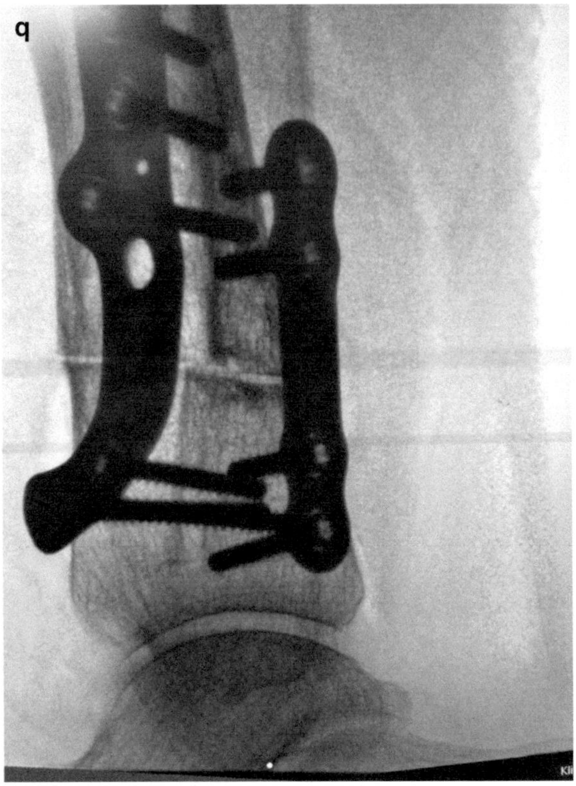

Fig. 8.4q Lateral view onto the osteotomy

- The length of the incision is approx. 7 cm
- Subcutaneous preparation and protection of the great saphenous vein and the saphenous nerve

  Note: The two structures often run anterior to the incision.
- Deep dissection until the periosteum of the medial tibia is reached
- Insertion of a Hohmann retractor anteriorly and posteriorly
- The proximal part of the tibialis posterior tendon sheath must often be slightly incised so that the soft tissues can be folded posteriorly
- The authors now use an 8 mm Hohmann retractor anteriorly and a so-called Eva hook posteriorly (wide hook, for better protection of the neurovascular, posteromedial bundle as well as the tendon structures)
- Once these steps have been completed, the tibia should be fully exposed
- A K-wire is placed under fluoroscopic control and inserted at the site of the osteotomy as planned
- A second wire is inserted at the preoperatively calculated angle to the first K-wire
- An oscillating saw is used to perform the osteotomy, which should only be incomplete (i.e. the lateral cortex of the tibia must not break)

- In addition to extensive irrigation, this always requires radiological control of the osteotomy depth
- It is possible to check manually whether the osteotomy is moving or not
- The second osteotomy is performed in the same way as the first.
- The wedge can be easily mobilized and removed with an osteotome (Fig. 8.1d)
- The tibia is now closed and the correction checked under X-ray control. (Fig. 8.1e)
- The construct is fixed medially with a plate and thus secured.

Asymmetric Osteoarthritis of the Upper Ankle Joint

Spherical or dome osteotomy [32–34]
Indications:
Varus or valgus deformity, i.e. talar tilt in the upper ankle joint with CORA at the level of the joint line
Target:
After determining the CORA, the osteotomy is planned so that the anatomical tibial axis passes through the center of the ankle joint.
Advantages:

- Maintains the length of the limb
- Allows multi-planar corrections.
- Sufficient bone contact
- Very large corrections possible

Disadvantage:

- Often only correction in one plane possible, although this is relative

Tips and tricks:
If a biplanar correction is to be made, the osteotomy can be widened ventrally with an osteotome and a bone wedge can be inserted (for extension malalignment in the sagittal plane) or rotated slightly dorsally (for flexion malalignment in the sagittal plane).
Technique (Figs. 8.2a and 8.2b):

- The patient is positioned supine. A cushion can be positioned under the ipsilateral buttocks.
- The incision is made centrally over the anterior upper ankle joint
- The length of the incision is approx. 10 cm
  Note: Do not use sharp hooks on the skin because this can injure the skin and promote wound healing problems
- Subcutaneous dissection and hemostasis
- Exposure of the extensor retinaculum

Note: The superficial peroneal nerve is visible at the distal end of the skin incision

- Incision of the extensor retinaculum along the lateral edge of the tibialis anterior tendon
- The fatty tissue can be recognized under the anterior tibial tendon, which is held away medially with a Langenbeck hook
- This is followed by deep dissection, whereby the vascular-nerve bundle is held away laterally

  Note: Dissection through the fatty tissue area often reveals large, crossing veins. These should be ligated.
- The soft tissue is now detached from the lower surface of the tibia using a blunt raspatory

  Note: The ankle joint does not need to be opened. It is important that the distal tibia is exposed.
- Insertion of two Hohmann hooks medially and laterally
- A 3.5 mm one-third tube plate is fixed centrally on the distal tibial plafond. The fixation should remain loose as the plate is used as a "compass" for the osteotomy.

  Note: Check that the screw does not perforate into the ankle joint.
- Using a 2.5 mm drill, a drill hole is now made step by step in a curved shape, very close to each other, from anterior to posterior

  Note: The drill must be positioned perpendicular to the anatomical tibial axis as seen on the lateral projection.
- A 5 mm and 10 mm Lambotte osteotome is used to complete the osteotomy
- A manual check is carried out to determine whether the osteotomy is or will be mobile
- Once the osteotomy is complete, the distal fragment can be rotated into the valgus or varus position
- The construct is secured via two 3.5 mm one-third tube plates—attached medially and laterally

Special Osteotomies

Plafondoplasty (Figs. 8.5a and 8.5b) [35–38]
Indications:
Intra-articular deformities involving the tibia, especially medially
Target:
Correction of the Tibial Plafonds
Advantage:

- Direct correction tibial plafond
- Relatively simple

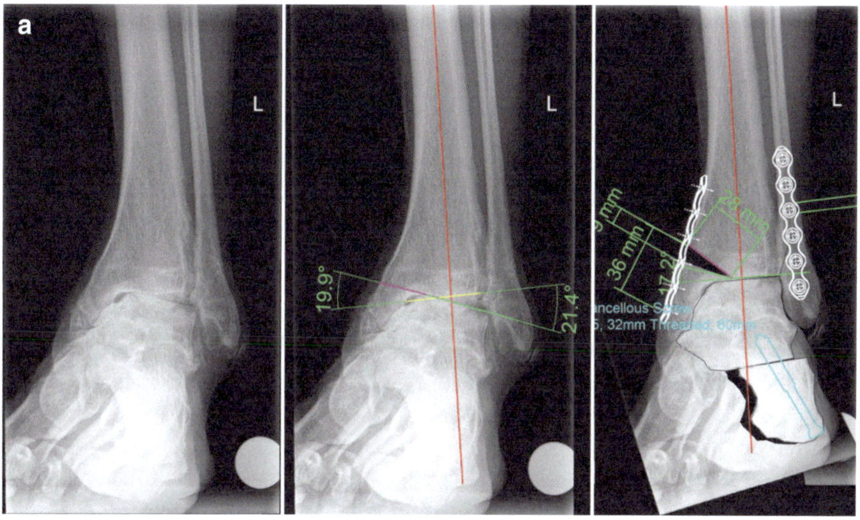

Fig. 8.5a This images show the ap radiographs of a varus ankle deformity with its apex at the level of the tibial plafond. In this case the medial plafond is distorted. In order to correct the deformity a virtual correction is made to simulate the re-alignment. As can be seen an osteotomy proximal to the medial malleolus is performed

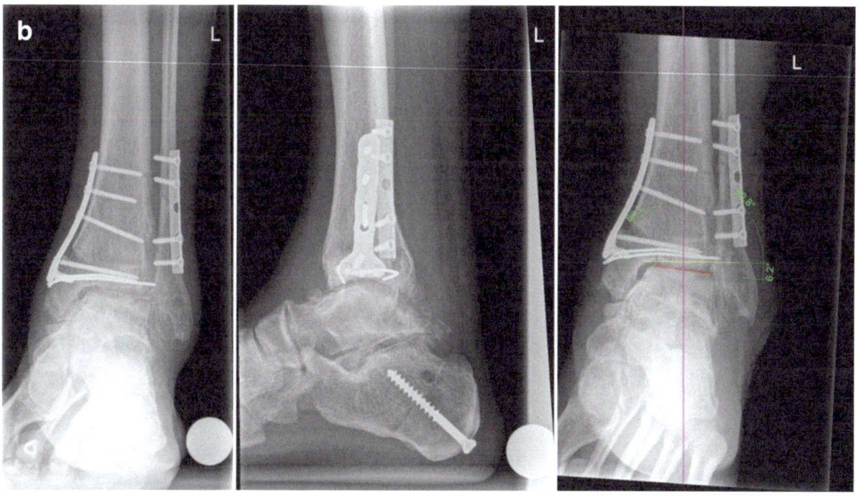

Fig. 8.5b The same patient as presented in Fig. 8.5a. A plafondoplasty has been made. Two K-wires have been inserted from medially to laterally in order to avoid a breakthrough of the osteotomy. A bony wedge has been inserted to fill the medial defect. A medial plate secures the construct. At the same time a shortening of the fibula and an inframalleolar osteotomy were added to achieve full correction

Disadvantage:

- Fixation sometimes difficult due to proximity to joint surface

Technique:

- The patient is positioned supine. The knee can be held slightly bent with the sandbag under the ipsilateral calf.
- The incision is made centrally over the medial malleolus
- The length of the incision is approx. 7 cm
- Subcutaneous preparation and protection of the great saphenous vein and the saphenous nerve
  Note: The two structures often run anterior to the incision.
- Deep dissection until the periosteum of the medial tibia is reached
- Insertion of a Hohmann retractor anteriorly and posteriorly
- Under fluoroscopic control, a K-wire is now inserted up to the lateral edge of the transition between the intra-articular step and the normal tibial plateau
- The wire is advanced approx. 45° from proximal-medial to distal-lateral
  Note: This is the wire that defines the osteotomy line
- Two additional wires, which are inserted parallel and almost subchondrally to the tibial plafond, are used to secure the osteotomy so that it does not break out intra-articularly
- The incomplete osteotomy is performed along the oblique wire using an oscillating saw
- The osteotomy is now distracted using a 15 mm osteotome
- The correction is completed under fluoroscopic control, i.e. the tibial plafond is parallel to the talar surface
- An allogenic or autologous bone graft is used to fill the gap
- The osteotomy is then secured with a 3.5 mm one-third tubular plate
- The two K-wires that were used to secure the tibial plafond can be cut and left in place

Fibular osteotomy [27, 28, 39–49]
Indications:
Additional correction in valgus or varus, depending on which osteotomy is used during the correction
Target:
Better adjustment of the talus
Advantage:

- Very simple

Technology in detail:

- The positioning depends on type of supramalleolar osteotomy
  - Lateral decubitus for lateral closing-wedge osteotomy
  - Supine for medial closing-wedge osteotomy

- The incision is made centrally over the fibula
- The length of the incision is approx. 5 cm
- Subcutaneous dissection and hemostasis
- Direct exposure of the lateral fibula cortex
- Insertion of two Hohmann hooks
- Perform an oblique osteotomy by using an oscillating saw
- Shortening or lengthening of the fibula, depending on what is to be corrected
- Fixation of the fibula with a 3.5 mm one-third tube plate

Inframalleolar osteotomy, calcaneal osteotomy (Figs. 8.6a, 8.6b, 8.6c, 8.6d, 8.6e, 8.6f, 8.6g, 8.6h, 8.6i, 8.6j, and 8.6k) [18, 50–52]

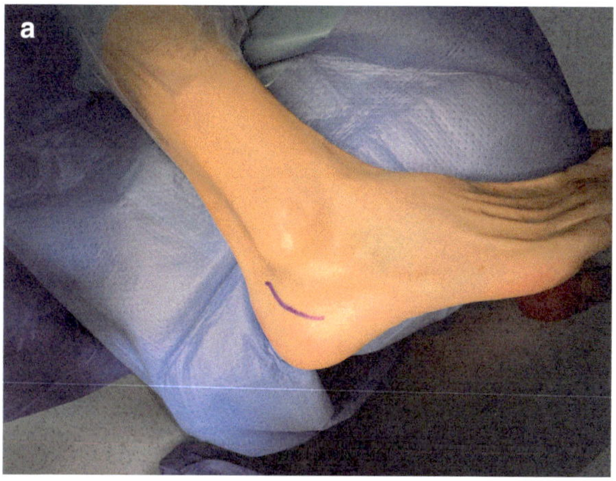

Fig. 8.6a Depicted is the slightly curved incision line for a calcaneal osteotomy

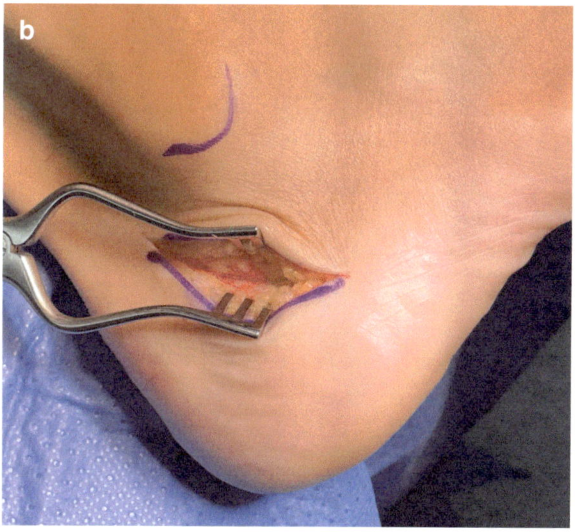

Fig. 8.6b The image depicts the subcutaneous preparation until reaching the bone

Fig. 8.6c After exposing the lateral cortex of the calcaneal tuberosity, two Hohmann retractors are inserted dorsally and plantarly

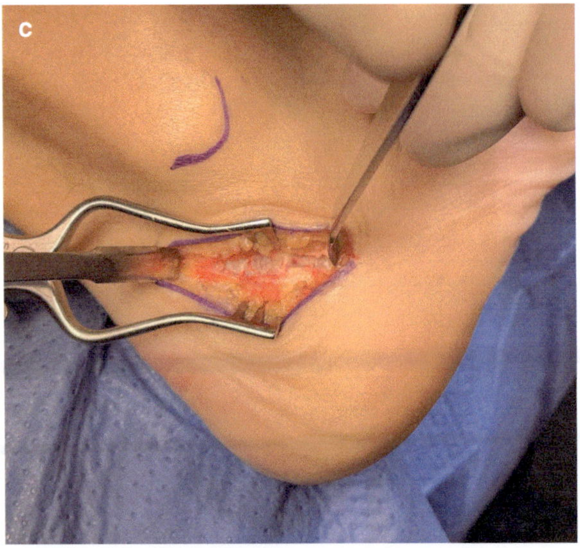

Fig. 8.6d By means of an oscillating saw the osteotomy is performed carefully. It is useful to take a wide fan-blade. The free hand should grab the entire hindfoot. This technique allows proper control of the osteotomy because it serves as control to note penetration of the saw blade on the medial side of the calcaneus

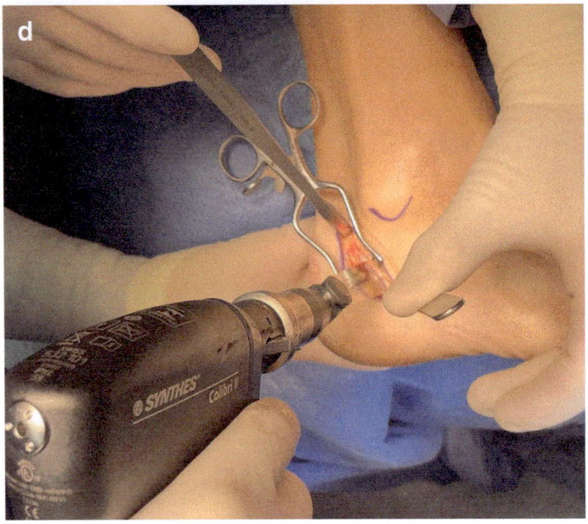

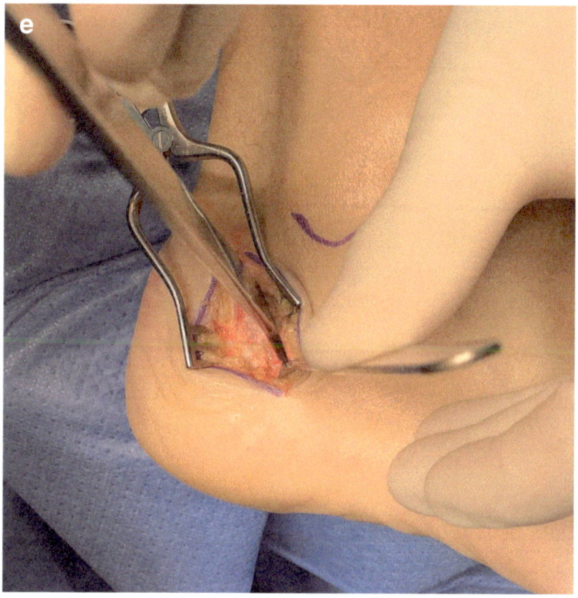

Fig. 8.6e An osteotome is inserted into the osteotomy line and then used to gently open the osteotomy

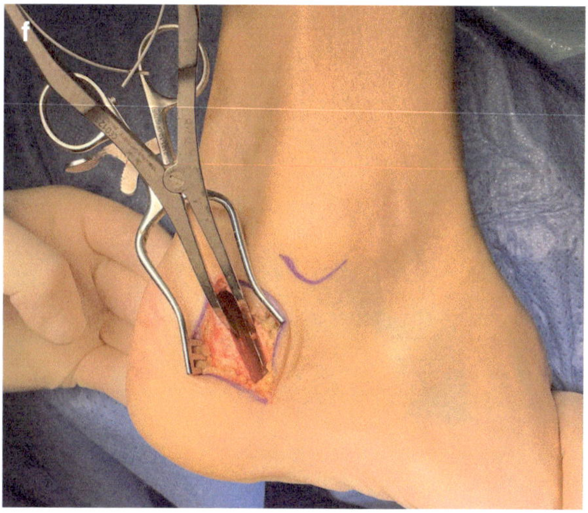

Fig. 8.6f The authors use a laminar spreader to help open the osteotomy while checking whether further releases of the periosteum or plantar ligament are needed

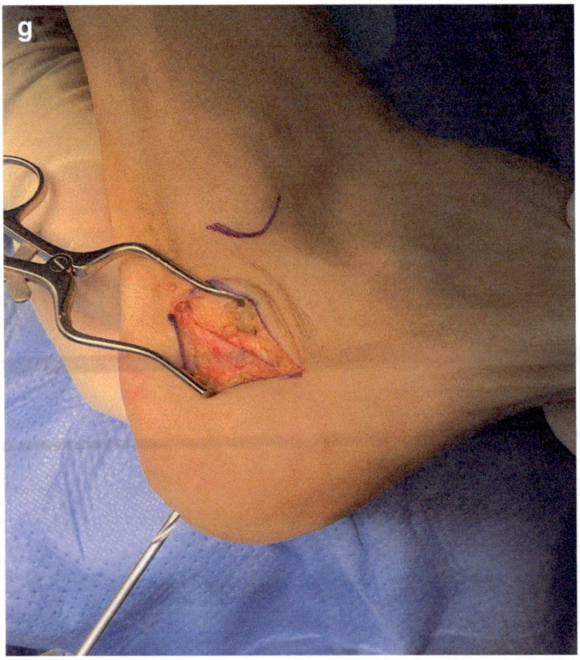

Fig. 8.6g The foot and knee are both flexed. By so doing the gastrocnemii become relaxed, allowing an easy shift of the calcaneal tuberosity into the desired position. The correction, i.e. the amount of shift, is checked and then the knee and foot extended. Dorsiflexion of the foot creates a tension band effect and secures the osteotomy in its corrected position. A guide wire is inserted into the calcaneal tuberosity

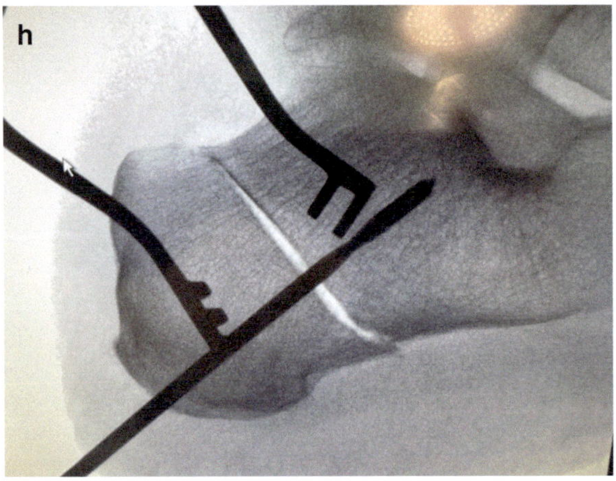

Fig. 8.6h Radiographic check of the K-wire position

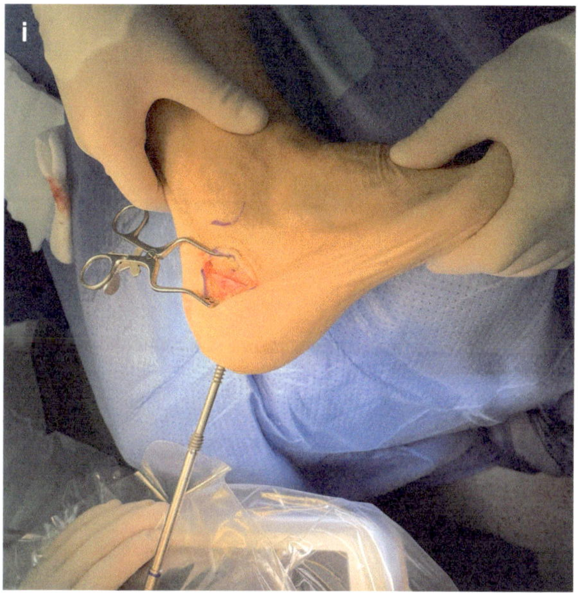

Fig. 8.6i A screw is inserted to fix the osteotomy. Please note how the foot is still held in maximal dorsiflexion

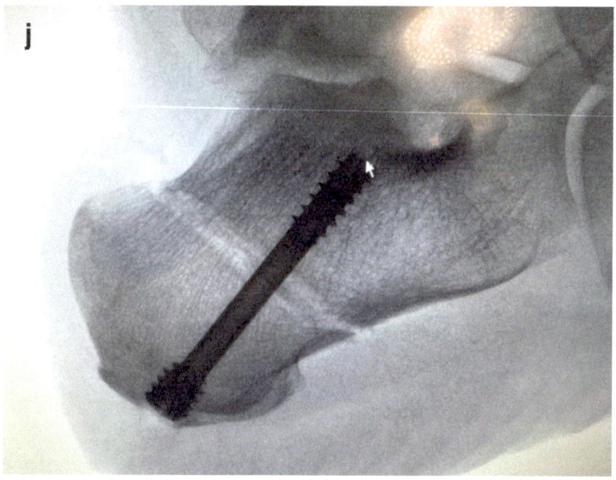

Fig. 8.6j Postoperative lateral view of the final calcaneal osteotomy

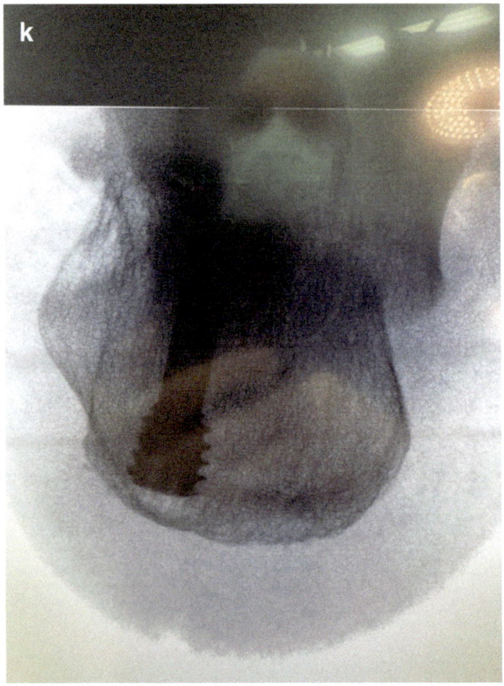

Fig. 8.6k Postoperative axial view of the calcaneus, demonstrating the shift and position of the screw

Indications:

Deformity lies below ankle joint

Remaining varus or valgus deformity after supramalleolar osteotomy

Target:

To normalize static overload and to re-align calcaneal tuberosity underneath the weight bearing axis.

Advantage:

- Very simple
- Quick

Potential problems

- Nonarthritic-convex shaped subtalar joint
- Subluxed subtalar joint

Complications

Among all complications that may occur after supramalleolar osteotomies progression of ankle osteoarthritis requiring total ankle replacement is found most frequently (average 3%), followed by recurrent deformity, under- or overcorrection (2.6%) [6].

Overcorrection and undercorrection may be the result from inappropriate planning, technical errors or loss of correction during the postoperative period. As mentioned before, in case of a too proximal CORA a lateral translational deformity will develop when using a valgus-directing osteotomy and a medial translational deformity will develop when using a varus-directing osteotomy. [11, 14] Thus, the site of osteotomy needs specific attention and should be calculated as best as possible.

Wound complications after surgery ranged 2.5% while superficial or deep infections were found to be quite low (1.3 and 0.4%) [6].

Nonunions and persisting pain have been reported to range about 2% and revisions needed where found to average 1.7%.

Acute tarsal tunnel syndrome may result in patients who undergo acute varus-to-valgus correction. If there is any doubt regarding the development of such a complication a prophylactic release might be indicated [53].

Progression of ankle osteoarthritis without further interventions and those requiring arthrodesis ranged around 1.2% [6, 29, 31, 47, 54–59].

Therefore, it could be stated that the risk of major complications is quite low when considering corrective osteotomies at the ankle.

History and Brief Overview of Results in the Scientific Literature

The first report of supramalleolar osteotomies dates back to Speed and Boyds paper published in 1936 [60]. The authors presented for the first time an operative reconstruction of 50 malunited fractures about the ankle joint and came to the conclusion that this type of surgery would be of greater benefit for the patients.

Since then a long time has passed without major interest in this kind of surgery. Most of the works regarding supramalleolar osteotomies were published in pediatric orthopaedics with specific regard on inborne deformities. Rehn, Schramm and Hierholzer, in 1968, first reported on the indication and technique of a so-called inversion osteotomy to correct malpositions after fractures of the lower limb [61].

This was followed by Janssen who published the technique of supramalleolar osteotomies following fractures of the ankle [62, 63]. Weber in 1977 published the technique of a supramalleolar valgus osteotomy in adults [64], which was then followed by his report in 1981 on lengthening osteotomies of the fibula to correct a widened mortise the ankle after fractures [65]. His work was based on a previously published Bernese scientific thesis of Bircher in 1973 [66].

However, all those works focused on how to correct malunions after fractures and none of them focused specifically on the topic of asymmetric ankle osteoarthritis.

In 1995 Takakura et al. published their results of a supramalleolar osteotomy for the correction of asymmetric ankle arthritis [10]. They were able to demonstrate that redirecting the forces across the ankle joint through limb realignment had a positive effect on fibrocartilage formation and slowed the progression of ankle joint arthritis.

Since this report several scientific studies were able to confirm those findings while providing evidence in terms of improved function, range of motion and low risk of complications [14, 18, 29–31, 46–48, 56–59, 67–83].

One of the largest studies performed by Krahenbuehl and coworkers showed that from a total of 294 patients 30 were converted into total ankle replacements and 8 received fusion after 5 years (range 2–16 years). The assessed overall survivorship was 88% after 5 years of follow-up. The radiographic parameters were normalized in most patients and the AOFAS scores improved significantly. Best outcomes were found in younger patient (less than 60 years) with moderate, asymmetric ankle arthritis [84]. Tanaka et al. found similar results thus stating that in advanced arthritis stages supramalleolar osteotomies might not be of benefit [76, 85]. Knupp and co-workers were also able to identify that a talar tilt of 7° or more was associated with a higher risk of failure [79].

Plafondoplasty has shown to be effective for smaller varus ankle corrections [35–37]. However, only little information is available in the literature and no true data is available regarding its influence on larger talar tilts. Mann et al. suggested a combination of a plafondoplasty and supramalleolar osteotomy in order to address major talar tilting [38].

On the other hand, calcaneal osteotomies themselves show a beneficial effect on tibiotalar load transmission [86–88]. A more recent, laboratory study by Flury et al. showed that a sliding calcaneal osteotomy had beneficial load-shifting capacities in ankles with neutral alignment or 5° of ankle varus malalignment [89]. Thus, the inframalleolar, adjunctive correction should be taken into consideration when correcting asymmetric ankle osteoarthritis.

More recently, patient-specific-instrumentation (PSI) has become a very valuable tool to provide most accurate corrections based on preoperative virtual planning [90, 91]. However, there are future scientific investigations needed to prove its cost-effectiveness and mid-to-long-term benefits [32, 92].

Two Illustrating Cases

Case 1

A 63-years old male presented with a posttraumatic varus deformity of the right hindfoot. In addition, the patient suffered from medially located ankle osteoarthritis, i.e. asymmetric osteoarthritis. This deformity was congruent with the apex of it lying quite proximal to the joint line. In an attempt to preserve the joint the decision was made to embark on joint sparing correction of the hindfoot. Figures 8.7a, 8.7b, 8.7c, 8.7d, 8.7e, 8.7f, and 8.7g illustrate step-by-step how the correction has been done.

Case 2

A 58-years old male patient presents with an asymmetric varus osteoarthritis of the left hindfoot. In contrast to case 1 the talus was found tilting and the talus subluxing anteriorly. Because most of the joint revealed intact cartilage the decision was made to solve the problem by supramalleolar osteotomy.

The case is illustrated in Figs. 8.8a and 8.8b.

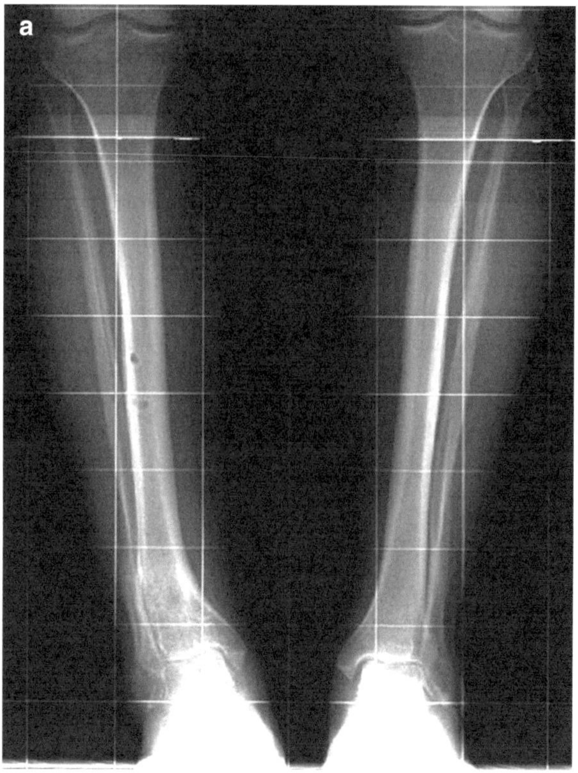

Fig. 8.7a Depicted is the lower leg of the patient mentioned in case 1. It is easy to realize the varus deformity of the right ankle

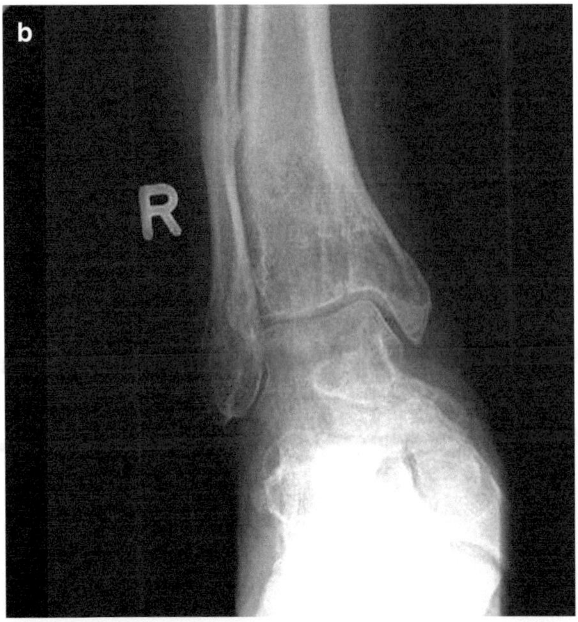

Fig. 8.7b Close-up view of the same patient. Note the congruent deformity type

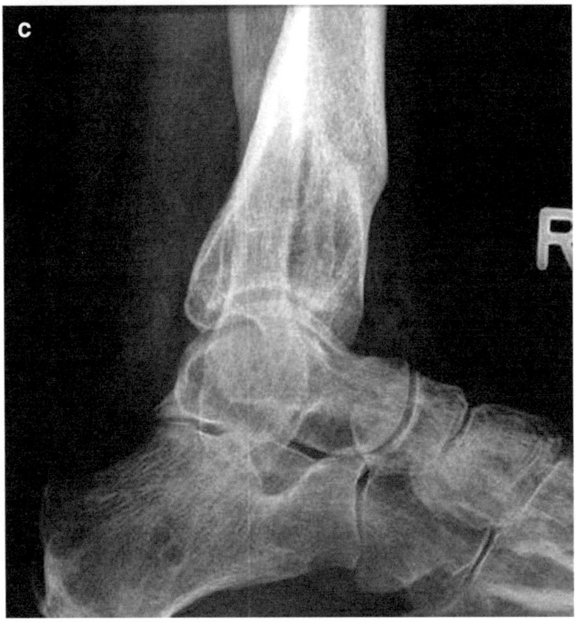

Fig. 8.7c Seen is the lateral view of the right ankle . The joint is still very well contained

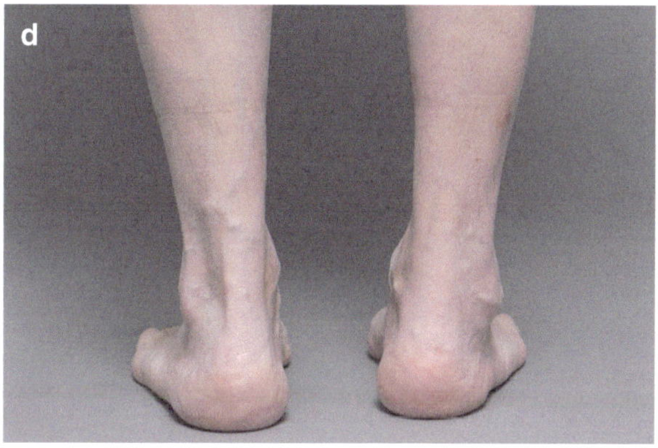

Fig. 8.7d The image shows the preoperative clinical deformity of the right hindfoot

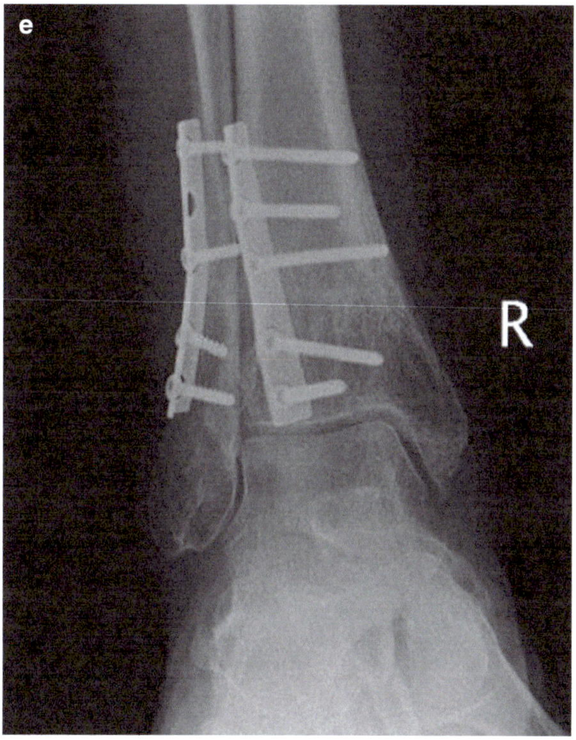

Fig. 8.7e Postoperative ap-view of the ankle after a lateral closing-wedge osteotomy. The ankle has been realigned

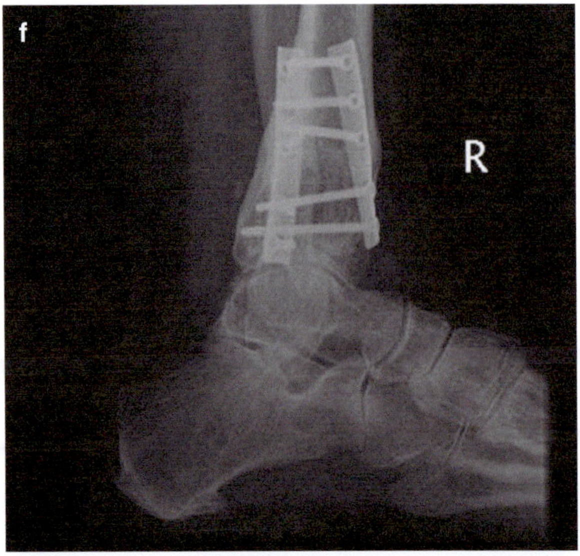

Fig. 8.7f Postoperative lateral view of the ankle after supramalleolar correction

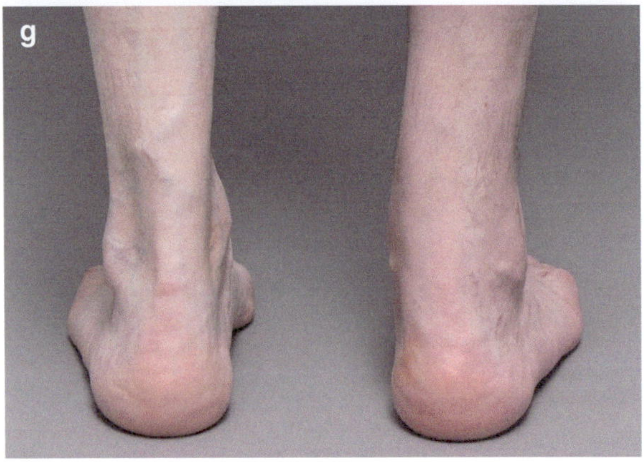

Fig. 8.7g The image shows the clinical result after bony correction. Please note the slight overcorrection, when compared with the contralateral left side

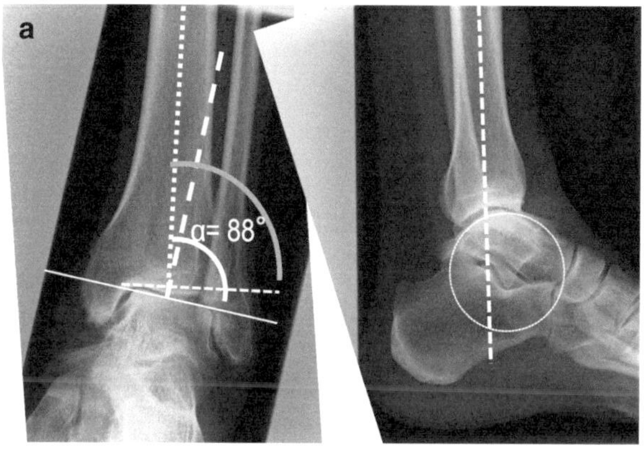

Fig. 8.8a Depicted are the preoperative ap and lateral radiographs of the patient mentioned as case 2. There is a varus tilt of the talus within the mortise. In addition to that the talus shows a visible anterior subluxation. The medial ankle joint reveals the existence of local degenerative changes

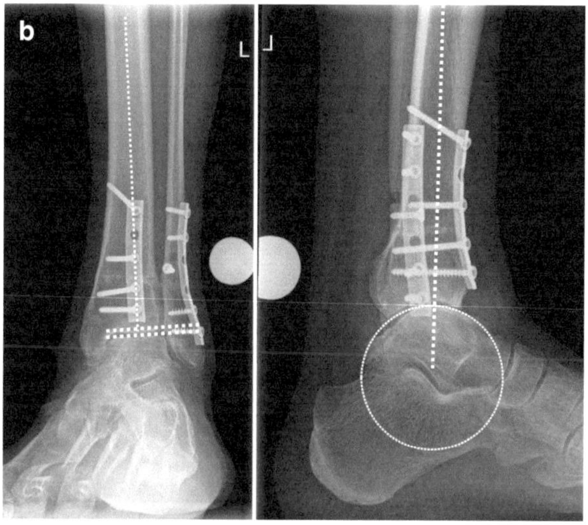

Fig. 8.8b The image demonstrates the postoperative radiographs of the same patient mentioned in Fig. 8.8a (Case 2). Note the re-alignment achieved through supramalleolar osteotomy and the centered talus underneath the tibia

Conclusion

Osteotomies around the ankle joint provide a useful and effective means to correct hindfoot alignments and to re-distribute trans-articular load transmissions in the presence of asymmetric ankle osteoarthritis. Surgeons need to be familiar with all techniques that could be applied and should also keep in mind that additional procedures often are necessary to provide a stable and well-functioning correction.

References

1. Valderrabano V, et al. Etiology of ankle osteoarthritis. Clin Orthop Relat Res. 2009;467(7):1800–6.
2. Pagenstert GI, et al. Realignment surgery as alternative treatment of varus and valgus ankle osteoarthritis. Clin Orthop Relat Res. 2007;462:156–68.
3. Choi S, et al. Correction target of supramalleolar osteotomy for early Varus ankle arthritis: is overcorrection necessary? Foot Ankle Int. 2024;46:10711007241300331.
4. Shah S, et al. Incidence and cost of ankle sprains in United States emergency departments. Sports Health. 2016;8(6):547–52.
5. Herrera-Perez M, et al. Ankle osteoarthritis aetiology. J Clin Med. 2021;10:19.
6. Mulhern JL, et al. Supramalleolar osteotomy: indications and surgical techniques. Clin Podiatr Med Surg. 2015;32(3):445–61.
7. Goetz JE, et al. A clinically realistic large animal model of intra-articular fracture that progresses to post-traumatic osteoarthritis. Osteoarthr Cartil. 2015;23(10):1797–805.
8. Knupp M. The use of osteotomies in the treatment of asymmetric ankle joint arthritis. Foot Ankle Int. 2017;38(2):220–9.
9. Sugimoto K, et al. Varus tilt of the tibial plafond as a factor in chronic ligament instability of the ankle. Foot Ankle Int. 1997;18(7):402–5.
10. Takakura Y, et al. Low tibial osteotomy for osteoarthritis of the ankle. Results of a new operation in 18 patients. J Bone Joint Surg Br. 1995;77(1):50–4.
11. Paley D. Pricinples of deformity correction. In: Berlin, Heidelberg. 3rd ed. New York: Springer; 2005.
12. Wagner E, Wagner P. Correction of sagittal plane deformity of the distal tibia. Foot Ankle Clin. 2022;27(1):129–44.
13. Keppler P. Treatment of rotational malalignment of the lower leg. Unfallchirurg. 2018;121(3):191–8.
14. Hintermann B, Knupp M, Barg A. Supramalleolar osteotomies for the treatment of ankle arthritis. J Am Acad Orthop Surg. 2016;24(7):424–32.
15. Saltzman CL, el-Khoury GY. The hindfoot alignment view. Foot Ankle Int. 1995;16(9):572–6.
16. Buck FM, et al. Hindfoot alignment measurements: rotation-stability of measurement techniques on hindfoot alignment view and long axial view radiographs. AJR Am J Roentgenol. 2011;197(3):578–82.
17. Reilingh ML, et al. Measuring hindfoot alignment radiographically: the long axial view is more reliable than the hindfoot alignment view. Skeletal Radiol. 2010;39(11):1103–8.
18. Hintermann B, et al. The use of Supramalleolar osteotomies in posttraumatic deformity and arthritis of the ankle. JBJS Essent Surg Tech. 2017;7(4):e29.
19. Stamatis ED, Cooper PS, Myerson MS. Supramalleolar osteotomy for the treatment of distal tibial angular deformities and arthritis of the ankle joint. Foot Ankle Int. 2003;24(10):754–64.
20. Stamatis ED, Myerson MS. Supramalleolar osteotomy: indications and technique. Foot Ankle Clin. 2003;8(2):317–33.
21. Haraguchi N, et al. Weight-bearing-line analysis in supramalleolar osteotomy for varus-type osteoarthritis of the ankle. J Bone Joint Surg Am. 2015;97(4):333–9.
22. Zhang S, et al. Changes in the subtalar joint alignment after supramalleolar osteotomy for varus ankle arthritis. Foot Ankle Surg. 2023;29(6):475–80.
23. Krahenbuhl N, et al. Morphologic analysis of the subtalar joint using statistical shape modeling. J Orthop Res. 2020;38:2625–33.
24. Hirschmann A, et al. Upright cone CT of the hindfoot: comparison of the non-weight-bearing with the upright weight-bearing position. Eur Radiol. 2014;24(3):553–8.
25. Fischer DR, et al. Therapeutic impact of [(18)F]fluoride positron-emission tomography/computed tomography on patients with unclear foot pain. Skeletal Radiol. 2010;39(10):987–97.
26. Bhure U, et al. Single-photon emission computed tomography/computed tomography arthrography of wrist, ankle, and knee joints. Nucl Med Commun. 2020;41(3):182–8.

27. Lee JM, et al. Prediction of prognosis in supramalleolar osteotomy with or without additional fibula osteotomy by approaching a biomechanical study: a finite element analysis. Biomed Eng Lett. 2024;14(5):1079–85.
28. Lee JM, Lee SJ, Park CH. Pressure change at ankle joint in supramalleolar osteotomy with or without fibular osteotomy according to different types of varus ankle. J Orthop Res. 2024;42(8):1771–9.
29. Barg A, Saltzman CL. Joint-preserving procedures in patients with varus deformity: role of supramalleolar osteotomies. Foot Ankle Clin. 2019;24(2):239–64.
30. Harstall R, et al. Supramalleolar lateral closing wedge osteotomy for the treatment of varus ankle arthrosis. Foot Ankle Int. 2007;28(5):542–8.
31. Krahenbuhl N, et al. Supramalleolar osteotomy in post-traumatic valgus ankle osteoarthritis. Int Orthop. 2020;44(3):535–43.
32. Faict S, et al. Correction of ankle varus deformity using patient-specific dome-shaped osteotomy guides designed on weight-bearing CT: a pilot study. Arch Orthop Trauma Surg. 2023;143(2):791–9.
33. Kim J, et al. Dome supramalleolar osteotomies for the treatment of ankle pain with opposing coronal plane deformities between ankle and the lower limb. Foot Ankle Int. 2022;43(4):474–85.
34. Easley ME, et al. Use of a locking plate and drill sleeves to guide dome-shaped supramalleolar osteotomy: technique tip. Foot Ankle Int. 2021;42(9):1185–90.
35. Zielli SO, et al. Indications, associated procedures, and results of ankle plafond-plasty for varus ankle osteoarthritis: a systematic review and meta-analysis. Foot Ankle Spec. 2024:19386400241236321.
36. Al-Nammari SS, Myerson MS. The use of tibial osteotomy (ankle plafondplasty) for joint preservation of ankle deformity and early arthritis. Foot Ankle Clin. 2016;21(1):15–26.
37. Kobayashi H, Kageyama Y, Shido Y. Treatment of varus ankle osteoarthritis and instability with a novel mortise-plasty osteotomy procedure. J Foot Ankle Surg. 2016;55(1):60–7.
38. Mann HA, Filippi J, Myerson MS. Intra-articular opening medial tibial wedge osteotomy (plafond-plasty) for the treatment of intra-articular varus ankle arthritis and instability. Foot Ankle Int. 2012;33(4):255–61.
39. Choi JY, Suh JS. Joint preserving procedures for Takakura stage IIIB varus ankle osteoarthritis. BMJ Case Rep. 2024;17(6)
40. Suh JW, et al. Outcomes of oblique supramalleolar osteotomy without fibular osteotomy for congruent- and incongruent-type medial ankle arthritis. Foot Ankle Surg. 2022;28(5):603–9.
41. Liang JQ, et al. Fibular osteotomy is helpful for talar reduction in the treatment of varus ankle osteoarthritis with supramalleolar osteotomy. J Orthop Surg Res. 2021;16(1):575.
42. Zhao H, et al. Supramalleolar osteotomy treatment of varus ankle osteoarthritis with or without fibular osteotomy. Zhongguo Xiu Fu Chong Jian Wai Ke Za Zhi. 2017;31(3):284–9.
43. Choi GW, et al. Effect of combined fibular osteotomy on the pressure of the tibiotalar and talofibular joints in supramalleolar osteotomy of the ankle: a cadaveric study. J Foot Ankle Surg. 2017;56(1):59–64.
44. Zhao H, et al. The role of fibular for supramalleolar osteotomy in treatment of varus ankle arthritis: a biomechanical and clinical study. J Orthop Surg Res. 2016;11(1):127.
45. Hongmou Z, et al. Supramalleolar osteotomy with or without fibular osteotomy for Varus ankle arthritis. Foot Ankle Int. 2016;37(9):1001–7.
46. Galli MM, Scott RT. Supramalleolar osteotomies: an algorithm for the deformed ankle. Clin Podiatr Med Surg. 2015;32(3):435–44.
47. Knupp M, Bolliger L, Hintermann B. Treatment of posttraumatic varus ankle deformity with supramalleolar osteotomy. Foot Ankle Clin. 2012;17(1):95–102.
48. Lee WC, et al. Supramalleolar osteotomy in patients with Varus ankle osteoarthritis. JBJS Essent Surg Tech. 2011;1(3):e13.
49. Lee WC, et al. Indications for supramalleolar osteotomy in patients with ankle osteoarthritis and varus deformity. J Bone Joint Surg Am. 2011;93(13):1243–8.

50. Stukenborg-Colsman C, et al. Conversion osteotomy for arthrosis of the ankle joint (supramalleolar and inframalleolar)—what can be expected? Critical review of the literature. Unfallchirurg. 2022;125(3):189–95.
51. Barg A, et al. Dwyer osteotomy: lateral sliding osteotomy of calcaneus. Oper Orthop Traumatol. 2015;27(4):283–97.
52. Hintermann B, Knupp M, Barg A. Osteotomies of the distal tibia and hindfoot for ankle realignment. Orthopade. 2008;37(3):212–23.
53. Paley D. The correction of complex foot deformities using Ilizarov's distraction osteotomies. Clin Orthop Relat Res. 1993;293:97–111.
54. Christidis P, et al. Supramalleolar osteotomies for ankle arthritis: a systematic review. Arch Orthop Trauma Surg. 2023;143(9):5549–64.
55. Lacorda JB, Jung HG, Im JM. Supramalleolar distal tibiofibular osteotomy for medial ankle osteoarthritis: current concepts. Clin Orthop Surg. 2020;12(3):271–8.
56. Colin F, et al. Supramalleolar osteotomy: techniques, indications and outcomes in a series of 83 cases. Orthop Traumatol Surg Res. 2014;100(4):413–8.
57. Hintermann B, Knupp M, Barg A. Joint-preserving surgery of asymmetric ankle osteoarthritis with peritalar instability. Foot Ankle Clin. 2013;18(3):503–16.
58. Myerson MS, Zide JR. Management of varus ankle osteoarthritis with joint-preserving osteotomy. Foot Ankle Clin. 2013;18(3):471–80.
59. Rush SM. Supramalleolar osteotomy. Clin Podiatr Med Surg. 2009;26(2):245–57.
60. Speed JB. HB, operative reconstruction of malunited fractures about the ankle joint. JBJS. 1936;18:270–86.
61. Rehn J, Schramm W, Hierholzer G. On the indication and technique of the inversion osteotomies because of malposition after fractures of the lower limbs. Arch Orthop Unfallchir. 1968;63(1):9–18.
62. Janssen G, Dietschi C. Supramalleolar corrective osteotomy after fractures of the leg (author's transl). Z Orthop Ihre Grenzgeb. 1974;112(3):444–9.
63. Janssen G. Proceedings: the supramalleolar correction osteotomy following fracture of the lower leg. Hefte Unfallheilkd. 1973;114:318–21.
64. Weber BG. Operative techniques for supramalleolar valgus osteotomy in adults (author's transl). Unfallheilkunde. 1977;80(5):191–3.
65. Weber BG. Lengthening osteotomy of the fibula to correct a widened mortice of the ankle after fracture. Int Orthop. 1981;4(4):289–93.
66. Bircher, I., Korrekturosteotomien der Fibula nach fehlverheilten Knochelbruchen. 1973.
67. Burssens A, et al. Supramalleolar osteotomy for ankle varus deformity alters subtalar joint alignment. Foot Ankle Int. 2022;43(9):1194–203.
68. Haraguchi N, et al. Supramalleolar lateral opening-wedge osteotomy in conjunction with progressive collapsing foot deformity reconstruction for PCFD with ankle instability. Foot Ankle Int. 2022;43(8):1070–83.
69. Alajlan A, Valderrabano V. Joint preserving surgery for valgus ankle osteoarthritis. Foot Ankle Clin. 2022;27(1):57–72.
70. Krahenbuhl N, et al. Extraarticular supramalleolar osteotomy in asymmetric Varus ankle osteoarthritis. Foot Ankle Int. 2019;40(8):936–47.
71. Chopra V, Stone P, Ng A. Supramalleolar osteotomies. Clin Podiatr Med Surg. 2017;34(4):445–60.
72. Krause F, Veljkovic A, Schmid T. Supramalleolar osteotomies for posttraumatic malalignment of the distal tibia. Foot Ankle Clin. 2016;21(1):1–14.
73. Colin F, et al. Effect of supramalleolar osteotomy and total ankle replacement on talar position in the varus osteoarthritic ankle: a comparative study. Foot Ankle Int. 2014;35(5):445–52.
74. Valderrabano V, et al. Joint-preserving surgery of valgus ankle osteoarthritis. Foot Ankle Clin. 2013;18(3):481–502.

75. Barg A, et al. Supramalleolar osteotomies for degenerative joint disease of the ankle joint: indication, technique and results. Int Orthop. 2013;37(9):1683–95.
76. Tanaka Y. The concept of ankle joint preserving surgery: why does supramalleolar osteotomy work and how to decide when to do an osteotomy or joint replacement. Foot Ankle Clin. 2012;17(4):545–53.
77. Siddiqui NA, Herzenberg JE, Lamm BM. Supramalleolar osteotomy for realignment of the ankle joint. Clin Podiatr Med Surg. 2012;29(4):465–82.
78. Knupp M, Hintermann B. Treatment of asymmetric arthritis of the ankle joint with supramalleolar osteotomies. Foot Ankle Int. 2012;33(3):250–2.
79. Knupp M, et al. Classification and treatment of supramalleolar deformities. Foot Ankle Int. 2011;32(11):1023–31.
80. Hintermann B, Barg A, Knupp M. Corrective supramalleolar osteotomy for malunited pronation-external rotation fractures of the ankle. J Bone Joint Surg Br. 2011;93(10):1367–72.
81. Knupp M, et al. Effect of supramalleolar varus and valgus deformities on the tibiotalar joint: a cadaveric study. Foot Ankle Int. 2011;32(6):609–15.
82. Swords MP, Nemec S. Osteotomy for salvage of the arthritic ankle. Foot Ankle Clin. 2007;12(1):1–13.
83. Savva N, Ramesh R, Richards RH. Supramalleolar osteotomy for unilateral tibial torsion. J Pediatr Orthop B. 2006;15(3):190–3.
84. Krahenbuhl N, et al. Mid- to long-term results of supramalleolar osteotomy. Foot Ankle Int. 2017;38(2):124–32.
85. Tanaka Y, et al. Low tibial osteotomy for varus-type osteoarthritis of the ankle. J Bone Joint Surg Br. 2006;88(7):909–13.
86. Krause F, et al. The effect of the mobile subtalar joint on calcaneal and supramalleolar osteotomies. Foot Ankle Int. 2021;42(12):1606–12.
87. Schmid T, et al. Ankle joint pressure changes in a pes cavovarus model: supramalleolar valgus osteotomy versus lateralizing calcaneal osteotomy. Foot Ankle Int. 2013;34(9):1190–7.
88. Krause FG, et al. Ankle joint pressure changes in a pes cavovarus model after lateralizing calcaneal osteotomies. Foot Ankle Int. 2010;31(9):741–6.
89. Flury A, et al. The unloading effect of supramalleolar versus sliding calcaneal osteotomy for treatment of osteochondral lesions of the medial talus: a biomechanical study. Orthop J Sports Med. 2023;11(10):23259671231176295.
90. Wirth SH, Espinosa N. The use of virtual planning and patient-specific guides to correct complex deformities of the foot and ankle. Foot Ankle Clin. 2020;25(2):257–68.
91. Weigelt L, et al. Three-dimensional correction of complex ankle deformities with computer-assisted planning and patient-specific surgical guides. J Foot Ankle Surg. 2017;56(6):1158–64.
92. Burssens A, Devos Bevernage B, Buedts K. Supramalleolar osteotomies in Cavovarus foot deformity: why patient-specific instruments make a difference. Foot Ankle Clin. 2023;28(4):843–56.

Chapter 9
Anterior Ankle Arthroscopy

C. Niek van Dijk

Introduction

Over the past 25 years, significant advancements have been made in the field of arthroscopic foot and ankle surgery, enabling procedures to be performed with fewer complications and faster recovery times for patients. The use of ankle arthroscopy has increased in recent years, outpacing other joint arthroscopies such as those of the shoulder, knee, and elbow [1].

A Medtech report forecasts that the volume of ankle arthroscopy will experience the most substantial growth, with the United States seeing an annual growth rate of over 6.5%, while the Asia-Pacific region is expected to grow by more than 11.5% annually [2].

In the past, fixed ankle distraction was the standard method for gaining access to the anterior ankle. However, current techniques involve performing anterior arthroscopy without fixed distraction. This so-called dorsiflexion approach enhances the volume of the anterior ankle joint, facilitating easier access to a variety of anatomical structures and resulting in more effective, safer procedures with fewer complications [3].

In the traditional fixed distracted position, the neurovascular structures are under tension, comparable to a bowstring, which prevents them from shifting aside when instruments make their way towards the joint (Fig. 9.1a). This increases the risk of iatrogenic injury. By contrast, in dorsiflexion, the anterior joint capsule and

C. N. van Dijk (✉)
Department of Orthopedic Surgery, University of Amsterdam, Amsterdam UMC Location AMC, Amsterdam, the Netherlands

FIFA Medical Centre of Excellence Ripoll-DePrado Sport Clinic, Madrid, Spain

FIFA Medical Centre of Excellence Clínica do Dragão Porto, Porto, Portugal

Orthopedic Department Casa di Cura San Rossore, Pisa, Italy

M. Bhatia (ed.), *Surgical Techniques of the Foot and Ankle*,
https://doi.org/10.1007/978-3-031-93742-2_9

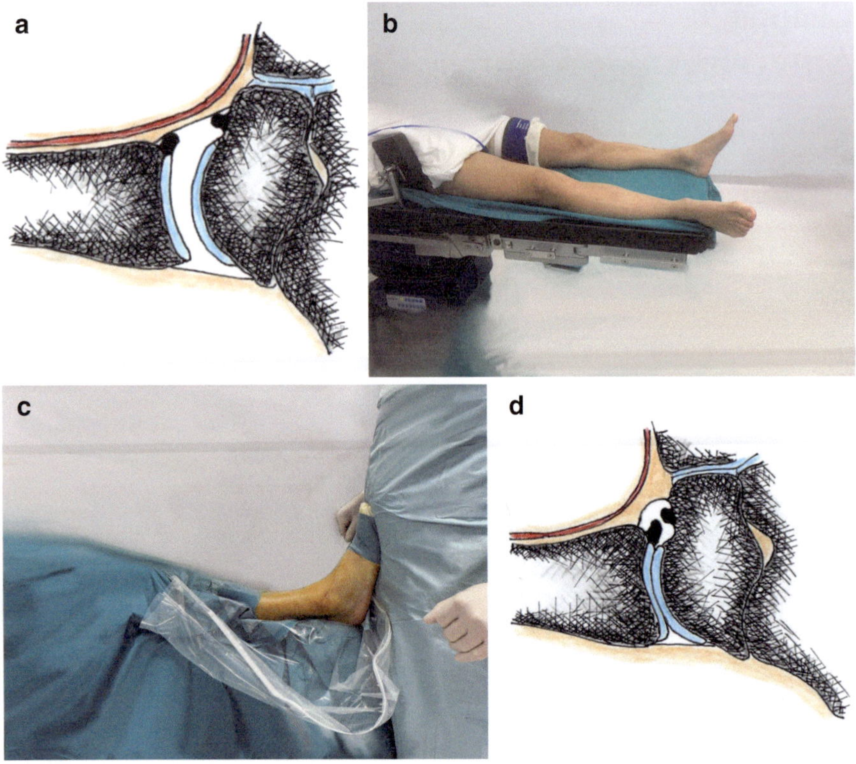

Fig. 9.1 (**a**) In fixed distraction the neurovascular structures (in red) are tight as a bowstring and therefore cannot move aside for a passing instrument. This makes them vulnerable for iatrogenic damage. In addition distraction pulls the deep peroneal nerve towards the joint which decreases the distance between nerve and joint thus increasing the risk of iatrogenic injury. (**b**) Anterior ankle arthroscopy is performed with the patient in a supine position, with slight elevation of the ipsilateral buttock to prevent external rotation of the foot. The heel is positioned at the very edge of the operating table to allow for both dorsiflexion and plantarflexion of the ankle as needed. (**c**) The dorsiflexion method finds it name in the dorsiflexion position in which the instruments shavers and scope are introduced into the joint. After introduction of the instruments—in dorsiflexion—the joint can be brought in any position for the surgical intervention. Each pathology—even each part of the procedure—has its own optimal position: dorsiflexion, neutral, plantar flexion, forced plantar flexion or distraction. (**d**) Dorsiflexion significantly enlarges the anterior joint space moving neurovascular structures (in red) away from the joint reducing the risk of iatrogenic damage. In addition in dorsiflexion the nerves are lax and thus easily pushed aside—in case they are close to the portal—by an instrument that is introduced into the joint, reducing the risk of accidental nerve damage. The talus is shielded within the joint, which protects the cartilage from potential iatrogenic damage

neurovascular structures are relaxed. They are naturally pushed aside by a blunt instrument that is introduced into the joint, reducing the risk of accidental damage to nerves or vessels (Fig. 9.1b, c). Small diameter instruments, such as shavers punches or arthroscope, have a more needle-like shape that increases the likelihood of inadvertent penetration of cartilage, nerves, or blood vessels. These small diameter instruments are more prone to bending or breakage. Larger instruments by their shape are more blunt, provide a clearer view, deliver more fluid into the joint and can more efficiently remove osteophytes and other impediments.

The dorsiflexion method finds its name in the dorsiflexion position in which the instruments (shavers and or scope) are introduced into the joint. Once saline is introduced into the joint, the anterior working area expands, allowing for safe insertion of the arthroscope and surgical instruments. In dorsiflexion, the talus is also shielded within the joint, which protects the cartilage from potential iatrogenic damage (Fig. 9.1c). After introduction of the instruments—in dorsiflexion—the joint can be brought in any position for the surgical intervention. Each pathology—and even each part of the procedure—has its own optimal position: dorsiflexion, neutral, plantar flexion, forced plantar flexion or distraction.

Ankle Pathology and Approach

Most pathologies affecting the ankle joint are located anterior or—in case of cartilage lesions—can be brought into this anterior working space for easier access during surgery [3] (Fig. 9.2). Joint distraction may be helpful to improve access to some posterior located OCD's. A non-invasive distraction device, attached to a sterile belt, allows the surgeon to easily transition between the dorsiflexed position and a distracted position as needed (Fig. 9.3).

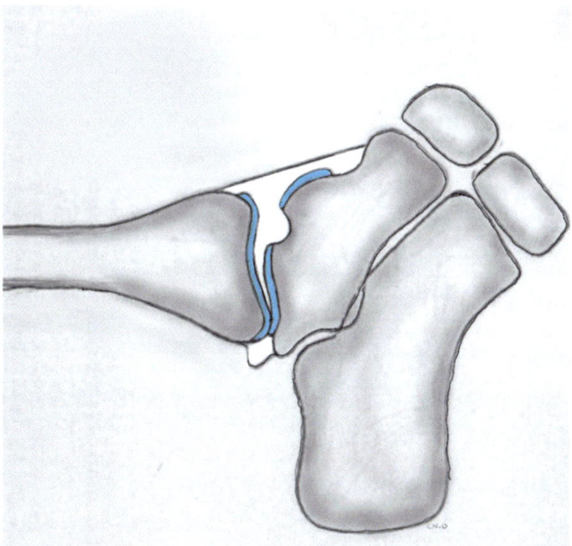

Fig. 9.2 In plantarflexion, the distance between the talus and the anterior tibial plafond widens automatically, providing access to posterior located osteochondral defects

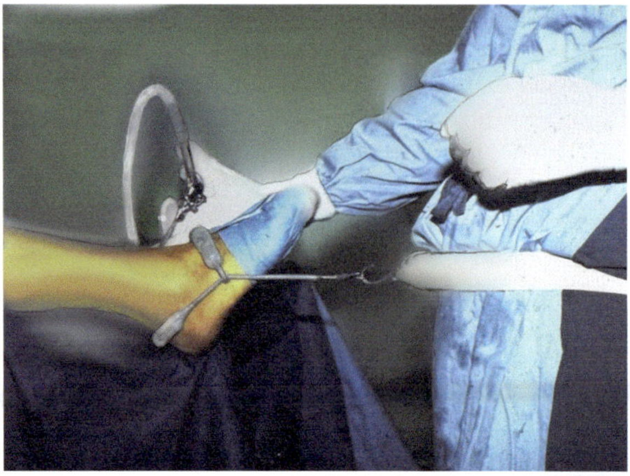

Fig. 9.3 A non-invasive distraction device, attached to a sterile belt, allows the surgeon to easily transition between the dorsiflexed position and a distracted position as needed

Evolution of Ankle Arthroscopy

Ankle arthroscopy was initially employed as a diagnostic tool, but over time, its role has evolved into a therapeutic and reconstructive technique. Recent research has supported its use for all-inside ligament reconstructions, the effective management of impingement syndromes, and the treatment of osteochondral lesions. The indications for ankle arthroscopy have expanded to include fracture management and arthrodesis [4].

This chapter summarizes the progression of ankle arthroscopy techniques over time, highlighting the shift from diagnostic to therapeutic approaches and a shift from fixed distraction to the dorsiflexion method.

Indications

Diagnostic Arthroscopy?

In the early stages of ankle arthroscopy, it was primarily employed as a diagnostic tool. Richard Ferkel reflects on this era, noting: "In 1984, Jim Guhl and I developed the fixed distraction system because we realized that we were missing a lot of pathology. Fixed non-invasive distraction allows the surgeon to see the entire joint, not just parts of it" [5]. This desire for comprehensive assessment led to the development of a methodical 21-point examination of the ankle [6]. At that time, non-invasive diagnostic tools were not as advanced, which made such thorough evaluations plausible.

However, diagnostic practices have evolved. Today, non-invasive imaging techniques are highly accurate and allow for precise diagnoses without the need for routine diagnostic arthroscopy. It is now widely accepted that there is no indication for routine diagnostic arthroscopy in any joint. A definitive diagnosis should always precede surgical intervention. This conclusion is supported by recent reviews, which state that ankle arthroscopy is now exclusively a therapeutic procedure [4].

The 21-point examination, once a standard, is no longer necessary and can increase the risk of iatrogenic cartilage damage when instruments are forced into difficult-to-reach areas unnecessarily. The current approach is more focused: identify the issue directly, address it, and remove the arthroscope.

This paragraph will focus on the role of diagnostic arthroscopy in specific cases, such as ankle fractures, in conjunction with arthroscopic ligament repair, as a second-look procedure after treating osteochondral defects (OCD), for diagnostic needle arthroscopy, and in the removal of asymptomatic osteophytes.

Diagnostic Arthroscopy in Ankle Fractures

Some surgeons advocate for diagnostic arthroscopy in all cases of ankle fractures, largely due to the high incidence of cartilage lesions associated with these injuries. Hintermann's landmark study, often cited in the literature, found that 80% of patients with ankle fractures also had cartilage damage [7]. A similar study by Howard found the rate to be 84% [8]. This led to the assumption that diagnostic arthroscopy should be performed routinely in ankle fractures.

However, interestingly, only about 1% of surgeons in the United States perform arthroscopy on ankle fractures [9]. Even in this small group, additional arthroscopic evaluation does not seem to make a significant clinical difference in outcomes [9].

A recent systematic review and meta-analysis confirmed that there was no difference in outcomes between ankle fracture patients with cartilage damage and those without [10]. From these findings, we can conclude that routine diagnostic arthroscopy in ankle fractures is not beneficial—it does not improve patient outcomes.

Diagnostic Arthroscopy in Chronic Ankle Instability Repair

The majority of patients with chronic ankle instability also present with asymptomatic cartilage damage. This has been shown in several studies [10, 11]. However, as with ankle fractures, research has demonstrated that there is no difference in clinical outcomes between patients with or without chondral lesions [12, 13].

Performing diagnostic arthroscopy at the time of ligament repair does not improve outcomes. In fact, it may lead to unnecessary surgical interventions. Superficial cartilage lesions in patients with ankle fractures or chronic instability mostly have no clinical consequences. Telling patients about or showing them these incidental findings can cause unnecessary concern without offering any real benefit (Fig. 9.4). Therefore, the focus should remain on treating the primary issue—instability or fracture—without being sidetracked by asymptomatic cartilage damage or asymptomatic spurs.

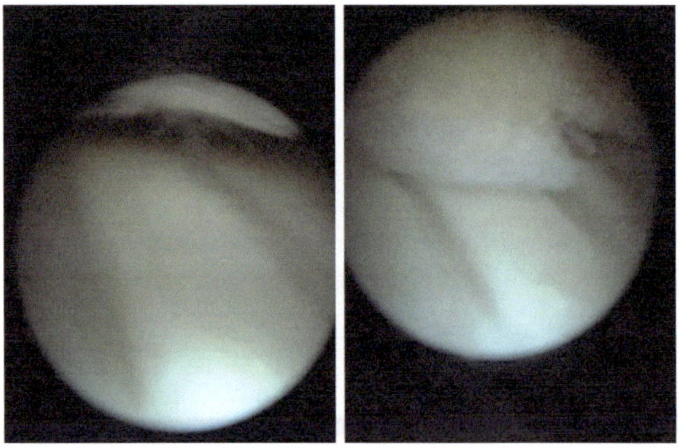

Fig. 9.4 Four tram track lesions as an accidental finding in left ankle of a professional football player. 17 years later no symptoms and no osteoarthritis

Second-Look Arthroscopy After OCD Treatment

Keun-Bae Lee conducted a second-look arthroscopy in 20 patients one year after undergoing microfracture for osteochondral defects (OCD). All 20 patients consented preoperatively to a follow-up arthroscopy to assess their cartilage treatment at 12 months post-surgery. At the time of the second-look procedure, 16 ankles (80%) still had visible cracks and fissures, and 7 ankles (35%) exhibited incomplete healing, classified as ICRS grade III [14]. Despite these findings, all patients showed clinical improvement, and the overall AOFAS scores demonstrated excellent or good results (over 80 points) in 90% of the cases.

A separate study followed 25 patients who underwent a second-look arthroscopy at an average of four years post-microfracture. Of these, 9 ankles (36%) showed incomplete healing with inferior quality of repair tissue, classified as ICRS grade III. However, all patients demonstrated significant clinical improvement from preoperative to latest follow-up ($p < 0.001$) [15]. Additionally, there were no changes in arthritic grading between the preoperative and latest follow-up radiographs.

These findings point to an important conclusion: While arthroscopy allows for evaluation of cartilage status, it is the condition of the subchondral bone that plays the key role in causing the patient's symptoms. Bone defects, such as those seen on MRI as bone marrow oedema or on CT as visible bone defects, correlate directly with symptoms. In contrast, irregularities in the cartilage without subchondral bone involvement do not typically lead to symptoms (Fig. 9.5).

Cartilage damage that does not affect the subchondral bone has little to no clinical significance.

For example, superficial cartilage damage is found in about 60% of patients with lateral ligament ruptures, yet this damage does not progress to osteoarthritis. This type of cartilage injury does not set off a cascade of degenerative changes leading to arthritis. Only very seldom these superficial lesions are the start of a Domino effect leading to joint destruction. On the contrary, treating superficial cartilage lesions may constitute unnecessary intervention that could potentially induce symptoms.

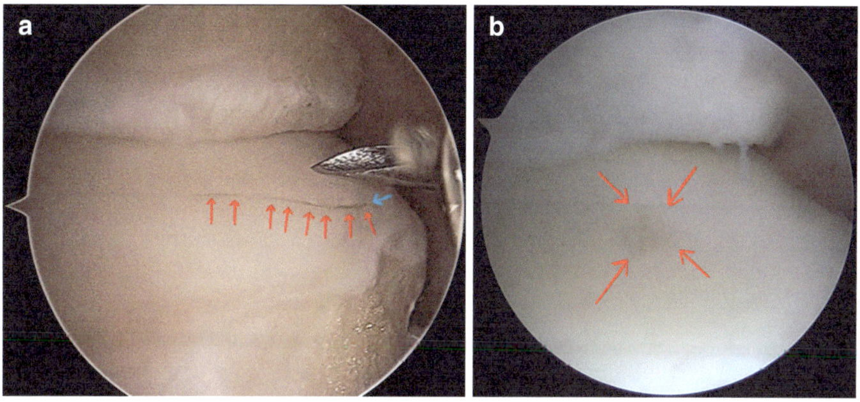

Fig. 9.5 (**a**) Iatrogenic cartilage damage (red arrows) caused by the introduction of a needle. The blue arrow points to the entry point of the needle in the cartilage. (**b**) Iatrogenic cartilage damage from an earlier arthroscopy with an estimated damaged area of 35 mm^2

Similarly, iatrogenic cartilage damage caused by the introduction of surgical instruments—such as mosquito forceps, arthroscopes, probes, shavers, or needles—should not be expected to result in deterioration. (Fig. 9.5).

I invite you to inspect the cartilage of talus and tibial plafond at the finish of any ankle arthroscopy. As for knee surgeons to inspect the condyles and tibia after a meniscectomy or meniscus repair. These iatrogenic cartilage lesions do not typically progress to arthritis, as long as the subchondral bone remains intact.

Needle Arthroscopy

Needle arthroscopy, also known as nanoscopy, is performed using a disposable 2.3 mm arthroscope (including the sheath) and is designed to be used without general anaesthesia, typically in an outpatient setting [16]. As early as the 1990s, it was shown that ankle arthroscopy could be performed effectively with excellent pain control and a high degree of patient satisfaction under local anaesthesia [17]. However, the prediction that we would increasingly rely on local anaesthesia for arthroscopy has not fully materialized [17], and it remains to be seen whether this new technology will change that trend.

If the goal of needle arthroscopy is to assess the status of the cartilage or demonstrate the standing of the cartilage to the patient, then we are heading down the wrong path. Consider the tram track lesions (Fig. 9.4). These lesions do not extend into the subchondral bone and have no clinical consequence. Showing these findings to patients may unnecessarily increase their anxiety. Questions like, "Doctor, is it really safe to walk without cartilage?" will arise. Similarly, performing a second-look needle arthroscopy after cartilage treatment may lead to unnecessary concern. A year after treatment, 80% of patients still show cartilage repair with cracks and fissures, despite achieving good clinical outcomes [14]. Even at four years, 35% of patients with satisfactory clinical results still have incompletely healed cartilage (ICRS grade III) and inferior-quality repair tissue [15]. This raises the inevitable question from patients: "Doctor, is this why my ankle sometimes feels a little stiff? Can you do something about it?"

The nanoscope has also been proposed for injecting substances like hyaluronic acid into the joint, but with less than 90% accuracy [18]. In this context, the single-use nanoscope seems more like a solution in search of an indication, rather than a device addressing a real problem. Moreover, the disposable nature of the nanoscope and its disposable instrument set presents environmental concerns [19], and its widespread use is likely to increase healthcare costs while also raising the risk of unnecessary interventions.

Asymptomatic Spurs and Osteophytes

Diagnostic arthroscopy may detect spurs or osteophytes in asymptomatic individuals, with the chance being approximately 20%. In fact, one in five asymptomatic people between the ages of 20–40 will have spurs or osteophytes [20]. Among patients with chronic ankle instability, 33% may have asymptomatic osteophytes, and up to 50% of those with talar osteochondral defects (OCD) have osteophytes [21].

What happens if these asymptomatic spurs or osteophytes are removed? While the post-operative X-ray may appear aesthetically pleasing, this does not last long. Spurs return over time [22, 23]. These asymptomatic spurs do no harm to the joint; in fact, they can be beneficial as they help stabilize the joint. In the rare event that they become symptomatic, they can always be removed at a later time.

Removal of asymptomatic osteophytes can lead to arthrofibrosis in case of joint immobilisation as for example osteophyte removal in combination with ligament repair. (Fig. 9.6).

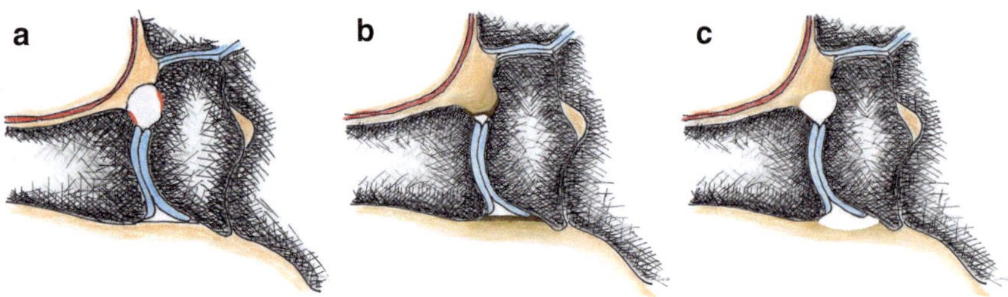

Fig. 9.6 (**a**) Removal of osteophytes (see Fig. 9.1d) leaves the distal tibia and talus with a bleeding bone surface. In order to prevent capsular adhesions and arthrofibrosis, it is important to stimulate early motion. (**b**) Arthrofibrosis results in restricted motion (**c**) Arthroscopic removal of the adhesions and capsule by combined anterior and posterior arthroscopy (See chapter on combined anterior and posterior ankle arthroscopy)

Anterior Ankle Impingement

Anterior ankle impingement syndrome is characterized by anterior ankle pain during physical activity. On clinical examination, recognisable tenderness is found on palpation of the anterior joint line.

If spurs or osteophytes are present, the diagnosis is "anterior bony impingement".

If no osteophytes are found, the diagnosis is "soft tissue impingement". Anterolateral impingement is typically due to soft tissue, whereas anterior and anteromedial impingement are more commonly related to bony involvement.

The pain associated with anterior impingement arises when synovial tissue becomes compressed or "caught" between the anterior margin of the tibia or fibula and the talar neck, particularly when the ankle is in dorsiflexion. Osteophytes reduce the anterior joint space, making it easier for the synovial tissue to become pinched, thereby causing the symptoms.

The rationale for removing osteophytes in these patients is to restore anterior joint space, reducing the likelihood of synovial tissue compression and preventing symptom recurrence.

Arthroscopic treatment involving the removal of osteophytes and/or soft tissue impediments has demonstrated favourable long-term outcomes, with 83% of patients achieving good to excellent results at 5–8 years follow-up for grade 0-I lesions. In patients with osteophytes secondary to arthritis (grade II lesions), the good/excellent result rate drops to 50% [22]. A recent systematic review confirmed an average success rate of 81% for arthroscopic removal of impingements, with patients returning to sports in an average of 8 weeks [25].

Despite a high 76–84% recurrence rate of osteophytes after resection, these patients most often report no recurrence of symptoms [22, 23]. This highlights that osteophytes play a role in joint stability. A study of 670 ankle specimens from individuals aged 20–40 found osteophytes in 21% of the samples, meaning that one in five asymptomatic individuals in this age range will have asymptomatic osteophytes [20].

Osteophytes and spurs typically form within the attachment of the joint capsule. On the talar side, osteophytes can be found just proximal to the talar neck notch. Both tibial and talar osteophytes are easily identifiable during arthroscopic procedures, particularly when the ankle is in dorsiflexion. Notably, the joint capsule does not need to be detached to locate and remove these osteophytes (Textbox 1).

Technical Tip: When removing osteophytes for impingement, a good technique is to identify the distal tibia above the osteophyte with your shaver and work towards the joint. For talar osteophytes, start in front of the spur and work towards the joint (Fig. 9.7).

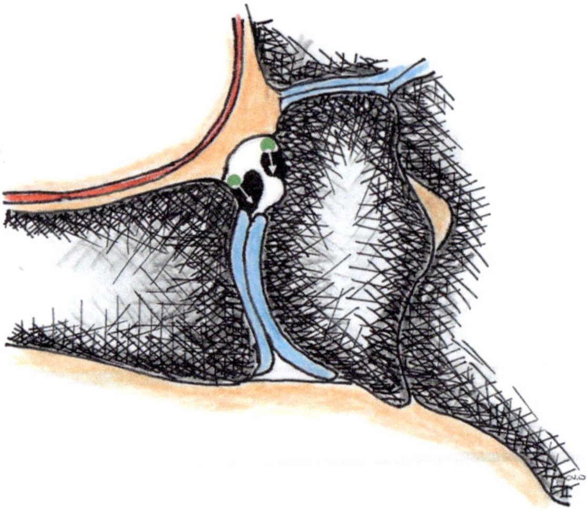

Fig. 9.7 When removing osteophytes identify the distal tibia proximal from the osteophyte with the shaver (blue icon) and use it as a reference as how much bone needs to be removed. For the talar osteophyte start with the shaver in front of the osteophyte and work towards the joint

Osteochondral Defects (OCD) of the Ankle

Overview

Osteochondral defects (OCD) of the talus are lesions that involve both the cartilage and subchondral bone, causing deep ankle pain during or after activity. The pain associated with OCD is perceived by the patient as deep ankle pain which cannot be touched, making it different from the superficial pain associated with anterior impingement. The fluid pressure within the cartilage plays a key role in the pain mechanism. Cartilage is mostly composed of water, and during weight bearing, this interstitial water is compressed through cracks in the subchondral bone into the underlying bone, stimulating the nerve endings and causing pain [26]. Over time, this repetitive fluid pressure can also result in bone resorption and cyst formation [27] (Fig. 9.8). This deep ankle pain is typically not reproducible by physical examination when the ankle is in a neutral position, which helps distinguish it from anterior ankle impingement. Additional diagnostic imaging is often required to confirm the diagnosis and plan treatment.

Surgical Approach and Preoperative Planning

The exact location and size of the lesion should be determined to guide surgical access. The choice of approach (anterior, posterior, combined or through a malleolar osteotomy) depends on the lesions location. A plantar flexed CT scan can assist with the decision making (Fig. 9.9). In my personal 35 years of experience with the treatment of talar OCD, I can roughly say that I have treated >95% with an anterior arthroscopic approach.

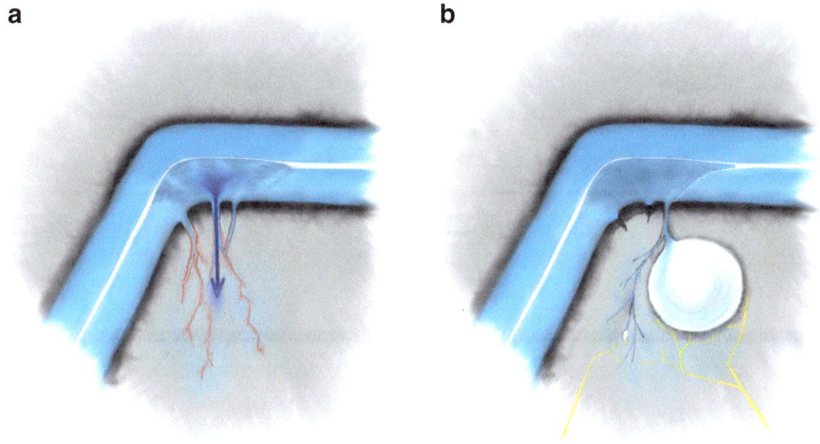

Fig. 9.8 (**a**) Acute injury resulting in damage to the talar cartilage, cracks in the subchondral bone plate and microfractures (red lines) in the subchondral bone. Cartilage is mostly composed of water (for this reason the cartilage is coloured blue in these drawings). During weightbearing, this fluid is compressed from the cartilage through cracks in the subchondral bone into the underlying bone leading to bone marrow oedema on T2 MRI images. When these subchondral bone plate cracks heal these microfractures have no long-term consequence. (**b**) In case a crack in the subchondral bone plate does not heal, then repetitive fluid pressure can cause bone resorption and cyst formation. Nerve endings (in yellow) in the subchondral bone are detected by this intermittent raise in pressure and perceived by the patient as deep ankle pain on activity

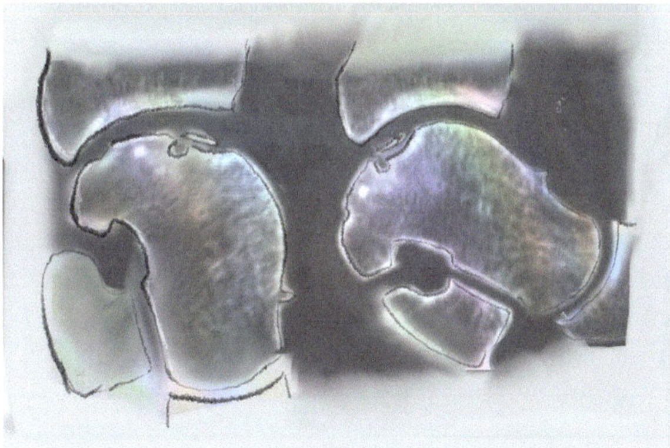

Fig. 9.9 Pre-operative sagittal CT scan with the ankle in plantarflexion, predicts if the lesion can be approached by anterior arthroscopy. Note the anterior widening between anterior distal tibia and talus

Current Evidence on the Treatment of Talar Osteochondral Defects

Microfracture for osteochondral defects (OCD) was first described by Steadman 25 years ago [28], though it was originally developed by Pridie [29]. Since then, numerous cartilage treatments have emerged, primarily aimed at regenerating hyaline cartilage. These treatments include biologic therapies such as Autologous

Chondrocyte Implantation (ACI), Matrix-induced Autologous Chondrocyte Implantation (MACI), Autologous Matrix-induced Chondrogenesis (AMIC), scaffolds, and morselized juvenile cartilage.

So, where do we stand today? Two recent reviews concluded that no single intervention outperforms the others clinically [30, 31]. The pooled success rate of 82% suggests that bone marrow stimulation (BMS) remains the first-line treatment [30]. A recent survey of 1800 surgeons indicated that 78% of them consider BMS their preferred approach [32]. BMS is a minimally invasive, cost-effective procedure that is technically simple, with low complication rates and favourable short- and long-term outcomes.

Long-Term Outcomes of Microfracture

Several studies have shown that the benefits of microfracture are maintained over time. Van Bergen reported 78% good-to-excellent results and an 88% return to sports at 8–20 years of follow-up, with joint space narrowing observed in only 4% of cases [33]. Similarly, Corr et al. reported a 93% survival rate and an 86% return to sport at 10–12 years of follow-up [34]. A study by Park et al. showed a 97% survival rate with 4.5% joint space narrowing at 10–19 years follow-up [35]. A review of six studies reported an average AOFAS score of 84 at a mean follow-up of 13 years, with 78% of patients participating in sports. Joint space narrowing was noted in 4% of patients [30, 36]. Asymptomatic osteophytes, which may have been present before surgery, were found in 30% of patients. While these spurs tend to recur in 84% of cases when removed, they are generally harmless and may even stabilize the joint. 50% of patients with untreated talar OCD have asymptomatic osteophytes [20, 21].

These findings suggest that the effects of microfracture endure over time, while other cartilage treatments lack similarly long-term data (10–20 years). It remains to be seen whether they will yield better results in the future.

Is There a Critical Size for Lesions?

Two foundational studies set a cutoff point for lesion size at 150 mm^2 [37, 38]. Kennedy's group recommends BMS for lesions no larger than 107 mm^2 (7 × 15 mm, or 8 × 13 mm, or 9 × 12 mm). However, the evidence supporting these recommendations is weak, as 24 out of 25 studies included in their review had poor methodology, and 22 of them demonstrated low levels of evidence [39].

A more recent study by Jin Woo Lee's group [35] analysed 202 patients with a mean follow-up of 14 years (ranging from 10 to 19 years). They concluded that clinical results remain stable regardless of lesion size, with no significant differences observed between small, large, or cystic lesions. Lesions smaller than 150 mm^2 had a survival rate of 97%, while lesions larger than 150 mm^2 had a survival rate of 83%. A recent survey of 1800 surgeons revealed that BMS is still the most common treatment for lesions larger than 150 mm^2 [32].

Chondrocyte Cultures and Scaffolds

Since Brittberg's pioneering work [40], large-scale randomized controlled trials (RCTs) have been conducted to compare Autologous Chondrocyte Implantation (ACI) with microfracture. Engebretsen's group, for example, found no significant difference between ACI and microfracture, even at 14 years of follow-up, with the ACI group experiencing twice as many total knee replacements [41].

In the case of ankle OCD, Imhoff reported a 26% rate of subsequent surgeries following AMIC, and Becher's group stopped using AMIC due to unsatisfactory results [42, 43]. They conducted an RCT comparing microfracture with or without AMIC for talar OCD in 32 patients with at least 5 years of follow-up and found no significant difference in outcomes [42]. A recent RCT with 63 patients comparing microfracture alone with microfracture plus a glycerol phosphate/blood implant showed no improvement in clinical or MRI outcomes with the addition of the implant [44].

Two recent systematic reviews concluded that adding cultured chondrocytes or scaffolds does not offer any clinical superiority over microfracture alone [30, 31]. Despite 30 years of research into cartilage repair, there has been little progress in improving outcomes for ankle OCD. Orthopedic treatment is largely about aligning mechanics and biomechanics to harness the body's remarkable natural healing capacity, with cartilage biological repair solutions only offering modest improvements over fibrocartilage.

Postoperative Care

- Weight Bearing: Evidence suggests that there is no significant difference in outcomes between early and delayed weight bearing after BMS. Patients typically begin to bear weight within 6 weeks and may return to sports within 5 months on average [45].
- Fibrocartilage Maturation: Studies show that the fibrocartilage that forms after microfracture continues to mature for up to 2 years post-surgery [46, 47]. As the fibrocartilage matures, patients may experience gradual improvements in pain and function.
- Follow-Up Imaging: Routine follow-up with MRI is generally not necessary unless complications are suspected. Studies have shown that bone marrow edema can persist for up to 2 years without causing symptoms [48].

Key Takeaways talar OCD Treatment

- BMS remains the gold standard for treating lesions up to 150 mm^2, with high success rates, low complications, and satisfactory long-term outcomes (Textbox 2)
- For larger lesions, other options such as fixation or OATS may be more appropriate.
- Biological augmentations like ACI or scaffolds have not shown superior outcomes compared to BMS.
- Routine MRI follow-up is not necessary unless there are concerns about complications.

Ankle Instability

Surgery is indicated for patients with mechanical ankle instability who do not improve after six months of conservative treatment. Anatomic repair involves shortening the elongated ligaments and can be done either through an open surgical approach or arthroscopically. It is currently the golden standard. Anatomic repair can be performed by open or arthroscopic surgery.

Laxity vs. Instability
An ankle with more than 2 mm of displacement on an anterior drawer test is considered lax. However, most lax ankles do not cause symptoms. Laxity is a sign, not a symptom. In contrast, instability is a symptom, specifically recurrent episodes of the ankle "giving way." Functional instability occurs in a stable ankle, while mechanical instability happens in a lax ankle. This paragraph will focus on mechanical instability.

Arthroscopic vs. Open Repair
Two meta-analyses in 2020 reported significant advantages for arthroscopic repair, including higher AOFAS scores, lower Visual Analog Scale (VAS) lower pain scores, and fewer wound complications compared to open repair [49, 50]. The most recent meta-analysis by Moorthy et al. further supported these findings, showing better AOFAS and Karlsson scores, lower pain scores, and fewer wound complications for arthroscopic repair, with similar stress X-ray results for both techniques [51].

Based on these findings, we can conclude that arthroscopic repair leads to better clinical outcomes and fewer complications than open repair. In open repair, both the anterior talofibular ligament (ATFL) and calcaneofibular ligament (CFL) are repaired, while in arthroscopic repair, only the ATFL is addressed. It has been shown that repairing just the ATFL can be sufficient, as de Vries demonstrated already in 2005 [52]. Since the ATFL and CFL are interconnected, tightening the ATFL through a more proximal fixation point on the fibula also tightens the CFL (Fig. 9.10).

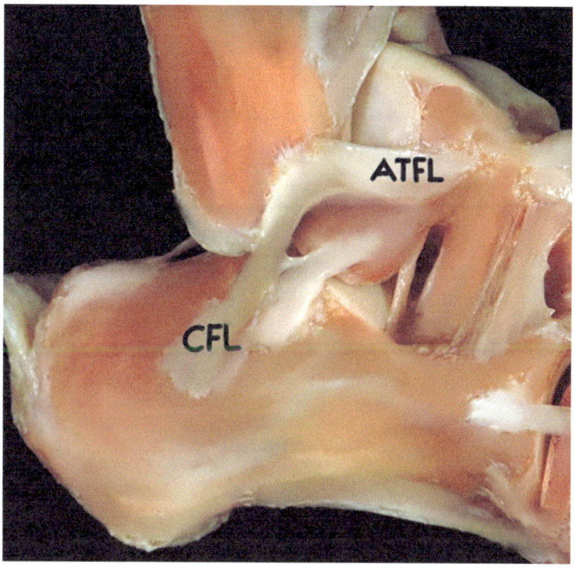

Fig. 9.10 Since the ATFL and CFL are interconnected, fixing the ATFL on a more proximal fixation point on the fibula also tightens the CFL

Operative Technique

Ankle arthroscopy has evolved significantly, and one of the key advancements is the preference for the dorsiflexion method over traditional fixed distraction. This section outlines the benefits of the dorsiflexion technique and compares it with routine distraction methods.

Dorsiflexion Method vs. Fixed Distraction (Textbox 3)

The arthroscopic dorsiflexion technique with distraction, at the discretion of the surgeon, is the current standard for ankle arthroscopy in most parts of the world. The rationale for using the dorsiflexion method for anterior ankle arthroscopy is related to the insertion of the anterior ankle joint capsule, which is located a distance from the articular surfaces (Fig. 9.1c). This provides a large, secure working area at the front of the ankle. Additionally, dorsiflexion helps reduce tension on the anterior neurovascular structures, moving them away from the ankle joint (Fig. 9.1c). This protects them from potential injury during the procedure. Studies have shown that dorsiflexion without distraction leads to a lower complication rate in ankle arthroscopy. In contrast, studies using fixed distraction report an average complication rate between 8% and 17% [53–55], with an overall average of 10%. A series of 1305 consecutive arthroscopic procedures using the dorsiflexion method found a complication rate of just 3% [3, 55], demonstrating a significant advantage of the dorsiflexion approach (Textbox 4). After introduction of the instruments in dorsiflexion, the joint can be positioned in neutral, in plantar flexion or remain in dorsiflexion. Each pathology and even each part of the surgical procedure has its own optimal position for treatment.

For the treatment of certain posteriorly located talar osteochondral defects (OCD), a soft tissue distractor can be applied [56] (Fig. 9.3). Alternative is to approach those lesions by means of a 2-portal posterior approach with the patient prone [57].

Instrumentation for Ankle Arthroscopy

In the past, the ankle joint was considered a small joint and was approached with a small-diameter arthroscope and fragile instruments. However, these days are behind us. The ankle is now regarded as a major joint, and like other major joints such as the knee and shoulder, ankle pathology can be effectively treated with instruments that match the size and capabilities of those used for these larger joints.

For routine ankle arthroscopy, a 4.0 mm arthroscope with a 30-degree oblique lens is commonly used. A smaller, 2.7 mm arthroscope sheath does not provide the same irrigation flow as the standard sheath, which can be a significant disadvantage when using motorized instruments, as these procedures benefit from a consistent and adequate flow of irrigation fluid.

Typically, gravity inflow is sufficient when fluid is introduced through the arthroscope sheath. Alternatively, an arthroscopic pumping device can be used for irrigation.

In addition to standard excisional and motorized instruments for treating osteophytes and ossicles, a 4 mm chisel and/or a small periosteal elevator are valuable tools. For treating osteochondral defects, essential instruments include a closed-cup curette, microfracture probes, and motorized tools for debridement and bone marrow stimulation (BMS).

The 5.5 mm bone cutter shaver is my primary tool [24], used in the majority of procedures, including the treatment of osteochondral defects (OCD). For OCD treatment in a tight ankle, I use a 4.5 mm bone cutter shaver.

Operative Setup for Anterior Ankle Arthroscopy

Anterior ankle arthroscopy is performed with the patient in a supine position, with slight elevation of the ipsilateral buttock to prevent external rotation of the foot. The heel should be positioned at the very edge of the operating table to allow for both dorsiflexion and plantarflexion of the ankle when needed (Fig. 9.1b). A tourniquet is placed on the upper leg. Due to the anterior capsule attachment being 6–8 mm from the articular surface, dorsiflexion of the ankle creates a large anterior working space. This position also allows for visualization of the anterior, medial, and lateral recesses, helping to identify and treat pathologies such as ossicles. Arthroscopic ligament repair and syndesmotic laxity testing can only be done effectively without distraction (Textbox 4).

An ankle harness may be attached to a sterile belt to apply variable distraction, enabling visualization of the tibiofibular recess and access to the posterior joint space [58] (Fig. 9.3). When the ankle is in forced plantarflexion, it allows access to osteochondral lesions (OCD) on the anterior half of the talar bone and beyond (Fig. 9.2). In plantarflexion, the distance between the talus and tibial plafond widens naturally in forced plantar flexion (Fig. 9.2). Providing access to more posteriorly located osteochondral defects. Pre-operative planning, including a CT scan with the ankle in plantarflexion, can help predict if the lesion can be approached via an anterior method (Fig. 9.9).

Portals

The anteromedial (AM) portal is created just medial to the tibialis anterior tendon, where the joint line is easily palpable during passive ankle range of motion (Figs. 9.11 and 9.12). This portal should be made with the ankle in dorsiflexion, as it allows the soft spot at the notch of Harty to be easily identified and helps protect the articular cartilage during the insertion of the curved mosquito forceps. In dorsiflexion, the anterior tibial tendon shifts to a more central position. This position is important for creation of the portal because the medial portal needs to be as centrally located as possible for optimal visualization of the lateral gutter and the attachment of the ATFL. If the joint is distracted or slightly plantar flexed, the anterior tibial tendon moves 1 cm medially, forcing the medial portal to shift to far medial, making visualisation of the lateral gutter and ATFL repair challenging or even impossible.

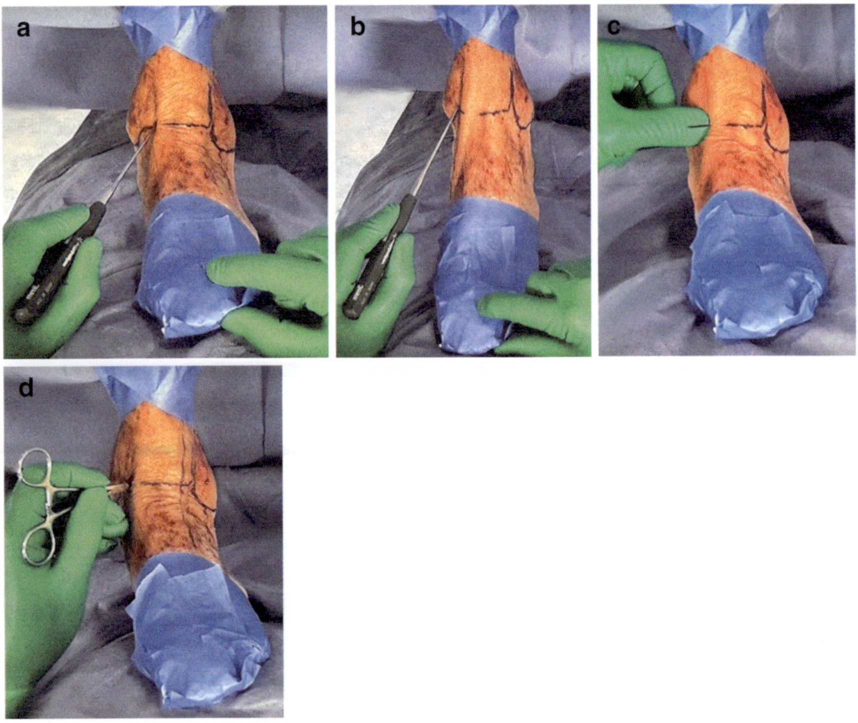

Fig. 9.11 For an adequate view of the lateral gutter and ATFL, the anteromedial portal must be as central as possible but still medial to the anterior tibial tendon ATT. In dorsiflexion the ATT moves lateral/central which facilitates the central location of this portal. (**a**) Left ankle in dorsiflexion. See how the probe moves the 'lax' ATT lateral/central. (**b**) With distraction the anterior tibial tendon moves medial, forcing the medial portal to shift away from the midline. This is undesirable (**c**) In dorsiflexion the joint line is easily palpable during passive ankle range of motion. When the thumb is "locked" in the soft spot at the notch of Harty the joint line is in the middle of the thumb: black line on the thumb is the level of the joint. (**d**) Introduction of a curved mosquito forceps into the joint with a knick and spread technique

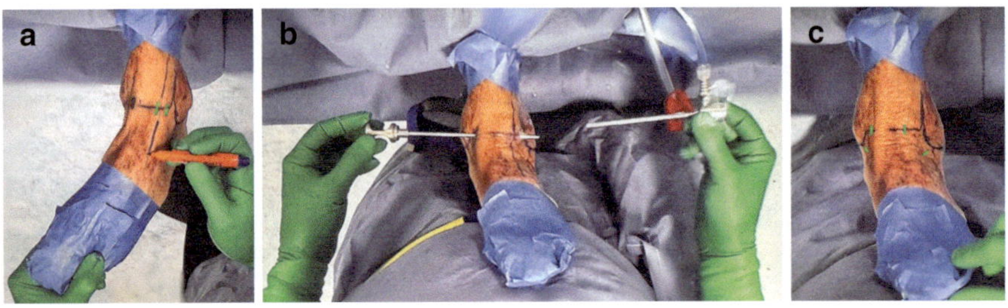

Fig. 9.12 (**a**) The superficial peroneal nerve (SPN), can be identified by bringing the foot in forced inversion-plantar flexion. In green the anterolateral (ALP)portal. The ALP portal is best placed just lateral to the extensor digitorum longus and peroneus tertius tendons and medial from the SPN. In case you want to make it lateral from the SPN then go >5 mm lateral from the marking since the nerve moves under the skin 4–5 mm in a lateral direction when the foot is brought back from inversion to neutral. Blunt dissection with mosquito forceps after skin incision. (**b**) The lateral portal can alternatively be made by an inside-out technique (**c**) the 2 standard portals are shown in green as well as the location of the accessory anteromedial and accessory anterolateral portals

The anterolateral (AL) portal is typically placed just lateral to the extensor digitorum longus and peroneus tertius tendons, using needle localization. However, it can be adjusted depending on the specific pathology being treated. Care must be taken to avoid the cutaneous branch of the superficial peroneal nerve (SPN), which can often be identified pre-operatively. Blunt dissection with mosquito forceps should be done after making the superficial skin incision. All instruments, including the mosquito forceps, blunt trocar, and shaver, should be introduced with the ankle in dorsiflexion. This position allows the neurovascular structures to relax and move out of the way, reducing the risk of iatrogenic damage. In contrast, when the ankle is in a distracted, slightly plantarflexed position, the neurovascular structures are tightly stretched and cannot move aside, making them more vulnerable to injury.

Using the dorsiflexion technique for debridement of anterior ankle impingement is safer and offers a larger working space compared to the ankle distraction method. Dorsiflexion significantly enlarges the anterior joint space while relaxing the anterior neurovascular structures and soft tissues away from the joint line [59] (Fig. 9.1c).

Once the working space is cleared of synovitis and anterior bony spurs, osteochondral talar defects become clearly visible when the ankle is moved in plantar flexion. Forced plantarflexion improves visualization of the cartilage up to the central talar dome (zones 4–6) and the anterior half of the posterior talar dome (zones 7–9). An arthroscopic probe can be used to detect unstable cartilage flaps or fissures (Fig. 9.13). Once the OCL is identified, a curette is used to remove unstable cartilage flaps until a stable rim is formed. Necrotic subchondral bone must be removed with a curette, although a bone shaver may be more effective in cases where the subchondral bone is hard and sclerotic. At this stage, the arthroscope and instruments can be exchanged between the AM and AL portals to achieve satisfactory debridement of the OCL, ensuring a stable rim of healthy cartilage.

Fig. 9.13 Technique of arthroscopic debridement and micro-fracturing for medial talar OCD. (**a**) Coronal CT showing the large and some smaller subchondral cysts. Note the defect in the subchondral bone plate which has lead for these cysts to occur. (**b–d**) 3 subsequent coronal slices from central (**b**) to Medial (**d**) Note the small cysts located anterior from the large cyst and the defect in the subchondral bone plate (**d**). In order to achieve the access as shown in Fig. 9.2 it is always needed to first perform a localised synovectomy opposite the medial OCD. This is done with the ankle in dorsiflexion. The technique is demonstrated in a left ankle with the scoop introduced through the anterolateral portal. (**e**) With the ankle in a semi neutral position the view on the medial malleolus is blocked by the synovitis opposite the medial talus with its OCD (**f**) Same view as in Fig. 9.13e but now with the ankle in plantar flexion. As can be clearly seen the access to the medial talus is completely blocked by the synovitis. (**g**) Ankle is brought back in dorsiflexion. A 5.5 mm bone cutter shaver is introduced through the anteromedial portal. Stay with the back of the shaver on the bone and let the suction do the work. Just a few turn of the shaver is enough to remove the synovitis in this area. (**h**) Clear medial view. Important now to advance the scope to a more medial position before you plantar flex (**i**) plantar flexion opens the anterior joint. The cartilage is intact but the slight elevation of the cartilage (red arrows) indicate the borders of the OCD. (**j**) Probing the soft cartilage (**k**) pushing the probe through the intact cartilage to reach the subchondral bone. (**l**) Lifting the cartilage from the subchondral bone which determines the exact extend and location of the OCD (**m**) Introducing the shaver over the centre of the OCD (**n** and **o**) Carefully pushing in the shaver into the cartilage and into the underlying cyst (**p**) The shaver has entered the large cyst. Red arrows mark the edge of the large cyst. Microfracturing of the cyst walls with a microfracture probe(**q**) Viewing the OCD from the AM portal—switching portals—provides a direct view into the OCD and must be done regularly during the procedure to check the progress and completeness of the debridement. Final view as seen from the anterolateral portal with ankle in a slightly plantar flexed position (**r**) Final view as seen from the anterolateral portal with ankle in a forced maximal plantar flexed position. Good correlation with preop CT scan. Stable cartilage rim. No bone graft applied. 1 = Distal tibia; 2 = Talus; 3 = Shaver (5.5 mm Bone cutter Shaver); 4 = Probe

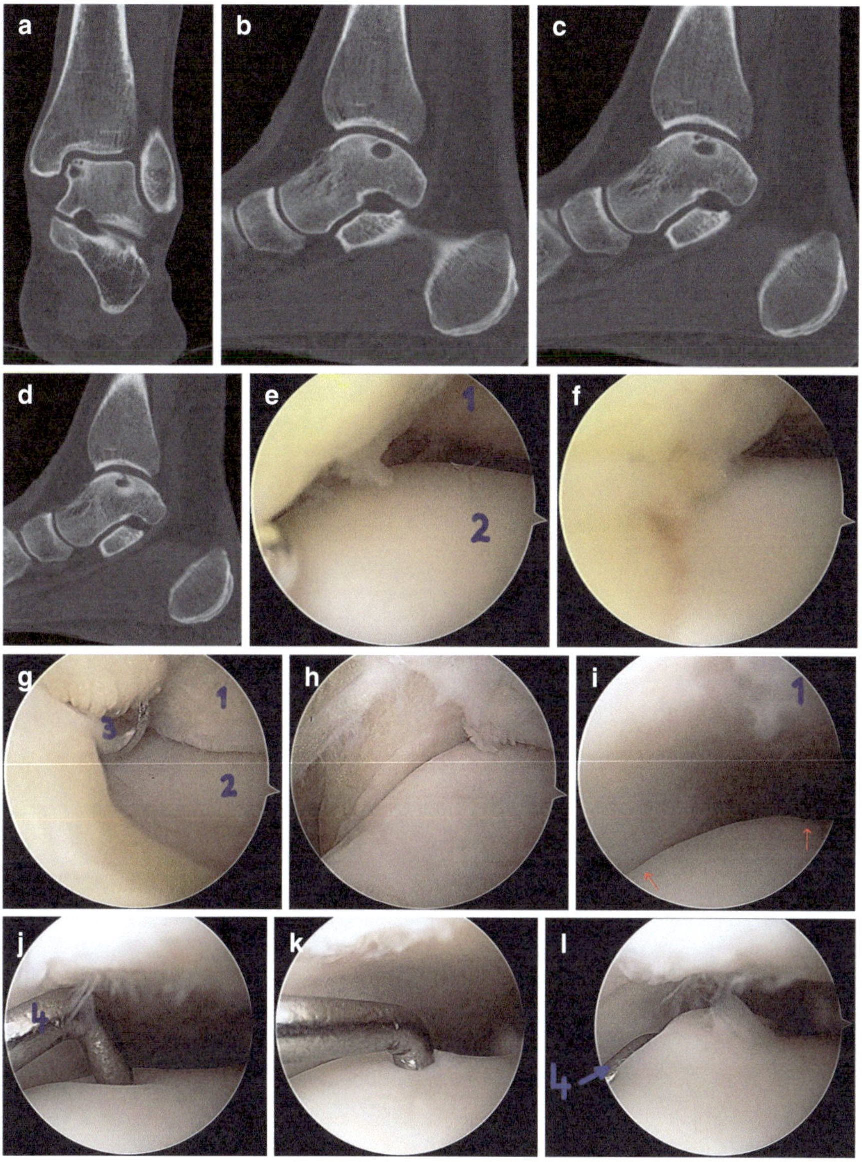

Fig. 9.13 (continued)

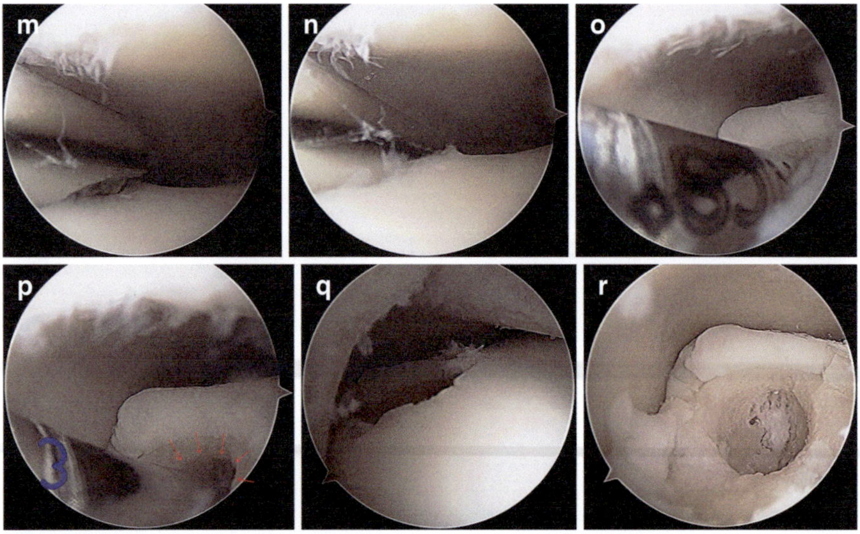

Fig. 9.13 (continued)

Conclusion

This chapter summarizes the progression of ankle arthroscopy techniques over time, highlighting the shift from diagnostic to therapeutic approaches and a shift from fixed distraction to the dorsiflexion method.

With the advancement of diagnostic tools like MRI and CT scans, the role of arthroscopy in diagnosis has become increasingly limited. Particularly in the ankle joint, various asymptomatic changes—such as spurs, ossicles, scar tissue, and cartilage damage—can coexist. A combination of patient history, physical examination, and additional diagnostic imaging is typically sufficient for making an accurate clinical diagnosis and determining the most appropriate surgical approach. Anterior pathologies, such as impingement syndromes, ossicles, loose bodies, and anterior osteochondral defects, can be effectively treated via a two-portal anterior approach [3, 22, 24]. Similarly, posterior ankle pathologies can be addressed with a two-portal hindfoot approach [57].

This highlights the importance of obtaining a diagnosis before proceeding. A proper diagnosis is essential for preoperative planning, allowing the surgeon to determine whether the lesions should be approached from the front, back, through a combined anterior and posterior arthroscopic approach, or via an open approach.

In the past, fixed ankle distraction was the standard method for gaining access to the anterior ankle. However, current techniques involve performing anterior arthroscopy without fixed distraction. This so called dorsiflexion approach enhances the volume of the anterior ankle joint, facilitating easier access to a variety of anatomical structures and resulting in more effective, safer procedures with fewer complications.

The dorsiflexion method finds its name in the dorsiflexion position in which the instruments (shavers and or scope) are introduced into the joint. After introduction of the instruments—in dorsiflexion—the joint can be brought in any position for the surgical intervention. Each pathology—even each part of the procedure—has its own optimal position: dorsiflexion, neutral, plantar flexion, forced plantar flexion or distraction.

This chapter discussed the main indications for anterior ankle arthroscopy and the techniques for effective and safe arthroscopic treatment.

Textbox 1: Anterior Ankle Impingement

- Clinical Presentation: A patient with anterior ankle impingement has anterior ankle pain during activity. Upon examination, recognisable tenderness is present on palpation at the anterior joint line.
- Pain Mechanism: The pain is caused by the compression of synovial tissue between the anterior tibial rim and the talar neck when the ankle is in a dorsiflexed position.
- Role of Osteophytes: Osteophytes reduce the anterior joint space, making it easier for synovial tissue to become compressed.
- Treatment Outcomes:
- Arthroscopic removal of osteophytes and soft tissue impediments leads to 83% good/excellent results, with these outcomes remaining stable over time.
- In patients with osteoarthritis, arthroscopic treatment of anterior ankle impingement yields 50% good/excellent results, which also persist over time.

Textbox 2: Guidelines for OCD Treatment

1. Asymptomatic/Low Symptomatic Lesion: Conservative management.
2. Symptomatic Lesion ≤150 mm^2: BMS (Debridement + Microfracture).
3. Symptomatic Lesions >150 mm^2: Fixation, Autograft or Allograft.
4. Large Cystic Lesions: Retrograde drilling and bone grafting.
5. Failed Primary Treatment: Osteochondral transplant, metal resurfacing, or calcaneal osteotomy.

Textbox 3: Considerations Favouring the Dorsiflexion Method

1. Better Visualization and Access:
   - The anterior joint space is enlarged when the ankle is dorsiflexed, allowing for optimal visualization of the anterior impingement lesions, ossicles, synovitis, and other anterior pathologies.
   - In dorsiflexion, the talar dome is protected from iatrogenic damage, as the joint is locked in a stable position, preventing loose bodies from migrating to the posterior compartment.
2. Neurovascular Protection:
   - The neurovascular structures in dorsiflexion are lax and easily moved aside for instrument insertion, preventing accidental injury. In contrast, distraction makes these structures taut and moves them also closer to the joint, increasing the risk of neurovascular damage.
3. Easier Instrument Handling:
   - Dorsiflexion provides more space to use larger diameter instruments, such as a 4.0 mm arthroscope and larger shavers. These instruments are more effective and less likely to break during use, especially in challenging cases such as osteochondral defect (OCD) treatment.
4. Ergonomics for the Surgeon:
   - Dorsiflexion offers a more ergonomic working position for the surgeon, who can stand at the foot of the table In contrast, with a distracted joint, the surgeon must stand beside the table, which is less ergonomic and more physically taxing.
5. For Posterior Talar OCD:
   - For posteriorly located OCD a soft tissue distractor can be used to create enough space for visualization and treatment [56]. In cases of an OCD located in the most posterior part of the talus, a 2-portal hindfoot approach can be used to access the posterior compartment effectively.

Textbox 4: Current Standard of Anterior Ankle Arthroscopy

- In the fully dorsiflexed position, the anterior working space expands, facilitating the treatment of conditions such as soft tissue and bony impingement, synovitis, loose bodies, and ossicles (Fig. 9.1c).
- The increased anterior working space provided by dorsiflexion allows for the use of a larger diameter arthroscope, which improves saline inflow. This, in turn,

enables the use of larger diameter instruments, which are more blunt and less prone to breakage compared to more fragile instruments.

- When the ankle is in forced plantarflexion, over 95% of talar osteochondral defects can be effectively addressed (Fig. 9.2).
- Smaller diameter instruments, such as shavers and scopes, are more likely to accidentally penetrate cartilage, nerves, or blood vessels. They are also more susceptible to bending or breaking.
- Joint distraction causes tightening of the anterior capsule and closure of the gutters, making it difficult to identify osteophytes, ossicles, loose bodies, and soft tissue obstructions (Fig. 9.1a).
- Arthroscopic ligament repair requires the absence of joint distraction, as distraction prevents the ligament from being tightened effectively.
- In the distracted position, the neurovascular structures are at a heightened risk of iatrogenic injury (Fig. 9.1a).

Bibliography

1. Werner BC, Burrus MT, Park JS, Perumal V, Gwathmey FW. Trends in ankle arthroscopy and its use in the management of pathologic conditions of the lateral ankle in the United States: a National Database Study. Arthroscopy. 2015;31(7):1330–7. https://doi.org/10.1016/j.arthro.2015.01.020. Epub 2015 Mar 12. PMID: 25771425
2. Medtech 360 June 2017 Markets for Arthroscopy Devices http://mrg.net/Products-and-Services/Syndicated)
3. van Dijk CN, van Bergen CJA. Advancements in ankle arthroscopy. J Am Acad Orthop Surg. 2008;16(11):635–46. https://doi.org/10.5435/00124635-200811000 00004.
4. Shah R, Bandikalla VS. Role of arthroscopy in various ankle disorders. Indian J Orthop. 2021;55(2):333–41. https://doi.org/10.1007/s43465-021-003602. eCollection 2021
5. Ferkel RD. Author reply to 'ankle arthroscopy: no-distraction and dorsiflexion technique is the key for ankle arthroscopy evolution'. Letter to the Editor. 2018;34(5):1382–3.
6. Ferkel RD, Ankle and foot arthroscopy. Contemporary approach to diagnosis and treatment. A small joint series technical guide. 2009 Smith & Nephew Inc. http://www.ankle-arthroscopy.co.uk
7. Hintermann B, Regazzoni P, Lampert C, Stutz G, Gächter A. Arthroscopic findings in acute fractures of the ankle. J Bone Joint Surg Br. 2000;82(3):345–51. https://doi.org/10.1302/0301-620x.82b3.10064. PMID: 10813167
8. Howard S, Hoang V, Sagers K, Brady C, Eudy A, Watson TS. Identifying intra-articular pathology with arthroscopy prior to open ankle fracture fixation. Arthrosc Sports Med Rehabil. 2021;3(1):e177–81. https://doi.org/10.1016/j.asmr.2020.08.020. PMID: 33615262; PMCID: PMC7879169
9. Yasui Y, Shimozono Y, Hung CW, Marangon A, Wollstein A, Gianakos AL, Murawski CD, Kennedy JG. Postoperative reoperations and complications in 32,307 ankle fractures with and without concurrent ankle arthroscopic procedures in a 5-year period based on a large U.S. healthcare database. J Foot Ankle Surg. 2019, ISSN 1067-2516,;58(1):6–9. https://doi.org/10.1053/j.jfas.2018.03.030.
10. Darwich A, Adam J, Dally FJ, Hetjens S, Jawhar A. Incidence of concomitant chondral/osteochondral lesions in acute ankle fractures and their effect on clinical outcome: a systematic review and meta-analysis. Arch Orthop Trauma Surg. 2021;141(1):63–74. Epub 2020 Oct 31. Erratum in: Arch Orthop Trauma Surg. 2021 Aug;141(8):1437–1438. PMID: 33128607;

PMCID: PMC8213566, doi:10.1007/s00402-020-03647-5, https://doi.org/10.1007/s00402-021-03985-y
11. Hintermann B, Boss A, Schäfer D. Arthroscopic findings in patients with chronic ankle instability. Am J Sports Med. 2002;30(3):402–9. https://doi.org/10.1177/03635465020300031601.
12. Okuda R, Kinoshita M, Morikawa J, Yasuda T, Abe M. Arthroscopic findings in chronic lateral ankle instability: do focal chondral lesions influence the results of ligament reconstruction? Am J Sports Med. 2005;33(1):35–42. https://doi.org/10.1177/0363546504271058.
13. Yasui Y, Murawski CD, Wollstein A, Kennedy JG. Reoperation rates following ankle ligament procedures performed with and without concomitant arthroscopic procedures. Knee Surg Sports Traumatol Arthrosc. 2017;25(6):1908–15. https://doi.org/10.1007/s00167-016-4207-x. Epub 2016 Jun 16. PMID: 27311448
14. Lee KB, Bai LB, Yoon TR, Jung ST, Seon JK. Second-look arthroscopic findings and clinical outcomes after microfracture for osteochondral lesions of the talus. Am J Sports Med. 2009;37(Suppl 1):63S–70S. https://doi.org/10.1177/0363546509348471. Epub 2009 Oct 20. PMID: 19843658
15. Yang H-Y, Keun-Bae-Lee. Arthroscopic microfracture for osteochondral lesions of the talus: second-look arthroscopic and magnetic resonance analysis of cartilage repair tissue outcomes. J Bone Joint Surg. 2019;102(1):1. https://doi.org/10.2106/JBJS.19.00208.
16. Stornebrink T, Emanuel KS, Shimozono Y, Karlsson J, Kennedy JG, Kerkhoffs GMMJ. A change in scope: redefining minimally invasive. Knee Surg Sports Traumatol Arthrosc. 2020;28(10):3064–5. https://doi.org/10.1007/s00167-020-05898-6. Epub 2020 Feb 11. PMID: 32047997
17. Eriksson E. Arthroscopic surgery and local anaesthesia, vol. 5. KSSTA; 1997. p. 205.
18. Stornebrink T, Stufkens SAS, Mercer NP, Kennedy, Kerkhoffs GMM. Can bedside needle arthroscopy of the ankle be an accurate option for intra-articular delivery of injectable agents? World J Orthop. 2022;13(1):78–86. https://doi.org/10.5312/wjo.v13.i1.78.
19. Egmond PW, Meester RJ, van Dijk CN. From big hands to green fingers: it is time for a change. JISAKOS. 2023;8(4):213–5. https://doi.org/10.1016/j.jisako.2023.04.005).
20. Talbot CE, Knapik DM, Miskovsky SN. Prevalence and location of bone spurs in anterior ankle impingement: A cadaveric investigation. Clin Anat. 2018;31(8):1144–50.
21. Wang DY, Jiao C, Ao YF, Yu JK, Guo QW, Xie X, Chen LX, Zhao F, Pi YB, Li N, Hu YL. Jiang D. Orthop J Sports Med. 2020;8(5):2325967120922821. https://doi.org/10.1177/2325967120922821. eCollection 2020 May. PMID: 32518802
22. van Dijk CN, Tol JL, Verheyen CC. A prospective study of prognostic factors concerning the outcome of arthroscopic surgery for anterior ankle impingement. Am J Sports Med. 1997;25(6):737–45. https://doi.org/10.1177/036354659702500603. PMID: 9397259
23. Walsh SJ, Twaddle BC, Rosenfeldt MP, Boyle MJ. Arthroscopic treatment of anterior ankle impingement: a prospective study of 46 patients with 5-year follow-up. Am J Sports Med. 2014;42(11):2722–6. https://doi.org/10.1177/0363546514550976. Epub 2014 Sep 26. PMID: 25261086
24. Van Dijk CN. Ankle arthroscopy: techniques developed by the Amsterdam foot and ankle school Springer 2014 ISBN-10: 3642359884 and ISBN-13: 978-3642359880.
25. Gianakos AL, Ivander A, DiGiovanni CW, Kennedy JG. Outcomes after arthroscopic surgery for anterior impingement in the ankle joint in the general and athletic populations: does sex play a role? Am J Sports Med. 2021;49(10):2834–42. https://doi.org/10.1177/0363546520980096. Epub 2021 Jan 5. PMID: 33400547
26. van Dijk CN, Reilingh ML, Zengerink M. Van Bergen CJA Osteochondral defects of the ankle: why painfull? KSSTA. 2010;18(5):570–80.
27. Gomoll AH, Madry H, Knutsen G, van Dijk N, Seil R, Brittberg M, Kon E. The subchondral bone in articular cartilage repair: current problems in the surgical management. Knee Surg

Sports Traumatol Arthrosc. 2010;18(4):434–47. https://doi.org/10.1007/s00167-010-1072-x. Epub 2010 Feb 4. PMID: 20130833; PMCID: PMC2839476
28. Steadman RJ, Rodkey WG, Singleton SB. Briggs KK Microfracture technique for full-thickness chondral defects: technique and clinical results. Oper Tech Orthop. 1997;7(4):300–4.
29. Martin R, Jakob RP. Review of K.H. Pridie (1959) on "a method of resurfacing osteoarthritic knee joints". J ISAKOS. 2022;7(1):39–46. https://doi.org/10.1016/j.jisako.2021.11.001. Epub 2021 Dec 6. PMID: 35543659
30. Dahmen J, Lambers KTA, Reilingh ML, van Bergen CJA, Stufkens SAS, Kerkhoffs GMMJ. No superior treatment for primary osteochondral defects of the talus. Knee Surg Sports Traumatol Arthrosc. 2018;26(7):2142–57. https://doi.org/10.1007/s00167-017-4616-5. Epub 2017 Jun 27. PMID: 28656457; PMCID: PMC6061466
31. Anwander H, Vetter P, Kurze C, Farn CJ, Krause FB. Evidence for operative treatment of talar osteochondral lesions: a systematic review. EFORT Open Reviews. 2022;7(7):460–9. https://doi.org/10.1530/EOR-21-0101.
32. Guelfi M, DiGiovanni CW, Calder J, Malagelada F, Cordier G, Takao M, Batista J, Nery C, Delmi M, Dalmau-Pastor M, Carcuro G, Khazen G, Vega J. Large variation in management of talar osteochondral lesions among foot and ankle surgeons: results from an international survey. Knee Surg Sports Traumatol Arthrosc. 2021;29(5):1593–603. https://doi.org/10.1007/s00167-020-06370-1. Epub 2020 Nov 22. PMID: 33221934
33. van Bergen CJ, Kox LS, Maas M, Sierevelt IN, Kerkhoffs GM, van Dijk CN. Arthroscopic treatment of osteochondral defects of the talus: outcomes at eight to twenty years of follow-up. J Bone Joint Surg Am. 2013;95(6):519–25. https://doi.org/10.2106/JBJS.L.00675. PMID: 23515986
34. Corr D, Raikin J, O'Neil J, Raikin S. Long-term outcomes of microfracture for treatment of Osteochondral lesions of the talus. Foot Ankle Int. 2021;42(7):833–40. https://doi.org/10.1177/1071100721995427. Epub 2021 Mar 10. PMID: 33719632
35. Park JH, Park KH, Cho JY, Han SH, Lee JW. Bone marrow stimulation for Osteochondral lesions of the talus: are clinical outcomes maintained 10 years later? Am J Sports Med. 2021;49(5):1220–6. https://doi.org/10.1177/0363546521992471. Epub 2021 Mar 4. PMID: 33661712
36. Rikken QGH, Dahmen J, Stufkens SAS, Kerkhoffs GMMJ. Satisfactory long-term clinical outcomes after bone marrow stimulation of osteochondral lesions of the talus. Knee Surg Sports Traumatol Arthrosc. 2021;29(11):3525–33. https://doi.org/10.1007/s00167-021-06630-8. Epub 2021 Jun 29. PMID: 34185110; PMCID: PMC8514351
37. Choi WJ, Park KK, Kim BS, Lee JW. Osteochondral lesion of the talus: is there a critical defect size for poor outcome? Am J Sports Med. 2009;37(10):1974–80. https://doi.org/10.1177/0363546509335765. Epub 2009 Aug 4. PMID: 19654429
38. Chuckpaiwong B, Berkson EM, Theodore GH. Microfracture for osteochondral lesions of the ankle: outcome analysis and outcome predictors of 105 cases. Arthroscopy. 2008;24(1):106–12. https://doi.org/10.1016/j.arthro.2007.07.022. Epub 2007 Nov 19. PMID: 18182210
39. Ramponi L, Yasui Y, Murawski CD, Ferkel RD, DiGiovanni CW, Kerkhoffs GMMJ, Calder JDF, Takao M, Vannini F, Choi WJ, Lee JW, Stone J, Kennedy JG. Lesion size is a predictor of clinical outcomes after bone marrow stimulation for osteochondral lesions of the talus: a systematic review. Am J Sports Med. 2017;45(7):1698–705. https://doi.org/10.1177/0363546516668292. Epub 2016 Nov 16. PMID: 27852595
40. Brittberg M, Lindahl A, Nilsson A, Ohlsson C, Isaksson O, Peterson L. Treatment of deep cartilage defects in the knee with autologous chondrocyte transplantation. N Engl J Med. 1994;331(14):889–95. https://doi.org/10.1056/NEJM199410063311401. PMID: 8078550

41. Knutsen G, Drogset JO, Engebretsen L, Grøntvedt T, Ludvigsen TC, Løken S, Solheim E, Strand T, Johansen O. A randomized multicenter trial comparing autologous chondrocyte implantation with microfracture: long-term follow-up at 14 to 15 years. J Bone Joint Surg Am. 2016;98(16):1332–9. https://doi.org/10.2106/JBJS.15.01208. PMID: 27535435
42. Becher C, Malahias MA, Ali MM, Maffulli N, Thermann H. Arthroscopic microfracture vs. arthroscopic autologous matrix-induced chondrogenesis for the treatment of articular cartilage defects of the talus. Knee Surg Sports Traumatol Arthrosc. 2019;27(9):2731–6. https://doi.org/10.1007/s00167-018-5278-7. Epub 2018 Nov 3. PMID: 30392029
43. Viehöfer AF, Casari F, Waibel FWA, Beeler S, Imhoff FB, Wirth SH, Ackermann J. Cartilage. 2021;13(1_suppl):1366S–72S. https://doi.org/10.1177/1947603520959405. Epub 2020 Sep 17. PMID: 32940049
44. Camurcu Y, Ucpunar H, Yapici F, et al. Clinical and magnetic resonance imaging outcomes of microfracture plus chitosan/blood implant vs microfracture for osteochondral lesions of the talus. Foot Ankle Int. 2020;41(11):1368–75. https://doi.org/10.1177/1071100720942173.
45. Song M, Li S, Yang S, Dong Q, Lu M. Is early or delayed weightbearing the better choice after microfracture for osteochondral lesions of the talus? A meta-analysis and systematic review. J Foot Ankle Surg. 2021;60(6):1232–40. https://doi.org/10.1053/j.jfas.2021.04.022. Epub 2021 May 10. PMID: 34215515
46. Wei M, Liu Y. Clinical effects of arthroscopic microfracture on osteochondral lesions of the talus. Zhongguo Gu Shang. 2017;30(8):751–4. https://doi.org/10.3969/j.issn.1003-0034.2017.08.014.
47. Kim TY, Song SH, Baek JH, Hwang YG, Jeong BO. Analysis of the changes in the clinical outcomes according to time after arthroscopic microfracture of osteochondral lesions of the talus. Foot Ankle Int. 2019;40(1):74–9. https://doi.org/10.1177/1071100718794944. Epub 2018 Aug 29. PMID: 30156871
48. van Dijk PAD, Murawski CD, Hunt KJ, Andrews CL, Longo UG, Mc Collum G, Simpson H, Sofka CM, Yoshimura I, Karlsson J; International Consensus Group on Cartilage Repair of the Ankle. Post-treatment Follow-up, Imaging, and Outcome Scores: Proceedings of the International Consensus Meeting on Cartilage Repair of the Ankle. Foot Ankle Int. 2018;39(1_suppl):68S–73S. Erratum in: Foot Ankle Int. 2021 Feb;42(2):248. PMID: 30215316. doi:10.1177/1071100718781861, https://doi.org/10.1177/1071100720967713
49. Zhi X, Lv Z, Zhang C, Kong C, Wei S, Xu F. Does arthroscopic repair show superiority over open repair of lateral ankle ligament for chronic lateral ankle instability: a systematic review and meta-analysis. J Orthop Surg Res. 2020;15(1):355. https://doi.org/10.1186/s13018-020-01886-1. PMID: 32843055; PMCID: PMC7448467
50. Brown AJ, Shimozono Y, Hurley ET, Kennedy JG. Arthroscopic versus open repair of lateral ankle ligament for chronic lateral ankle instability: a meta-analysis. Knee Surg Sports Traumatol Arthrosc. 2020;28(5):1611–8. https://doi.org/10.1007/s00167-018-5100-6. Epub 2018 Aug 14. PMID: 30109370
51. Moorthy V, Sayampanathan AA, Yeo NEM, Tay KS. Clinical outcomes of open versus arthroscopic Broström procedure for lateral ankle instability: a meta-analysis. J Foot Ankle Surg. 2021;60(3):577–84. https://doi.org/10.1053/j.jfas.2020.10.001. Epub 2020 Oct 7. PMID: 33509712
52. De Vries J, Struijs PA, Raaymakers EL, Marti RK. Long-term results of the Weber operation for chronic ankle instability: 37 patients followed for 20–30 years. Acta Orthop. 2005;76(6):891–8. https://doi.org/10.1080/17453670510045552. PMID: 16470448
53. Ferkel RD, Heath DD, Guhl JF. Neurological complications of ankle arthroscopy. Arthroscopy. 1996;12:200–8. https://doi.org/10.1016/S0749-8063(96)90011-0.
54. Galla M, Lobenhoffer P. Technique and results of arthroscopic treatment of posterior ankle impingement. Foot Ankle Surg. 2011;17:79–84. https://doi.org/10.1016/j.fas.2010.01.004.

55. Zengerink M, van Dijk CN. Complications in ankle arthroscopy. Knee Surg Sports Traumatol Arthrosc. 2012;20(8):1420–31. https://doi.org/10.1007/s00167-012-2063-x. Epub 2012 Jun 5. PMID: 22669362; PMCID: PMC3402678
56. Dalmau-Pastor M, Vega J. Ankle arthroscopy: no-distraction and dorsiflexion allows advanced techniques. Arthroscopy. 2019;35(12):3171–2. https://doi.org/10.1016/j.arthro.2019.10.013. PMID: 31785741
57. van Dijk CN, Scholten PE, Krips R. A 2-portal endoscopic approach for diagnosis and treatment of posterior ankle pathology. Arthroscopy. 2000;16(8):871–6. https://doi.org/10.1053/jars.2000.19430. PMID: 11078550
58. Van Dijk CN, Verhagen RA, Tol HJ. Technical note: Resterilizable noninvasive ankle distraction device. Arthroscopy. 2001;17(3):E12. https://doi.org/10.1053/jars.2001.19453. PMID: 11239363
59. de Leeuw PA, Golanó P, Clavero JA, van Dijk CN. Anterior ankle arthroscopy, distraction or dorsiflexion? Knee Surg Sports Traumatol Arthrosc. 2010;18(5):594–600. https://doi.org/10.1007/s00167-010-1089-1. Epub 2010 Mar 9. PMID: 20217392; PMCID: PMC2855029

Chapter 10
Posterior Arthroscopy of Ankle and Subtalar Joints

Xavier Martin Oliva

Introduction

For many years, ankle arthroscopy has played a role in foot and ankle surgery. However, since 2000, when Van Dijk et al. [1] introduced the 2-portal posterior approach for hindfoot arthroscopy with the patient in the prone position, an important change has taken place in the surgical treatment of ankle and subtalar pathology. In contrast to anterior ankle pathology, most structures of the hindfoot have a deep location that makes direct access more difficult. Until 2000, posterior soft tissue and bone impingement and tendonitis of the flexor hallucis longus (FHL) were only treated by open surgery. Further, subtalar arthrodesis was performed using an open lateral approach, mini-open treatments, or lateral arthroscopic procedures. Hindfoot endoscopy by means of this two portal approach with the patient in the prone position allows the treatment of posterior hindfoot pathologies reducing morbidity, such as fewer soft tissue complications. This is optimal for patients who are smokers and those with diabetes or vascular diseases.

Anatomy

For us the concept of peritalar joint is very important in the function of the hindfoot and it is an anatomical functional structure formed by the ankle joint, subtalar joint and talo-navicular joint. This joint is mainly stabilized by different ligament structures.

X. Martin Oliva (✉)
Foot and ankle Unit, H.M. Hospital, Barcelona, Catalonia, Spain

Anatomy Department, Barcelona University, Barcelona, Catalonia, Spain

M. Bhatia (ed.), *Surgical Techniques of the Foot and Ankle*,
https://doi.org/10.1007/978-3-031-93742-2_10

1. Lateral ligament complex, formed by the anterior talofibular ligament, calcaneofibular ligament (Fig. 10.1), and posterior talofibular ligament.
2. Medial ligament complex (deltoid ligament), formed by the superficial deltoid ligament with 4 fascicles (tibiospring tibionavicular, tibiocalcaneal and superficial posterior tibiotalar) and the deep deltoid ligament with 2 fascicles (deep anterior tibiotalar and deep posterior tibiotalar).
3. Anterior Syndesmotic ligaments. The tibiofibular joint is ensured in its anterior part by the anterior tibiofibular ligament and the interosseous membrane, forming the anterior syndesmosis.
4. Posterior Syndesmotic ligaments. In this anatomical region, covering the posterior part of the ankle joint capsule we find the Rouvière-Canela ligament (fibulotalocalcaneal ligament). Anterior to this ligament and the joint capsule, we find the posterior tibiofibular ligament that is generally found with two fascicles, one proximal that runs from the tibia to the posterior part of the fibula (superficial fascicle) and the most distal fascicle that is inserted into a canal posteriorly on the lateral malleolus (posterior deep tibiofibular ligament also called transverse ligament) (Fig. 10.2) [2]. Both stabilize the posterior syndesmosis. As Van Dijk described, the best way to visualize this ligament is by anterior arthroscopy

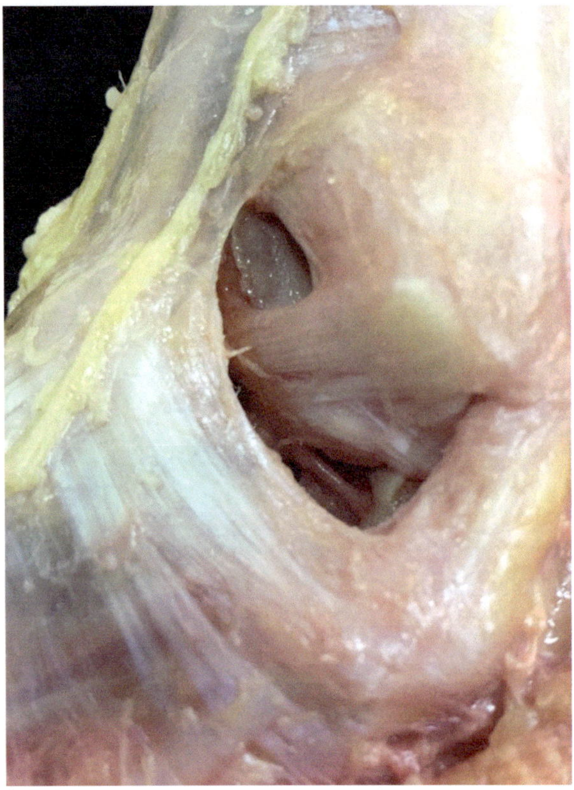

Fig. 10.1 Lateral ligament complex, formed by the anterior talofibular ligament, calcaneofibular ligament

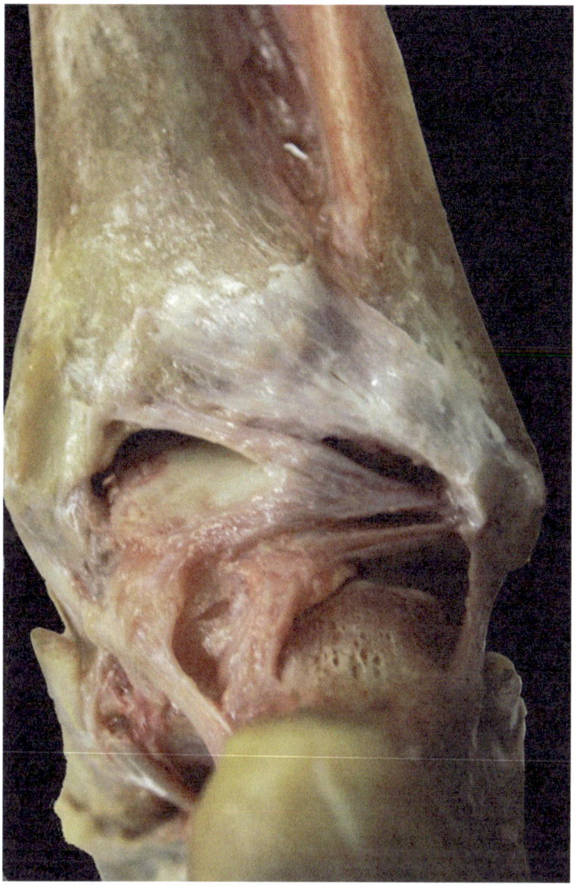

Fig. 10.2 Posterior tibiofibular ligament, with two fascicles, one proximal that runs from the tibia to the posterior part of the fibula (superficial fascicle) and the most distal fascicle that is inserted into a canal posteriorly on the lateral malleolus (posterior deep tibiofibular ligament also called transverse ligament)

when we look at the anterior capsule. More distally, we find the intermalleolar ligament. Another ligamentous structure we mentioned earlier when referring to the lateral complex of the ankle is the posterior talofibular fascicle, which we see in the posterior arthroscopy inserting in the posterolateral tubercle of the talus at the level of the FHL groove (Fig. 10.3).

5. Subtalar joint ligaments. We describe different ligaments that stabilize the subtalar joint, divided into intrinsics and extrinsics. The intrinsic ligament is composed of the interosseous talocalcaneal ligament (ITCL), cephalic ligament (CL) and the anterior capsular ligament (ACaL). The extrinsic ligament is composed of the 3 components of the inferior extensor retinaculum (IER), lateral, medial and intermediate. However, we must consider the CFL because it is the only ligament crossing both the tibiotalar and subtalar joints. Despite having a major role on the stability of the tibiotalar joint, this ligament is fundamental to the subtalar stability. The CL is the only subtalar ligament easily visualized in the anterior part of the tarsal sinus, whereas the ITCL, ACaL, and IER are difficult

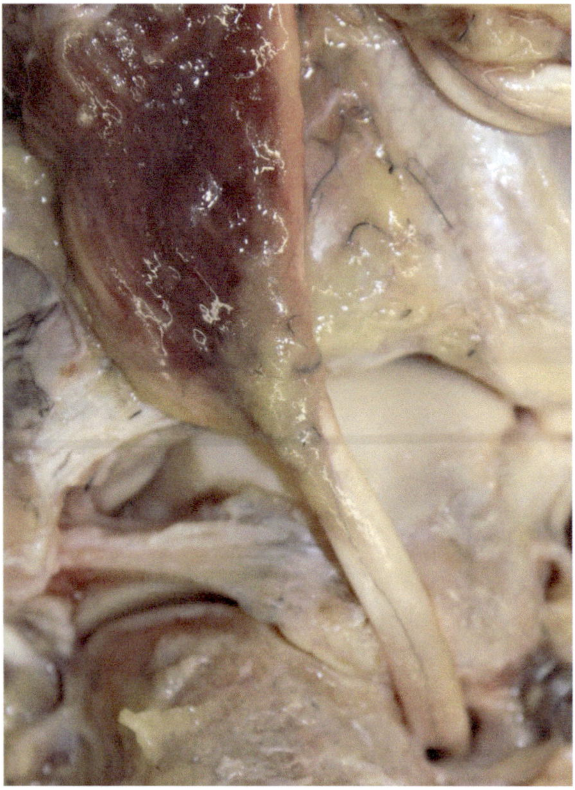

Fig. 10.3 FHL, running by the Talus groove. Also Postero lateral tubercle and the insertion of the post talo fibular ligaments

to assess because they remain in the posterior part of the tarsal sinus.Perhaps, this may be the cause for the different descriptions, location, and nomenclature found in the literature about the subtalar ligaments.

The CL can be described as a thin structure in the tarsal sinus in front of the IER. This ligament has been found wider than the ATFL and ITFL and located anterior to the IER. This ligament has an intimate relation to the posterior surface of the calcaneus-navicular joint capsule. Both footprints of the CL are in the tarsal sinus. The calcaneus footprint is located at the superior anterolateral surface of the calcaneus while the talus footprint is located at the medial surface of the talus neck approximately 2.8 mm posterior to the talonavicular joint [3] cartilage.

The ACaL runs vertically to the calcaneus surface. It has been described as a rectangular bundle when found in the anterior part of the posterior subtalar joint capsule, at the level of the anterior border of this [4] joint. However, conflicting reports of its prevalence remain in the literature. The ITCL remains anterior to the ACaL has been described in a Y and V shape located in the tarsal canal running in an oblique direction with a length varying [3] from 10.7 to 11 mm.

The CFL is the only ligament that crosses the tibiotalar and subtalar joint. The CFL acts as a restraint to anterolateral ankle laxity with assistance of the lateral talocalcaneaL ligament. The CFL provides stability to the subtalar joint when the ankle is neutral dorsiflexion-plantarflexion and restricts the adduction when the ankle is in neutral position and in [5] dorsiflexion. The IER is found in the lateral surface of the Chopart joint. Three divisions of the IER can be described: medial, intermediate, and lateral root.

The lateral root can be found attached to the lateral border of the tarsal sinus running to the calcaneus superolateral facet. Medial to the lateral root lays the intermediate root and medial to it lays the medial root. The medial root runs from the IER to the tarsal sinus, it penetrates the tarsal canal, and it finally inserts in the talus and calcaneus, almost in contact with the ITCL insertion on the talus and [6] calcaneus. The medial root insertion on the calcaneus has a V-shape inside the tarsal canal. This insertion is reported as constant meanwhile the talus insertion has a 75% incidence. The layout described for this root is fundamental in stabilizing the subtalar joint as well as its dynamic roll due to the extensor tendons action.

Indications of Posterior Arthroscopic Procedures: Osteochondral Lesions

In our clinical practice, when there is a suspicion of an osteochondral lesion of the talus, we always perform X-ray and MRI studies, which allow us to confirm the diagnosis and assess associated injuries. Finally, with a CT scan, we achieve the planning of our surgery. When we diagnose a primary osteochondral lesion with a surface area of less than 1.5–2 cm, the technique of arthroscopic debridement, curettage, and microfractures to penetrate the subchondral plate without penetrating the subchondral bone and respecting the surrounding cartilage, is our gold standard indication.

Elias, in his MRI study, achieved a topographic description of the lesions, dividing the talar dome into 9 anatomical zones.

When the lesion affects zones 7, 8, and 9, which are very difficult to treat with anterior arthroscopic approaches, posterior approaches provide us with excellent visualization and treatment options.

Insertional Achilles Tendonitis Secondary to Haglund

Arthroscopic treatment of insertional Achilles tendinitis secondary to a Haglund deformity, which causes compression on the distal area of the Achilles tendon, is an alternative to the open resection of the posterior tuberosity of the calcaneus through a lateral incision. Using posterior arthroscopic approaches, we can identify the insertion of the Achilles tendon and resect the pre-Achilles bursa and the posterior tuberosity of the calcaneus.

Posterior Bone and Soft Tissue Impingement

To explain this clinical scenario, it is important to know the anatomy of the posterior area of the talus, with its two tubercles, the posterolateral, is where Shepherd's fractures occur. In some cases, we also find the accessory bone, os trigonum, and the Stieda process, which cause impingement with the flexor hallucis longus (FHL) tendon. and posteromedial tubercles, where we find Cedell's fractures. It is also important to note that the posterior talofibular ligament (PTFL) inserts at the posterolateral tubercle of the talus. These tubercles delimit the groove through which the tendon of the flexor hallucis longus (FHL) runs. This tendon originates from the posterior area of the fibula and the interosseous membrane, and at the level of the posterior part of the subtalar joint, it runs through the groove between the two posterior tubercles of the talus.

Pain is caused by an abnormal movement between the os trigonum and talus, compression of a thickened joint capsule with os trigonum or postero lateral talus apophysis, scar tissue between the os trigonum and the posterior tibial rim or some fibrosis or postero lateral apophysis contact with flexor hallucis longus tendon. Flexor hallucis longus tendinitis is often present in patients with posterior ankle impingement syndrome, with the pain located posteromedially.

The main procedures to be performed are resection of an os trigonum, reduction of a prominent posterior talar process, resection of the intermalleolar ligament or liberation of Flexor hallucis longus tendon fibrosis. All these conditions could be affiliated as probable cause and also related to a Flexor Hallucis Longus (FHL) tendonitis [7].

During examination there is pain at palpation of the posterior aspect of the talus. The posterior talar process can be palpated posterolaterally between peroneal tendons and the Achilles tendon. On the posteromedial side, the neurovascular bundle and flexor tendons cover the talus. Posteromedial pain on palpation therefore does not automatically indicate impingement pain. The passive forced plantar flexion test is most important. With this test the examiner performs repetitive quick passive forced plantar hyperflexion movements [8].

We always confirm the diagnosis with XRay and MRI study and finally a postero lateral anesthesic infiltration could confirm our diagnosis.

Release of the FHL tendon can be performed by resection of the flexor retinaculum, removal of adhesions, and release of the flexor tendon sheath.

Overuse injuries associated with posterior impingement often occur in ballet dancers and runners, whereas acute symptoms result from a hyperplantarflexion or supination trauma, predominantly in soccer players.In one study posterior ankle impingement caused by overuse seemed to have a better prognosis [9]. An os trigonum is usually not the cause of impingement on its own.

Van Dijk's group's research into retired dancers is interesting.They analysed the average length of ballet dancers careers that spanned 37 years. All of the dancers had been dancing en pointe. None of these dancers had suffered a posterior ankle impingement syndrome. A hypertrophic posterior talar process or an os trigonum (Fig. 10.4) was present in 18 of the 38 investigated ankle joints. The presence of an os trigonum itself therefore does not seem to be relevant. This anatomic anomaly must be combined with a traumatic event such as supination trauma, dancing on hard surfaces, or pushing beyond anatomic limits. The pain is caused by an abnormal movement between the os trigonum and talus or compression of a thickened joint capsule / scar tissue between the os trigonum and the posterior tibial rim [10].

Conservative treatment (physical therapy, antiinflammatory drugs, local injection) is effective in approximately 60% of the patients according to Hedrick and McBryde [11]. If, after 3–6 months, conservative treatment fails to correct the symptoms, the adequate choice would be hindfoot endoscopic surgery.

Fractures

Literature has shown without doubt that anatomic restoration of the calcaneal shape and joint congruity predict greater functional scores [12, 13] and a lower incidence of post-traumatic subtalar arthritis [14].

There are common significant risks of wound problems with open reduction and internal fixation of a calcaneus fracture, with reported rates of deep infection of 8–25%, with superficial infection occurring in 40% and wound necrosis in around 14%.

Calcaneal fractures with little displacement and a fragment that allows mobilization, an arthroscopic reduction and fixation with minimal incision can be attempted

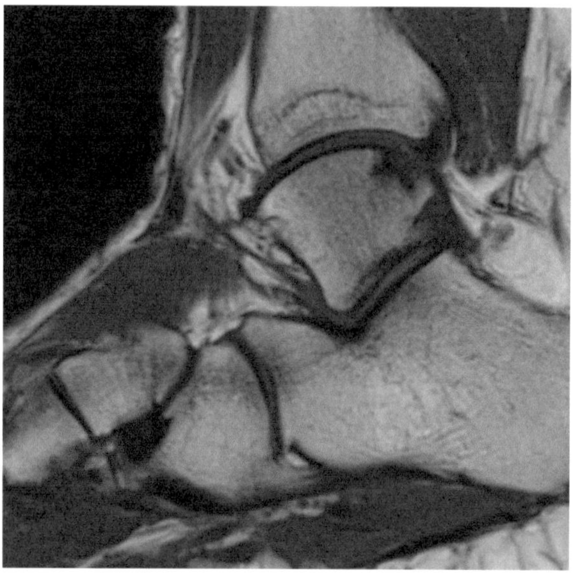

Fig. 10.4 A hypertrophic posterior talar process

[15]. This can be achieved by elevating the depressed posterior facet percutaneously under image intensifier guidance and at the same time performing an arthroscopy using 2 sinus tarsi portals and often a third posterolateral portal.

Subtalar Arthrodesis

Isolated subtalar joint fusion is usually preferred rather than triple arthrodesis to preserve transverse tarsal joint motion and decrease the potential for degenerative joint disease in the ipsilateral periarticular joints. Is a well documented and accepted procedure for surgical treatment of subtalar joint pathology presenting with pain, instability and deformity that does not respond to conservative treatment. The main indications are calcaneal fracture nonunions, malunions, primary, inflammatory or post-traumatic subtalar joint arthritis, painful talocalcaneal coalitions, and neuromuscular/tendon disorders that lead to subtalar joint instability [16].

In patients with soft tissues problems, the arthroscopic arthrodesis is a very good option that almost completely avoids wound complications [17]. In the subtalar arthrodesis by posterior ankle approaches the contra-indications are: severe varus or valgus deformities of the hindfoot such as some sequels of calcaneal fractures [18, 19], single or multi-plane deformities [20], failed arthrodesis which require an open approach and extended debridement [21].

Subtalar arthroscopy is a more demanding procedure, but offers a less invasive surgery with many potential advantages over traditional open methods [22], like preservation of blood supply, faster recovery, less pain, preservation of foot proprioception and fewer complications [23, 24]. However if a moderate hindfoot deformity exists subtalar arthrodesis can't be addressed by an arthroscopic procedure. Many authors are beginning to use the posterior portals for subtalar arthrodesis with a high union rate and less complications [25].

Posterior Ankle Arthroscopy Technique and Our Tricks

The patient is placed in the prone position with the foot hanging off the operating table and a support under the tibia, to allow plantar and dorsiflexion, eversion and inversion of the ankle joint. This position is preferred to the lateral position. Skin traction is avoided.

The equipment necessary to complete the procedure is:

- 4 mm arthroscope.
- 2.7 mm arthroscope for tight joints or in selected cases
- Curettes.
- Chisels.

- Drill.
- Shaver

All procedures are performed under general or regional anaesthesia. A tourniquet is used and prophylactic antibiotics are administered. Patients are placed prone with the foot outside the operating table edge. We never use traction.

The prone position helps us create a working space between the Achilles tendon and the posterior area of the tibiotalar and subtalar joint.

We use two posterior arthroscopic portals while other authors recommend 3 portals, specially in subtalar arthrodesis technique [26]. Precise placement of portals is important in order to avoid neuro-vascular bundle injury and to allow proper articular access. Sural nerve is at an average of 9.7 mm from the postero lateral approach (Fig. 10.5) and the posterior tibial nerve and vascular structures are at an average distance of 7.27 mm and 11.4 mm respectively from the postero medial approach [27] (Fig. 10.6).

The posterolateral portal is first made 1 cm proximal to the distal point of the lateral malleolus and adjacent to the lateral edge of the Achilles tendon. The posteromedial portal is made at the same level on the medial edge of the Achilles.

Fig. 10.5 Sural nerve are at an average of 9,7 mm. from the postero lateral approach

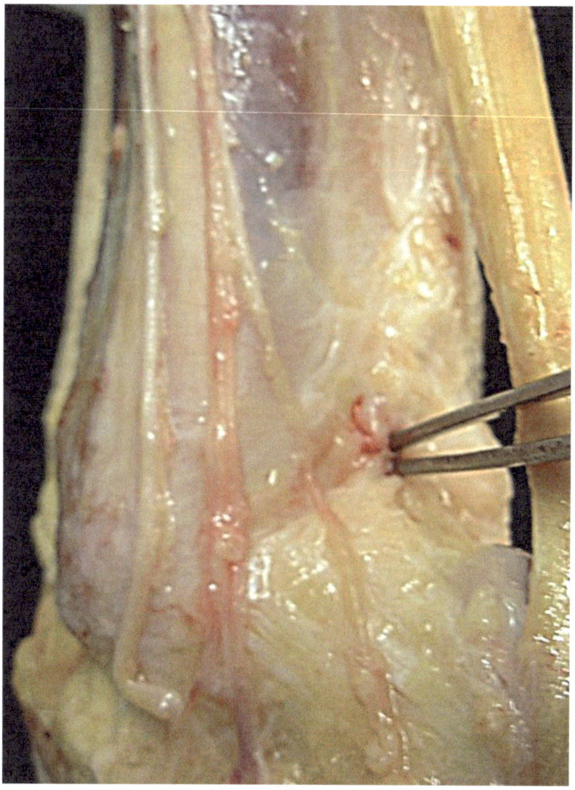

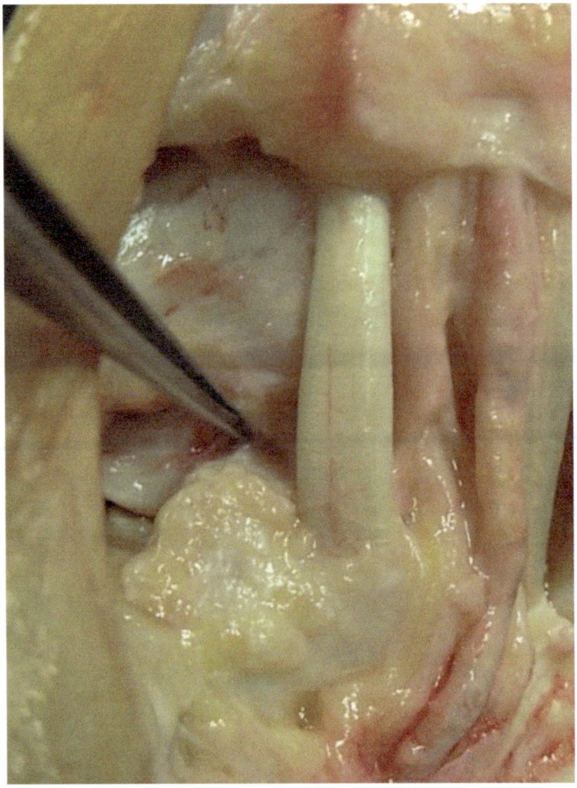

Fig. 10.6 Post tibial nerve and vascular structures are at an average distance of 7,27 mm and 11,4 mm respectively from the postero medial approach

The scope (4.5-mm 30° optic athroscope) is introduced through the posterolateral portal directed towards the second metatarsal, until the posterior part of the talus bone can be felt. If the instruments are introduced through the posteromedial portal in the same direction, damage to the posterior tibial nerve is very probable (Fig. 10.7).

To avoid this complication, the blunt trocar is introduced through the posteromedial incision and after reaching the Achilles tendon, it is turned 90° laterally, until the sheath of the optical device can be felt (Fig. 10.8). Keeping this metallic contact we slide the trocar along the sheath until reaching the posterior part of the tibio talar articulation or the talus (Fig. 10.9) as was described by Martin Oliva [28].

When portals are placed close to the Achilles tendon, instruments introduced in the correct direction (pointing the middle) and using the FHL as a medial boundary marker, posterior portals are safe [29].

The crural fascia in the posterior area of the ankle is called the Rouvière ligament. This structure must be resected in order to access the posterior processes of the talus.

Clear vision of the posterior part of the ankle joint is often obstructed with abundant fatty tissue and it is important to spend time clearing it away with a shaver and blunt trocar using gentle movements. The main objective is to visualize the FHL

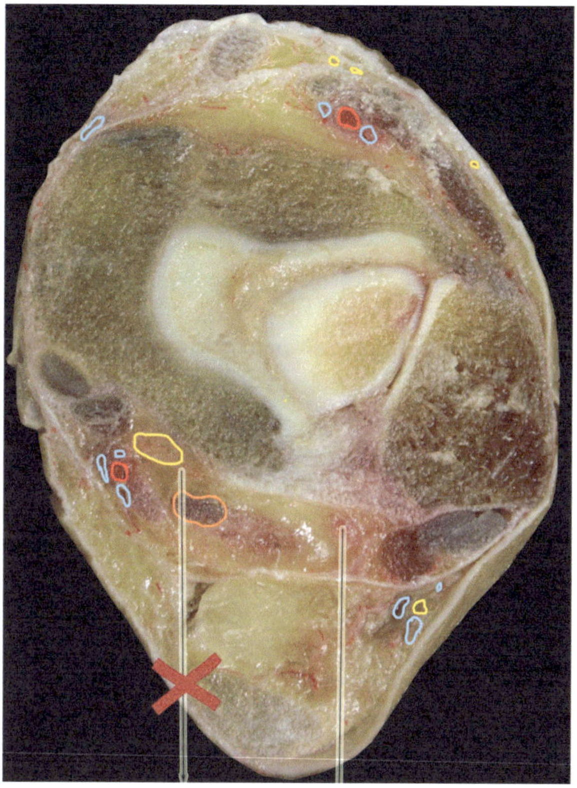

Fig. 10.7 The scope is introduced through the posterolateral portal directed towards the second metatarsal, until the posterior part of the talus bone can be felt. If the instruments are introduced through the posteromedial portal in the same direction, damage to the posterior tibial nerve is very probable

tendon, the posterior intermalleolar ligament, the posterior tibio peroneal ligament and tibiotalar and subtalar articular surfaces. It is important to stay lateral to the FHL tendon because that way we can protect the posterior tibial neurovascular bundle, that we find just medial to the tendon. Lifting the posterior intermalleolar ligament using the probe we observe the ankle joint.

The resection of the talo calcaneal ligament allows visualization of the subtalar articular surfaces.

Having identified the articular structures and the FHL, we are able to perform a careful resection of the Os trigonum, and in other patients a resection of an enlarged Stieda's process. During these procedures, in some cases, we use an elastic vessel loop to separate the FHL tendon and avoid damaging it.

Also we perform with a radiofrequency wand a release of the FHL in cases of chronic tendinitis (sometimes the cause is post-traumatic) or we can also use a punch for the release and if necessary identify better some structures and open subtalar joint. Occasionally we resect the Intermalleolar ligament in case it causes a conflict of space.

If we perform a subtalar arthrodesis, we carry out the same approach that we described earlier. We start with decortication with removal of cartilage and 2 mm of subchondral bone [30]. For this we use a shaver, burr, chisel or curette. We start the

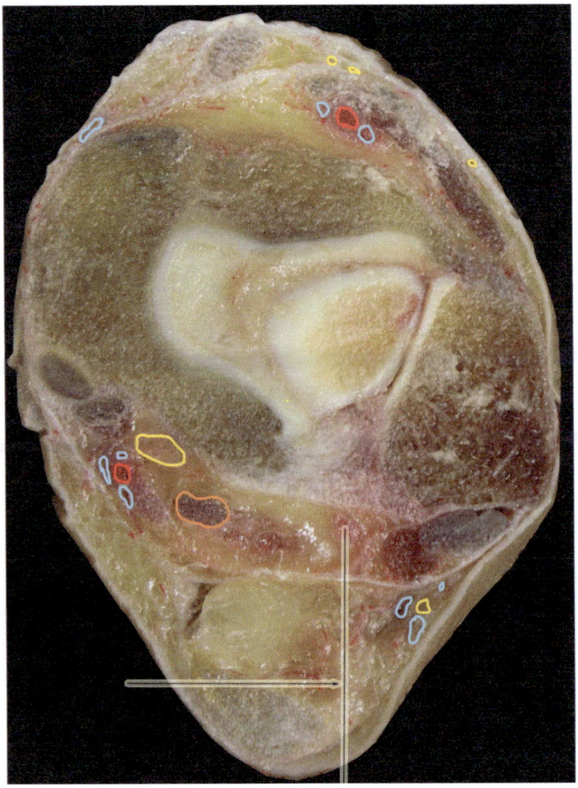

Fig. 10.8 To avoid this complication, the blunt trocar is introduced through the posteromedial incision and after reaching the Achilles tendon, it is turned 90° laterally, until the sheath of the optical device can be felt

resection of the articular surfaces with the shaver and also with chisel (Fig. 10.10), and when we have enough space, we use a burr or a curette and progress until we arrive to the anterior edge of the posterior subtalar facet (Fig. 10.11).

A complete cartilage resection of the articular surfaces must be carried out . The most critical part is the medial and lateral edges of the posterior subtalar joint in order to achieve optimum surface contact for the correct consolidation of the fusion. Some authors recommend a lateral accessory portal [31], in order to introduce instrumentation with the aim of mobilising the articulation and to facilitate the arthrodesis technique. We used it on a few occasions. During manipulation in the sinus tarsi space be careful to avoid damage in this anatomic area.

Only the posterior facet is prepared. Anterior limit is the interosseous ligament. Once we achieve normal bone counter (so we don't provoke a deformity) fixation is done with 2 percutaneous 6.5 mm screws from calcaneus to talus (posterior and plantar to anterior and dorsal) (Fig. 10.12) [32]. Screws are inserted in a parallel configuration with fluoroscopy. No bone graft or bone substitute is used. Skin incisions are closed and a plaster boot is applied.

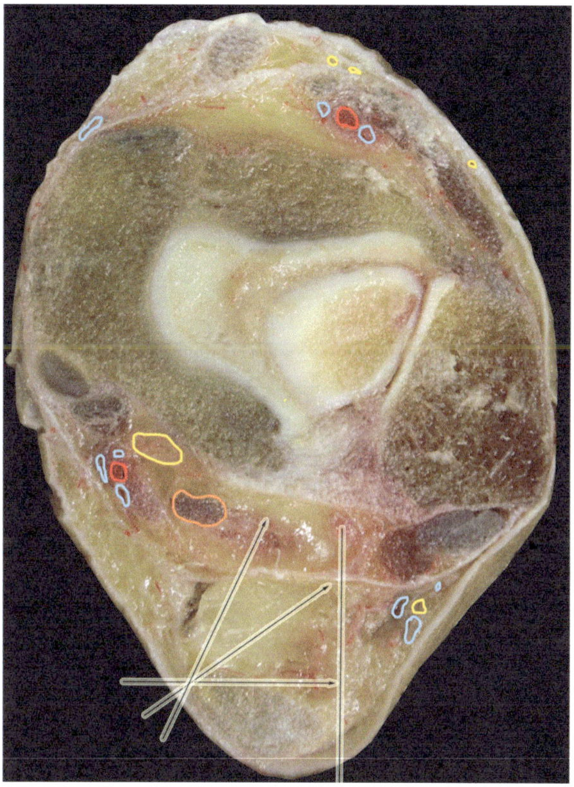

Fig. 10.9 Keeping this metallic contact we slide the trochar along the sheath until reaching the posterior part of the tibio talar articulation or the talus

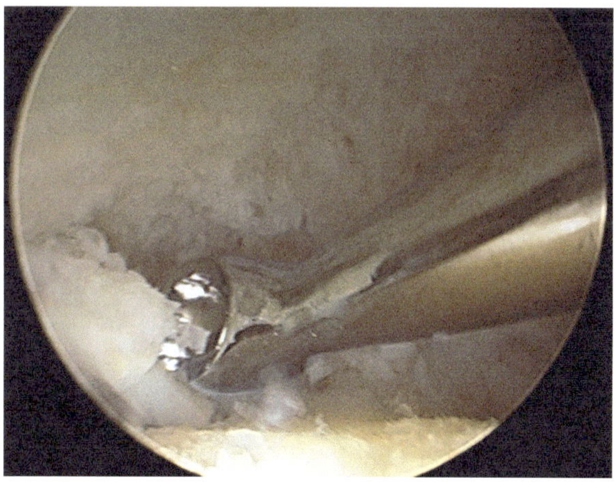

Fig. 10.10 Resection of the articular surfaces with the shaver and also with chisel

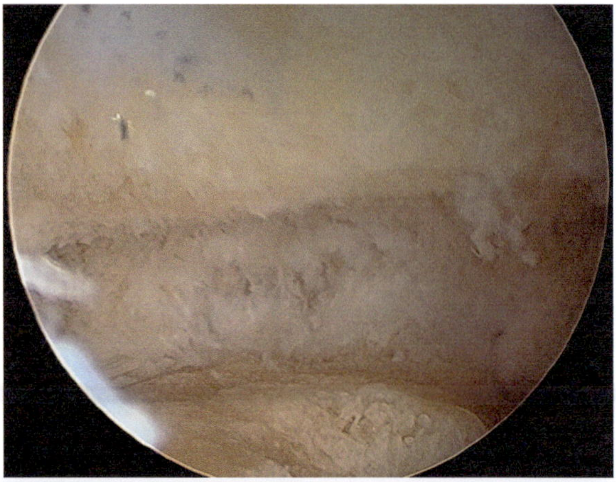

Fig. 10.11 A complete cartilage resection of the articular surfaces must be carried out

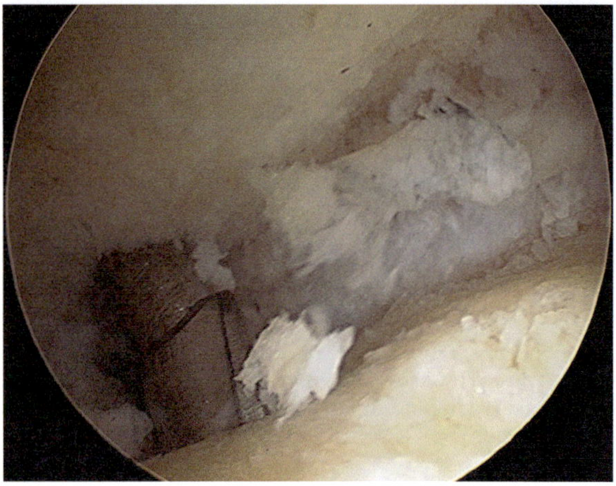

Fig. 10.12 Fixation is done with 2 percutaneous 6.5 mm screws from calcaneus to talus (posterior and plantar to anterior and dorsal)

De Carbo et al. compared the use of single Vs two screws construct and found no differences on the union rate [33]. However there are several concerns about the rotational stability of the single screw construct. When a two screw fixation is used different screw configurations have been reported. Recently Bavornrit Chuckpaiwong and colleagues compared single screw, double parallel screws and double divergent screws configuration in cadaver specimens. They concluded that double diverging screws confer the highest compression, the greatest torsional stiffness, and the least joint rotation [34].

We do not usually use bone graft owing to the fact that studies available do not show better results for the rate of fusion in comparison to patients not using bone graft.

Our post operative protocol for arthroscopic subtalar arthrodesis consists of a 4 week immobilization of the ankle joint, and non weight bearing for approximately 6 weeks. After this period, the patient can start with partial and progressive weight bearing. In our series we have an average time until complete fusion of 8–9 weeks (range of 7–15 weeks), similar to the publications of Tasto [35], and Perez Carro [36].

Complications in Ankle Arthroscopic Procedures

There are some common complications in the arthroscopic treatment of this joint. Nickisch and colleagues [37] studied 186 hindfoot arthroscopies with 8.5% of complications that included 4 plantar numbness, 3 sural nerve dysesthesia, 4 Achilles tendon tightness, 2 complex regional pain syndrome and 2 infections, and 1 cyst at the posteromedial portal. Finally, 1 case each of plantar numbness and sural nerve injury that could not be resolved. We are aware of the incidence of nerve damage, to avoid it we have to be especially careful with our approaches and maneuver in a delicate manner when performing articular resection and releasing structures. In their systematic review Donnenwerth and Roukis [38] reported complications in 3.8% of 452 patients who underwent hindfoot endoscopy. These included wound-healing problems, recurrent symptoms, neuritis of the medial calcaneal nerve, transient incision anesthesia, traumatic sural neuroma and transient superficial peroneal neuritis; only 1.8% required additional treatment or operative intervention.

In a revision of our patients treated by posterior ankle arthroscopy we found 3.4% of complications. These included medial calcaneal nerve dysesthesia, spontaneously solved at 6 months, and wound healing problems.

Zengerink reported 1,8% complications in 315 consecutive hindfoot procedures [39].

All these studies revealed a low frequency of complications after hindfoot endoscopy but a high rate of neurologic injuries among the complications that occurred [40]. All these peripheral nerve complications could be avoided, by making a posterolateral portal just lateral to the Achilles tendon and being guided by a thorough understanding of the regional anatomy.

Van Dijk et al. reported 0,15% of deep infections. We think it could be useful to administer prophylactic antibiotics. Ferkel [41] has summarized to prevent infections in ankle arthroscopy, prophylactic antibiotics and immobilization. In this article he wrote that the most common complication is neurologic injury. The overall complication rate is 9%. Most complications associated with foot and ankle arthroscopy are transient and tend to resolve within 6 months. The only complication that persisted at 10 years followup was a neurologic injury, specifically, numbness at the incision site. Because the difficulty of procedures has increased, so has the complication rate.

We never use immobilization in our patients after an ankle arthroscopic procedure. We like active mobilization same day of the surgery. For us this is one of the great advantages of the arthroscopic technique. Also we try to limit the debridement of the subcutaneous fat in the portal site.

Pearls

Always think about the direction of the scope, and check if your view is lateral.

The direction of the scope must be to the first and second intermetatarsal space.

When we begin to use the instruments, we should never go beyond the FHL tendon medially until we are very clear about our intra-articular situation.

Curettes are very useful for resecting the joint surfaces, especially at the medial and lateral ends.

Before placing the 2 osteosynthesis screws in the subtalar arthrodesis, check the alignment of the hindfoot.

For the correct stabilization of the arthrodesis, two cannulated screws is the best option.

The main limitation to the use of posterior arthroscopic techniques in subtalar arthrodesis is that the patient must not present severe varus/valgus deformity.

References

1. Van Dijk CN, Scholten PE, Krips R. A 2-portal endoscopic approach for diagnosis and treatment of posterior ankle pathology. Arthroscopy. 2000;16:871–6.
2. Margarida M, Ivan MC, Monica AS, Alejandro GH, Xavier MO. Posteroinferior tibiofibular ligament – A cadaveric study Carla Fernandes Martinsa. Foot and Ankle Surgery. 2021;27:296–300.
3. Michels F, Matricali G, Vereecke E, et al. The intrinsic subtalar ligaments have a consistent presence, location and morphology. Foot Ankle Surg. 2021;27(1):101–9.
4. Kelikian A. Sarrafian's anatomy of the foot and ankle: descriptive, topographic, and functional. Philadelphia: Lippincott Williams & Wilkins; 2011.
5. Pereira BS, Andrade R, Espregueira-Mendes J, et al. Current concepts on subtalar instability. Orthop J Sport Med. 2021;9(8):232596712110213.
6. Martinsa CF, Mirandab M, Corteganac IM, Sanchezd MA, Harpee AG, Oliva XM. Posteroinferior tibiofibular ligament – a cadaveric study. Foot Ankle Surg. 2021;27:296–300.
7. Leeuw D, Peter AJ, van Sterkenburg MN, van Dijk CN. Arthroscopy and endoscopy of the Ankle and Hindfoot. Sports Med Arthrosc Rev. 2009;17(3):175–84. https://doi.org/10.1097/JSA0b013e3181a5ce78.
8. van Dijk N. Ankle arthroscopic. Springer; 2014.
9. Stibbe AB, van Dijk CN, Marti RK. The Os trigonum syndrome. Acta Orthop Scand. 1994;Suppl 262:59–60.
10. Van Dijk CN, Lim LS, Poortman A, Strubbe EH, Marti RK. Degenerative joint disease in female ballet dancers. Am J Sports Med. 1995;23:295–300.

11. Hedrick MR, Mcbryde AM. Posterior ankle impingement. Foot Ankle Int. 1994;15:2–8.
12. Thordarson DB, Krieger LE. Operative vs non-operative treatment of intra-articular fractures of the calcaneus: a prospective randomized trial. Foot Ankle Int. 1996;1:2–9.
13. Sanders R. Displaced intra-articular fractures of the calcaneus. J Bone Joint Surg Am. 2000;82:225–50.
14. Rammelt S, Amlang M, Barthel S, Gavlik JM, Zwipp H. Percutaneous treatment of less severe intraarticular calcaneal fractures. Clin Orthop Relat Res. 2010;468:983–90.
15. Pastides P, Milnes L, Rosenfeld P. Percutaneous arthroscopic calcaneal Osteosynthesis: a minimally invasive technique for displaced intra-articular calcaneal fractures. J Foot Ankle Surg. 2015:1–7. https://doi.org/10.1053/j.jfas.2014.12.033.
16. Daniel S, Markus K, André SR, Tiago MG, Xavier MO. Outcomes of posterior arthroscopic subtalar arthrodesis for medial facet talocalcaneal coalition. Foot and ankle int, Vol 42(12).
17. Roster B, Kreulen C, Giza E. Subtalar joint arthrodesis open and arthroscopic indications and surgical techniques. Foot Ankle Clin N Am. 2015;20:319–34.
18. Tasto JP, Mcginty JB, Burkhart SS, Jackson RW, et al., editors. Subtalar arthroscopy: operative arthroscopy. 3rd ed. New York: Lippincott Williams & Wilkins; 2003. p. 944–52.
19. Ferkel RD. Subtalar arthroscopy. In: Ferkle RD, Whipple TL, editors. Arthroscopic surgery: the foot and ankle. Philadelphia: Lippincott-Raven; 1996. p. 231–54.
20. Radnay C, Clare M, Sanders R. Subtalar fusion after displaced intra-articular calcaneal fractures: does initial operative treatment matter? J Bone Joint Surg Am. 2010;92(Suppl 1, Pt 1):32–43.
21. Lijkele Beimers Æ, de Leeuw PAJ, van Dijk CN. A 3-portal approach for arthroscopic subtalar arthrodesis. Knee Surg Sports Traumatol Arthrosc. 2009;17:830–4.
22. Albert A, Deleu PA, Leemrijse T, Maldague P, Devos BB. Posterior arthroscopic subtalar arthrodesis: ten cases at one-year follow-up. Orthop Traumatol Surg Res. 2011;97(4):401–5.
23. Muraro GM, Carvajal PF. Arthroscopic arthrodesis of subtalar joint. Foot Ankle Clin N Am. 2011;16:83–90.
24. Lee KB, Park CH, Seon JK, Kim MS. Arthroscopic subtalar arthrodesis using a posterior 2-portal approach in the prone position. Arthroscopy. 2010;26(2):230–8.
25. Oliva XM, Falcão P, Cerqueira RF, Rodrigues-Pinto R. Posterior arthroscopic subtalar arthrodesis. Our experience with 18 cases. J Foot Ankle Surg. 2017;
26. Lee KB, Saltzman CL, Suh JS, Wasserman L, Amendola A. A posterior 3 portal arthroscopic approach for isolated subtalar arthrodesis. Arthroscopy. 2008;24:1306–10.
27. Oliva XM, López JMM, Planella MM, Bravo A, Rodrigues-Pinto R. Anatomical relations of anterior and posterior ankle arthroscopy portals: a cadaveric study. Eur J Orthop Surg Traumatol. 2015;25(3):577–58.
28. Martin X. Arthroscopic Subtalar arthrodesis. In: Stone JW, Kennedy JG, Glazebrook M, editors. The foot and ankle: AANA advanced arthroscopic surgical techniques; 2015.
29. Sitler DF, Amendola A, Bailey CS, et al. Posterior ankle arthroscopy: an anatomic study. J Bone Joint Surg Am. 2002;84:763–9.
30. Amendola A, Lee KB, Saltzman CL, et al. Technique and early experience with posterior arthroscopic subtalar arthrodesis. Foot Ankle Int. 2007;28(3):298–302.
31. Beimers L, De Leeuw P, Van Dijk N. A 3-portal approach for arthroscopic subtalar artrodesis. Knee Surg Sports Traumatol Arthrosc. 2009;17:830–4.
32. Gómez J, Musatadi M, Martínez J. Artrodesis subastragalina artroscópica. Revista Española de Cirugía Osteoarticular. 2010;45(241):1–4.
33. De Carbo WT, Berlet GC, Hyer CF, Smith WB. Single-screw fixation for subtalar joint fusion does not increase nonunion rate. Foot Ankle Spec. 2010;3:164–6.
34. Chuckpaiwong B, Easley ME, Glisson RR. Screw placement in subtalar arthrodesis: a biomechanical study. Foot Ankle Int. 2009;30(2):133–41.
35. Tasto JP. Arthroscopic subtalar arthrodesis. Tech Foot Ankle Surg. 2003;2:122–8.

36. Perez Carro L, Golanó P, Vega J. Arthroscopic subtalar arthrodesis: the posterior approach in the prone position. Arthroscopy. 2007;23:445.
37. Nickisch F, Barg A, Saltzman CL, et al. Postoperative complications of posterior ankle and hindfoot arthroscopy. J Bone Joint Surg Am. 2012;94(5):439–46.
38. Donnenwerth MP, Roukis TS. The incidence of complications after posterior hindfoot endoscopy. Arthroscopy. 2013;29(12):2049–54.
39. Zangerinh M, Van Dijk CN. Complications in ankle arthroscopy. Knee Surg Sports Traumatol Arthrosc. 2012;20:1420–3.
40. Miyamoto W, Takao M, Matsushita T. Hindfoot endoscopy for posterior ankle impingement syndrome and flexor Hallucis longus tendon disorders. Foot Ankle Clin N Am. 2015;20:139–47.
41. Ferkel RD. Complications in foot and ankle arthroscopy. Clin Orthop Relat Res. 2001;391(391):89–104.

Chapter 11
Combined Anterior and Posterior Ankle Arthroscopy

C. Niek van Dijk

Introduction

Most ankle and hindfoot pathology can be treated by arthroscopy with excellent results.

A diagnosis must be established before the surgery. By means of pre-operative planning it has to be decided to approach the ankle by means of a two portal anterior approach in supine position, by means of a two portal hindfoot approach in a prone position or by means of a combined approach. In some cases we can decide for an open procedure with or without an osteotomy or ligament turn down. Nowadays with highly accurate non-invasive diagnostics it is always possible to decide for the correct approach pre-operatively. In this chapter we discuss in detail the three most relevant combined arthroscopic approaches.

The Three Main Combined Approaches and Indications

For a combined arthroscopic approach there are several possibilities. The main options are a proper 2-portal anterior arthroscopy with an auxiliary posterolateral portal in which the patient remains in the supine position, a proper 2-portal posterior arthroscopy with an auxiliary anterior portal in which the patient remains in the

C. N. van Dijk (✉)
Department of Orthopedic Surgery, University of Amsterdam, Amsterdam UMC Location AMC, Amsterdam, the Netherlands

FIFA Medical Centre of Excellence Ripoll-DePrado Sport Clinic, Madrid, Spain

FIFA Medical Centre of Excellence Clínica do Dragão Porto, Porto, Portugal

Orthopedic Department Casa di Cura San Rossore, Pisa, Italy

M. Bhatia (ed.), *Surgical Techniques of the Foot and Ankle*,
https://doi.org/10.1007/978-3-031-93742-2_11

prone position or a proper 2-portal anterior arthroscopy in supine position followed by a proper 2-portal posterior scope in the prone position.

Apart from these approaches several other approaches have been described. These include anterior + posterior access by means of a lateral decubitus position approach and a technique in which a supine anterior approach is combined with a posterior upside down approach with a 90 degree flexed knee position (Fig. 11.1).

For most cases of combined anterior and posterior pathology my advice is to use a proper anterior 2 portal approach supine, finish the procedure, suture the portals, apply an initial bandage, turn the patient, apply new draping and perform a proper 2 portal posterior approach.

A high volume with a procedure provides a better outcome. Combining a proper 2 portal anterior approach supine with a proper 2 portal posterior approach prone, has a better chance of success for a surgeon who employs both these 2 approaches on a regular basis when compared to a low volume procedure such as a combined anterior and posterior approach in a lateral decubitus position.

Key Box 11.1 The Main Combined Approaches Which Are Described in this Chapter

1. 2 portal hindfoot approach prone with an additional anterior portal.
2. 2-portal anterior approach supine with an additional posterolateral portal.
3. 2-portal anterior approach supine combined with a 2-portal posterior prone.

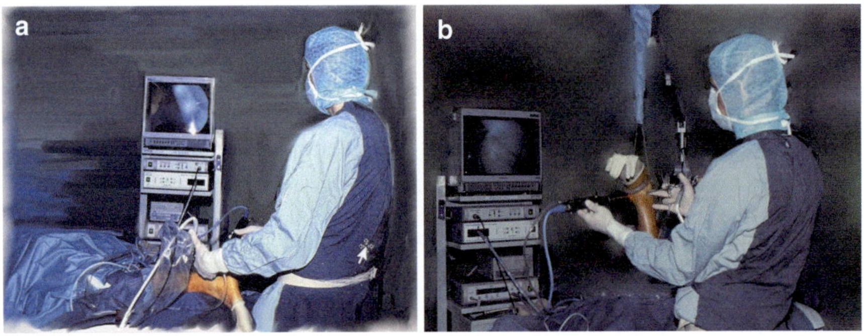

Fig. 11.1 A supine anterior approach is combined with a posterior upside down approach with a 90 degree flexed knee position in a left ankle (**a**) posterior approach with scope in the posterolateral portal and shaver in the posteromedial portal. (**b**) patient remains supine, with the knee flexed in a 90 degree position. The foot and lower leg are lifted by means of a traction device connected to a standard shoulder holder. Scope is in the anterolateral portal and the shaver in the anteromedial portal

2 Portal Hindfoot Approach Prone with an Additional Anterior Portal

For this approach the patient is in a prone position and the main 2 portals are the posterior portals. The anterior portal is mainly used as an auxiliary working portal to assist the surgery which is mainly performed from posterior.

Indications

The main indications for adding an anterior portal to a 2-portal posterior ankle arthroscopy approach are subtalar arthrodesis and treatment of lateral talar process fracture/non-union.

Subtalar Arthrodesis and Ankle Arthrodesis

After posterior ankle arthroscopy has been introduced, this approach has subsequently also been applied to perform posterior arthroscopic subtalar arthrodesis [1–4]. Arthroscopic subtalar arthrodesis has become a widely used procedure during the last decade, as evidenced by the large amount of studies and reviews that have been published since then *(See the Chapter by Molund M. on subtalar arthrodesis in this book).* The posterior arthroscopic approach with an accessory anterolateral portal has become the most frequently used arthroscopic technique [5–8].

A third portal in the sinus tarsi is helpful for introduction of a 4 mm trocar which is “forced“into the joint (Fig. 11.2). The trocar serves as a “distractor” which facilitates the removal of cartilage and denudes the joint surfaces though the posterior portals. This anterolateral portal can also be used to approach the anterior part of the joint for removal of cartilage of the anterior part of the posterior joint facet [4].

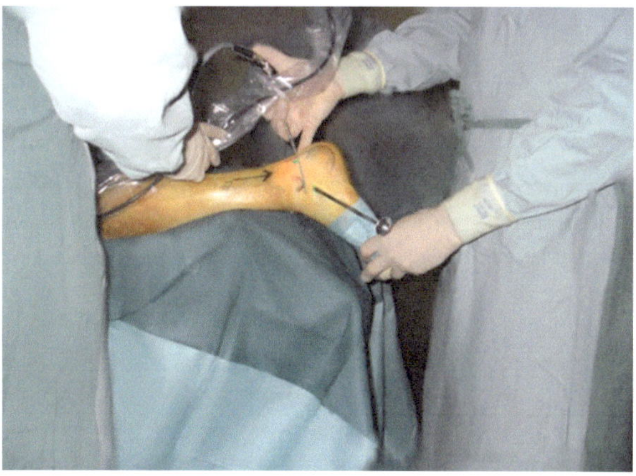

Fig. 11.2 Arthroscopic Subtalar arthrodesis in a left ankle by means of a 2-portal hindfoot approach. A 4 mm trocar is “forced“into the subtalar joint through a third portal in the sinus tarsi which serves as a “distractor” to facilitate the removal of cartilage though the posterior portals

Arthroscopic subtalar arthrodesis yields clinical outcomes comparable to the open technique and a fusion rate of approximately 95%. The risk of wound complications is very low *(See the Chapter by Molund M. on subtalar arthrodesis in this book).*

For an arthroscopic ankle arthrodesis the approach can be from anterior but also be from posterior. With the 2-portal posterior ankle arthroscopy approach a 100% fusion rate has been reported [9] The addition of an anteromedial portal facilitates the procedure. Through this portal a 4 mm trocar is "forced "into the joint. The trocar serves as a "distractor" which facilitates the removal of cartilage and denuding of the joint surfaces though the posterior portals. This anteromedial portal can also be used to approach the anterior part of the joint for removal of cartilage in this anterior area.

Lateral Talar Process Fracture/Non-union

Arthroscopic treatment of a non-union of a lateral talar process fracture can be performed by several portals. It demands a combination of anterior and posterior portals (Fig. 11.3).

2-Portal anterior Approach (Supine) with an Additional Posterolateral Portal

For this approach the patient is in supine position and the main 2 portals are the anterior portals. The posterior portal is mainly used as an auxiliary working portal to assist the surgery which is mainly performed from anterior (Fig. 11.4). In combination with a small diameter arthroscope this portal is important for flow management.

Indications

The main indication for adding a posterolateral portal to a routine 2 portal anterior arthroscopy -with the patient in a supine position- is removal of a loose body from the posterior ankle joint or a simple synovectomy of the posterior ankle.

For more complex procedures such as posterior impingement treatment, FHL release or transfer, Cedell fracture treatment, tarsal tunnel release and more extensive synovectomies or chondromatosis treatment it is better and more safe to use a 2 portal hindfoot approach in the prone position.

In the past routine application of an additional posterolateral portal was advocated when a small diameter arthroscope was used for a 2 portal anterior arthroscopy with continuous distraction [10, 11]. The routine addition of a posterolateral portal was advocated for better flow management and for diagnostic purposes [12]. Adding a posterolateral portal made it also possible to perform a routine diagnostic

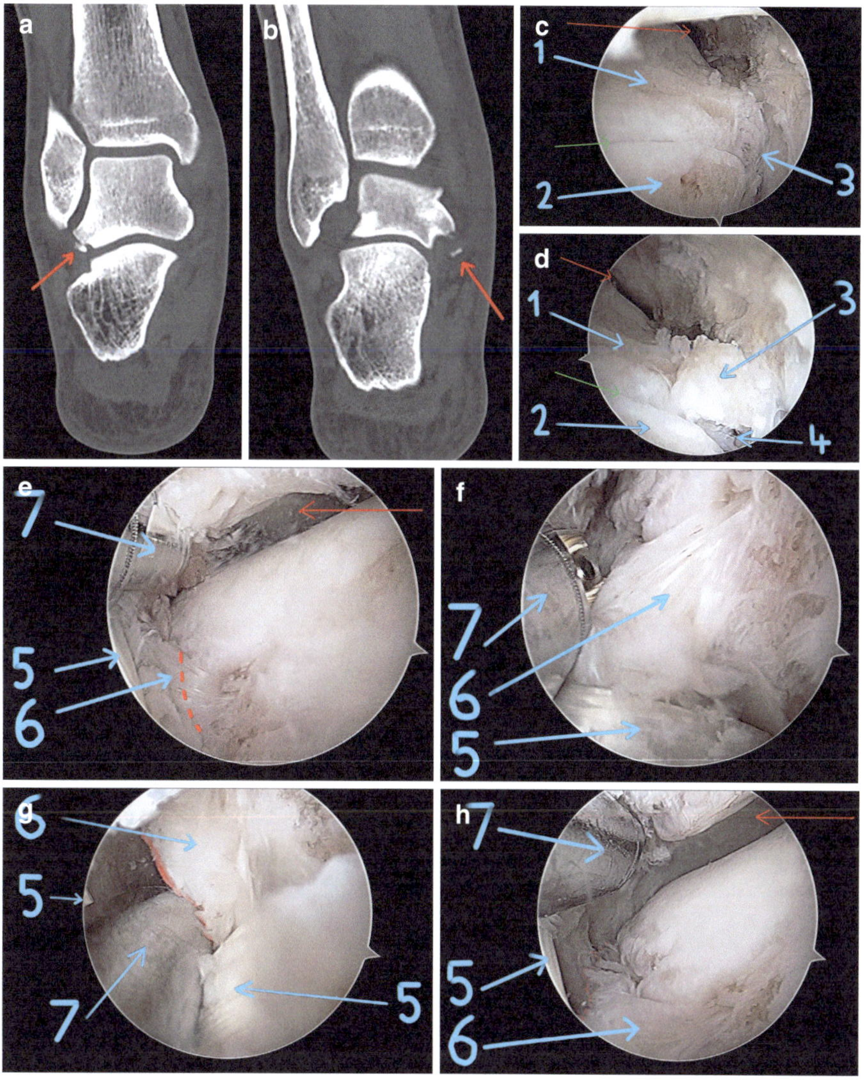

Fig. 11.3 Patient with painful non-union of a lateral talar process fracture combined with a posteromedial Cedell fracture (avulsion/calcification of the deep portion of deltoid ligament). Both fragments are removed by this 2-portal posterior arthroscopy with scope in the posteromedial portal and instruments in the additional sinus tarsi portal. (**a**) Coronal CT scan with red arrow pointing at the lateral talar process fragment (**b**) Coronal CT scan with red arrow pointing at the posteromedial Cedell fragment (**c** and **d**) Small fragment periosteal elevator which separates and lifts the avulsion from the talus. (**e**)The shaver is initially used as a 'probe' to push the FHL medial out of from its gliding channel thus disclosing the anterior insertion of the flexor retinaculum (FR) on the posteromedial talar process. The Cedell avulsion/calcification is located just anterior from this FR insertion. In order to remove the Cedell fragment, the FR needs to be cut along the red dotted line by means of a punch or shaver. Just anterior from the tip of the shaver we see articular synovitis which is removed first by a few turns of the shaver. (**f**) Moving the shaver downwards along the red dotted line, taking care not to damage the FHL. (**g** and **e**) Complete detachment of the FR (Red markings). Following this, the shaver is moved 5–15 mm forward, to remove the Cedell fragment/calcification. 1 = Talus, 2 = Calcaneus, 3 = Non-union fragment lateral talar process. 4 = Small fragment periosteal elevator, 5 = FHL, 6 = Flexor retinaculum (FR), 7 = 5.5 mm bone-cutter shaver. Red arrow = ankle joint and green arrow = subtalar joint

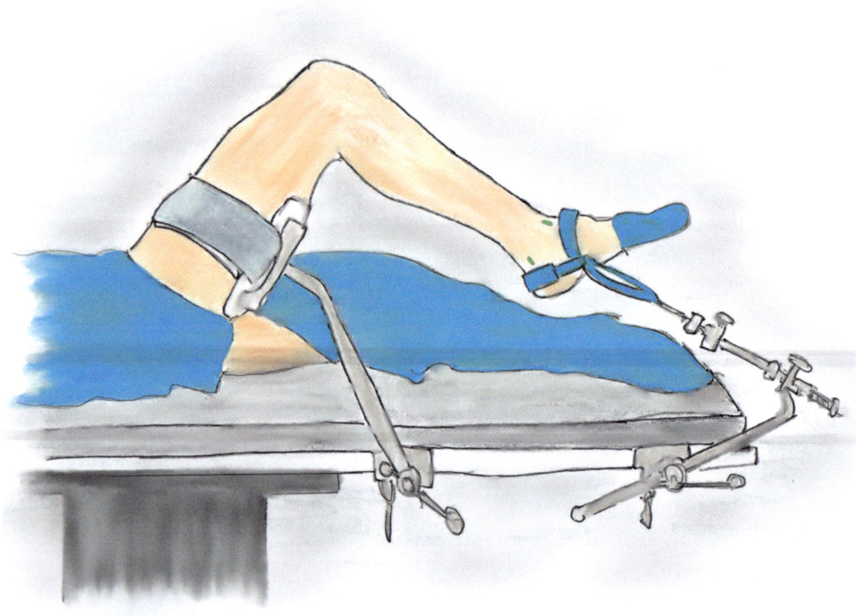

Fig. 11.4 The standard setup for a 2-portal anterior approach with an additional posterolateral portal and a fixed distraction system attached to the operating table. The patient is in supine position and the main 2 portals are the anterior portals. The anterolateral and posterolateral portals are marked in green

21-point examination of the ankle [13]. With the development of more accurate non-invasive diagnostics, better flow management and the development of a safe 2-portal posterior arthroscopy prone position approach for therapeutic purposes, the routine application of this additional posterolateral portal to an anterior arthroscopy has diminished.

Diagnostic Arthroscopy

In the early days arthroscopy was used as a diagnostic tool. Richard Ferkel phrases it as follows: "In 1984, Jim Guhl and I developed the fixed distraction system because we realized that we were missing a lot of pathology. Fixed non-invasive distraction provides the surgeon the opportunity to see the whole joint, not just part of it" [11]. In order to provide complete access to the joint, three portals were routinely established, the anterolateral, the anteromedial, and the posterolateral portal. A diagnostic arthroscopy was indicated in patients whose ankle problems include unexplained pain and stiffness. Diagnostic arthroscopy was also advocated to detect the extent of articular surface damage [10, 13].

In these early days non-invasive diagnostics were less sophisticated. But this has changed. Noninvasive diagnostics are highly accurate and enable us to make a diagnosis. Most of us would agree that currently there is no indication for routine diagnostic arthroscopy of any joint. We need a diagnosis before we start! That is also the conclusion from this recent review: ankle arthroscopy is now exclusively used as a therapeutic tool [14].

Although there are regional differences the 3 portal fixed distraction method including diagnostic arthroscopy is still in use today mainly in USA [15].

In this chapter we consider diagnostic arthroscopy in ankle fractures, in combination with arthroscopic ligament repair, as second look after OCD treatment, diagnostic needle arthroscopy and asymptomatic osteophyte removal.

Diagnostic Arthroscopy in Ankle Fractures

Some advocate a diagnostic arthroscopy in ankle fractures. As was shown by Hintermann- in his often cited classic paper- 80% of patients with an ankle fracture also have cartilage lesions [16]. Howard found a similar 84% [17]. Initially this has led to the assumption that each ankle fracture should get a diagnostic arthroscopy.

Interestingly enough only 1% of surgeons in the US scope an ankle fracture [18].

And even in this 1% the additional scoping does not make a clinical difference [18].

A recent systematic review and meta-analysis confirmed that there was no difference in outcome between ankle fracture patients with cartilage damage and ankle fracture patients without cartilage lesions [19]. From both these studies we can conclude that a diagnostic arthroscopy in an ankle fracture is not useful. It does not make the patient better and it adds to the complexity of the surgery.

Diagnostic Arthroscopy in Adjunction with Chronic Ankle Instability Repair

The majority of patients with chronic ankle instability also have asymptomatic cartilage damage. This was shown by several authors [19, 20]. But similar as with ankle fractures, it has been shown that there is no difference in outcome between patients with or without these chondral lesions [21, 22]. A diagnostic arthroscopy at the time of repair does not make the patient better. It can only lead to unnecessary interventions.

Superficial cartilage lesions in patients with an ankle fracture or in patients with chronic instability have no consequences. You'll only frighten your patient when you tell or show them the damage, and for no good reason.

Second Look Arthroscopy After OCD Treatment

Keun-Bae Lee performed a second-look arthroscopy in 20 ankles 1 year after microfracture treatment. All 20 patients preoperatively agreed to undergo this second-look arthroscopy to evaluate their cartilage repair at 12 months postoperatively. Sixteen ankles (80%) still had macroscopic cracks and fissures and 7 (35%) showed abnormal and incomplete healing ICRS gr III. Nevertheless all patients achieved improvements in terms of clinical outcomes and overall AOFAS scores revealed excellent or good results of over 80 points in 90% of the patients [23].

Twenty five patients underwent a second-look arthroscopy at a mean of 3.6 yrs. after microfracture. Nine ankles (36%) were incompletely healed ICRS gr III, with inferior quality of repair tissue, but all patients had significant clinical improvement between preoperative and latest Follow-up ($p < 0.001$) [24]. In addition all 25 patients showed no change in arthritic grade between the preoperative and latest follow-up radiographs.

So what is the explanation of all these findings? In fact it tells us what we already know. The pain comes from the bone and not from the cartilage. With the arthroscope we can determine the status of the cartilage. But it is the status of the subchondral bone that matters. A defect in the subchondral bone plate makes the patient symptomatic. Bone marrow oedema on MRI or a defect seen on CT correlates with symptoms, not an irregularity in the cartilage. Cartilage damage without subchondral bone involvement has no consequences. This is not the start of a cascade of events leading to arthrosis when left untreated. On the contrary, treatment of these superficial lesions is unnecessary treatment which can potentially induce symptoms.

Superficial cartilage damage is known to occur in 60% of patients with an acute lateral ligament rupture. One such event does not deteriorate to arthrosis. And what to think of the iatrogenic cartilage damage due to the introduction of a mosquito forceps, an arthroscope, probes, shavers or needles (Fig. 11.5). I invite you to check the cartilage at the end of an ankle arthroscopy (Fig. 11.6), or for knee surgeons after a meniscectomy or a meniscal repair. We all assume that iatrogenic superficial cartilage lesions do not deteriorate. These lesions are limited in size and do not extend through the subchondral bone plate. They are not the initiators of a cascade of events leading to arthrosis.

Needle Arthroscopy

Needle arthroscopy, also known as nanoscopy, is performed with a disposable 2.3 mm (including sheath) arthroscope that is proposed to be used without general anaesthesia, in an outpatient setting [25].

As was already shown in the 90's, arthroscopic surgery of the ankle can be performed with very good pain control and a high degree of patient satisfaction under local anaesthesia [26]. The prediction that we would all be turning more and more to local anaesthesia for arthroscopy in the future however, never came true [26]. Time will show if with this new technology it will.

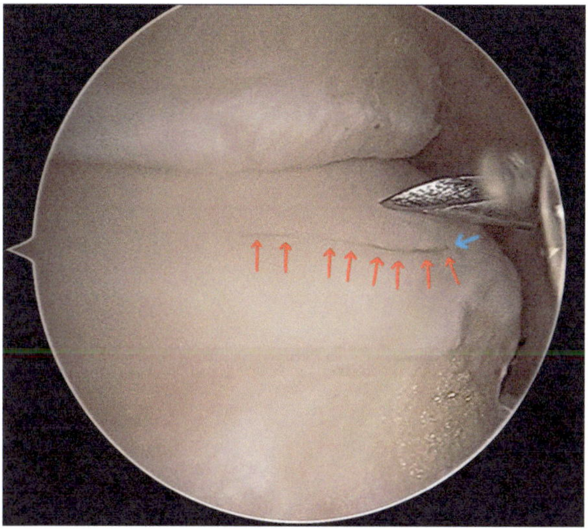

Fig. 11.5 Iatrogenic cartilage damage (red arrows) caused by the introduction of a needle. The blue arrow points to the entry point of the needle in the cartilage

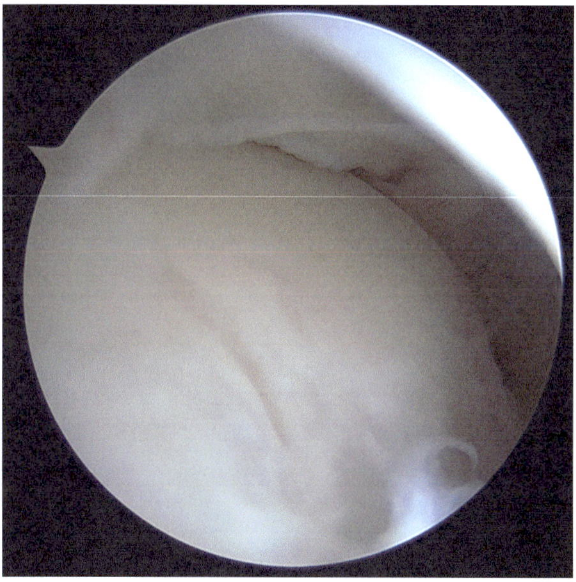

Fig. 11.6 Arthroscopic image in a patient who had arthroscopic surgery 2 years before. Multiple areas of iatrogenic superficial cartilage damage are visible

If this nanoscope is used to demonstrate the patient the status of his/her cartilage then we are on the wrong track. Consider these tram track lesions (Fig. 11.7). They have no consequences since they don't extend into the subchondral bone. You will only make your patient extremely worried when you show them these bare tracks in their ankle. "Doktor is it really safe to walk without cartilage?" Same for a second look needle scope after cartilage treatment. At 1 year in 80% of patients the repair cartilage does not look nice, with cracks and fissures in spite of a clinical good outcome [23]. At 4 years 35% of satisfied patients still have incompletely healed

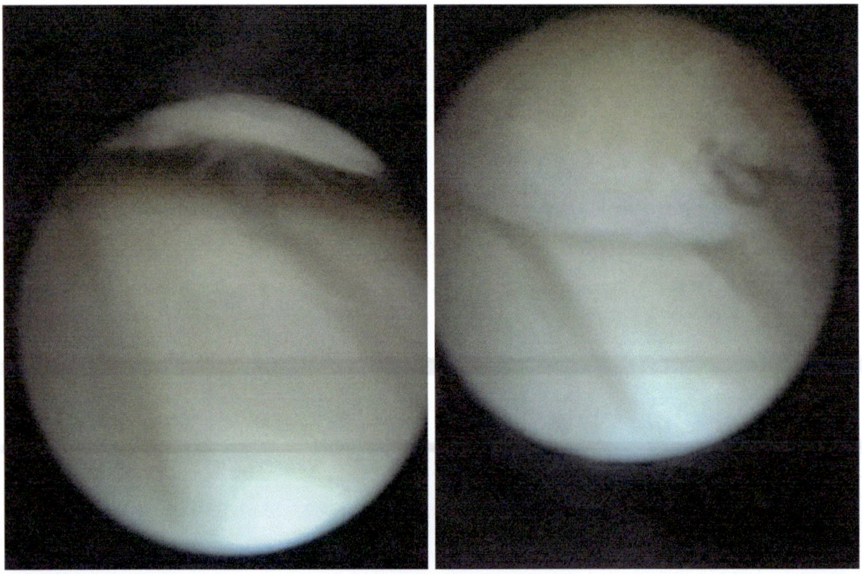

Fig. 11.7 Four tram track lesions as an accidental finding in left ankle of a professional football player. 17 years later no symptoms and no osteoarthritis

cartilage ICRS gr III, with inferior quality of repair tissue. You can already hear the patient ask: Doktor is that the reason why my ankle sometimes feels a little stiff? Can you do something about it?

Use of the nanoscope has been advocated to deliver injectables such as hyaluronic acid into the joint. And even then with <90% accuracy [27]. The single-use nanoscope is an example of a device looking for an indication rather than of a problem looking for a solution.

The single-use nanoscope which comes with a complete disposable instrument set and is certainly not environmentally friendly [28]. It will likely raise the cost of healthcare with the additional risk of unnecessary interventions.

Asymptomatic Spurs and Osteophytes

The chance that a diagnostic arthroscopy will detect a spur or osteophyte in a healthy asymptomatic individual is 20%. One in five asymptomatic persons in the age 20–40 years have spurs or osteophytes [29]. One in three patients (33%) with chronic ankle instability and one in two patients (50%) with a talar OCD have asymptomatic osteophytes [30].

What happens if we remove these asymptomatic spurs or osteophytes?

Removal of spurs and osteophytes results in a nice looking postoperative X-Ray. But not for long since these spurs return [31, 32].

These asymptomatic spurs do no harm, they are even beneficial. They stabilize the joint. In the unlikely case that they become symptomatic they can be removed in the future. Removal of asymptomatic spurs and osteophytes can lead to arthrofibrosis in case of postoperative joint immobilization as for example spur removal in combination with ligament repair (Fig. 11.8).

Conclusion

In the early days when non-invasive diagnostics were less sophisticated, arthroscopy was used as a diagnostic tool. But evidently this has changed. Noninvasive diagnostics are highly accurate and enable us to make a diagnosis. Most of us will agree that currently there is no indication for routine diagnostic arthroscopy of any joint. We need a diagnosis before we start! A methodical 21-point examination of the ankle is not needed and can only create iatrogenic cartilage damage by forcing scopes or probes into difficult to reach areas. As was shown in several

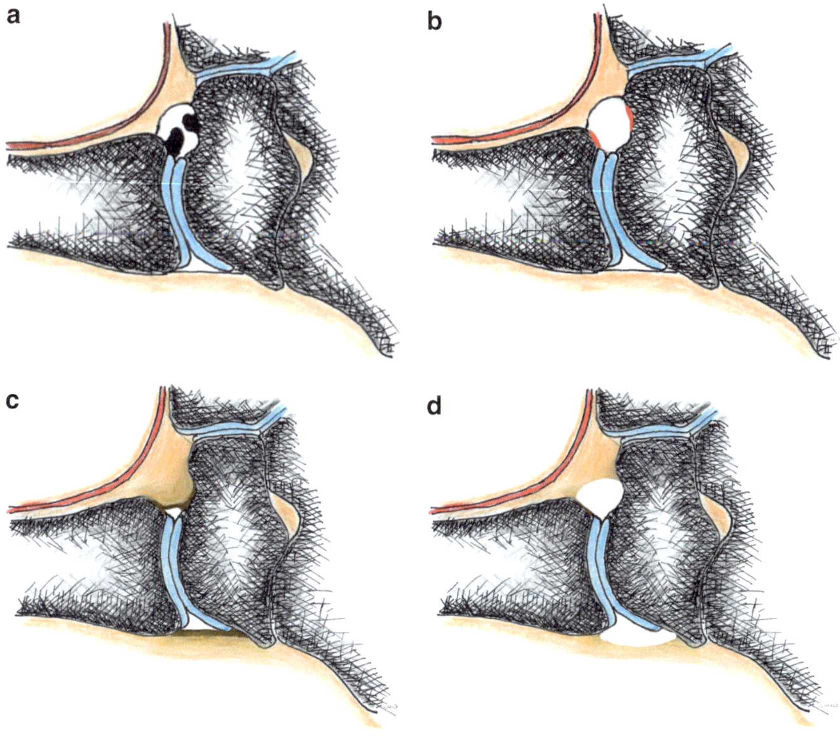

Fig. 11.8 (**a** and **b**) Removal of osteophytes leaves the distal tibia and talus with a bleeding bone area. In order to prevent arthrofibrosis it is important to stimulate early motion. (**c**) Arthrofibrosis resulting in restricted motion (**d**) Arthroscopic removal of the adhesions and capsule by combined anterior and posterior arthroscopy

articles a diagnostic arthroscopy in ankle fractures or in combination with arthroscopic ligament repair does not make the patient better. Patients do not benefit from asymptomatic osteophyte removal. Asymptomatic cartilage changes as seen after OCD treatment or with a diagnostic needle arthroscopy should be left untouched. Only when these lesions extend into the subchondral bone they might warrant further monitoring. But there are certainly better and non-invasive methods to do this.

2-Portal Anterior Supine Approach Combined with a 2-Portal Posterior Prone Approach

For most cases of combined anterior and posterior pathology my advice is to use a proper anterior 2 portal approach supine, finish the procedure, suture the portals apply an initial bandage, turn the patient into the prone position, apply new draping and perform a proper 2 portal posterior approach.

It is possible to change the order and start prone with the posterior approach, turn the patient and perform the anterior arthroscopy supine but this demands extra precautions for the anterior approach. In order to prevent infection the freshly sutured posterior portals should not be in direct contact with the operating table. This needs a support under the lower leg.

Indications

A combined arthroscopic approach can be indicated in patients with more extensive anterior as well as posterior ankle or hindfoot pathology.

Coexistence of any of the following pathologies can be an indication for a combined arthroscopic approach.

For a proper 2 portal anterior ankle arthroscopy these include anterior ankle impingement, OCD, loose bodies, synovitis, ATFL ligament repair, syndesmotic stabilization and arthrodesis.

The main indication for a 2-portal posterior arthroscopic procedure are osteochondral defects in the posterior 1/3 of the talus, osteochondral defects in the posterior tibial plafond, posterior ankle impingement, treatment of synovial chondromatosis, reduction of posterior tibial RIM osteophytes, FHL release or transfer and tarsal tunnel release [33]. The same 2 portal hindfoot approach is used for ankle arthrodesis, subtalar arthrodesis or arthroscopic pantalar. arthrodesis. More seldom indications include the treatment of a Cedell fracture, treatment of avulsions of the posterior talofibular ligament (PTFL) and treatment of posterior impingement after total ankle prothesis [34–36].

By means of tendoscopy pathology in the peroneal tendons, posterior tibial tendons and Achilles tendons can be treated. Indications include retrocalcaneal bursitis and insertional achilles tendinopathy, peroneal tenosynovectomy, groove deepening for recurrent peroneal tendon dislocation, posterior tibial synovectomy and treatment of Achilles (para)tendinopathy [37].

Apart from coexistence of any of these anterior and posterior pathologies there are some specific indications for a combined proper 2 portal anterior supine with a proper 2-portal prone approach. These include arthrofibrosis, synovial chondromatosis and a total synovectomy. Another frequent combined indication is posterior impingement in a patient with chronic ankle instability (Fig. 11.9).

Synovial Chondromatosis

A growing pool of evidence is emerging to suggest favorable outcomes for arthroscopic treatment of Synovial chondromatosis of the ankle joint [38]. This is confirmed by a systematic review of 15 articles [39].

A proper synovectomy of the anterior as well as the posterior compartment can only be done with such a combined approach (Fig. 11.10). For a total synovectomy it is important to exactly see and visualise what your shaver or radiofrequency probe is doing. The detection of multiple loose bodies likewise demands a proper visualisation. The procedure must be done without distraction in order not to lose the loose bodies through the joint anterior or posterior.

Arthrofibrosis

Arthrofibrosis is defined as joint pain and stiffness that does not allow functional range of motion and is commonly due to adhesions, scarring, and contracture of the joint [40].

In the ankle, this condition is mostly posttraumatic. More than 50% of ankle fractures report diminished range of motion and ankle stiffness [41].

Limitation of ankle motion can also occur after supination trauma or after ankle surgery (Fig. 11.8c). Clinically, arthrofibrosis is characterized by pain, diminished range of motion, stiffness, and difficulty with performing daily activities due to impaired gait and abnormal ankle function. On clinical investigation there is tenderness to palpation of the joint margins anterior as well as posterior. Typical magnetic resonance (MR) imaging findings consist of capsular and pericapsular thickening. Ultrasonography demonstrates hypoechoic capsular thickening and pericapsular scars. Arthroscopic treatment with removal of scar tissue and adhesions as well as capsular release has been reported by various authors [42–44] (Fig. 11.8d).

Lui et al. [45] found that the mean dorsiflexion increased from 1 to 19 degrees and plantarflexion increased from 16 to 39 degrees following combined anterior and posterior arthroscopic debridement and release, whereas Cui et al. [46].

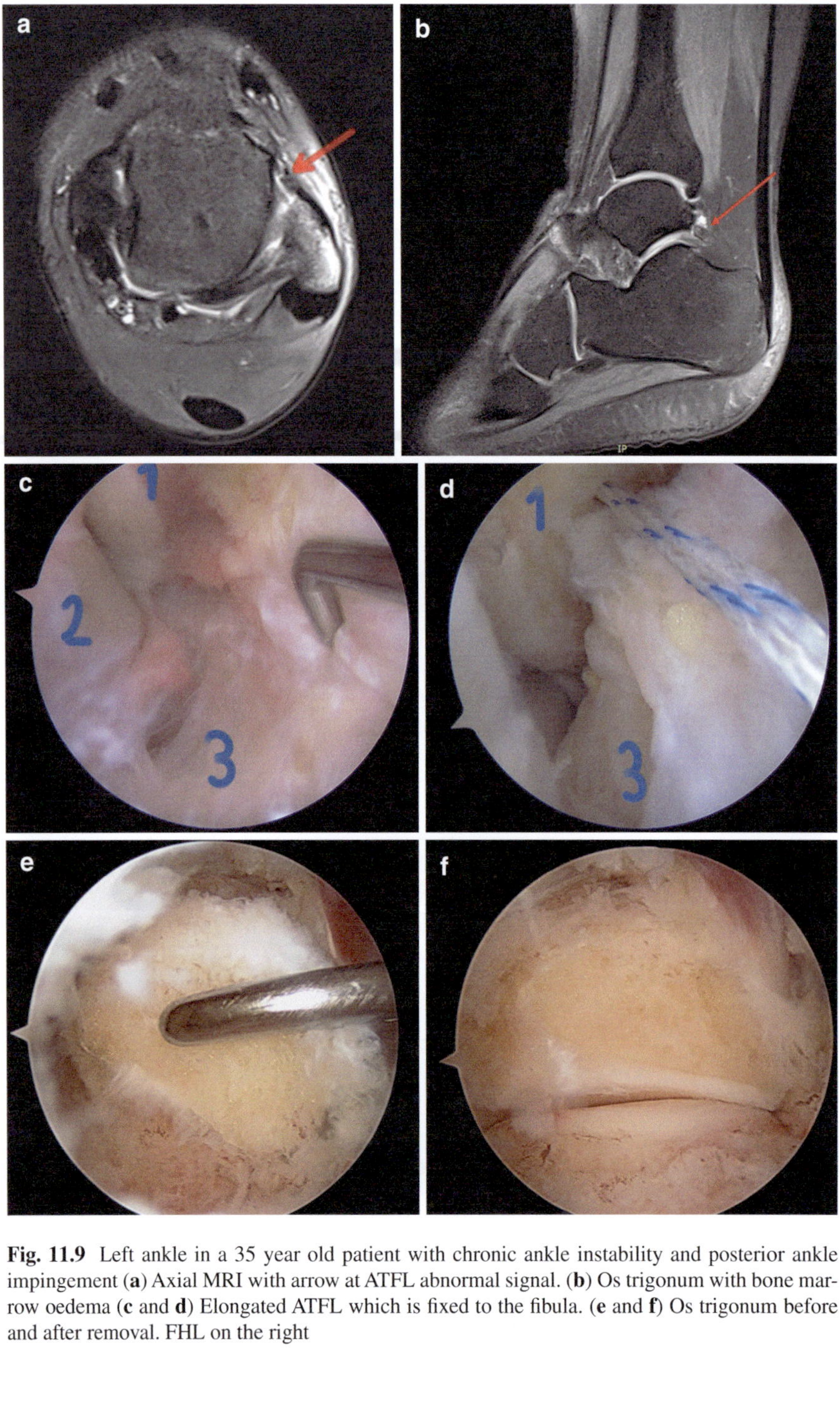

Fig. 11.9 Left ankle in a 35 year old patient with chronic ankle instability and posterior ankle impingement (**a**) Axial MRI with arrow at ATFL abnormal signal. (**b**) Os trigonum with bone marrow oedema (**c** and **d**) Elongated ATFL which is fixed to the fibula. (**e** and **f**) Os trigonum before and after removal. FHL on the right

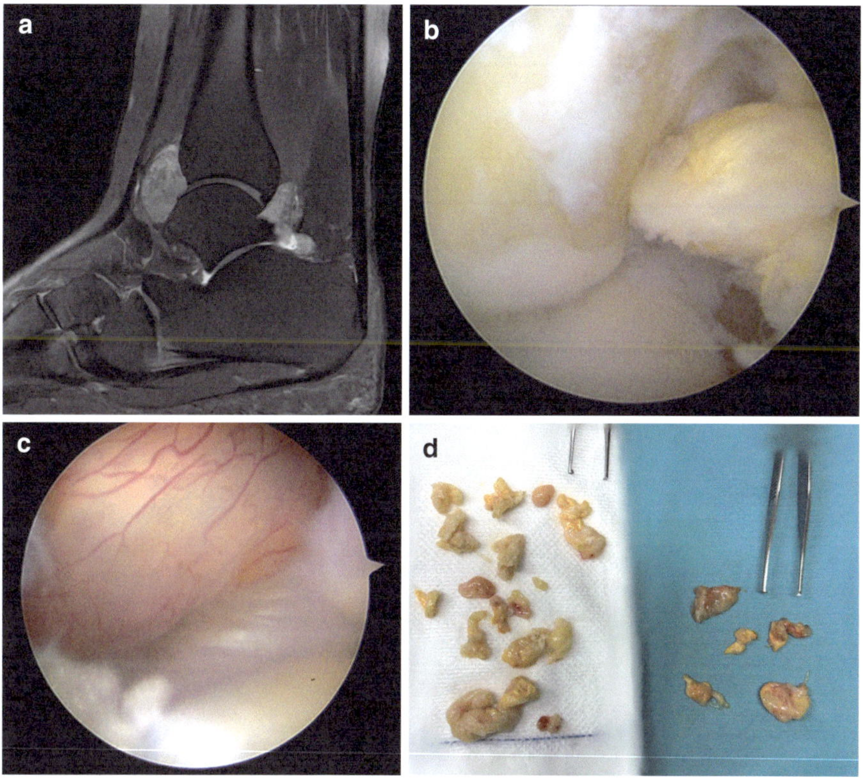

Fig. 11.10 47 year female with pain and swelling anterior as well as posterior and swelling of the left Ankle. (**a**) MRI compatible with chronic synovitis or giant cell tumor. (**b** and **c**) Pathologic tissue visible in the anterior compartment and in the posterior compartment. (**d**) On white dressing the tissue removed from anterior compartment and on the green dressing from posterior. Histologic analysis confirmed a rare presentation of Giant Cells Tumor

found that range of motion increased by 6.7 degrees and an improvement in patient outcome scores including American Orthopaedic Foot & Ankle Society (AOFAS) scores (63.8–88.6) and Foot Function Index scores.

Arthrofibrosis must be differentiated by other causes of limitation of motion in both dorsiflexion and plantar flexion (Fig. 11.11).

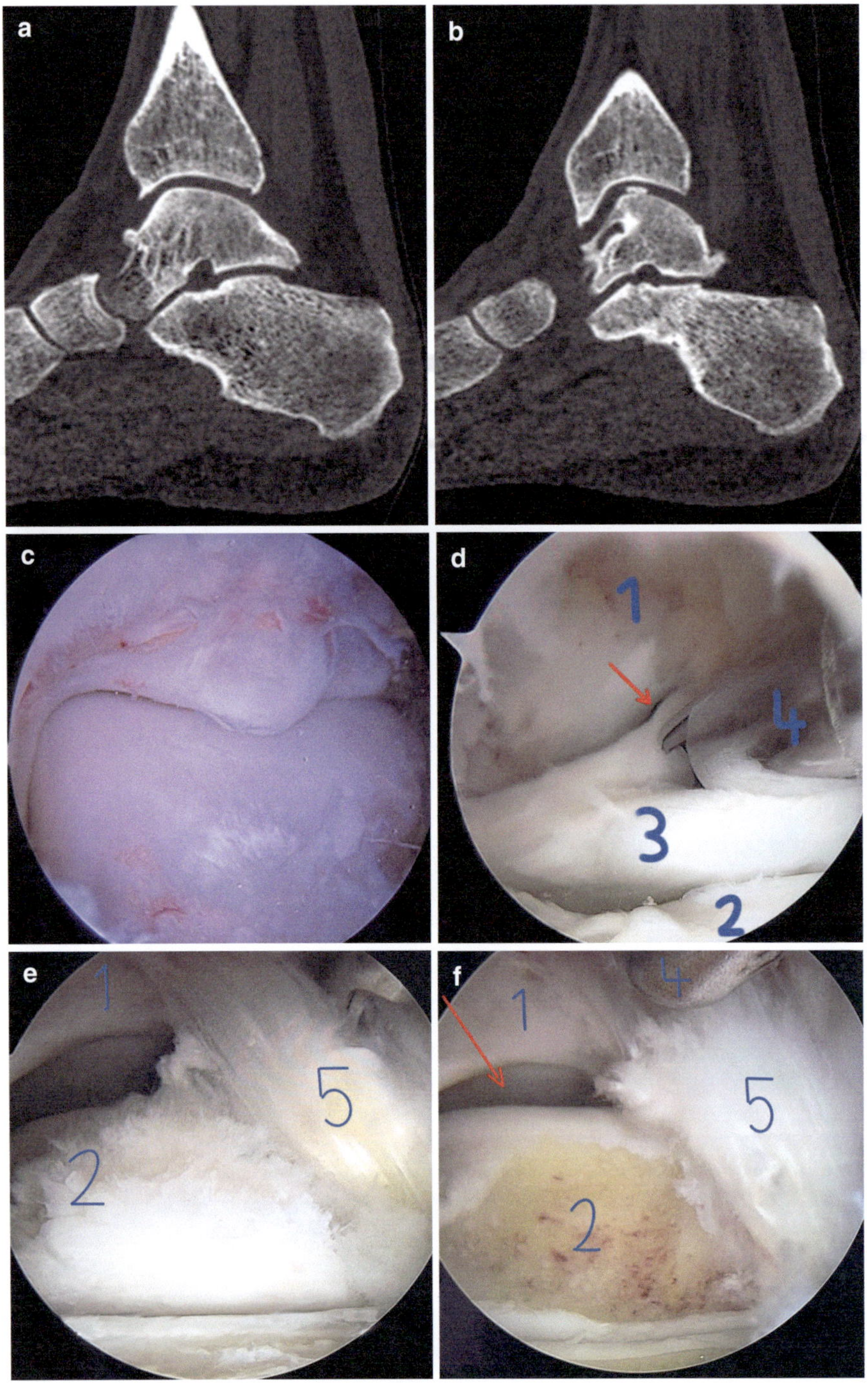

Fig. 11.11 (continued)

Some Technical Aspects of Anterior and Posterior Approaches

In the past fixed ankle distraction was routinely used to access the anterior ankle. However, nowadays, anterior arthroscopy is done in dorsiflexion as this increases the anterior ankle joint volume, providing easy access to various anatomical structures and allowing for procedures to be performed better, more effective and with less complications [47] (Fig. 11.12a). In a fixed distracted position the neurovascular structures are tight as a bowstring and therefore cannot move aside for any passing instrument. This makes them much more vulnerable for iatrogenic damage. This is especially valid for the superficial peroneal nerve in relation to the anterolateral portal and the sural nerve in relation to the posterolateral portal. But also the deep peroneal nerve is pulled like a bowstring towards the joint with distraction, whereas in dorsiflexion the deep peroneal nerve and anterior tibial artery move away from the joint and remain lax [48] (Fig. 11.12b). In dorsiflexion the distance between the distal tibia and neurovascular structures is 3.7 mm while in distraction the distance is 1.7 mm [49]. Distraction compromises the safety for anterior arthroscopy significantly.

In dorsiflexion the neurovascular structures are lax and they will be pushed aside by a blunt instrument which is accidentally introduced right on top of such a nerve or vessel. Small diameter instruments, shavers and scopes by their "needle shape" are more likely to accidentally penetrate cartilage nerves or vessels. They are also more prone to instrument breakage. Large diameter scoop and shaver are more blunt, provide better view, can deliver more fluid and remove osteophytes and other impediments quicker and more efficiently.

After introduction of saline the anterior working area opens up thus allowing for safe introduction of arthroscopes and instruments. In the dorsiflexed position the talus is concealed in the joint, thereby protecting the cartilage for potential iatrogenic damage.

Fig. 11.11 21-year-old female dancer presented with locking and anterior+ posterior left ankle pain. Posterior ankle pain on plantar flexion. Recognizable tenderness on palpation anterior joint line. Posterior impingement test positive and recognizable tenderness over the FHL. Slightly limited motion of the ankle joint in both directions. Stable ankle. (**a** and **b**) 2 sagittal CT with anterior osteophytes on the distal tibia as well as talar neck, a loose body intra articular and an irregular enlarged posterior talar process. (**c**) Anterior arthroscopic view showing the osteophyte on the distal tibia. Anteromedial Talar osteophyte already removed. On the left (3 o'clock position) the medial malleolus. (**d**) Thickened intermalleolar ligament with longitudinal split. (**e** and **f**) Posterior view before (**e**) and after (**f**) removal of the pathological intermalleolar ligament, posterior talar process and release of the flexor retinaculum. Note there is some fraying of the FHL. This has no consequence as long as the flexor retinaculum has been fully released. 1 = distal tibia. 2= talus with the superior border of the posterolateral talar process. 3 = thickened intermalleolar ligament with longitudinal split. 4 = 5.5 mm bone-cutter shaver. 5 = FHL. Red arrow points at the ankle joint

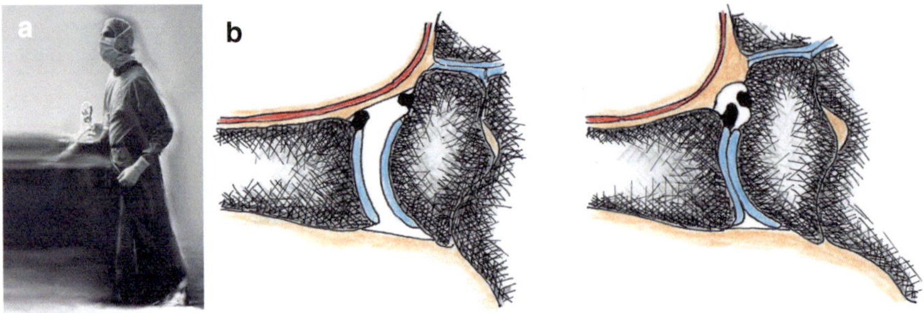

Fig. 11.12 (**a**) Setup for anterior ankle arthroscopy with the dorsiflexion method. Instruments must always be introduced in this position to avoid iatrogenic damage to nerves and cartilage. (**b**) In a fixed distracted position the neurovascular structures (in red) are tight as a bowstring and therefore cannot move aside for a passing instrument. This makes them much more vulnerable for iatrogenic damage. This is especially valid for the superficial peroneal nerve in relation to the anterolateral portal. But also the deep peroneal nerve is pulled like a bowstring towards the joint with distraction, (**b**) whereas in dorsiflexion the deep peroneal nerve and anterior tibial artery move away from the joint and remain lax. In dorsiflexion the distance between the distal tibia and neurovascular structures is 3.7 mm while in distraction the distance is 1.7 mm. *(Tonogai I 2018)* Distraction compromises the safety for anterior arthroscopy

Most of the pathology is located in the anterior aspect of the ankle joint or -in case of a talar OCD- can be brought into this anterior working area by means of (forced) plantar flexion [47]. In my personal 35 years of experience with operative treatment of talar OCD, I can roughly say that I have treated >95% of my microfracture cases by an anterior arthroscopic approach and <5% by means of a posterior arthroscopic approach. The anterior approach has always been without fixed distraction. Osteochondral defects can be brought into the anterior working area by means of forced plantar flexion (Fig. 11.13). There are cases in which joint distraction eases access to the OCD. A non-invasive device that enables the surgeon to quickly change from the dorsiflexed position to the distracted position and vice versa can then be used (Fig. 11.14).

The technique of anterior ankle arthroscopy as well as for a 2-portal posterior ankle arthroscopy has been well described in Chapters 106–109 and 116–117. For a step-by-step instruction in text, pictures and instructional videos visit the free assessable Ankleplatform website [50].

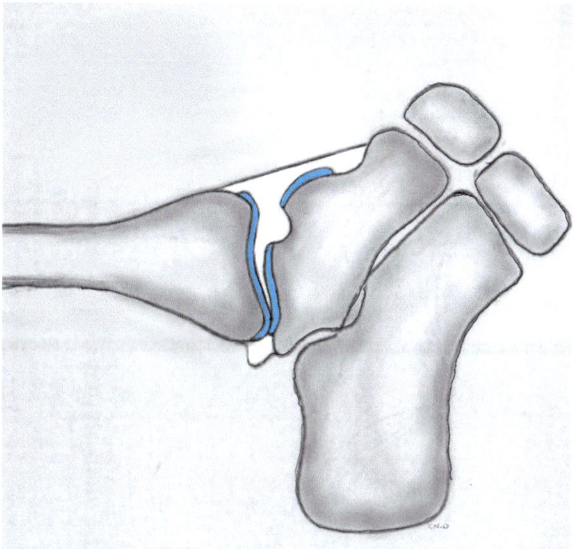

Fig. 11.13 Osteochondral defects are brought into the anterior working area by forced plantar flexion. In plantarflexion, the distance between the talus and anterior tibial plafond widens automatically, providing access to posterior located osteochondral defects

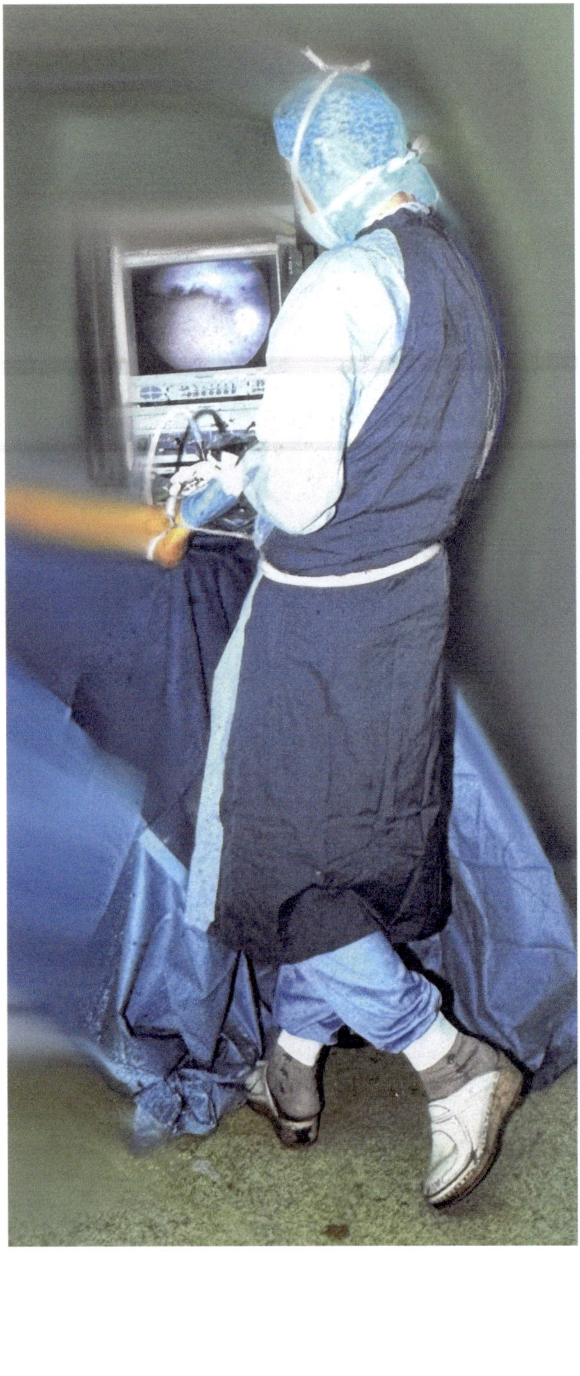

Fig. 11.14 A non-invasive distraction device, attached to a sterile belt, allows the surgeon to easily transition between the dorsiflexed position and a distracted position as needed

Technique Combined 2-Portal Anterior Supine Approach with a 2-Portal Posterior Prone Approach

We start with a proper anterior 2 portal approach with the patient supine, finish the procedure, suture the portals, apply an initial bandage, turn the patient, apply new draping and subsequently perform a proper 2 portal posterior approach with the patient in a prone position.

The patient is supine with slight elevation of the ipsilateral buttock and a support against the contralateral pelvis (Fig. 11.15a). The heel of the affected ankle is placed on the very end of the operating table. By leaning against the foot sole the surgeon can fully dorsiflex the ankle. Routine anterior portals are the anteromedial and anterolateral portal. A soft-tissue distraction device can be used when indicated. With the ankle in the plantarflexed position, one can reach osteochondral lesions in the anterior half of the talar bone [6]. In the forced plantarflexed position the anterior ankle joint opens up. This provides access to the more posterior located osteochondral defects.

At the end of the procedure the portals are sutured, covered and bandaged with a sterile bandage. The instruments, arthroscope, shaver and radiofrequency probes are kept sterile by a sterile nurse on a sterile side table (Fig. 11.15b).

The patient is turned, keeping the lower leg sterile.

The bandage is removed and the leg is newly prepared with iodine or chlorhexidine. New sterile drape is applied and the elevation of the ipsilateral buttock and a support against the pelvis are adjusted if needed. The foot should be positioned just over the edge of the table with a small support placed under the lower leg allowing dorsiflexion of the ankle (Fig. 11.15c).

It is important that the 2 anterior freshly sutured anterior portals are not pressing on the support. They must be free from pressure in order to prevent infection. In case they make contact with the drape covering the support bacteria can easily be rubbed inside by the continuous ankle movements which inevitably take place during the arthroscopy.

When starting the combined procedure with the 2-portal posterior approach prone and finishing with the 2-portal anterior approach supine it is important to keep the 2 freshly sutured posterior portals/incisions free from rubbing on the operating table. This means that a support must be placed under the lower leg proximal to the ankle joint. This to prevent contact between the fresh wounds and the operating table. Performing an anterior ankle arthroscopy with such a support under the lower leg is suboptimal since it does not allow maximal forced plantar flexion for OCD treatment. For this reason it is my advice to start anterior, flip the patient and end with the posterior approach.

The portals and technique for the 2-portal hindfoot approach are shown in (Fig. 11.16).

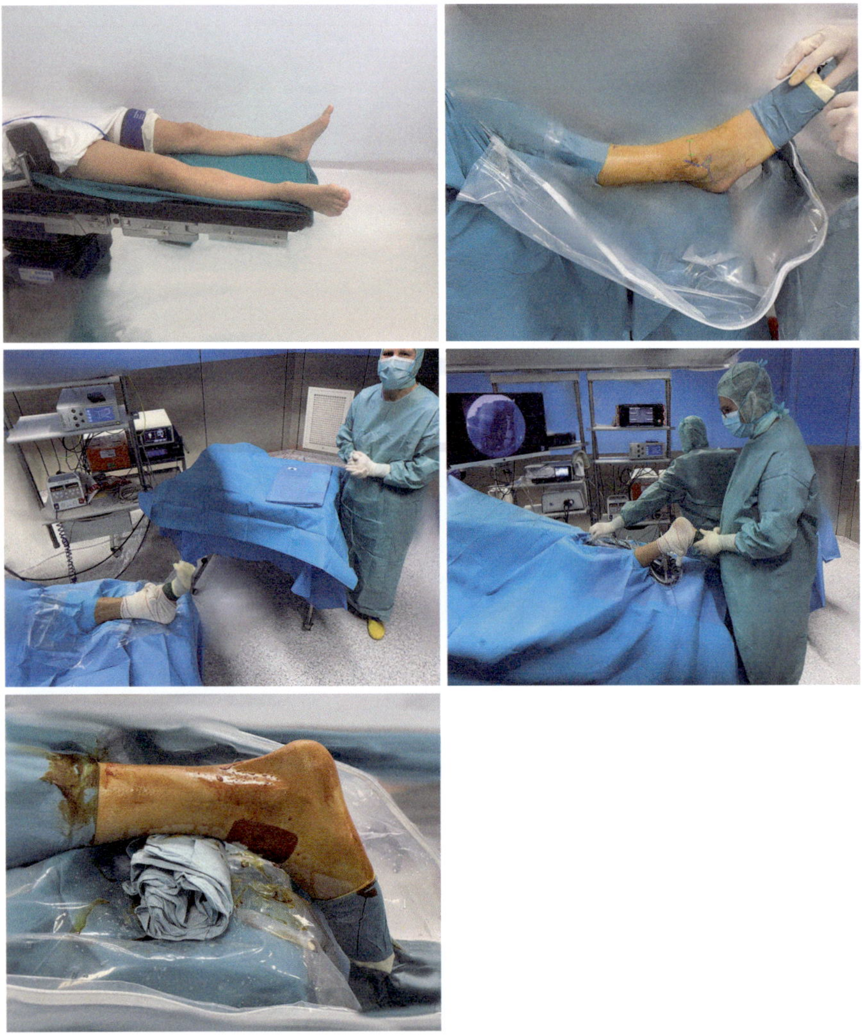

Fig. 11.15 (**a**) Patient position for an anterior 2 portal approach with the patient supine with slight elevation of the ipsilateral buttock and a support against the contralateral pelvis. The heel of the affected ankle is placed on the very end of the operating table. By leaning against the foot sole the surgeon can fully dorsiflex the ankle (See fig. 11.12a). (**b**) Routine anterior portals are the anteromedial and anterolateral portal. These portals are marked in green including the additional inferior anterolateral portal which is used for ligament repair. The contours of fibula, tibia, and location of ATFL and CFL are marked on the skin. (**c**) After suturing of the 2 anterior portals and application of a sterile bandage, the instruments, arthroscope, shaver and radiofrequency probes are kept sterile by a sterile nurse on a sterile side table. (**d**) Following this, the patient is then turned keeping the lower leg sterile. The instruments are brought back to the operating field. (**e**) The bandage is removed and the leg is newly prepared with iodine or chlorhexidine. New sterile drape is applied and the elevation of the ipsilateral buttock and a support against the pelvis are adjusted if needed. The foot must be positioned just over the edge of the table with a small support placed under the lower leg allowing dorsiflexion of the ankle. It is important that the 2 anterior freshly sutured anterior portals are not pressing on the support. They must be free from pressure in order to prevent infection. In case the make contact with the drape covering the support bacteria can easily be rubbed inside by the continuous ankle movements which inevitably take place during the arthroscopy

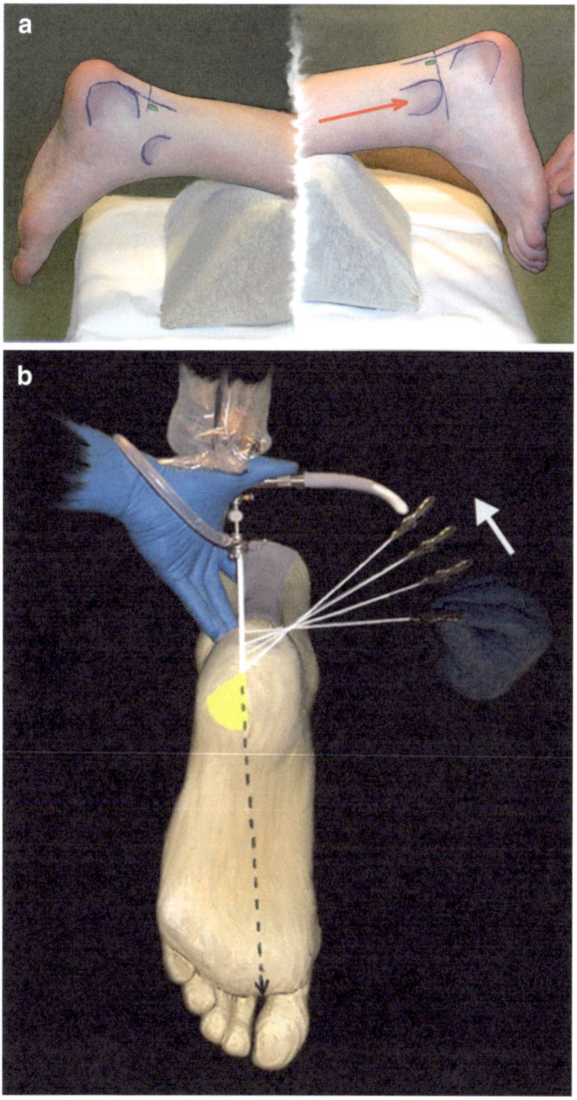

Fig. 11.16 (**a**) The portals and technique for the 2-portal hindfoot approach are shown on a left foot. Marked on the skin are the fibula the calcaneus and Achilles tendon. The red arrow points at the fibula. The tip of the fibula is the landmark for the 2 posterior portals. Their precise location is determined as follows. (1) Bring the foot in a neutral 90 degree position. (2) Draw a line through the tip of the fibula parallel to the foot sole. (3) The posterolateral portal is marked on the skin in green: 7–8 mm anterior and parallel to the Achilles tendon, extending from the line upward. (4) The posteromedial portal is marked on the skin in green. It is located opposite the anterolateral portal. (**b**) After making the skin incision, enter with a curved Mosquito forceps into the direction of the webspace between the first and second toe (black dotted line arrow) Exchange the forceps for 4 mm scope pointing in same direction with the 30 degree direction of view to the lateral side. A skin incision is now made posteromedial and the forceps is introduced at a 90 degree angle towards the scope. Once the shaft it reached, use the shaft as a guide towards the tip of the scope. Leave the forceps in this position (don't move it) and pull back the scope slightly, angulate it and now you will see the tip of the forceps. Do the same with a shaver. Start shaving on the lateral side to first disclose the subtalar joint. Move over the posterolateral talar process towards the FHL. For full technique see www.ankleplatform.com

Conclusion

For a combined arthroscopic approach there are several possibilities. The main options are a proper 2-portal supine anterior arthroscopy with an auxiliary posterolateral portal, a proper 2-portal prone posterior arthroscopy with an auxiliary anterior portal or a proper 2-portal anterior scope supine followed by a proper 2-portal posterior scope prone.

For most cases of combined anterior and posterior pathology it is advisable to use a proper anterior 2 portal approach supine, finish the procedure, suture the portals, apply an initial bandage, turn the patient, apply new draping and perform a proper 2 portal posterior approach.

The indications include all combined anterior and posterior pathologies. Specific indications are Arthrolysis for Arthrofibrosis and synovectomy for chondromatosis.

Acknowledgements Fig. 9 and 10, Dr. H Pereira, Póvoa de Varzim, Portugal
Fig 11, Dr. Gonen Haba, Israel

References

1. Amendola A, Lee KB, Saltzman CL, Suh JS. Technique and early experience with posterior arthroscopic subtalar arthrodesis. Foot Ankle Int. 2007;28:298–302. https://doi.org/10.3113/FAI.2007.0298.
2. Carro LP, Golanó P, Vega J. Arthroscopic subtalar arthrodesis: the posterior approach in the prone position. Arthrosc J Arthrosc Relat Surg. 2007;23:445.e1–4. https://doi.org/10.1016/j.arthro.2006.07.049.
3. Lee KB, Saltzman CL, Suh JS, Wasserman L, Amendola A. A posterior 3-portal arthroscopic approach for isolated subtalar arthrodesis. Arthrosc J Arthrosc Relat Surg. 2008;24:1306–10. https://doi.org/10.1016/j.arthro.2006.01.025.
4. Beimers L, De Leeuw PAJ, Van Dijk CN. A 3-portal approach for arthroscopic subtalar arthrodesis. Knee Surg Sports Traumatol Arthrosc. 2009;17:830–4. https://doi.org/10.1007/s00167-009-0795-z.
5. Rungprai C, Phisitkul P, Femino JE, Martin KD, Saltzman CL, Amendola A. Outcomes and complications after open versus posterior arthroscopic Subtalar Arthrodesis in 121 patients. J Bone Joint Surg Am. 2016;98:636–46. https://doi.org/10.2106/JBJS.15.00702.
6. Vilá-Rico J, Mellado-Romero MA, Bravo-Giménez B, Jiménez-Díaz V, Ojeda-Thies C. Subtalar arthroscopic arthrodesis: technique and outcomes. Foot Ankle Surg. 2017;23:9–15. https://doi.org/10.1016/j.fas.2015.11.007.
7. Loewen A, Ge SM, Marwan Y, Berry GK. Isolated arthroscopic-assisted subtalar fusion: a systematic review. JBJS Rev. 2021;9
8. Rungprai C, Jaroenarpornwatana A, Chaiprom N, Phisitkul P, Sripanich Y. Outcomes and complications of open vs posterior arthroscopic subtalar arthrodesis: a prospective randomized controlled multicenter study. Foot Ankle Int. 2021;42:1371–83. https://doi.org/10.1177/10711007211047239.
9. de Leeuw PA, Hendrickx RP, van Dijk CN, Stufkens SS, Kerkhoffs GM. Midterm results of posterior arthroscopic ankle fusion. Knee Surg Sports Traumatol Arthrosc. 2016;24(4):1326–31. https://doi.org/10.1007/s00167-015-3975-z. Epub 2016 Jan 12

10. Guhl J. Ankle arthroscopy. Schlack Inc; 1992. ISBN-10 0387985115
11. Ferkel RD. Author reply to 'Ankle arthroscopy: no-distraction and dorsiflexion technique is the key for ankle arthroscopy evolution'. Letter to the Editor. 2018;34(5):1382–3.
12. Ferkel RD. Foot and ankle arthroscopy. 2nd ed. Wolters Kluwer; 2017. ISBN 9780781783415
13. Ferkel RD. Ankle and foot arthroscopy, contemporary approach to diagnosis and treatment. Smith & Nephew Inc.; 2009. http://www.ankle-arthroscopy.co.uk
14. Shah R, Bandikalla VS. Role of arthroscopy in various ankle disorders. Indian J Orthop. 2021;55(2):333–41. https://doi.org/10.1007/s43465-021-00360-2. Connelly J, Ferkel RD. Ankle arthroscopy: correct portals and noninvasive distraction. Arthroscopy. 2023;7(4):1066–7. https://doi.org/10.1016/j.arthro.2021.02.023.
15. Connelly J, Ferkel RD. Ankle arthroscopy: correct portals and noninvasive distraction. Arthroscopy. 2021;37(4):1066–7. https://doi.org/10.1016/j.arthro.2021.02.023.
16. Hintermann B, Regazzoni P, Lampert C, Stutz G, Gächter A. Arthroscopic findings in acute fractures of the ankle. J Bone Joint Surg Br. 2000;82(3):345–51. https://doi.org/10.1302/0301-620x.82b3.10064. Howard S et al. Arthrosc Sports Med Rehabil. 2021
17. Howard S, Hoang V, Sagers K, Brady C, Eudy A, Watson TS. Identifying intra-articular pathology with arthroscopy prior to open ankle fracture fixation. Arthrosc Sports Med Rehabil. 2021;3(1):e177–81. https://doi.org/10.1016/j.asmr.2020.08.020.
18. Yasui Y, Shimozono Y, Hung CW, Marangon A, Wollstein A, Gianakos AL, Murawski CD, Kennedy JG. Postoperative reoperations and complications in 32,307 ankle fractures with and without concurrent ankle arthroscopic procedures in a 5-year period based on a large U.S. Healthcare Database. J Foot Ankle Surg. 2019., ISSN 1067-2516;58(1):6–9. https://doi.org/10.1053/j.jfas.2018.03.030.
19. Darwich A, Adam J, Dally FJ, Hetjens S, Jawhar A. Incidence of concomitant chondral/osteochondral lesions in acute ankle fractures and their effect on clinical outcome: a systematic review and meta-analysis. Arch Orthop Trauma Surg. 2021;141(1):63–74. https://doi.org/10.1007/s00402-020-03647-5. Epub 2020 Oct 31. Erratum in: Arch Orthop Trauma Surg. 2021;141(8):1437–1438. https://doi.org/10.1007/s00402-021-03985-y.
20. Hintermann B, Boss A, Schäfer D. Arthroscopic findings in patients with chronic ankle instability. Am J Sports Med. 2002;30(3):402–9. https://doi.org/10.1177/03635465020300031601.
21. Okuda R, Kinoshita M, Morikawa J, Yasuda T, Abe M. Arthroscopic findings in chronic lateral ankle instability: do focal chondral lesions influence the results of ligament reconstruction? Am J Sports Med. 2005;33(1):35–42. https://doi.org/10.1177/0363546504271058.
22. Yasui Y, Murawski CD, Wollstein A, Kennedy JG. Reoperation rates following ankle ligament procedures performed with and without concomitant arthroscopic procedures. Knee Surg Sports Traumatol Arthrosc. 2017;25(6):1908–15. https://doi.org/10.1007/s00167-016-4207-x. Epub 2016 Jun 16
23. Lee KB, Bai LB, Yoon TR, Jung ST, Seon JK. Second-look arthroscopic findings and clinical outcomes after microfracture for osteochondral lesions of the talus. Am J Sports Med. 2009;37 Suppl 1:63S–70S. https://doi.org/10.1177/0363546509348471. Epub 2009 Oct 20
24. Yang H-Y, Keun-Bae-Lee. Arthroscopic microfracture for osteochondral lesions of the talus: second-look arthroscopic and magnetic resonance analysis of cartilage repair tissue outcomes. J Bone Joint Surg. 2019;102(1):1. https://doi.org/10.2106/JBJS.19.00208.
25. Stornebrink T, Emanuel KS, Shimozono Y, Karlsson J, Kennedy JG, Kerkhoffs GMMJ. A change in scope: redefining minimally invasive. Knee Surg Sports Traumatol Arthrosc. 2020;28(10):3064–5. https://doi.org/10.1007/s00167-020-05898-6. Epub 2020 Feb 11
26. Eriksson E. Editorial: Arthroscopic surgery and local anaesthesia. 1997;5:205. KSSTA.
27. Stornebrink T, Stufkens SAS, Mercer NP, Kennedy J, Kerkhoffs GMM. Can bedside needle arthroscopy of the ankle be an accurate option for intra-articular delivery of injectable agents? World J Orthop. 2022;13(1):78–86. https://doi.org/10.5312/wjo.v13.i1.78.
28. Egmond PW, Meester RJ, van Dijk CN. From big hands to green fingers: it is time for a change. JISAKOS. 2023;8(4):213–5. https://doi.org/10.1016/j.jisako.2023.04.005.

29. Tonogai I, Hayashi F, Tsuruo Y, Sairyo K. Distance between the anterior distal Tibial edge and the anterior Tibial artery in distraction and nondistraction during anterior ankle arthroscopy: a cadaveric study. Foot Ankle Int. 2018;39(1):113–8. https://doi.org/10.1177/1071100717732550. Epub 2017 Oct 27
30. Wang DY, Jiao C, Ao YF, Yu JK, Guo QW, Xie X, Chen LX, Zhao F, Pi YB, Li N, Hu YL, Jiang D. Orthop J Sports Med. 2020;8(5):2325967120922821. https://doi.org/10.1177/2325967120922821. eCollection 2020 May
31. van Dijk CN, Tol JL, Verheyen CC. A prospective study of prognostic factors concerning the outcome of arthroscopic surgery for anterior ankle impingement. Am J Sports Med. 1997;25(6):737–45. https://doi.org/10.1177/036354659702500603.
32. Walsh SJ, Twaddle BC, Rosenfeldt MP, Boyle MJ. Arthroscopic treatment of anterior ankle impingement: a prospective study of 46 patients with 5-year follow-up. Am J Sports Med. 2014;42(11):2722–6. https://doi.org/10.1177/0363546514550976. Epub 2014 Sep 26
33. van Dijk CV, Vuurberg G, Batista J, et al. Posterior ankle arthroscopy: current state of the art. JISAKOS. 2017;2:269–77.
34. van Dijk CN, de Leeuw PA, Scholten PE. Hindfoot endoscopy for posterior ankle impingement. Surgical technique. J Bone Joint Surg Am. 2009;91(Suppl 2):287–98.
35. van Dijk CN, Kort N. Tendoscopy of the peroneal tendons. Arthroscopy. 1998;14(5):471–8. https://doi.org/10.1016/s0749-8063(98)70074-x.
36. Steenstra F, van Dijk CN. Achilles tendoscopy. Foot Ankle Clin. 2006;11(2):429–38, viii. https://doi.org/10.1016/j.fcl.2006.02.001.
37. van Dijk CN, van Dyk GE, Scholten PE, Kort NP. Endoscopic calcaneoplasty. Am J Sports Med. 2001;29(2):185–9. https://doi.org/10.1177/03635465010290021101.
38. Bojanic I, Bergovec M, Smoljanovic T. Foot Ankle Int. 2009;30(11):1120–3. https://doi.org/10.3113/FAI.2009.1120.
39. Farii HA, Doyle-Kelly C, Marwan Y, Volesky M, Turcotte R. Arthroscopic management of synovial chondromatosis of the ankle joint: a systematic review of the literature. JBJS Rev. 2020;8(9):e2000045. https://doi.org/10.2106/JBJS.RVW.20.00045.
40. Linklater JM, Fessa CK. Imaging findings in arthrofibrosis of the ankle and foot. Semin Musculoskelet Radiol. 2012;16(3):185–91. https://doi.org/10.1055/s-0032-1320059.
41. Utsugi K, Sakai H, Hiraoka H, Yashiki M, Mogi H. Intra-articular fibrous tissue formation following ankle fracture: the significance of arthroscopic debridement of fibrous tissue. Arthroscopy. 2007;23(1):89–93. https://doi.org/10.1016/j.arthro.2006.07.055.
42. Amendola A, Petrik J, Webster-Bogaert S. Ankle arthroscopy: outcome in 79 consecutive patients. Arthroscopy. 1996;12(5):565–73.
43. Parisien JS, Vangsness T. Operative arthroscopy of the ankle. Three years' experience. Clin Orthop Relat Res. 1985;199:46–53.
44. Kim JH, Gwak HC, Park DH, Lee CR, Jung SH, Kim JG, Lee SJ. Second-look arthroscopic findings and clinical outcomes after management of intra-articular lesions in acute ankle fractures with arthroscopy. Foot Ankle Surg. 2021;27(7):799–808. https://doi.org/10.1016/j.fas.2020.10.010. Epub 2021 Jan 14
45. Lui TH, Chan WK, Chan KB. The arthroscopic management of frozen ankle. Arthroscopy. 2006;22(3):283–6. https://doi.org/10.1016/j.arthro.2005.12.012.
46. Cui Q, Milbrandt T, Millington S, Anderson M, Hurwitz S. Treatment of posttraumatic adhesive capsulitis of the ankle: a case series. Foot Ankle Int. 2005;26(8):602–6. https://doi.org/10.1177/107110070502600805.
47. van Dijk CN, van Bergen CJA. Advancements in ankle arthroscopy. J Am Acad Orthop Surg. 2008;16(11):635–46. https://doi.org/10.5435/00124635-200811000-00004.
48. de Leeuw PA, Golanó P, Clavero JA, van Dijk CN. Anterior ankle arthroscopy, distraction or dorsiflexion? Knee Surg Sports Traumatol Arthrosc. 2010;18(5):594–600. https://doi.org/10.1007/s00167-010-1089-1. Epub 2010 Mar 9
49. Talbot CE, Knapik DM, Miskovsky SN. Prevalence and location of bone spurs in anterior ankle impingement: A cadaveric investigation. Clin Anat. 2018;31(8):1144–50.
50. www.ankleplatform.com

Chapter 12
Flatfoot Reconstruction

Manuel Monteagudo

Introduction

Flatfoot deformity is one of the most common disorders in our practice. Progressive collapse of the medial arch ends up causing peritalar pain and dysfunction. Patients may be asymptomatic for years until compensation mechanisms are lost and present with tenderness and feeling of giving way medially. Clinical gait analysis with patient barefeet is fundamental to address the type of deformity which may vary from isolated hindfoot valgus to different and complex combined hindfoot- midfoot-forefoot deformities. Forefoot varus can be estimated with the patient seated and the hindfoot positioned into slight valgus. In some severe, long-standing cases, ankle valgus and medial ankle instability are also present. Weightbearing x-rays of both feet and ankles may be misleading if the patient is still able to heel rise, as compensation mechanisms will allow for "good-looking" radiographs that do not match with visual gait analysis. Other image studies—CT, MRI, WBCT—permit to complete the picture of associated pathologies that should be considered for surgical planning. Most patients will improve function and get pain relief with the use of the correct insoles if the heel posted into varus prevents foot collapse in the transition from the first to the second rockers of gait. Surgery should be individualized as many factors may influence our choice of surgical techniques. Classically, osteotomies with soft tissue reconstruction are indicated in flexible deformities and arthrodesis in rigid deformities. However, other factors—age, body weight, occupation—may influence the surgical strategy. Although outcomes following flatfoot reconstruction are good in most cases, realistic expectations mean most

M. Monteagudo (✉)
Foot and Ankle Unit—Trauma & Orthopaedics—Hospital Universitario Quironsalud, Madrid, Spain

Department of Medicine, Faculty of Medicine, Health and Sports, European University of Madrid, Madrid, Spain

M. Bhatia (ed.), *Surgical Techniques of the Foot and Ankle*,
https://doi.org/10.1007/978-3-031-93742-2_12

patients will need a long time to recover with some not fully recovering. Collapsing progressive foot deformity is challenging and bespoke solutions are needed for most patients. In this chapter I will focus on surgical techniques available for flatfoot deformities and will try to provide the reader with some of the tips and tricks I have learned through years of success and failure.

Background/Pathogenesis/Classifications

Over the years, the concept of flatfoot has changed from considering progressive degeneration of the posterior tibial tendon as the predisposing factor leading to longitudinal arch collapse, to believing that it is a multifactorial process [1, 2]. Progressive weakness of subtalar ligaments and other concomitant disorders ultimately progress to a painful and poorly functioning flatfoot causing damage to medial soft tissues, including posterior tibial tendon [3]. Most soft tissue damage seems to be a consequence rather than the cause of foot collapse. Classification systems allow us to identify the severity of the condition and try to provide guide treatment plans [4–6]. Over the past few years, a better understanding of the biomechanics and the progression of flatfoot led to a new classification system and newly accepted terminology of progressive collapsing foot deformity which acknowledges the involvement of soft tissue structures and joint alignment of the hindfoot, midfoot, forefoot, and ankle [7, 8].

Key Points in Examination

The combination of a thorough physical examination including visual gait analysis should allow us to make the diagnosis of collapsing foot deformity.

Clinical examination—*visual gait analysis and deformities.*

I routinely ask the patient to walk barefeet in my clinic to start with visual gait analysis. Each case may present with different deformities which should be addressed to plan for the surgical strategy. Some cases present with isolated valgus hindfoot with no midfoot/forefoot abduction, and no forefoot supination. In some other cases, abduction is also observed in combination with a valgus heel ("too many toes" sign) [9–11]. Forefoot varus/supination is better examined with the patient seated with manual correction of hindfoot into slight valgus position and it can be flexible or rigid. When forefoot supination is an issue for considering plantarflexion of the first ray within reconstructive surgery, it is common to find pain around the cuboid and on the plantar base of the first metatarsal, corresponding to a swollen and overloaded peroneus longus tendon. Tenderness over the posterior tibialis tendon around the medial malleolus and lateral subtalar/peroneal pain due to impingement are common clinical findings. Strength of posterior tibial tendon and flexibility of deformity is assessed with single and double heel rise tests. A fixed valgus deformity will not correct into heel varus on heel rise. Ankle is also tested for medial instability to complete the clinical picture.

Imaging studies—*Less is more.*

Weight bearing radiographs of both feet provide most of the information necessary to complete the diagnosis of progressive collapsing foot deformity when all compensation mechanisms are lost. But we should beware of the interpretation of weight bearing x-rays when the patient is still capable of performing a single heel rise test with a flexible foot as they may be misleading. A dissociation can frequently be observed between bone disposition on the x-rays and visual gait analysis [12]. In that scenario, surgical planning should be done on deformities assessed on visual gait analysis rather than on the weight bearing x-rays. Some of my failures have had this origin. MRI allows us to address soft tissue damage and bone oedema, and CT helps us with the diagnosis of osteoarthritis in neighbouring joints. WBCT imaging has improved our understanding of the three-dimensional deformity of flatfoot [13, 14]. Other tests such as SPECT-CT scintigraphy can also help to assess subtle associated arthritic lesions in hindfoot and midfoot joints.

Management

Conservative treatment should be considered before surgery regardless of the type of arthritis, pain, or stage of the condition.

Non-operative Treatment

Mechanical foot problems need mechanical-based solutions. The use of insoles with a supinatory wedge (varus heel posting) may work in most patients [15]. Flexible deformities tend to respond better to insoles than rigid deformities. Several studies have demonstrated good results in 67–90% of cases using conservative treatment [16]. When the ankle is painful and/or presents with medial instability the addition of an ankle-foot orthosis (AFO) may help in controlling instability and pain. If orthotics and braces do not provide relief, surgery should be considered.

Operative Treatment

Surgical goals include relief of pain, obtaining a stable plantigrade foot, and the maintenance of the integrity and motion of as many joints as possible [17]. Insoles and bracing should ideally be discontinued after surgery. There are some general considerations common to most surgical procedures when treating flatfoot deformity. The author prefers to perform flatfoot surgery with a thigh tourniquet inflated to 300 mm Hg. Patients receive a popliteal block followed by spinal or general anaesthesia and surgery is done under fluoroscopic guidance. Postoperatively, a bulky dressing and splint are applied. Patients are usually discharged on the day following surgery. A week from surgery the splint is discontinued, and a walking boot is used to protect the reconstruction. Sutures are removed in 3 weeks. Weight Bearing is allowed at around 3 weeks after osteotomies and 6 weeks after an arthrodesis. Soft tissue reconstruction should be regarded as an adjunct to the joint preserving bony procedures. There are many different surgical procedures to be considered. My preferred techniques are presented in this chapter. In a book on surgical techniques the detail of each procedure is important, but the combination of indication and the different techniques remains the choice of each surgeon.

Flexible Deformities

The combination of osteotomies and soft tissue repair is of choice in flexible deformities in the young. Advanced age, high body mass index and physically demanding occupations may favour arthrodesis even in the presence of flexible non-arthritic joints. The different scenarios may present different indications.

Hindfoot Valgus—No Abduction, No Forefoot Varus

Patients with an isolated hindfoot valgus are good candidates for a medial sliding calcaneal osteotomy [18]. With the patient in lateral decubitus and a thigh tourniquet, a lateral approach to the posterior tuberosity of the calcaneus is made. An 8- to 10 cm longitudinal incision is centred along the posterior calcaneal tuberosity. A full-thickness flap is made to avoid skin problems. Soft tissue structures are protected over the superior and inferior aspects of the calcaneus. The osteotomy is created using irrigation to avoid thermal injury to bone. The cut is carried out until the opposite cortex is reached, and care is taken to progressively debilitate the distal cortex to end up with a single clean cut. Failure to do so will cause difficulties in displacing the osteotomy medially. A 10 mm medial slide is performed and a 3- to 4 cm incision in the heel allows for the introduction of two parallel k-wires to hold the osteotomy in place. Fluoroscopy is used to confirm position of the wires and to measure the length of the screws to be inserted. Two parallel, short thread 6.5- or 7.0-mm cannulated screws are used to maintain displacement of the osteotomy (Fig. 12.1). Either headless or headed screws may be selected because the goal of the screws is not compression (as in an arthrodesis) but maintenance of the obtained displacement. Once the osteotomy has been fixed, the edge of the osteotomy is crushed until flush with the lateral wall of the posterior tuberosity of the os calcis thus avoiding lateral prominence that might be uncomfortable with shoewear. Regardless of the approach and/or implants, this type of osteotomy is primarily

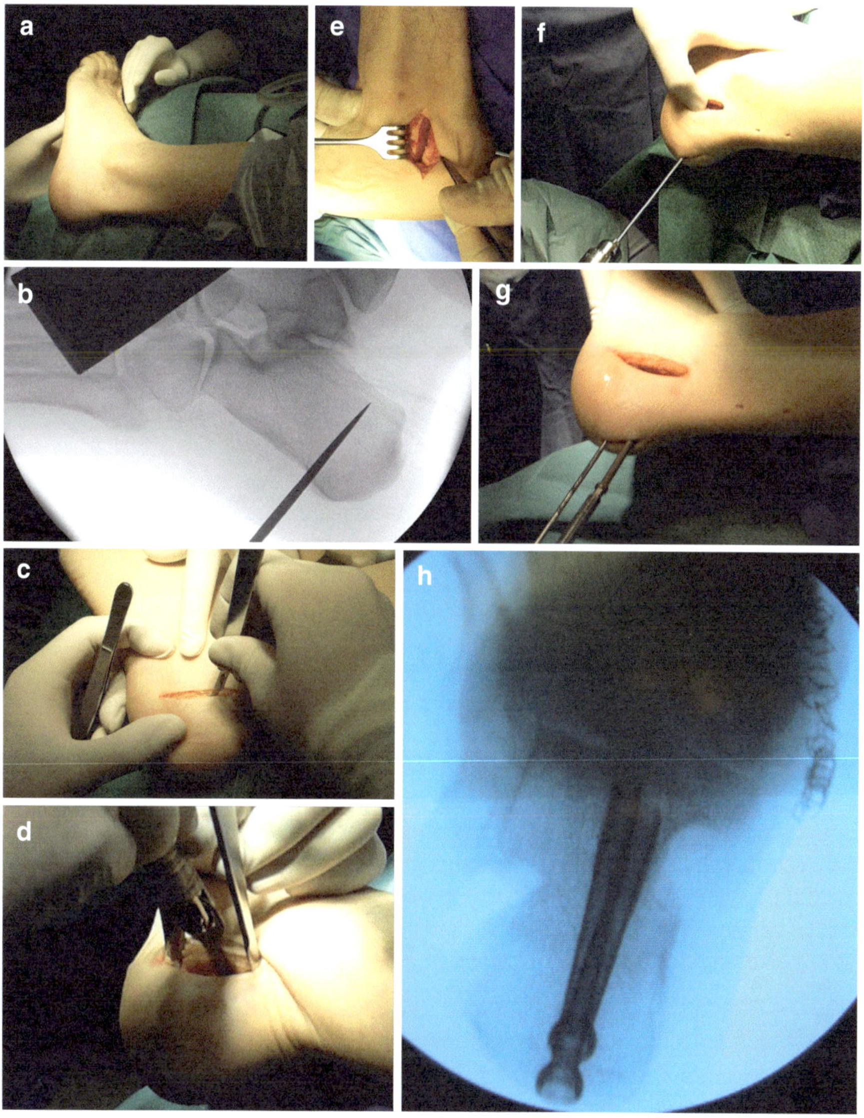

Fig. 12.1 Medial sliding calcaneal osteotomy is the most performed procedure in the reconstruction of a flexible flatfoot. (**a**) Patient in lateral decubitus with the calcaneal prepared for the osteotomy. (**b**) Fluoroscopy helps to correctly placing the cut perpendicular to the long axis of the calcaneus. (**c**) Lateral approach is relatively free of anatomical dangers. (**d**) With the soft tissues protected with Hohmann retractors, a single cut is performed. (**e**) A 10 mm slide is enough in most patients. (**f**) Parallel K-wires are inserted into the bone to guide cannulated screws. (**g**) Two 6.5 mm cannulated screws are inserted. (**h**) Axial view with fluoroscopy showing medial displacement of the osteotomy

stable enough to allow almost immediate protected weight bearing in a walking boot. Step-plates and other implants are also used for this type of osteotomy. Over the last years, minimally invasive approaches have been used to perform medial displacement calcaneal osteotomies.

Tip

To effectively maintain the desired medial displacement of the osteotomy I place one of my thumbs in the lateral aspect of the posterior tuberosity (Fig. 12.2). Should correction be lost while inserting the screws repositioning of the wires and screws is advisable. This happens when the screw contacts the distal inner lateral wall of the calcaneus causing lateral shifting of the posterior tuberosity.

Hindfoot Valgus with Abduction—No Forefoot Varus

Midfoot and forefoot abduction is best assessed with visual gait analysis. Isolated abduction (without hindfoot valgus) and forefoot varus is present in some patients. Although lengthening of the lateral column is controversial, this type of osteotomy has been shown to restore height of the medial arch and correct hindfoot valgus and midfoot/forefoot abduction [19, 20]. With the patient in lateral decubitus and a thigh tourniquet a lateral approach to the sinus tarsi and the anterior tuberosity of the calcaneus is made. A 3- to 5 cm longitudinal incision is centred along the anterior aspect of the lateral subtalar joint. Dissection is carried out from the joint to expose the lateral wall of the calcaneus around 3–4 cm proximal to the calcaneocuboid joint. Peroneal tendons and sural nerve are carefully retracted plantarly with a Hohmann retractor positioned around the plantar aspect of the bone. With a saw blade, the osteotomy is created taking care to position it between the articular facets of the subtalar joint. The cut is carried out until the medial cortex is reached, and care is taken to progressively debilitate the distal cortex without completely cutting it, so osteoclasia can be made to open the osteotomy laterally. With the use of two saw blades/osteotomes and a lamina spreader

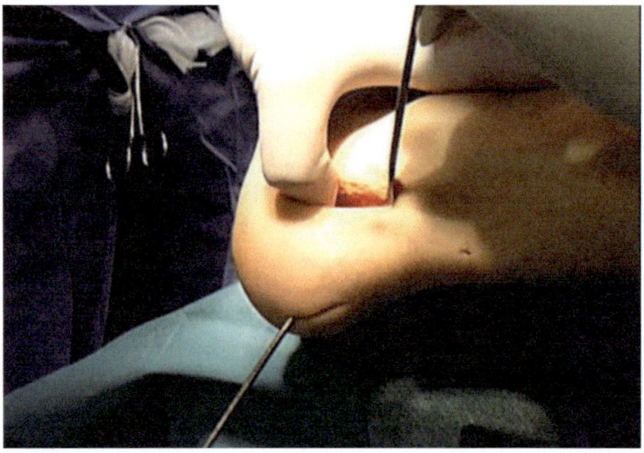

Fig. 12.2 To effectively maintain the desired medial displacement of the osteotomy the thumb of the surgeon placed over the lateral aspect of the posterior calcaneal tuberosity should notice potential loss of correction while inserting the wires and screws. Should correction be lost, repositioning of the wires and screws is mandatory

the osteotomy is wedged open to correct abduction. The distance of the opening is measured, and the appropriate trial of the wedge is selected. Once the trial is inserted the saw blades/osteotomes are carefully removed. Correction is checked both visually and under fluoroscopy. A specific Evans-type titanium wedge is inserted and rechecked for position and stability. The wedge (or graft) usually measures between 6 and 10 mm in width (Fig. 12.3). Overcorrection frequently results in painful lateral column overload and eventually in calcaneocuboid arthritis. Other implants like plate and screws or even allografts may also be used. Lateral lengthening calcaneal osteotomy is a powerful tool to correct foot abduction but at the price of exerting forefoot varus/supination. Should this secondary forefoot varus not be flexible to easily and passively take the forefoot into a plantigrade position, a plantarflexion osteotomy of the first cuneiform should be performed. Titanium wedges provide great primary stability that allow early protected weightbearing in a boot [21].

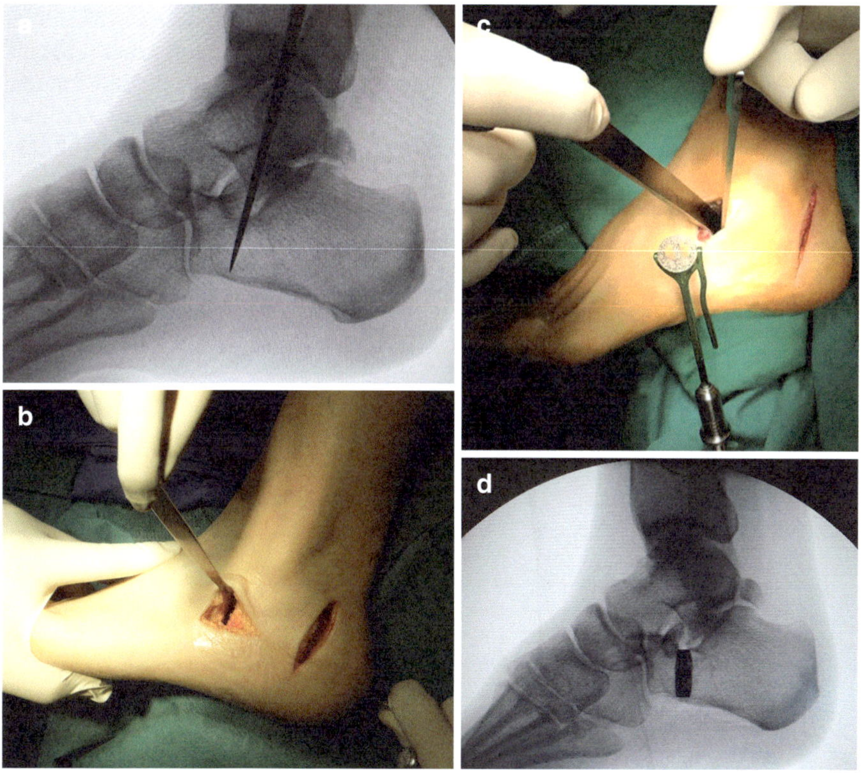

Fig. 12.3 Lateral lengthening osteotomy starts with (**a**) the location of the cut under fluoroscopy. (**b**) Lateral approach for the Evans-type osteotomy that in this patient was made in combination with a medial sliding calcaneal osteotomy. (**c**) A porous titanium wedge is about to be introduced in the osteotomy site. (**d**) Fluoroscopic control after wedge insertion allows us to check the wedge is not protruding into the subtalar joint

Tip A k-wire is inserted to provisionally fix the anterior tuberosity of the calcaneus to the cuboid so that cranial migration of the tuberosity is avoided while the wedge is inserted. Even in the event of migration and asymmetrical joint disposition on fluoroscopy, the calcaneocuboid joint is usually permissive and very uncommonly symptomatic. Compression forces are usually a concern so lengthening over 10 mm should not be done, otherwise calcaneocuboid arthritis may develop (Fig. 12.4). Children may admit lengthening procedures of even double that figure as their bony and soft tissue structures readapt overtime. Beware of lengthening over 10 mm in adolescents as they do not have the same capacity of readapting the rest of the foot.

Hindfoot Valgus with Abduction and Forefoot Varus

Some patients present with isolated forefoot varus, but it is usually observed in combination with hindfoot valgus and midfoot/forefoot abduction as the result of a long-standing hindfoot deformity that adapts the midtarsal joints and forefoot to rotate and cause supination/varus in the forefoot. Forefoot varus causes difficulties in gait progression because of a weakened propulsion during the third rocker of gait. When the three deformities are found—hindfoot valgus, abduction, and forefoot varus—all three should be corrected in reconstructive surgery. The most common technique to restore plantar positioning of the forefoot is Cotton osteotomy [22, 23]. Cotton osteotomy is a medial cuneiform opening wedge osteotomy with the wedge based dorsally that aims to plantarflex the medial column to correct forefoot supination. Following calcaneal osteotomies, the patient is placed supine, and the surgeon may evaluate the position of the medial column and residual forefoot varus. My threshold to perform Cotton osteotomy in the context of a multiplanar deformity is

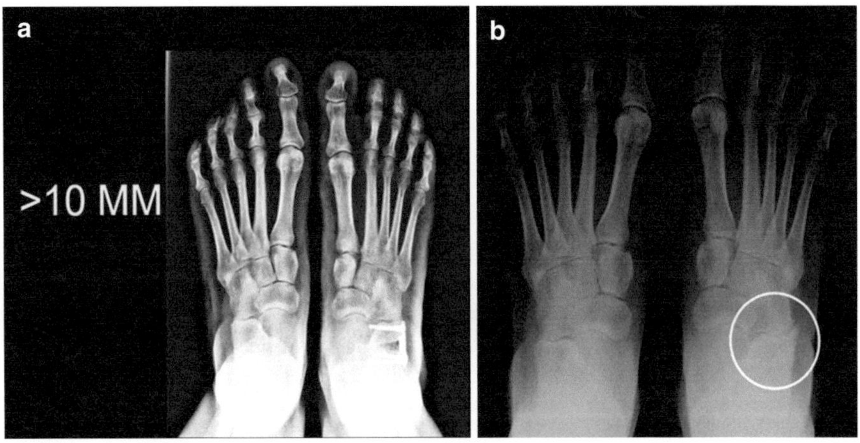

Fig. 12.4 Postoperative x-rays after lateral lengthening osteotomy with 11 mm wedging. (**a**) 6 months after surgery. (**b**) 2 years after surgery and after plate removal, calcaneocuboid joint is arthritic and symptomatic

lower than at the beginning of my surgical career. I prefer a 4- to 5 cm dorsomedial incision over the medial cuneiform. Careful dissection avoids damaging the medial dorsal cutaneous nerve and the saphenous nerve and vein. Capsulotomy is placed just medial to the extensor hallucis longus tendon, taking care not to disrupt the dorsal ligaments of the adjacent joints. Tibialis anterior tendon will lay medial and plantar to the planned cut of the osteotomy. I use fluoroscopy to identify the orientation of the osteotomy to ensure it remains extra-articular. Then I insert 25- or 27-gauge needles into the first metatarsocuneiform, the naviculocuneiform, and the second metatarsocuneiform joint. I prefer to place the cut just proximal to the level of the second metatarsocuneiform joint to avoid invading the joint which might require revision surgery. A transverse osteotomy is then created with a sagittal saw from dorsal to plantar parallel to the first metatarsocuneiform joint. I use a smooth wide lamina spreader to gently lever the site open until the forefoot is plantigrade. I use porous titanium wedges to maintain correction as an alternative to plates or allografts. With the appropriate sizer inserted fluoroscopy helps in checking that the future implant will not invade the second metatarsocuneiform joint. With a specific impactor the specific Cotton-type titanium wedge is seated into position by tapping gently with a hammer and rechecked for position and stability. The wedge (or graft) usually measures between 6 and 8 mm in width (around 1–2 mm less than the Evans wedge when both procedures are simultaneously performed) (Fig. 12.5). Overcorrection may result in second rocker metatarsalgia under the first metatarsophalangeal joint. Plates and screws and freeze-dried wedged allografts may also be

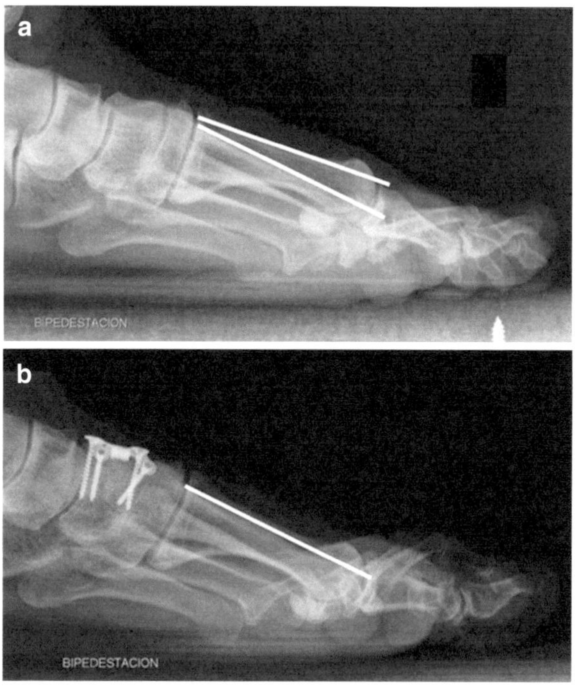

Fig. 12.5 Plantar flexion of the first ray allows for the correction of forefoot varus. (**a**) Preoperative lateral view weightbearing x-ray showing forefoot varus with divergent dorsal cortices of the first and second metatarsals. (**b**) 6 months after forefoot varus correction with Cotton osteotomy, both cortices are parallel

used for Cotton osteotomies. Grafts and titanium wedges are usually primarily stable without the need for additional fixation, but an additional screw, staple, wire, may be used. Lapicotton or Lapidus procedures may be considered in the presence of first metatarsocuneiform arthritis with the same effect of correction for the forefoot varus [24].

Tip Extreme care should be taken to ensure reaching but preserving the medial cuneiform's plantar cortex. I always check the lateral and medial edges of the medial cuneiform to ensure both cortices are cut and that I have reached the plantar cortex prior to attempting to open the osteotomy. Should one of these cortices fail to be cut or the cut insufficient, the plantar hinge may fracture into the distal or proximal joints when opening the osteotomy (Fig. 12.6).

The combination of the three osteotomies—calcaneal medial slide, lengthening, and plantarflexion of the first cuneiform is a common procedure in the young active patient with a dysfunctional flexible flatfoot deformity (Fig. 12.7).

Soft Tissue Reconstruction

Posterior tibialis tendon debridement and reinforcement combined with medial displacement calcaneal osteotomy has been the gold standard for flexible flatfoot deformity for a long time [3]. Repair of the soft tissues is now understood as adjunct procedures to the bony reconstruction. Not all surgeons perform the repair of the medial soft tissues. In most of my flexible cases treated with osteotomies, I prefer tendoscopic debridement and thinning of the diseased tendon with the conviction that bony correction will mechanically be enough [25–28] (Fig. 12.8). For those who repair the posterior tibial tendon, exposure through a medial perimalleolar incision is followed by debridement as needed and tendon transfer. The flexor digitorum longus tendon is dissected distal to the knot of Henry and divided. A 4.5 mm drill hole is made in the navicular tuberosity and the flexor digitorum longus tendon is

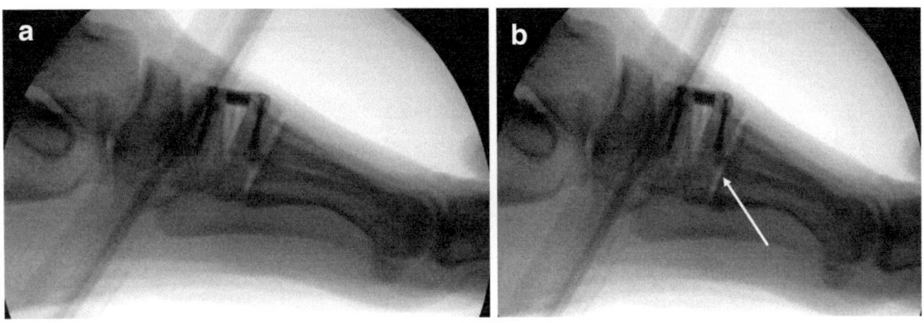

Fig. 12.6 Intraoperative fluoroscopic images showing Cotton osteotomy fixed with plate and screws. (**a**) We all tend to pay our attention to the correction and the wedging that seem correct. (**b**) But a closer look allows for the diagnosis of an intraoperative fracture of the cuneiform (arrow) because of an insufficient cut that did not reach the plantar cortex

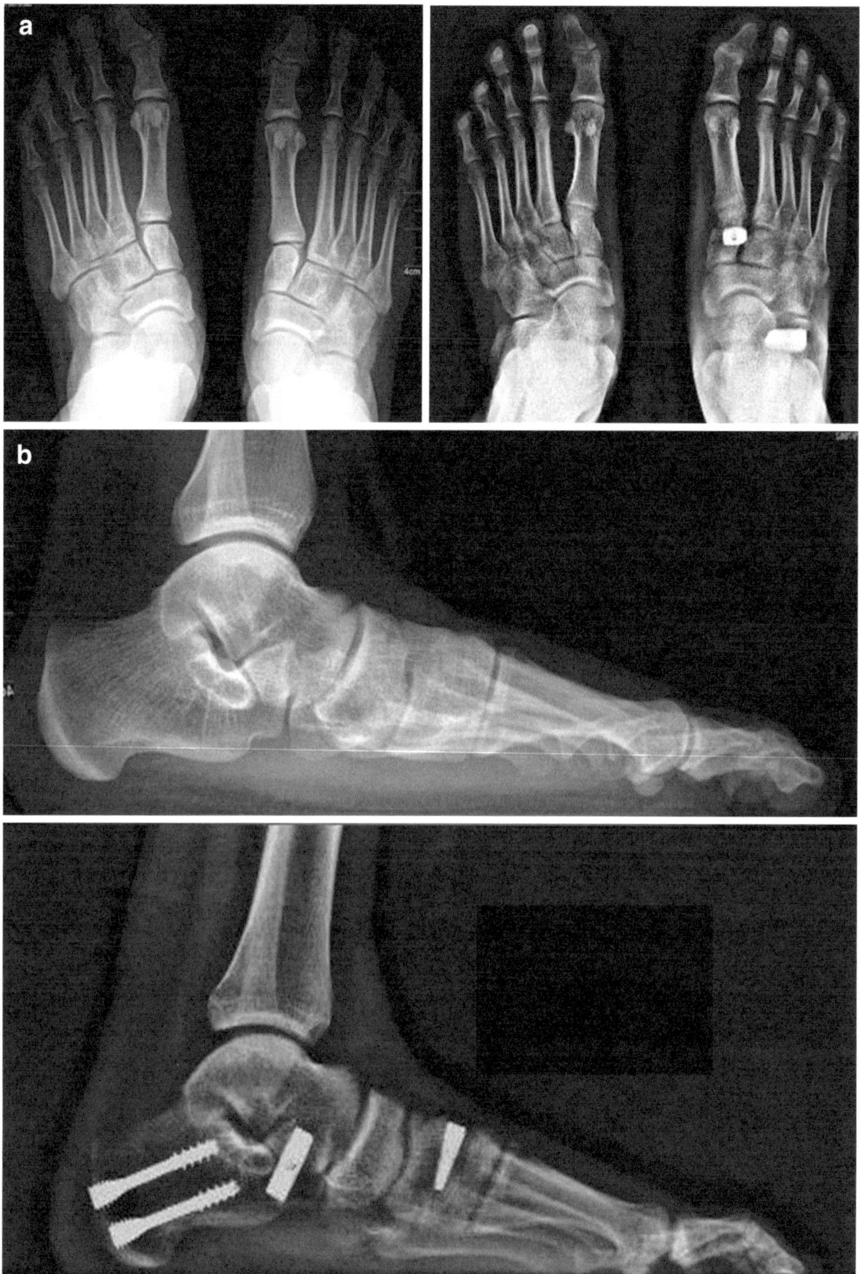

Fig. 12.7 The combination of medial sliding, lateral lengthening calcaneal osteotomies and plantarflexion osteotomy of the first cuneiform is a common combination in the reconstruction of a flexible deformity in the young active patient. (**a**) Dorsoplantar views of weightbearing of x-rays preoperative and postoperative 12 months after surgery showing changing in bony alignment. (**b**) Lateral views of the same case with visible restoration of medial arch height

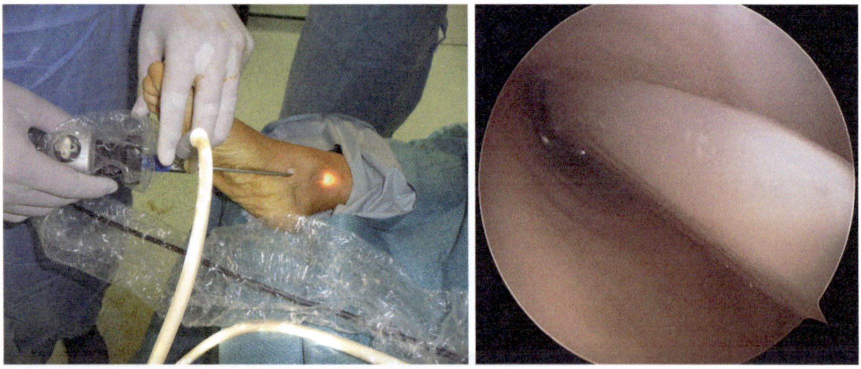

Fig. 12.8 Posterior tibial tendoscopy may be an alternative to open soft tissue reconstruction in many flexible flatfoot cases. (**a**) Working through a portal placed close to the navicular insertion allows for the inspection of the full length of the tendon. (**b**) Tendoscopic view of a posterior tibial tendon with no structural damage, a typical scenario in the young patient with flexible deformity

passed from plantar to dorsal through the hole with the help of a grasping suture. Tensioning of the transfer should be done once the bony reconstruction has been completed. The tendon is secured back into itself with nonabsorbable sutures. An interference screw may also be used to fix the transferred tendon to the navicular tunnel (Fig. 12.9). Spring ligament may be reconstructed with direct sutures or with reinforcement with one of the many synthetic ligament augmentation systems. Tendo Achilles lengthening or gastroc-soleus lengthening may be necessary to correct equinus if present at the end of the reconstruction [29]. Tendo Achilles lengthening can be done percutaneously or with a mini open technique.

Other Procedures in Flatfoot Reconstruction

Several sinus tarsi techniques have been used to limit excessive subtalar pronation and prevent foot arch collapse [30–32]. These techniques—Grice-type subtalar block arthrodesis, arthroereisis, calcaneo-stop—are minimally invasive and a block of bone or an implant is used to limit or block subtalar motion after a reduction manoeuvre to restore the anatomical relationships between the talus and the calcaneus.

Rigid Deformities

Arthrodesis for the treatment of flatfoot deformity is indicated in the presence of rigid deformities or flexible deformities with arthritis [33, 34]. The more severe the deformity the more segments will have to be included in the arthrodesis. Fusion procedures for collapsing progressive foot deformity include subtalar, naviculocuneiform, double, triple, tibiotalocalcaneal, and pantalar. Limited isolated fusions are

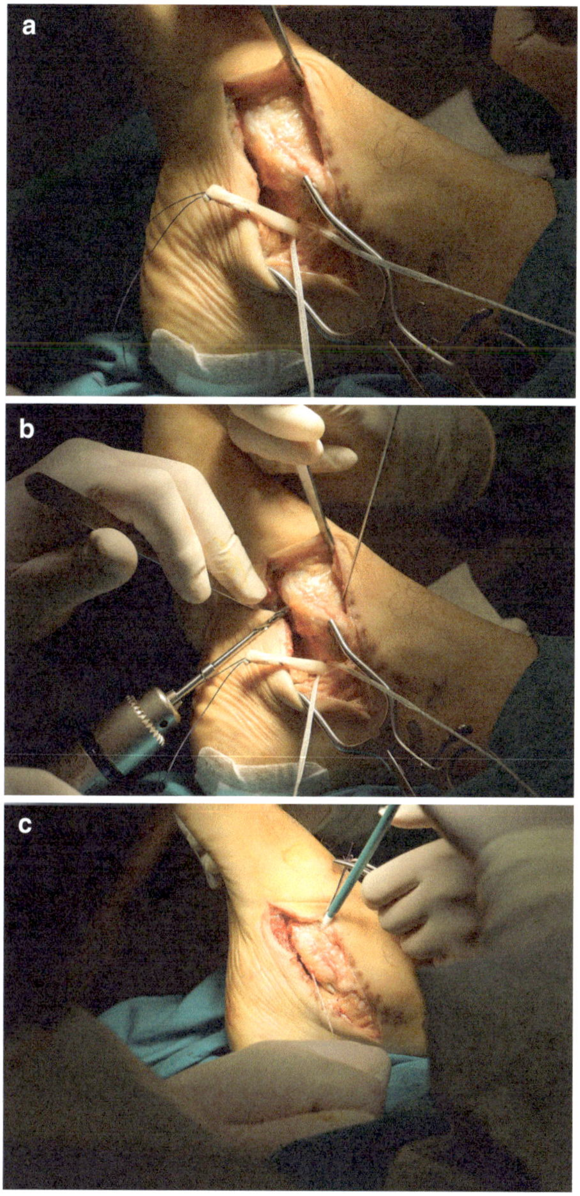

Fig. 12.9 Flexor digitorum longus transfer has been classically used as an adjunct procedure for bony reconstruction in flexible flatfoot deformity. (**a**) Harvesting of the flexor digitorum tendon. (**b**) Drilling of the tunnel in the navicular. (**c**) Fixation of the transferred tendon into the navicular with the use of an interference screw

indicated when there is moderate deformity with arthritis. Isolated naviculocuneiform, talonavicular, or subtalar arthrodesis may limit pain and improve function in flatfoot with joint involvement [35]. In the presence of severe deformity, a more extensive remodelling arthrodesis is needed to fully correct the fixed deformity. Double or triple arthrodesis, medial column arthrodesis are of choice when the ankle joint can be salvaged or repaired. Triple arthrodesis allows for reconstruction of almost any flatfoot deformity and position of the forefoot may be adjusted to the midfoot and hindfoot. Surgical techniques for these arthrodeses are not the focus of this chapter and are described in other chapters in this book.

Hindfoot/Ankle Valgus With/Without Ankle Arthritis

Some patients with severe foot collapse present with medial ankle instability with or without tibiotalar arthritis. A wide variety of combinations of techniques may be performed depending on the affected joints [36]. Reconstruction with a combination of osteotomies and soft tissue repair including deltoid ligament augmentation is preferable to arthrodesis. Sometimes fusion of different hindfoot/midfoot segments is performed and a total ankle replacement is added on top of the subtalar/doble/triple arthrodesis. Tibiotalocalcaneal or pantalar arthrodesis are indicated when deformity is severe, and bone stock is limited.

Outcomes

Different studies have focused on outcomes after flatfoot reconstruction [37–39]. Most patients are satisfied with the results and report life-changing improvements, but many also experienced prolonged pain and difficulty after surgery with difficulty or inability to return to their preoperative maximum level of physical activity [40].

Conclusions

The correct management of progressive collapsing foot deformity starts with a careful clinical examination including visual gait analysis. Nonoperative management with the use of insoles and braces is recommended as initial treatment regardless of the stage of the disorder or the type of deformity. Surgical management should be individualised and foot flexibility, age, occupation, may condition surgical decision-making. In the absence of arthritis, the combination of deformities may be corrected with the use of different osteotomies—medial displacement calcaneal, lateral lengthening, plantarflexion of the medial cuneiform—and soft tissue procedures—tendon transfers, ligament repair—with the goal of a plantigrade pain-free foot. In the presence of arthritis and/or rigid deformities, a variety of arthrodesis may be utilized to restore medial arch height. Individualization of surgical procedures is paramount to obtain a good outcome.

Ethical Statement **Not applicable for this article.**

Conflict of Interest **There are no conflicts for interest for the authors of this article.**

Funding No financial support.

References

1. Rodrigues-Fonseca J. Pe plano. Oporto: Estudo dinâmico. Lab Bial; 1984.
2. Johnson KA, Strom DE. Tibialis posterior tendon dysfunction. Clin Orthop Relat Res. 1989;239:196–206.
3. Myerson MS. Adult acquired flatfoot deformity: treatment of dysfunction of the posterior tibial tendon. Instr Course Lect. 1997;46:393–405.
4. Bluman EM, Title CI, Myerson MS. Posterior tibial tendon rupture: a refined classification system. Foot Ankle Clin. 2007;8(3):637–45.
5. Raikin SM, Winters BS, Daniel JN. The RAM classification: a novel, systematic approach to the adult-acquired flatfoot. Foot Ankle Clin. 2012;17(2):169–81.
6. Abousayed MM, Tartaglione JP, Rosenbaum AJ, et al. Classifications in brief: Johnson and Strom classification of adult-acquired flatfoot deformity. Clin Orthop Relat Res. 2016;474(2):588–93.
7. Myerson MS, Thordarson DB, Johnson JE, et al. Classification and nomenclature: progressive collapsing foot deformity. Foot Ankle Int. 2020;41(10):1271–6.
8. Monteagudo M, Martínez-de-Albornoz P. Progressive collapsing foot deformity. Is there really a Johnson and Strom stage I? Foot Ankle Clin. 2021;26(3):443–63.
9. Deland JT. Adult-acquired flatfoot deformity. J Am Acad Orthop Surg. 2008;16:399–406.
10. Lee MS, Vanore JV, Thomas JL, et al. Clinical practice guideline adult flatfoot panel. Diagnosis and treatment of adult flatfoot. J Foot Ankle Surg. 2005;44(2):78–113.
11. Smyth NA, Aiyer AA, Kaplan JR, et al. Adult-acquired flatfoot deformity. Eur J Orthop Surg Traumatol. 2017;27(4):433–9.
12. Sutter R, Pfirrmann CW, Espinosa N, et al. Three-dimensional hindfoot alignment measurements based on biplanar radiographs: comparison with standard radiographic measurements. Skeletal Radiol. 2013;42(4):493–8.
13. de Cesar NC, Shakoor D, Dein EJ, et al. Influence of investigator experience on reliability of adult acquired flatfoot deformity measurements using weightbearing computed tomography. Foot Ankle Surg. 2019;25(4):495–502.
14. Barbachan Mansur NS, Lalevée M, Lee HY, et al. Influence of weightbearing computed tomography in the progressive collapsing foot deformity classification system. Foot Ankle Int. 2023;44(2):125–9.
15. Pascual-Huerta J, Ropa JM, Kirby KA, et al. Effect of 7-degree varus and valgus rearfoot wedging on rearfoot kinematics and kinetic during the stance phase of walking. J Am Podiatr Med Assoc. 2009;99(5):415–21. https://doi.org/10.7547/0990415.
16. Vulcano E, Deland JT, Ellis SJ. Approach and treatment of the adult acquired flatfoot deformity. Curr Rev Musculoskelet Med. 2013;6(4):294–303.
17. Sangeorzan BJ, Hintermann B, de Cesar NC, et al. Progressive collapsing foot deformity: consensus on goals for operative correction. Foot Ankle Int. 2020;41(10):1299–302.
18. Schon LC, de Cesar NC, Day J, et al. Consensus for the indication of a medializing displacement calcaneal osteotomy in the treatment of progressive collapsing foot deformity. Foot Ankle Int. 2020;41(10):1282–5.
19. Schleunes SD, Campbell SN, Jones JM, et al. Radiographic analysis of the lateral column lengthening procedure in stage II adult acquired flatfoot deformity. J Foot Ankle Surg. 2022;61(6):1293–8.

20. Thordarson DB, Schon LC, de Cesar NC, et al. Consensus for the indication of lateral column lengthening in the treatment of progressive collapsing foot deformity. Foot Ankle Int. 2020;41(10):1286–8.
21. Stamatos NJ, Murasko MJ, Richardson K, et al. Radiographic outcomes of titanium augment vs bone graft in lateral column lengthening for adult-acquired flatfoot deformity. Foot Ankle Orthop. 2023;8(2):24730114231176554.
22. Gross CE, Jackson JB 3rd. The importance of the medial column in progressive collapsing foot deformity: osteotomies and stabilization. Foot Ankle Clin. 2021 Sep;26(3):507–21.
23. Johnson JE, Sangeorzan BJ, de Cesar NC, et al. Consensus on indications for medial cuneiform opening wedge (cotton) osteotomy in the treatment of progressive collapsing foot deformity. Foot Ankle Int. 2020;41(10):1289–91.
24. de Cesar NC, Ehret A, Walt J, et al. Early results and complication rate of the LapiCotton procedure in the treatment of medial longitudinal arch collapse: a prospective cohort study. Arch Orthop Trauma Surg. 2023;143(5):2283–95.
25. van Dijk CN, Knort N, Scholten PE. Tendoscopy of the posterior tibial tendon. J Arthroscopic Rel Surg. 1997;13(6):692–8.
26. Gianakos AL, Ross KA, Hannon CP, et al. Functional outcomes of tibialis posterior tendoscopy with comparison to magnetic resonance imaging. Foot Ankle Int. 2015;36(7):812–9.
27. Monteagudo M, Maceira E. Posterior tibial tendoscopy. Foot Ankle Clin. 2015;20(1):1–13.
28. Monteagudo M, de Albornoz PM. Posterior Tibial Tendoscopy in flexible acquired flatfoot deformity. J Foot Ankle Surg (Asia Pacific). 2022;9(3):123–7.
29. Chang SH, Abdelatif NMN, Netto CC, et al. The effect of gastrocnemius recession and tendoachilles lengthening on adult acquired flatfoot deformity surgery: a systematic review. J Foot Ankle Surg. 2020;59(6):1248–53.
30. Caravaggi P, Rogati G, Leardini A, et al. Clinical and multi-segment kinematic analysis of a modified Grice arthrodesis to correct type II adult-acquired flat-foot. Gait Posture. 2023;100:268–75.
31. Viladot A, Fontecilla N, Serrá JA, et al. Results of subtalar arthroereisis for posterior tibial tendon dysfunction stage IIA1. Based on 35 patients. Foot Ankle Surg. 2018;24(1):28–33.
32. Galán-Olleros M, Del Baño BL, Figueroa MJ, et al. Outcomes of the "Calcaneo-stop" procedure for treating symptomatic flexible flatfoot in children: a systematic review and meta-analysis of 2394 feet. Foot Ankle Surg. 2024;30(7):535–45.
33. Johnson JE, Yu JR. Arthrodesis techniques in the management of stage II and III acquired adult flatfoot deformity. Instr Course Lect. 2006;55:531–42.
34. Tao X, Chen W, Tang K. Surgical procedures for treatment of adult acquired flatfoot deformity: a network meta-analysis. J Orthop Surg Res. 2019;14(1):62.
35. Hintermann B, Deland JT, de Cesar NC, et al. Consensus on indications for isolated subtalar joint fusion and naviculocuneiform fusions for progressive collapsing foot deformity. Foot Ankle Int. 2020;41(10):1295–8.
36. Monteagudo M, Martínez-de-Albornoz P, Bhatia M. Pes plano valgus. In: Essentials of foot and ankle surgery. CRC Press; 2021. p. 102–12.
37. Chadwick C, Whitehouse SL, Saxby TS. Long-term follow-up of flexor digitorum longus transfer and calcaneal osteotomy for stage II posterior tibial tendon dysfunction. Bone Joint J. 2015;97-B(3):346–52.
38. Conti MS, Garfinkel JH, Ellis SJ. Outcomes of reconstruction of the flexible adult-acquired flatfoot deformity. Orthop Clin North Am. 2020;51(1):109–20.
39. Goss M, Stauch C, Lewcun J, et al. Natural history of 321 flatfoot reconstructions in adult acquired flatfoot deformity over a 14-year period. Foot Ankle Spec. 2020:1938640020912859. https://doi.org/10.1177/1938640020912859.
40. Fuller RM, Eble SK, Day J, et al. Return to physical activity following flatfoot reconstruction. Foot Ankle Int. 2022;43(6):772–82.

Chapter 13
Pes Cavovarus Reconstruction

Nicholas Cullen and Shelain Patel

Introduction

Pes cavovarus is a pathological foot deformity characterised by an excessively high medial longitudinal arch that remains when loaded, hindfoot varus, equinus, and clawed toes. It results from an imbalance between intrinsic and extrinsic foot musculature, and is commonly due to neurological conditions such as Charcot-Marie-Tooth disease (also known as hereditary motor sensory neuropathy), spinal cord disorders, or after trauma. In some cases, the etiology is idiopathic. The deformity disrupts normal weight-bearing biomechanics, leading to progressive pain, instability, and difficulty with ambulation.

Patients with pes cavovarus often experience lateral ankle instability due to increased stress on the lateral foot structures, predisposing them to recurrent ankle sprains. The rigid deformity also results in excessive pressure on the lateral border of the foot, increasing the risk of stress fractures, callosities, and ulcerations, particularly in neuropathic patients. Additionally, claw toe deformities contribute to metatarsal overload and painful plantar keratoses.

If left untreated, pes cavovarus can lead to progressive joint degeneration, severe gait impairment, and chronic pain. Over time, compensatory changes in the knee and hip may develop, further affecting mobility. Early recognition and intervention are critical in preventing irreversible damage. Treatment ranges from orthotic management in flexible deformities to surgical reconstruction for rigid or progressive cases, aiming to restore alignment, stability, and function.

Concerning each segment, the ankle typically develops an equinus deformity secondary to gastrocnemius-soleus contracture. In severe deformity, the talus can displace into a varus alignment relative to the tibial plafond. Meanwhile, the hindfoot deviates into supination, which manifests as a varus heel and adduction and/or

N. Cullen (✉) · S. Patel
Royal National Orthopaedic Hospital, Stanmore, UK

M. Bhatia (ed.), *Surgical Techniques of the Foot and Ankle*,
https://doi.org/10.1007/978-3-031-93742-2_13

supination across the Chopart joints. The net result is 'over coverage' of the talonavicular joint which is the opposite finding commonly seen in progressive collapsing foot deformity where the talonavicular joint is 'uncovered'. The midfoot is variably involved, although plantar flexion of the metatarsals is common, which contributes to the classic forefoot finding of clawed toes.

As a rule, the authors tend to correct deformity from proximal to distal, enabling reduction of the distal deformity relative to an optimally aligned proximal anatomy which is used as a reference.

Patient Positioning

The combination of neuropathy, the effect of deformity correction surgery that stretches tissue on the medial side of the foot and potentially concertinaing skin on the lateral side of the foot, use of orthopaedic implants and often prolonged surgical time, means that prophylactic parenteral antibiotics should be administered according to local protocols to minimise the risk of infection. General or regional anaesthesia is recommended to ensure adequate relaxation of the limb relaxation during the procedure.

The patient is positioned supine on the operating table, with a sandbag placed under the ipsilateral buttock. It is often necessary to over-correct the position initially with internal rotation of the foot to allow adequate access to the lateral hindfoot whilst undertaking either peroneal tendon transfer and/or calcaneal osteotomy surgery. The sandbag can then be removed later when medial sided surgery is needed to be performed, since removal enables the hip to externally rotate. A thigh tourniquet is used to provide a dry bloodless field, and inflated prior to the first skin incision. The leg is prepared up to the tourniquet allowing for surgical drapes to be placed above the knee since the alignment of the foot requires a proximal reference point to ensure a patient will stand and walk with an appropriate foot progression angle.

Surgical Technique—Tendo-Achilles Lengthening

The most commonly encountered deformity at the level of the ankle is an equinus deformity secondary to a tight Achilles tendon. Reducing the tibo-talar joint to a plantigrade/neutral position is the first step of pes cavovarus deformity correction since it acts as a reference point for the hindfoot. Careful evaluation of the lateral radiograph will guide the amount of lengthening that needs to be achieved; namely the calcaneal pitch should be restored within the normal range otherwise over lengthening will result in the heel adopting a high pitch which causes heel pain and difficulty in standing and walking.

It is the authors' experience that most equinus ankle deformities will correct with a percutaneous triple hemisection of the Achilles tendon which was first described by Hoke in 1931 [1].

The leg is elevated and the ankle is dorsiflexed by a surgical assistant to produce tension within the Achilles tendon. The procedure utilises three longitudinal 'stab' incisions made using a No. 15 surgical blade in the midline of the Achilles tendon spaced throughout the tendon. The incisions can be marked out to ensure they are not inadvertently made too close together that will otherwise increase the risk of a full thickness rupture (Fig. 13.1).

The initial incision is made 3–5 cm above the insertion of the Achilles tendon through the skin and then tendon. Resistance to the blade will decrease as it exits through the anterior surface of the Achilles tendon. The blade is then angled inferiorly using the skin layer as a pivot point to extend the incision with the tendon only. This allows space for the blade to be rotated 90 degrees. Due to the spiral pattern of the tendon fibres, the inferior hemisection incision is directed medially using the skin as the pivot point, the middle hemisection is directed laterally and the proximal hemisection is again directed medially. All this is performed with constant tension on the tendon through both maintaining a dorsiflexion force at the ankle, and additionally with a finger placed on the skin applying gentle pressure towards the direction of the scalpel blade. This allows for controlled division of the tendon fibres, as well as tactile feedback on when a gap is produced in the tendon. 50% of the width of the tendon should be preserved and not sectioned (Figs. 13.2, 13.3, and 13.4).

This technique is repeated with the middle and proximal incisions, ensuring the direction of hemisection is alternated as described earlier. After the third hemisection, the knee is extended and a controlled dorsiflexion force is applied to the foot. The tendon is typically felt to slowly lengthen, with manipulation stopping once the ankle achieves a position of between 5 and 10 degrees of dorsiflexion. Rapid, aggressive and uncontrolled force to the foot is more likely to result in a full thickness rupture.

Percutaneous techniques may not be effective in severe fixed equinus deformity. In this case, open Z-lengthening of the Achilles tendon can be used. The leg is moved into a 'figure of 4' position and longitudinal incision made paramedial to the Achilles tendon which respects angiosomes. The incision is made from the insertion of the tendon to the musculotendinous junction through the skin, subcutaneous tissue and paratenon of the Achilles tendon. This creates a full thickness flap and avoids undermining the skin and subcutaneous tissue which can otherwise result in delayed wound healing or dehiscence.

A longitudinal, midline incision begins 1 cm inferior to the musculotendinous junction and continues distally to approximately 4 cm above the insertion of Achilles tendon. Again the blade must go through the anterior border of the tendon. The tenotomy is then completed by making the transverse limbs of the tenotomy. Distally this will occur laterally and proximally this will occur medially which minimises the risk of sural nerve injury. A controlled dorsiflexion force is applied to the foot which is usually sufficient to reduce it to plantigrade. The tendon is repaired in a

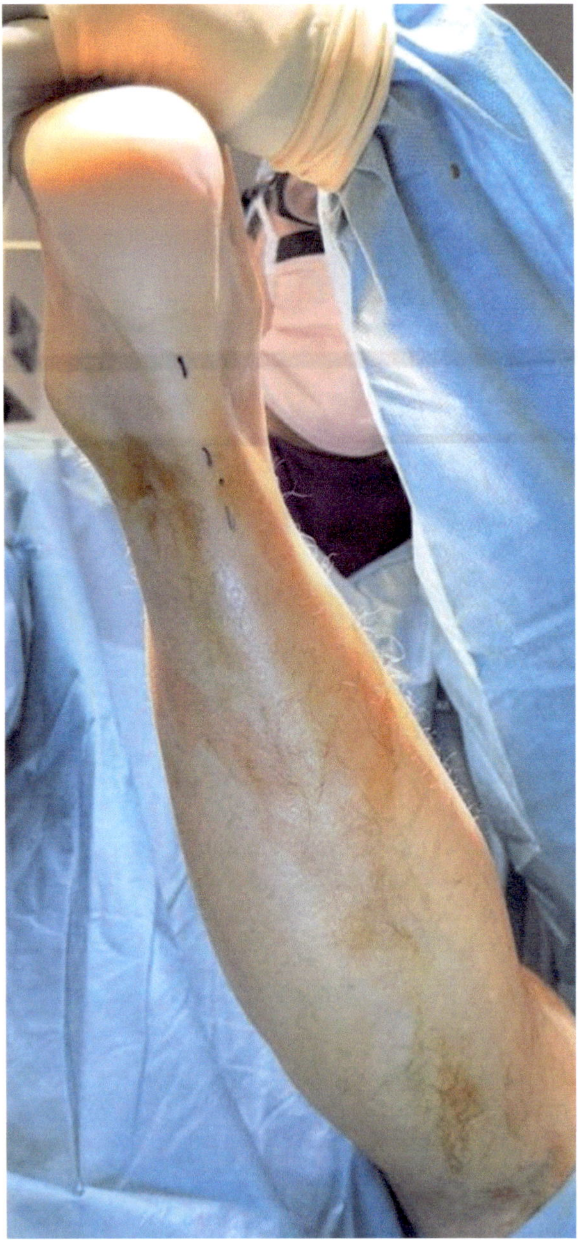

Fig. 13.1 Posterior view of the leg showing a surgical assistant applying dorsiflexion force to the foot resulting in tension of the Achilles tendon. Markings have been made on the skin to ensure incisions are made centrally and with sufficient spacing

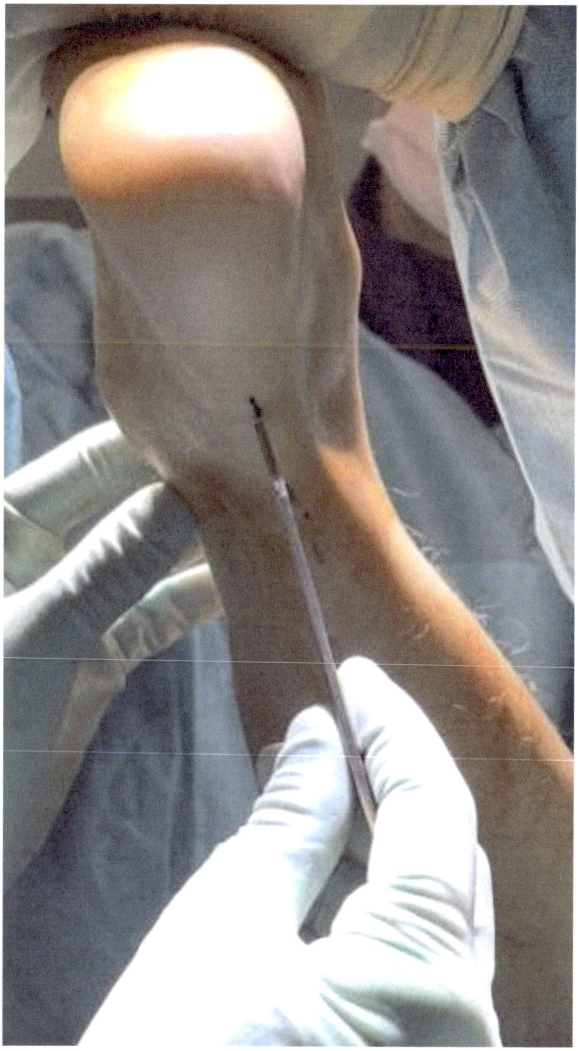

Fig. 13.2 A longitudinal incision is initially made in the inferior Achilles tendon

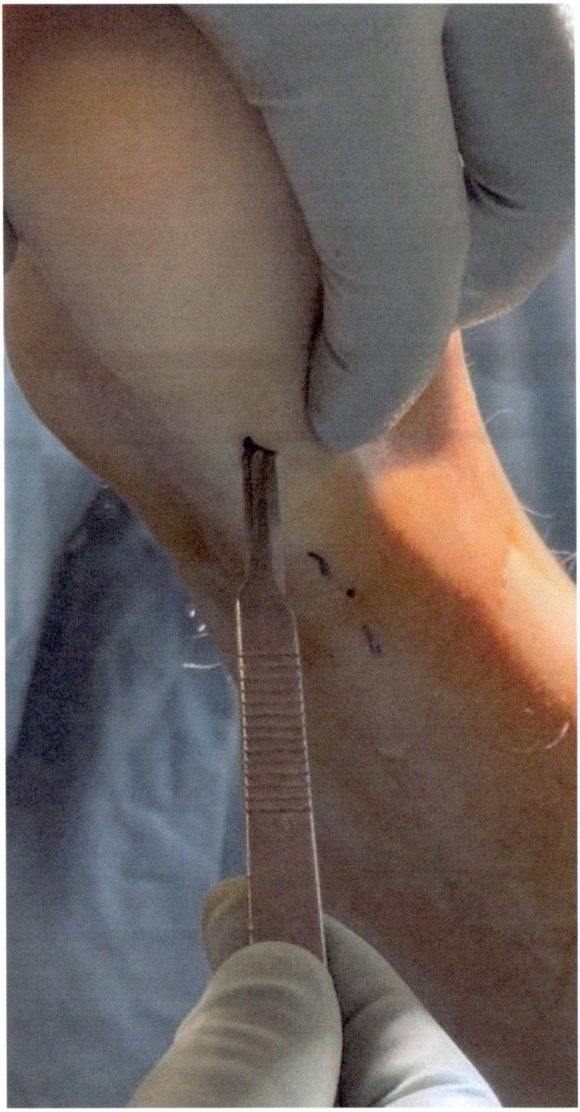

Fig. 13.3 The scalpel is directed medially and a surgeon's finger applies counter pressure to the direction of the blade

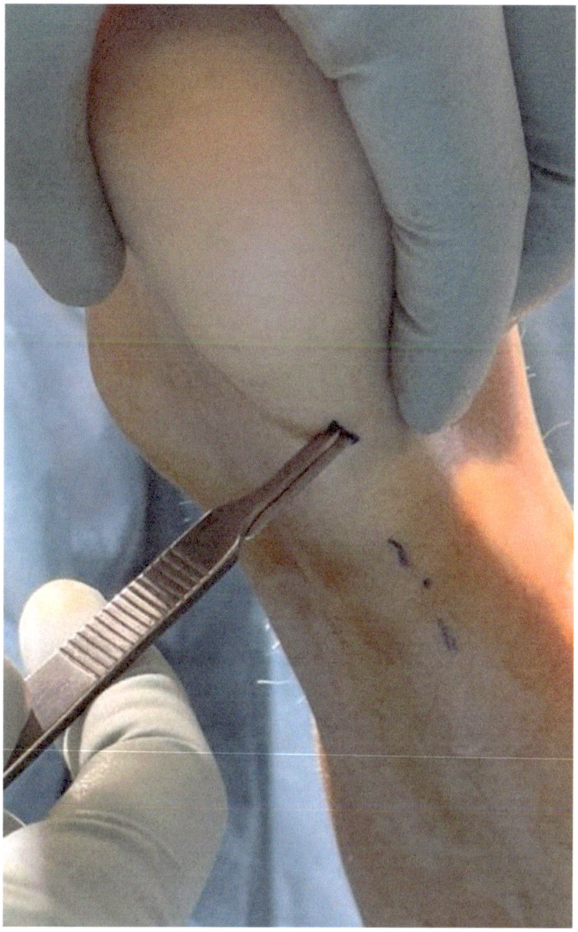

Fig. 13.4 The tenotomy is typically complete when the scalpel is perpendicular to its original position and gap is felt in the tendon

side to side fashion using a No.1 absorbable suture ensuring the foot is plantigrade and resists dorsiflexion or more than 10 degrees.

A common pitfall is making the incision and the longitudinal cut in the tendon too small. If there is inadequate length of the longitudinal cut of the tenotomy, there will be a loss of contact between the two ends of the Achilles tendon step cut when the foot is brought to plantigrade.

Surgical Technique—Calcaneal Osteotomy

Lateralizing calcaneal osteotomy is indicated in flexible hindfoot varus deformity. The aim of this is to place calcaneal tuberosity underneath the mechanical axis of the leg thereby improving mechanical stability and also moving the vector of action of the Achilles tendon laterally, such that it ceases to become a deforming force which reduces the risk of recurrence. Osteotomy will be less effective in fixed deformity, in which case corrective subtalar or other hind foot fusions may be required.

The osteotomy can be made either through an extended lateral approach, direct lateral approach or minimally invasive approach. Whilst the direct lateral approach is the most straightforward, the incision passes over the distribution of the sural nerve and its branches such that it is at risk of injury which can result in painful neuromas. Minimally invasive approaches are increasingly popular but do rely on some shortening of the calcaneus to aid the translation, and it is anecdotally more difficult to achieve lateral translation than medial translation.

For these reasons, the extended lateral approach is the authors' preferred approach which respects the angiosome of the peroneal artery [2]. The foot is kept plantar flexed for the preparation and displacement of the osteotomy since this relaxes the skin and de-tensions the Achilles tendon. The skin incision is made by two straight incisions meeting at the lateral side of the heel at an angle of no less than 100 degrees. The horizontal incision starts distally at the base of the fifth metatarsal and passes posteriorly along the junction of glabrous and non-glabrous skin finishing 2 cm anterior to the heel. The vertical limb then passes proximally aiming towards the posterior midline which preserves the angiosomes and avoids injury to the sural nerve (Fig. 13.5).

A full thickness flap is developed down to the lateral wall of the calcaneus. The flap is carefully dissected subperiosteally off the lateral cortex of the calcaneus using a combination of sharp dissection and periosteal elevation (Fig. 13.6). Care should be taken to avoid injury to the peroneal tendons which are located in the distal part of the wound.

Mini Hohmann or Trethowan bone retractors are positioned over the superior and plantar cortices in line with the planned osteotomy, and the alignment of the oblique osteotomy can be marked out if required (Fig. 13.7). It starts 2 cm anterior to the Achilles tendon and is angled at 30–45 degrees relative to the plane of the foot exiting distal to the origin of the plantar fascia. Maintaining an oblique rather than vertical osteotomy confers stability and reduces the risk of superior translation.

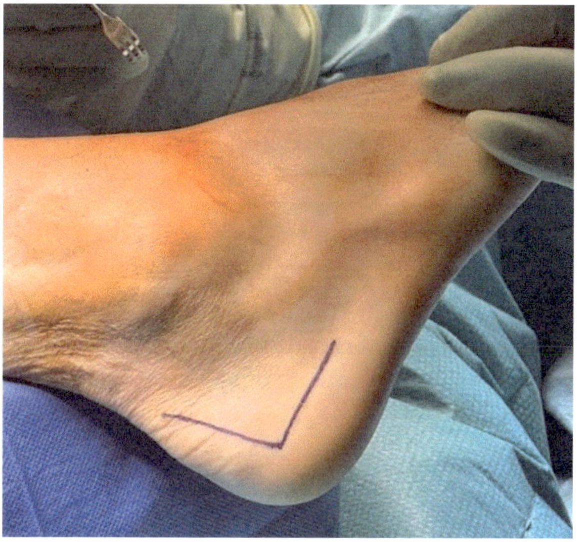

Fig. 13.5 An incision is made on the lateral side of the heel ensuring an angle of at least 100 degrees between its two limbs

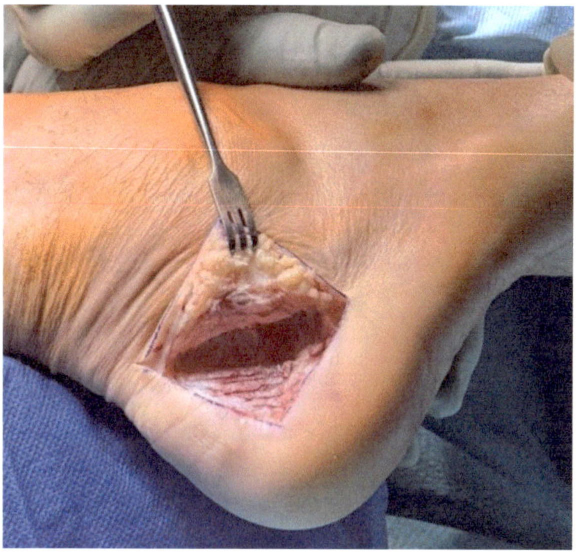

Fig. 13.6 A full thickness flap allows adequate exposure of performing the calcaneal osteotomy

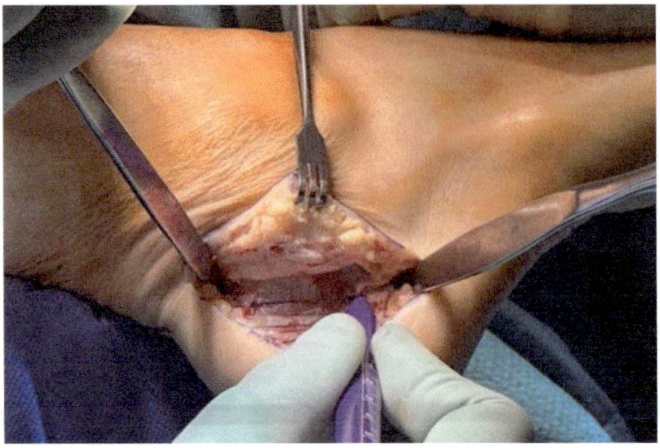

Fig. 13.7 A sterile marker is used to confirm the direction of the osteotomy

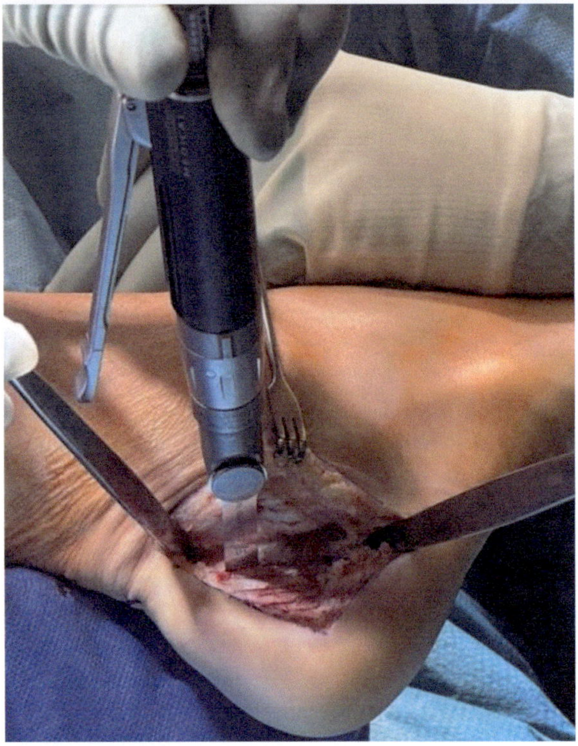

Fig. 13.8 A saw is used to initiate the osteotomy

The osteotomy is initiated with a saw applied to the lateral wall (Fig. 13.8) but a straight osteotome is then used to complete the cut through the medial wall (Fig. 13.9). This allows the surgeon to take care in avoiding iatrogenic injury to the medial soft tissues including the terminal branches of the tibial nerve.

Lateral displacement osteotomy of the calcaneus is typically more resistant to translation due to the tension induced within the plantar fascia. It is therefore vital

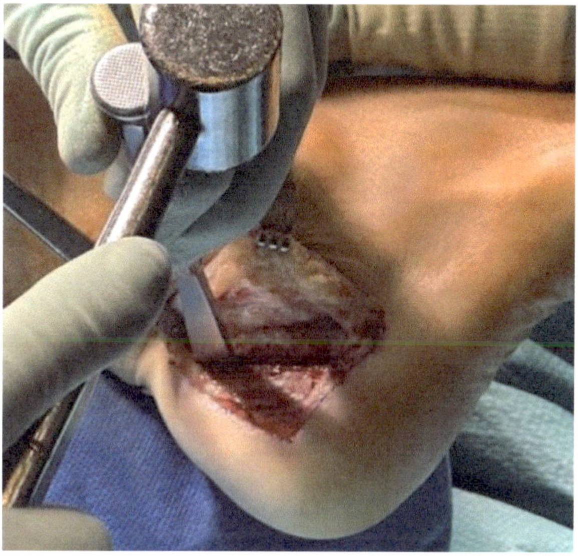

Fig. 13.9 The osteotomy is completed with an osteotome applied to the medial wall

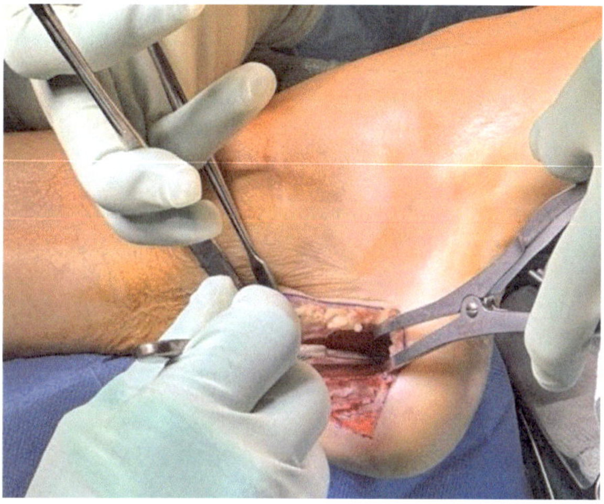

Fig. 13.10 The osteotomy is distracted with a laminar spreaded whilst a periosteal elevator clears the medial soft tissues

to ensure the plane of the osteotomy does not lengthen the calcaneus as translation is performed or else the amount of displacement will be insufficient.

A laminar spreader is then placed across rather than into the osteotomy, which would otherwise crush the cancellous bone present in the middle of the osteotomy (Fig. 13.10). A periosteal elevator is passed through the distracted bone parts to clear soft tissue away from the medial side of the osteotomy, create a pocket to allow displacement, and reduce the risk of nerve compression or entrapment when the osteotomy is displaced.

An alternative to a translational displacement osteotomy is the Dwyer closing wedge osteotomy is created by removing a laterally based wedge from the

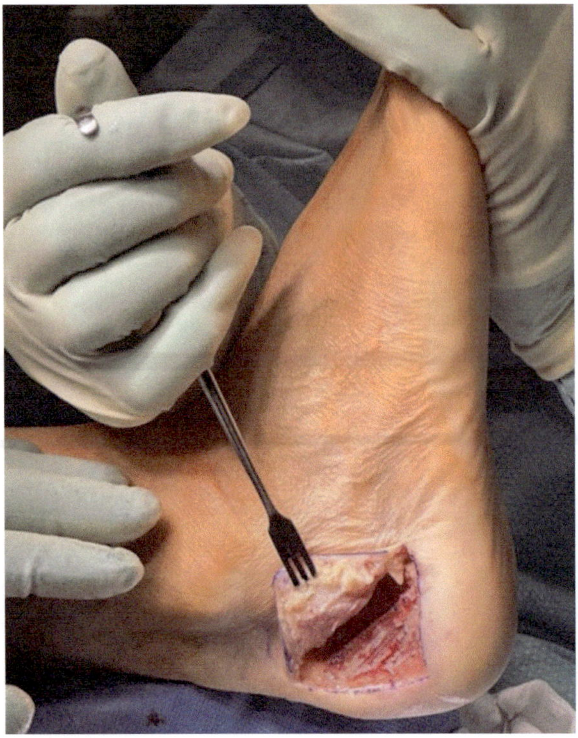

Fig. 13.11 Maximal dorsiflexion of the foot locks the osteotomy and prevents displacement whilst fixation is performed

calcaneum [3]. The alignment of the primary cut is developed in the same plane as the displacement osteotomy, and the second cut to create the wedge is performed more proximally, and is aimed to transect the primary cut at the level of the medial cortex. A combination of translation and closing wedge can be used in more severe deformity.

The tuberosity fragment is then manually displaced with the foot maintaining a plantar flexed attitude. To lock the displacement, the foot is then maximally dorsiflexed which tensions the Achilles tendon and plantar fascia simultaneously (Fig. 13.11).

Fixation can then be achieved with either staples, plates or screws. The authors' preference for fixation are screws. An adequate displacement might result in only 50% of bony overlap at the osteotomy so the entry point for screws will need to be in the medial half of the tuberosity fragment perpendicular to the osteotomy. One or two parallel guide wires are passed through the heel aiming towards the anterior crease of the ankle with their position confirmed on fluoroscopy. Screws are inserted and used in line with each manufacturer's individual technique.

Once the calcaneal osteotomy has been stabilised, a prominent step in the bone created by the displacement is tamped down with a bone punch that improves the contour of the lateral calcaneus and reduces tension on the wound (Fig. 13.12). The skin flap is then closed in layers.

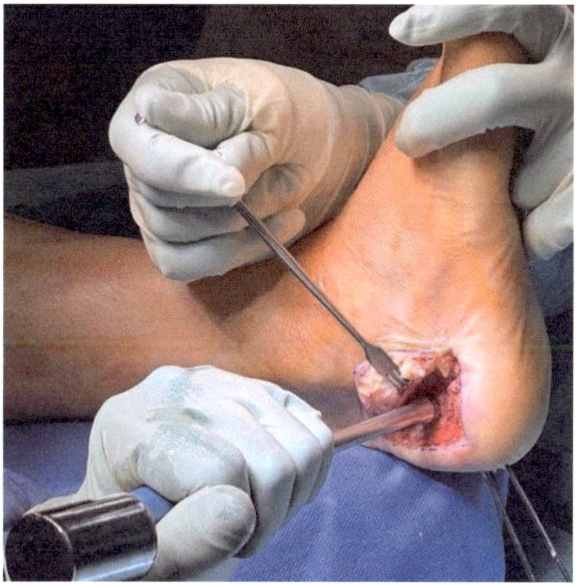

Fig. 13.12 A bone punch is used to soften the sharp edge of the osteotomy

Surgical Technique—Midfoot Osteotomy and Tarsectomy

There are multiple patterns of deformity with the pes cavovarus foot creating variability in the centre of rotation and angulation of deformity. Where it occurs across the mid-tarsal joints, it may be necessary to undertake correction at this level. There are broadly three described techniques:

- Cole wedge tarsectomy [4]: Dorsally based wedge excision of the naviculocuneiform joints and central body of the cuboid. This technique is occasionally called the Meary wedge tarsectomy who popularised this technique in France.
- Jahss wedge tarsectomy [5]: Dorsally based wedge across the tarsometarsal joint.
- Japas osteotomy [6]: V-shaped osteotomy with the apex sited within the navicular, and one limb exiting through the medial cuneiform and other through the cuboid. This technique is designed to be both bone and joint sparing.

The authors perform a Cole osteotomy although utilise dorsal and lateral incisions rather than the medial and lateral incisions that were originally described. The dorsal incision is made between extensor hallucis longus and tibialis anterior tendons taking care to avoid branches of the deep peroneal nerve. Subperiosteal dissection is made to the dorsal surface of the navicular and cuneiforms followed by a separate lateral incision over the cuboid extending from the distal calcaneus to the base of the fourth and fifth metatarsals.

The size of the wedge to be removed will depend on the severity of the deformity although typically a dorsal based wedge of between 1 and 1.5 cm is needed. An initial k-wire is passed from dorsal to plantar through the medial cuneiform stopping at the level of the plantar fascia. A further wire is passed through the distal navicular at a pre-planned distance converging the tip towards the tip of the initial wire. This will create a truncated wedge rather than a triangular wedge utilising the tension within the plantar fascia. Further wires are then passed under image guidance across the planned osteotomy and a saw used to perform the tarsectomy.

The initial bone resection can be conservative with further bone taken as required. This will avoid gaps in the osteotomy and prevent overcorrection. Closure of the osteotomy across the navicular-cuneiform joints will be prevented by the cuboid, so a cuboid osteotomy is required to aid both dorsiflexion and abduction. Guide wires are again passed from dorsal to plantar to create a truncated wedge. The width of the bone removed from the dorsum of the cuboid is approximately 0.75 cm and this is extended as required. The osteotomy is closed with dorsal and abduction forces, and thereafter stabilised with either staples or locking plates.

Surgical Technique—Dorsiflexion Osteotomy of the First Metatarsal

One of the most common deformities encountered in pes cavovarus is plantar flexion of the first metatarsal (Fig. 13.13). The Jones procedure [7] involving transfer of the extensor hallucis longus tendon to the first metatarsal and interphalangeal fusion of the hallux, is effective in the juvenile, flexible pes cavus, but is rarely powerful enough on its own in established adult deformity. In these cases, a dorsiflexion osteotomy of the base of the first metatarsal is an effective way of correcting this deformity.

The base of the first metatarsal is approached with a dorsal longitudinal incision from the first tarsometatarsal joint to the mid-diaphysis. Subperiosteal dissection is performed medially and laterally, and mini Hohmann retractors are used to protect

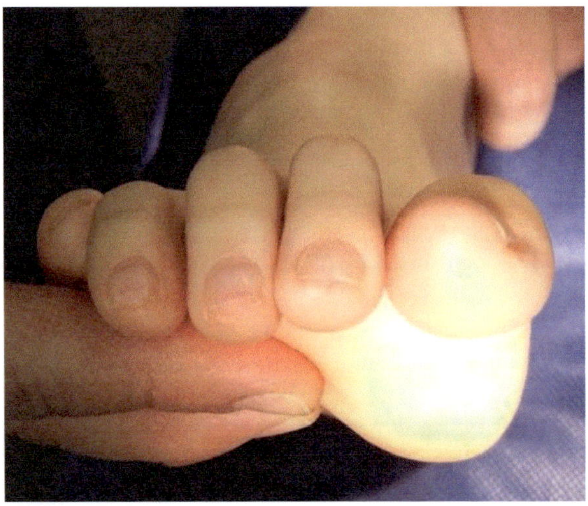

Fig. 13.13 The head of the first metatarsal can be seen to be much lower than lesser metatarsal heads

the soft tissues including the extensor hallucis longus tendon laterally. A saw is then used to make an osteotomy 1 cm distal to the tarsometarsal joint, taking care not to violate the plantar cortical surface which will act as a hinge. A further saw cut is then made to create a dorsally based closing wedge. Gentle pressure is applied under the head of the first metatarsal to close the osteotomy. If the apex of the wedge is too dorsal, the osteotomy will not close. In this case, light passes of the saw blade to feather the plantar cortex will facilitate controlled closure of the gap. Adequate wedge resection is confirmed when the first metatarsal head lies at the level of the lesser metatarsal heads. Fixation can be achieved with either screws, plates or staples with no one method being more advantageous than any other.

Surgical Technique—Hallux Interphalangeal Joint Fusion and Extensor Hallucis Longus Tendon Transfer

The clawed hallux has a number of effects. Firstly it provides traction on the plantar fascia that activates the windlass mechanism, which exacerbates the high arch and plantar flexion of the first ray seen in pes cavovarus. Secondly, the dorsiflexed proximal phalanx acts as a "plunger" to further depress the first metatarsal leading to increased pressure under the first metatarsal head, which can clinically manifest as pain in this region, plantar callosities or ulceration. Clawing at the interphalangeal joint meanwhile may create pressure in the toe box of a shoe leading to a callosity or pressure sore on the dorsum of the joint.

The surgery of choice to address these issues is corrective arthrodesis of the interphalangeal joint of the hallux, and transfer of the extensor hallucis longus tendon to the neck of the first metatarsal. The combination of these two procedures is known as a Jones procedure, and can be used in conjunction with the dorsiflexion osteotomy of the first metatarsal described earlier.

A longitudinal incision is made at the junction of proximal and middle thirds of the first metatarsal on the medial border of the extensor hallucis longus tendon. It is extended distally to the interphalangeal joint of the hallux where the incision can be turned perpendicular to be in line with the joint. The tendon is exposed and crucially the extensor hallucis brevis which is lying laterally is then identified and protected.

The extensor hallucis longus tendon is divided at the level of the interphalangeal joint. The tendon tends to be adherent to its sheath over the phalanx and so these attachments and vinculae are dissected until the tendon is free to the proximal edge of the wound. The distal end of the tendon is prepared with a whipstitch to allow it to be tensioned and easily passed through the metatarsal head.

To aid exposure of the interphalangeal joint is exposed, the medial and lateral collateral ligaments are divided with sharp dissection. Once exposed, the proximal and distal surfaces are excised with a saw, taking sufficient bone to correct the claw toe. Fixation is achieved with a 4 mm compression screw inserted through the distal end of the hallux.

There are various methods to attach the extensor hallucis longus tendon to the first metatarsal head. The authors' preferred method is to pass the tendon through the metatarsal and secure it to itself. This is performed by making an appropriately sized drill hole from the medial cortex to the lateral cortex of the metatarsal head. A suture passer or similar device is used to pass the whipstitch through the medial eminence and exit laterally. Traction on the whipstitch then will pull the tendon in the same direction and once the tendon has been tensioned adequately with the foot in dorsiflexion relative to the ankle, it can be sutured back onto itself using No. 1 absorbable suture (Fig. 13.14).

Clawing of the lesser toes can be corrected through a combination of osseous and soft-tissue procedures which will be covered elsewhere in this book.

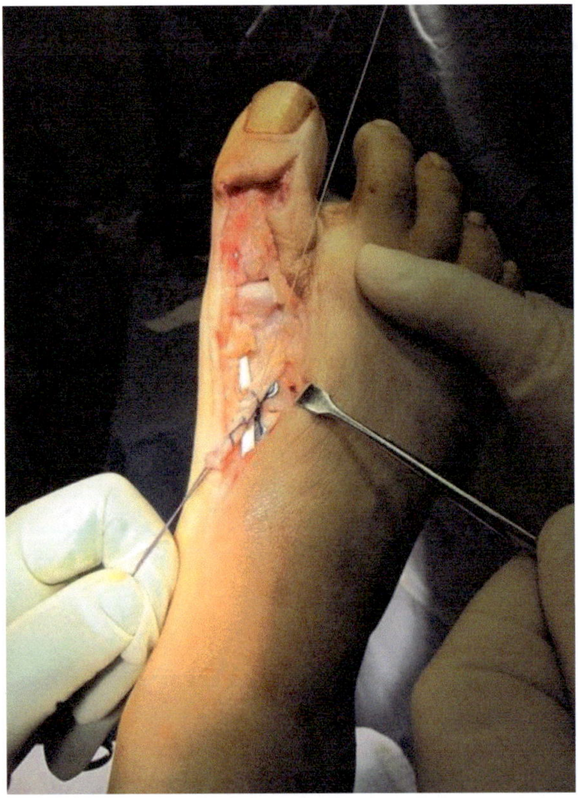

Fig. 13.14 The extensor hallucis longus tendon will be sutured back onto itself at the appropriate tension after passing through the first metatarsal

Surgical Technique—Tendon Transfers

Most cases of pes cavovarus deformity requiring surgery will have an underlying neurological condition. Charcot Marie Tooth disease is the most common cause and this frequently but not always leads to weakness in the tibialis anterior and peroneus brevis muscles.

Whilst the osseous surgical techniques described thus far will correct deformity, failure to balance the foot will impair function and increase the risk of recurrent deformity.

Peroneus longus to brevis tenodesis: This is indicated in patients with pes cavovarus who have a weak peroneus brevis but strong peroneus longus. This transfer has the dual effect of aiding eversion and reducing the plantar flexion moment at the first metatarsal.

A 5 cm incision is made on the posterior border of the fibula proximal to the superior peroneal retinaculum. The peroneal tendon sheath is identified and care is taken to identify and protect the superficial peroneal nerve which passes through the sheath anteriorly to supply sensation to the dorsum of the foot. Incision of the sheath will facilitate access to both peroneal tendons with the peroneus brevis lying anterior to the longus tendon adjacent to the bone. Recognising each tendon can be confirmed by using a tendon hook to apply traction; pulling the peroneus brevis should reproduce a force on the base of the fifth metatarsal. The peroneus longus tendon is then pulled proximally with the foot dorsiflexed and everted to allow maximal excursion and the tendon is then sectioned as far distal as possible. The brevis tendon is then retrieved and the longus tendon is weaved through the brevis tendon with the foot dorsiflexed and everted. The longus tendon is tensioned by being pulled inferiorly and then tenodesed to the brevis as low as possible on the peroneus brevis tendon with No. 1 absorbable sutures.

Tibialis posterior tendon transfer: Weakness in dorsiflexion and eversion can be aided by transfer of a strong tibialis posterior. Tendon transfer also weakens the deforming force on the hindfoot thereby reducing the risk of recurrence of pes cavovarus deformity.

Harvesting the tibialis posterior tendon can be helped by removing the sandbag that may have been placed at the start of the surgery. A 6 cm longitudinal incision is made over the medial border the navicular tuberosity. The tendon will have flattened as it inserts onto the navicular so identification of the tendon is easiest at the proximal end of the wound. Once the tibialis posterior tendon sheath is opened the tendon should be inspected to ensure that it is intact and healthy (Fig. 13.15).

The tendon can then be transected at its insertion and whipstitched if desired now or later. A further incision is made 10–15 cm proximal to the medial malleolus in line with the posteromedial edge of the tibia. The saphenous nerve and vein are at risk so careful dissection is required to avoid iatrogenic injury. Once the fascia is incised, the flexor digitorum longus muscle belly and tendon is first encountered. This can be confirmed by dorsiflexion of the lesser toes, and these are retracted

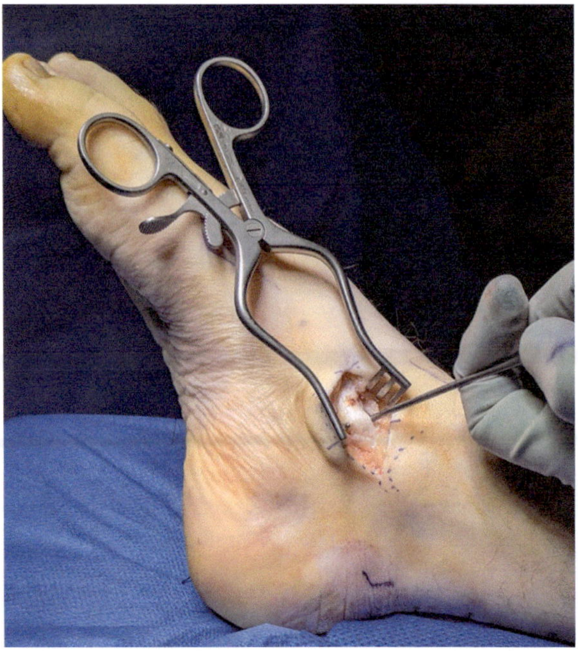

Fig. 13.15 The tibialis posterior tendon is identified inserting onto the navicular tuberosity

posteriorly to expose the proximal end of the tibialis posterior tendon (Fig. 13.16). This can be corroborated by applying traction to the end of the detached tendon.

The tendon needs to be delivered through the proximal wound but it is common to encounter difficulty in passing the distal tendon around the medial malleolus. Dilating the tendon sheath both proximally and distally with McIndoe scissors can help. Once cleared, the tendon is retrieved using Carroll tendon tunnelling forceps (Fig. 13.17).

The options for tibialis posterior tendon are now either:

- Transfer to the dorsum of the foot.
- Transfer to the peroneus brevis tendon.
- Split transfer to the tibialis anterior and peroneus brevis tendons.

If the tendon is transferred to the dorsum of the foot then it is passed through the interosseous membrane, under the extensor retinaculum and to either the intermediate of lateral cuneiform. Fixation options include passing it through the bone and using a biotenodesis screw or securing it to the bone surface using a suture loaded bone anchor.

If a split transfer is performed, then the tendon needs to be divided into two limbs before each is individually whipstitched and fed through the interosseous membrane towards their respective targets.

With transfer to the peroneus brevis, the tibialis posterior tendon is fed through to the peroneal compartment and a separate incision over the peroneal tendons at the level of the ankle (Fig. 13.18). The tibialis posterior tendon is then passed

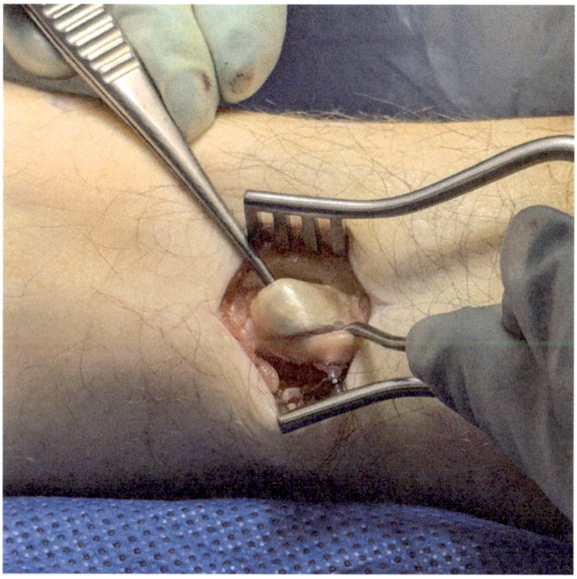

Fig. 13.16 The tibialis posterior tendon is identified after the flexor digitorum longus is retracted with a tendon hook

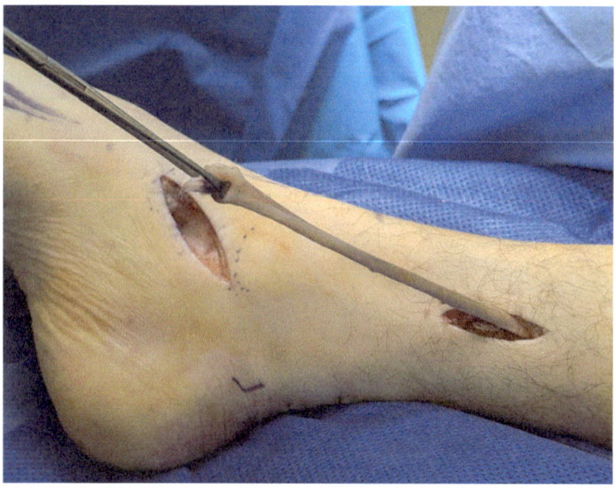

Fig. 13.17 The tibialis posterior tendon has been harvested and is now ready to be passed through the interosseous membrane

subcutaneously to the inferior wound (Fig. 13.19) where it is either weaved through the peroneus brevis and secured, or tenodesed with a side to side repair. Crucially this should be performed whilst the foot is everted and with the transferred tendon under maximal tension and secured as inferior as possible to the peroneus brevis.

A variety of other tendon transfers are available but are used less frequently including the Bridle procedure, split tibialis anterior transfer and Hibbs tendon transfer.

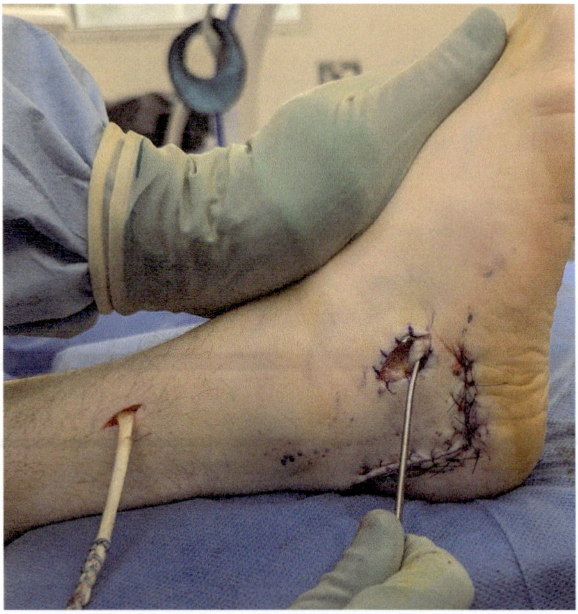

Fig. 13.18 The tibialis posterior tendon is seen passing from the posterior compartment out anterolaterally, whilst the peroneus brevis is exposed at the level of the ankle

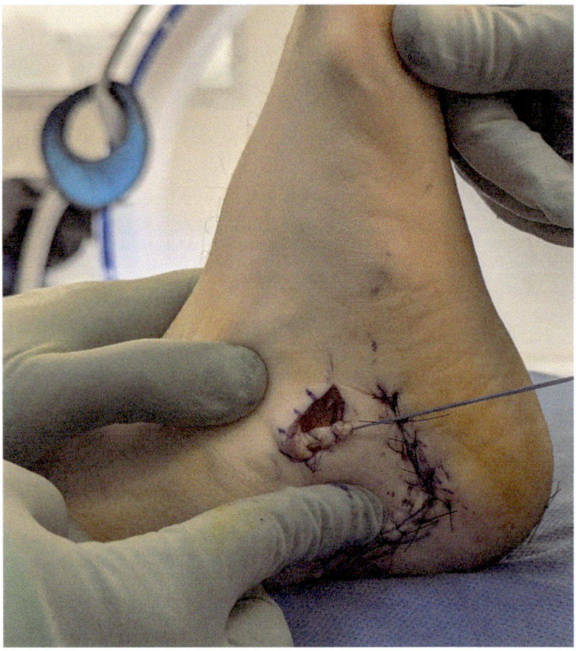

Fig. 13.19 The tibialis posterior tendon is passed subcutaneously ready to be stitched to the peroneus brevis

Post-operative Care

Surgery to correct pes cavovarus deformity is at high risk of complication. It is therefore preferable to immobilise the foot for at least 6 weeks in a cast depending on the osteotomies and the tendon transfers employed. Weight bearing supervised by a physiotherapist is encouraged after 6 weeks to allow early functional rehabilitation of any tendon transfers.

Controversies

The authors have not described plantar fascia release since there is debate about its role in pes cavovarus deformity correction. Specifically the authors do not believe that division aids functional outcome. Whilst the plantar fascia will be tight in pes cavovarus, this arises from dorsiflexion of the lesser toes at the metatarsophalangeal joints which in effect tightens the windlass mechanism. Division of the plantar fascia may hinder the mechanical ability of the foot and consequently correcting the dorsiflexion deformity of the toes at the level of the metatarsophalangeal joints could be a safer and more important part of deformity correction.

Summary

Pes cavovarus deformity correction is a complex surgery that should be individualised to the patient's foot shape and underlying disorder. Surgery starts from proximal to distal, using each corrected proximal segment as a new reference point. A combination of osseous and soft tissue procedures are frequently required in a single surgery, and it is vital to correct muscle imbalance or else recovery will be compromised and the patient will be at a higher risk of recurrent deformity.

References

1. Hoke M. An operation for the correction of extremely relaxed flat feet. J Bone Joint Surg Am. 1931;13:773–83.
2. Freeman BJ, Duff S, Allen PE, Nicholson HD, Atkins RM. The extended lateral approach to the hindfoot. Anatomical basis and surgical implications. J Bone Joint Surg Br. 1998;80:139–42. https://doi.org/10.1302/0301-620x.80b1.7987.
3. Dwyer FC. Osteotomy of the calcaneum for pes cavus. J Bone Joint Surg Br. 1959;41-B:80–6. https://doi.org/10.1302/0301-620X.41B1.80.

4. Cole WH. The treatment of claw-foot. J Bone Joint Surg Am. 1940;22:895–908.
5. Jahss MH. Tarsometatarsal truncated-wedge arthrodesis for pes cavus and equinovarus deformity of the fore part of the foot. J Bone Joint Surg Am. 1980;62:713–22.
6. Japas LM. Surgical treatment of pes cavus by tarsal v-osteotomy. J Bone Joint Surg Am. 1968;50:927–44.
7. Jones R. III. The soldier's foot and the treatment of common deformities of the foot. Br Med J. 1916;1:749–53. https://doi.org/10.1136/bmj.1.2891.749.

Chapter 14
Achilles Tendinopathy

Nuno Côrte-Real, João Caetano, and Maneesh Bhatia

Background

Achilles tendinopathy is usually an overuse lesion that can be divided into two different conditions: the mid-portion (or non-insertional) and the insertional tendinopathy. This distinction has diagnostic and therapeutic implications.

Mid-portion tendinopathy is usually related with sports activities, especially recreational running. Insertional tendinopathy can also be sports-related but there is an important group of patients with this condition with different characteristics, namely middle-aged overweight women. The location of tenderness in the tendon can help us determine the type of tendinopathy the patient has. Additionally, the location of swelling provides the same information [1, 2]. In non-insertional tendinopathy, tenderness and thickness, if noticeable, are found 2–8 cm from the insertion at the calcaneus.

Although these situations can have an acute outset, the evolution to chronicity is usual. The differential diagnosis of chronic tendinopathy and chronic rupture must be done. The ability to do one-legged heel rise, although painful, would be in favor of tendinopathy, ruling out chronic rupture [3].

Tendinopathy is primarily treated with conservative methods, such as eccentric loading exercises, shockwave therapy, or physiotherapy [1]. Shoes modification and

N. Côrte-Real (✉)
Department of Orthopedics, Hospital de Cascais, Dr. José de Almeida, Cascais, Portugal

J. Caetano
Department of Orthopedics, Hospital da Luz Lisboa/Torres de Lisboa, Lisbon, Portugal

M. Bhatia (✉)
Consultant Orthopaedic Foot Ankle Surgeon, University Hospitals Leicester, Spire Hospital Leicester and Nuffield Health Leicester, Leicester, UK

Associate Professor, University of Leicester, Leicester, UK

Professor, DeMontfort University Leicester, Leicester, UK

M. Bhatia (ed.), *Surgical Techniques of the Foot and Ankle*,
https://doi.org/10.1007/978-3-031-93742-2_14

changes in training conditions can also be effective. However, there is a group of patients who will not improve with this type of treatment and may benefit from surgical intervention. This group is more significant in terms of percentage in insertional tendinopathy and is quite rare in the mid-portion type. Surgical treatment should only be considered after a well-conducted course of conservative treatment for at least 3 months.

With the emergence and development of arthroscopic and endoscopic techniques in ankle surgery, which have well documented benefits in terms of morbidity and recovery duration, some endoscopic modalities have been proposed to treat these conditions. We will discuss these treatment strategies separately for each condition.

Mid Portion Tendinopathy

There is some controversy regarding the pathophysiology of this tendinopathy, and particularly concerning the physical factors that generate pain in this condition. The most widely accepted opinion is that the pain is related to increased vascularization and neo neurogenesis, particularly on the ventral aspect of the tendon, and the pathology may be centered on the paratenon [2].

The plantaris tendon has also been related with the onset of this condition by some authors, as it can develop tendinopathy or have a mechanical effect directly on the Achilles tendon, causing chronic dysfunction of this tendon. Therefore, plantaris tenotomy can be an important accessory gesture in this context [4].

The traditional open surgical treatment of non-insertional tendinopathy consisted of excision of the degenerated tendon tissue. This approach could be effective, but it has a relatively high complication rate (4.7–11.6%) [5]. However, it does not directly address the most widely accepted origin of the pain—the increased vascularization and neo neurogenesis.

The endoscopic approach was developed to specifically target adhesions, neovessels, and nerves. It can be less aggressive, with fewer complications and faster return to activity, and, at least, provides results as good as the open procedure [5].

Endoscopic Achilles Debridement—Surgical Technique

The patient is placed in the prone position with a tourniquet at the root of the limb. A small pillow placed under the contralateral pelvis may help keeping the lower leg in a neutral position. The foot can overhang the edge of the table to allow free mobilization of the ankle. Standard arthroscopic instruments are used.

A lateral visualizing portal is made 1 cm above the insertion of the tendon. A mosquito clamp is introduced through the portal creating space for the endoscope, both on the dorsal and ventral sides of the tendon. This can be complemented with the introduction of a blunt trocar, trying to identify the space between the tendon and the paratenon, releasing adhesions. The arthroscope can be introduced through the distal portal. Extreme care should be used to ascertain that the scope is placed between the tendon and the paratenon.

A second portal is made on the medial side of the tendon, 2–4 cm above the thickened part of the tendon, using a needle or transillumination. This portal can be used for the introduction of instruments (shaver, probe, etc.). A shaver is introduced through the proximal portal, and, with direct vision and triangulation, the remaining adhesion and neovascularization are removed from all around the tendon, starting distally and moving proximally. Portals can be changed if needed (Fig. 14.1). Extreme care should be taken when working on the lateral side of the tendon to avoid injuring the sural nerve.

The medial or lateral position of the portals can be changed if more convenient in the case at hand.

After careful removal of the paratenon, the plantaris tendon (if present) can be identified on the medial side of the Achilles tendon. If there are signs of impingement or degenerative changes, the tenotomy of plantaris can be performed using the shaver blade. (Figs. 14.2 and 14.3).

Depending on the severity of the case, some vertical "cuts" can be made on the tendon body, at the degenerative foci, using the arthroscopy hook or a small retro knife, the so-called scarification.

Fig. 14.1 Achilles tenoscopy

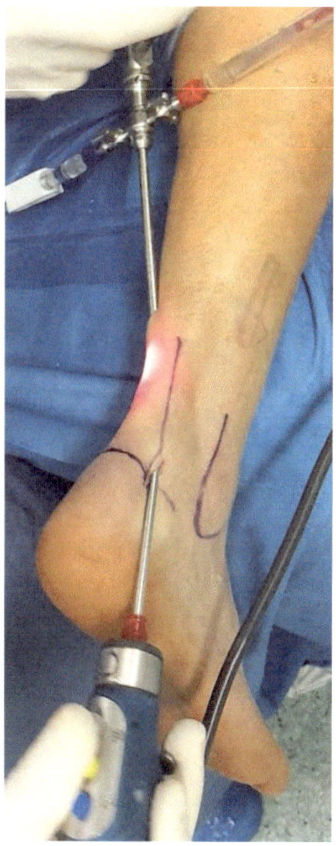

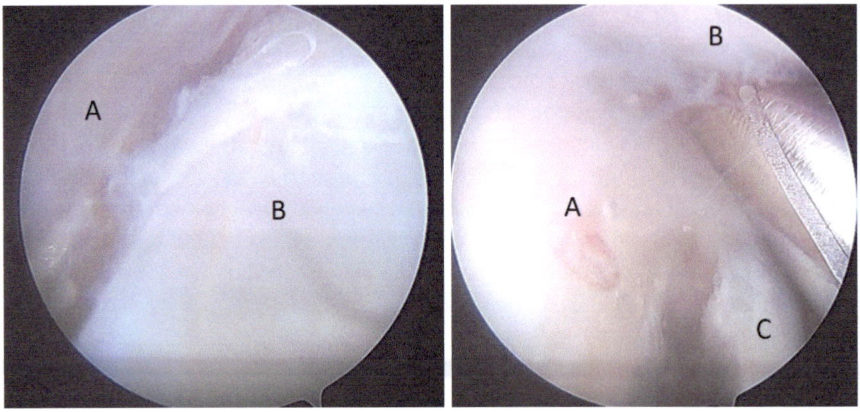

Fig. 14.2 Endoscopic view of the Achilles tendon: A—Achilles tendon; B—Paratenon; C—plantaris tendon

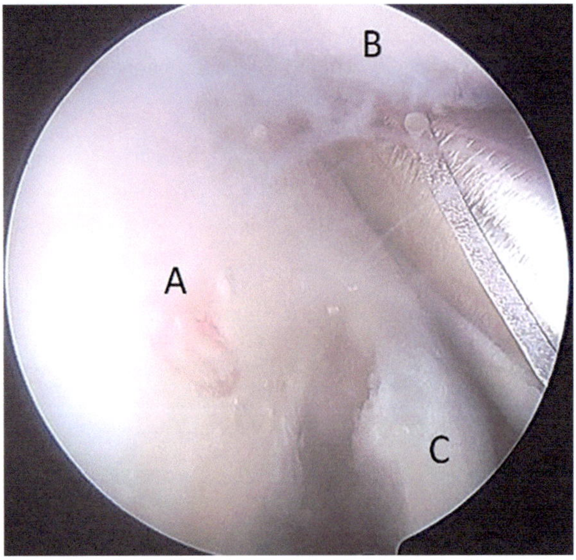

Fig. 14.3 Debridement of the Achilles (A) with a shaver. A—Achilles tendon; B—Paratenon; C—plantaris tendon

The endoscopic procedure can be supplemented with other surgical (minimal invasive) or non-surgical procedures. These are usually techniques already in use for the treatment of this condition, such as, the release of the medial gastrocnemius (described at the end of the chapter) or the injection of substances like PRP. These are adjuvant procedures of the main intervention that is the release of adhesion and destruction of the neo vascularization and innervation.

As the endoscopic transfer of FHL has shown good results in the treatment of chronic Achilles tendon rupture, this technique has been also used to treat insertional tendinopathy (as we will see in the next section) and mid-portion afflictions. However, the limited number of cases makes it difficult to assess the results.

Postoperative Care

A soft dressing is applied, and immediate active mobilization of the ankle is allowed as tolerated by pain. Partial weight-bearing is permitted on the second day and prolonged for 2 weeks. Physiotherapy can be started as soon as tolerated.

After 14 days full, weight bearing is allowed, and physiotherapy is intensified. If any condition is suspected to be the cause of the tendon dysfunction, it should be corrected.

Insertional Tendinopathy

As previously discussed, insertional tendinopathy is an overuse injury caused by repetitive activity. It has a bimodal incidence, affecting both athletes (especially uphill runners) and sedentary, middle-aged, overweight individuals [6]. This condition is characterized by pain and swelling at the insertion of the Achilles tendon. A hallmark feature of insertional tendinopathy is the painful protuberance on the posterior aspect of the heel, adjacent to the tendon insertion, often referred to as the "hump-bump".

This condition typically has three features [7]:

1. Bony component:
    - Prominent posterosuperior corner of the calcaneus
    - Bone edema
2. Tendon component:
    - Degeneration
    - Calcification and bone spurs
3. Soft tissue component:
    - Retrocalcaneal bursitis

These three components are usually present, though they vary in severity depending on the case. In some patients, the impairment may be primarily tendinous, while in others, the bone component or soft tissue alterations may be the main issue. Additionally, combinations of these components may occur. The severity of these components and the location of the degenerative changes have clear implications for treatment options.

As with mid-portion tendinopathy, the treatment for insertional tendinopathy is primarily conservative, involving eccentric loading exercises, shockwave therapy, physiotherapy, and shoe modifications [8]. Most patients respond well to this treatment approach. However, the presence of significant calcification or bone spurs may negatively impact adherence to the non-surgical program. For this reason, along with patient characteristics and specific features of the condition, the reported efficacy of conservative measures for insertional tendinopathy is generally lower than that for mid-portion tendinopathy [8, 9]. The success rate of non-surgical treatment for insertional tendinopathy is typically reported to be 50–70% [8], though recent studies show efficacy rates approaching those seen in non-insertional tendinopathy, with success rates just over 80%. Despite this, clinical experience suggests that insertional tendinopathy often requires more surgical intervention compared to non-insertional cases.

When discussing operative treatment for insertional tendinopathy, distinguishing between calcified and non-calcified tendons may have therapeutic implications. As a result, endoscopic techniques are more commonly considered for non-calcified tendons [10].

Another important feature is the presence of a prominent posterosuperior corner of the calcaneus, known as Haglund's deformity or disease. While the presence of this deformity typically does not influence the choice of approach (open or arthroscopic, as both can be used), it may affect the treatment modality. In the presence of a Haglund's deformity, there may be a tendency to favor a surgical option. When surgery is chosen, the protocol typically includes the removal of the prominent bone [9].

The degree of tendon degeneration is an important factor, particularly with the occurrence of partial ruptures, and it has therapeutic implications [11]. If these partial ruptures involve more than 50% of the tendon thickness, a pre-rupture state is considered, and most would opt for an open procedure or tendon transfer, as discussed below.

The technique described here is for non-calcific insertional tendinopathy with Haglund's deformity and limited tendon degeneration, commonly referred to as calcaneoplasty.

Endoscopic Calcaneoplasty (Haglund Excision)—Surgical Technique

With the patient under general or spinal anesthesia, a tourniquet is placed on the calf, and the patient is positioned prone, with the feet just over the edge of the operative table. A small pillow is placed beneath the ankle to allow free movement of the foot. Additionally, a pillow may be placed under the contralateral hip to position the foot vertically, rather than in its normal resting position with slight external rotation.

At the beginning of the learning curve, using an image intensifier to verify the correct positioning of the instruments and the amount of bony removal can be extremely helpful. Therefore, a C-arm should be positioned to provide a lateral view of the operated calcaneus (Fig. 14.4). To improve visualization without moving the ankle, the opposite leg should be lowered, if possible. Standard arthroscopic instruments are used.

For this procedure, two portals are required on each side of the Achilles tendon. In regular posterior ankle arthroscopy, the tip of the distal fibula is used as a

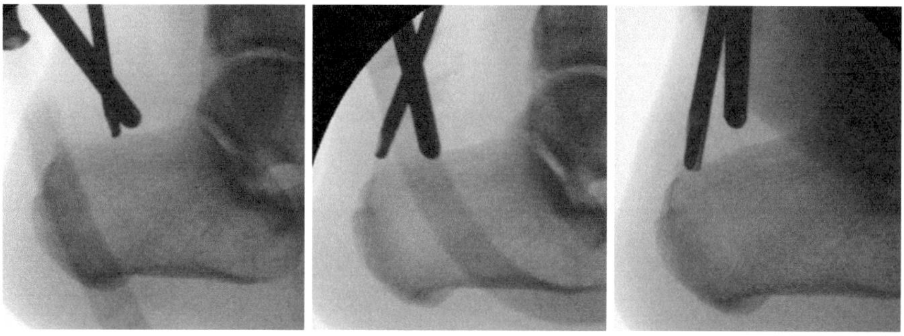

Fig. 14.4 Controlling instruments position and Haglund removal with fluoroscopy

landmark. A horizontal line is drawn from the tip of the fibula, parallel to the sole of the foot, extending towards the Achilles tendon. The portals are placed just posteromedial and posterolateral to the tendon. For endoscopic calcaneoplasty, the portals should be placed 15–20 mm below this line, immediately above the bone (Fig. 14.5).

The lateral portal is made first, the retrocalcaneal bursa is accessed with a blunt trocar creating the space for the scope to operate. A 4.5 mm 30° arthroscope is introduced and the bursa is inspected. The second portal is made just medial to the tendon at the same level and the entrance to the instrument is made with a mosquito clamp.

Soft tissues are removed with a shaver, including the remains of the retrocalcaneal bursa, creating a working space. The dorsal aspect of the calcaneus is clear of soft tissues, exposing the bone. In most cases, the use of a radiofrequency wand is necessary.

Care should be taken to ensure that all the prominent bone is exposed up to the insertion of the Achilles tendon, which is located on the posterior wall of the calcaneus. At this point, fluoroscopy can be used to confirm that the instruments have passed over the top of the Haglund deformity (Fig. 14.6). The tendon fiber can be seen at this point on the posterior part of the operating field.

To ensure complete exposure of the prominence, the interchangeable use of the portals is typically necessary. During the procedure, the foot should be kept in plantar flexion. A bone-cutter shaver is used to remove all the prominent bone from the tendon insertion forward. Extreme care should be taken to ensure that the cutting face of the shaver remains directed only at the bone. Switching portals again may be helpful to ensure that all the bone is removed. Additionally, fluoroscopy can be useful to confirm the amount of bone removal (Figs. 14.7 and 14.8).

A gentle excision of the anterior paratenon can be done on the most distal part of the tendon.

With this procedure, the bony and soft tissue components of the condition are addressed. If the tendinous involvement is not too severe, there is a good chance of improvement with this operation.

In cases of calcified or pre-rupture tendons, an open procedure is typically preferred. In selected cases, an endoscopic option can be considered, consisting of calcaneoplasty, as described above, complemented by endoscopic transfer of the

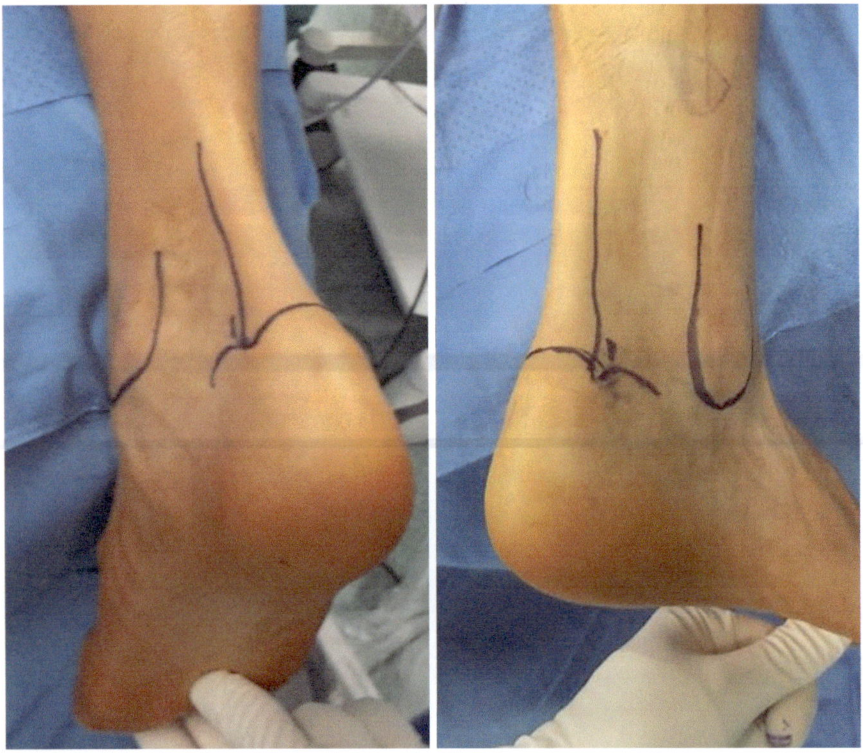

Fig. 14.5 Position of the posterior endoscopic portals for endoscopic calcaneoplasty, just near the deformity

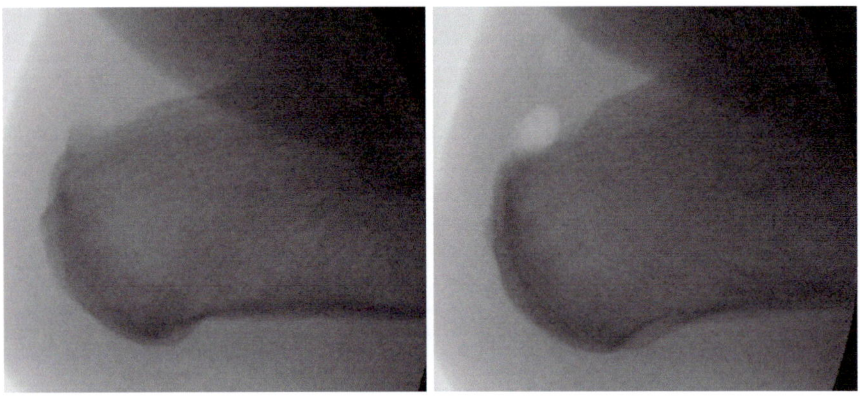

Fig. 14.6 Comparing initial deformity with the final result (Fluoroscopy)

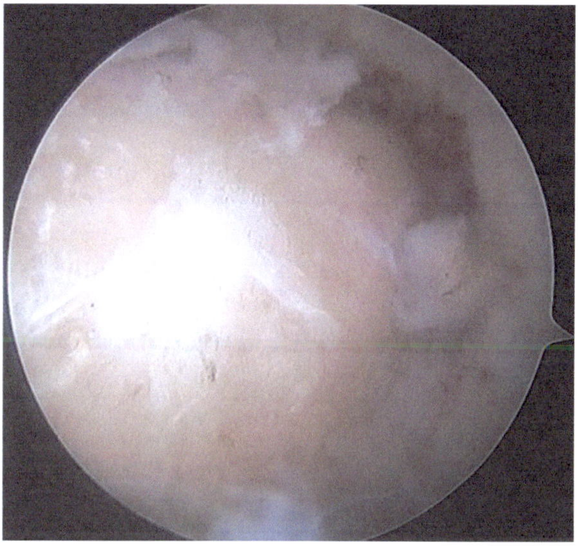

Fig. 14.7 Prominent calcaneal eminence on the left

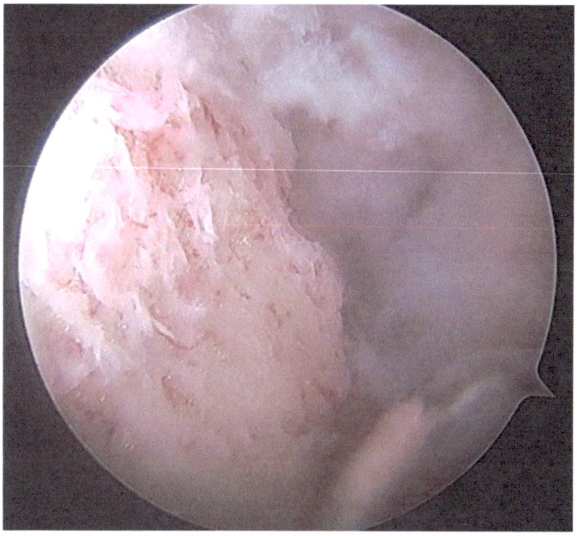

Fig. 14.8 Final result after removal of the eminence with a bone shaver

Flexor Hallucis Longus (FHL), as detailed in a subsequent section. The transfer provides mechanical support to the impaired Achilles tendon, with the FHL muscle belly placed in contact with the degenerative tendon. These two interventions may promote the healing of the degenerated tendon [12].

Postoperative Care

A soft dressing is applied and partial weight bearing is allowed as tolerated. Active range of motion exercises are also encouraged, as tolerated. A normal shoe can be used as soon as possible. Some physiotherapy may be required, especially if there is a limited range of motion. Running is allowed from 4 weeks post-surgery and return to play is typically authorized within 2 months.

Chronic Achilles Tendon Rupture

Background

The Achilles tendon is the largest and most commonly ruptured tendon in the human body. Chronic Achilles tendon rupture (CATR) usually results from a neglected acute rupture (i.e., a rupture left untreated for more than 4 weeks) or from re-ruptures after surgical treatment [13, 14]. CATR usually evolves with the separation of the tendon stumps, creating a gap that causes loss of mechanical efficiency of the triceps surae complex [15] (Fig. 14.9). This results in functional impairments such as weakness in the push-off component of gait, difficulty in going up or down stairs, and inability to tiptoe.

Even though conservative management of CATR is possible, surgical repair is usually recommended, with the goal being to restore continuity of the tendon [15]. Depending on the size of the gap and amount of scar tissue present, direct

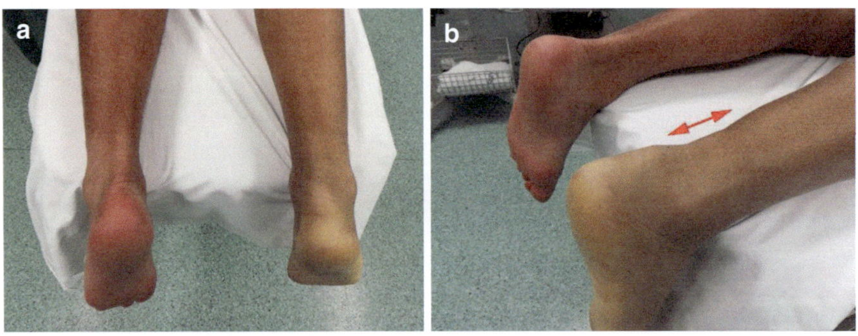

Fig. 14.9 Pre-operative CATR—Achilles tendon rupture on right ankle neglected for 3 months. Note the loss of resting plantar flexion (**a**) and a clearly externally visible tendon gap (**b**—red double arrow)

end-to-end repair of the tendon might be possible. However, defects larger than 2–4 cm tend to require other types of procedure, such as "V-Y" plasty, turndown flaps, or tendon transfers. Various tendons can be used for transfer, but the Flexor Hallucis Longus (FHL) is usually the choice, due to it being a strong plantar flexor, with a well vascularized ventral muscle, and located adjacent to the triceps surae complex, with which it has in-phase muscle and shares the same line of contraction [16]. Outcomes of isolated FHL transfer for the treatment of CATR are typically successful, with full integration and hypertrophy of the FHL, leading to normal walking and allowing patients to return to their pre-injury activities, including those with high demands.

Although open-surgery FHL transfer can be performed with a single incision (described in the next section), this technique requires an extensive surgical field in a vulnerable location, with associated risk of infection and soft tissue healing problems. More recently, however, endoscopic transfer of FHL (ETFHL) techniques have been with good outcomes [17–19]. Endoscopic treatment has important advantages over open techniques, requiring a lesser degree of soft tissue dissection and leading to faster healing and lower risk of infection, as well as a more cosmetically desirable outcome [20].

In open techniques, often the scarred portion of the Achilles tendon is excised at the time of FHL transfer, as it is thought that altered gene expression by the ruptured Achilles tendon, particularly greater amounts of type III collagen [21], might interfere with recovery. However, in a study by Vega et al. [19], it has been shown that with ETFHL, where the scarred tissue was not excised, postoperative MRIs indicated the presence of a normal or close-to-normal Achilles tendon in the previously affected areas. This is thought to be due to the high vascular density of the FHL muscle belly, which was placed in contact with the scarred area (Fig. 14.10), bringing increased perfusion to the affected area [19]. We have thus opted for not performing Achilles tendon debridement in our technique.

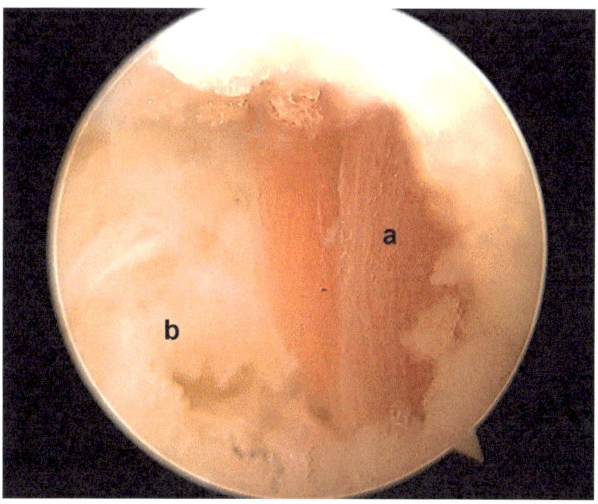

Fig. 14.10 FHL muscle belly—The image shows a low position of the FHL muscle belly, thus helping with perfusion of the affected area (a—FHL muscle belly; b—calcaneus)

There is a generalized belief that FHL transfer impacts toe function, as this tendon is responsible for flexion of the hallux, as its name indicates. However, studies show that the reduction in flexion strength might be small and not noticeable to the patient [22]. This technique was first described by Gonçalves e Corte-Real in 2015 [18].

Endoscopic Transfer of Flexor Hallucis Longus to the Calcaneus—Surgical Technique

The patient lies prone, and a 2-portal technique using the posterolateral and posteromedial portals is performed. The posterolateral portal is primarily used as the viewing portal, and the posteromedial portal is used as the instrumentation portal. The FHL tendon is identified after debridement and clearing using a shaver and a radiofrequency wand (Fig. 14.11); it lies medial to the talus and is clearly visible until entering the fibro-osseous tunnel. The FHL tendon is pierced with a suture passer, and a lasso loop-type suture is tied using a non-absorbable suture; this provides traction on the tendon. While the hallux is flexed and the foot is held in maximum plantar flexion (Fig. 14.12a), the traction suture is grasped and gently pulled; the tendon is cut as deep as possible on the retromalleolar groove using arthroscopic scissors (Fig. 14.12b) and, if necessary, completed with a radiofrequency wand, aiming to obtain the maximum length of tendon possible.

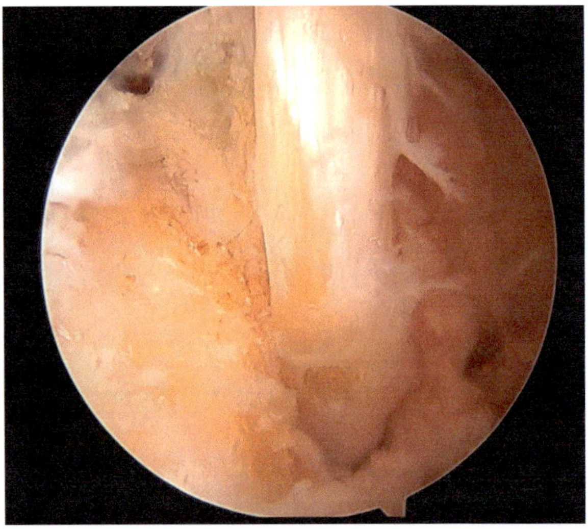

Fig. 14.11 Isolated FHL tendon

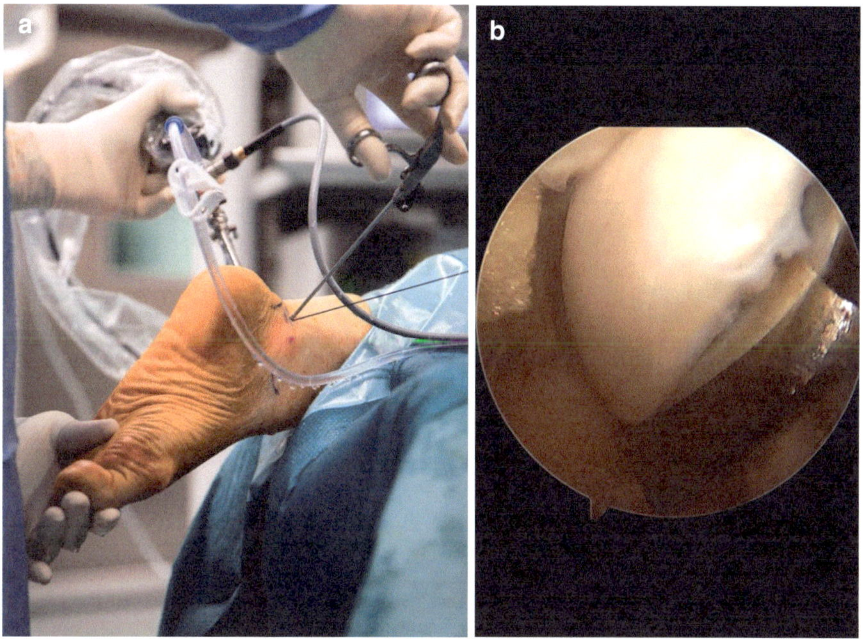

Fig. 14.12 EFHLT procedure—FHL tendon cut—Moment the FHL is cut, with the foot held in plantar flexion. (B) The tendon is cut using arthroscopic scissors

The free end of the FHL tendon is exteriorized through the medial portal using the traction suture. A Krackow-type suture with a non-absorbable wire is applied on the distal end of the FHL and will allow for its shuttling through the calcaneal tunnel (Fig. 14.13), as well as adequate grasping for tensioning before final fixation.

The intended footprint for the calcaneus tunnel placement is cleared to the bone; a medial insertion site is chosen to closely resemble the Achilles tendon anatomic footprint on the medial aspect of the middle facet of the calcaneal tuberosity. It is important to advance the suture-passing wire in a medial to lateral direction and at an approximately 15° angle to the plantar aspect of the foot (Fig. 14.14a). This direction of the planned tunnel placement provides adequate bone coverage for graft integration. The cannulated reamer (of the same width of the harvested tendon) is then advanced through the medial portal, sliding over the suture-passing wire. A

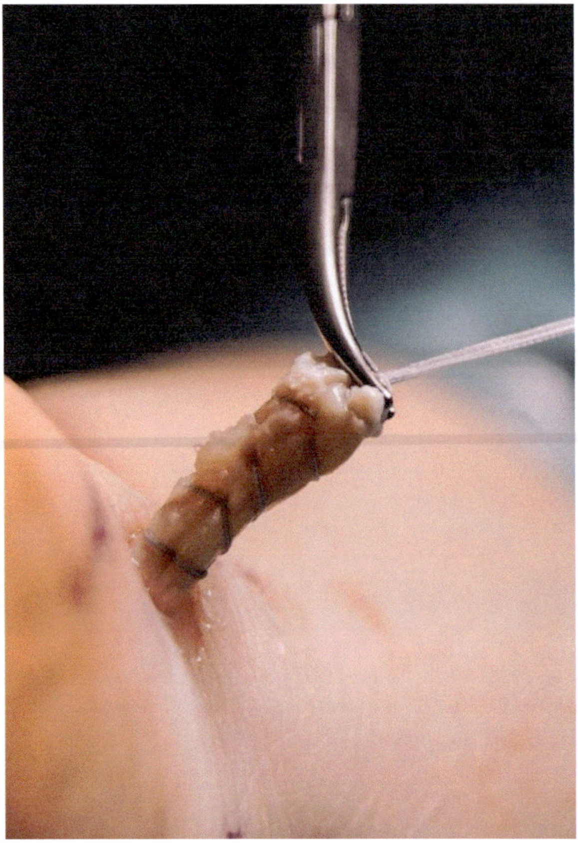

Fig. 14.13 FHL distal end preparation—Non-absorbable wire is applied to the FHL stump, which will allow it to shuttle through the calcaneal tunnel

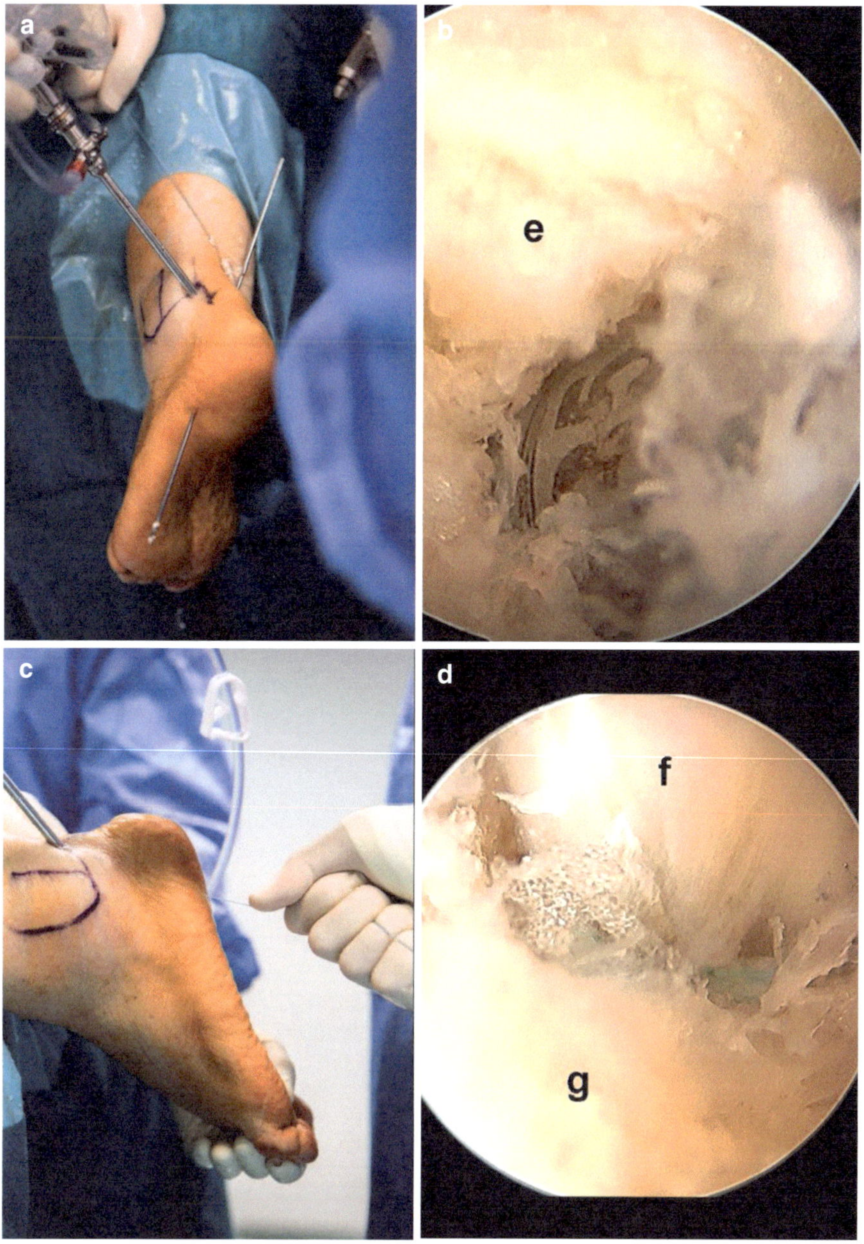

Fig. 14.14 EFHLT procedure—Calcaneus fixation. (**a**) Medial to lateral direction of the suture-passing wire. (**b**) Tunnel drilling. (**c**) Suture ends pulled, advancing the FHL tendon through the tunnel to its final position (**d**) (e—calcaneus; f—FHL tendon; g—calcaneus)

tunnel is drilled to a depth of 30–35 mm deep (Fig. 14.14b). After the reamer is removed, with care taken to avoid removing the suture-passing wire, the free ends of the Krackow suture are passed through the eyelet and the wire is fully advanced to the plantar aspect of the foot (Fig. 14.14c and d). Moving the foot through its range of motion permits the surgeon to select adequate tension before final fixation so that the foot is resting in a neutral position or slight dorsiflexion. The tendon is fixed with an interference screw (Figs. 14.15 and 14.16).

The Achilles tendon is not directly visualized, and no debridement is performed.

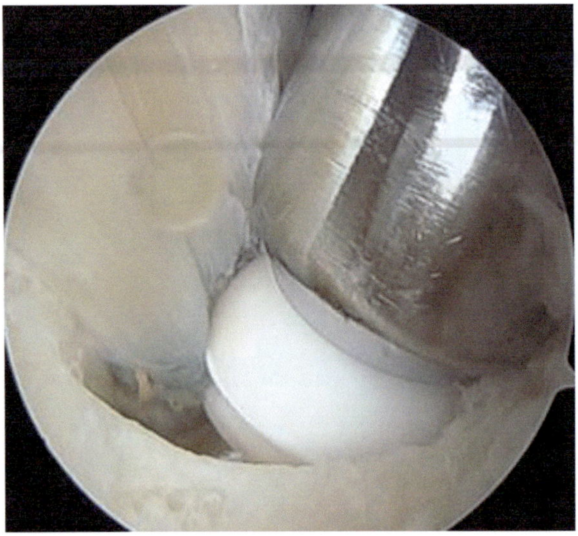

Fig. 14.15 Interference screw fixing the FHL in its final position

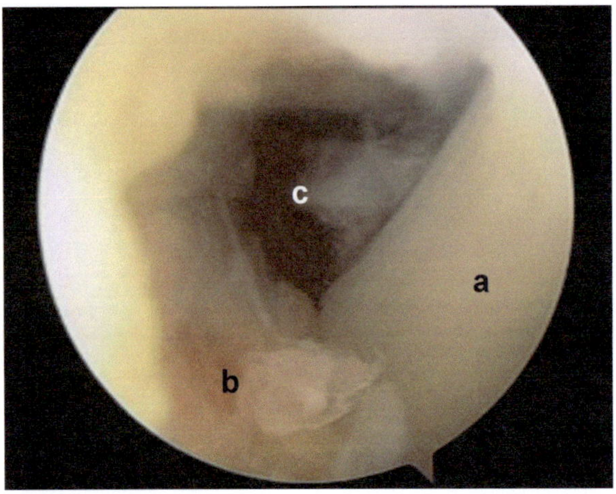

Fig. 14.16 EFHLT procedure—Final result—FHL tendon fixed with an interference screw (a—FHL tendon; b—calcaneus; c—interference screw)

Post Operative Care

An equinus posterior splint immobilization is applied for 4 weeks postoperatively. Sutures are removed in 2 weeks if the wounds are completely healed. At this stage, the splint can be replaced by a boot with wedges but only toe-touch weight-bearing is allowed till 4 weeks. After this period, weight bearing is permitted and a progressive reduction of equinus is undertaken.

Physiotherapy begins at 6 weeks with exercises for progressively increase the strength and range of motion. Walking with no support can be expected by the two-month mark. The aim is for the patient to walk with no limp and have normal push-off during gait within the first 3–5 weeks of physiotherapy.

At this point of time, the patient will regain ability for single-leg heel rise and near normal push-off power. After 3 months, exercises like running and jumping can be introduced. At the 6-month mark, a full recovery can be expected (Fig. 14.17).

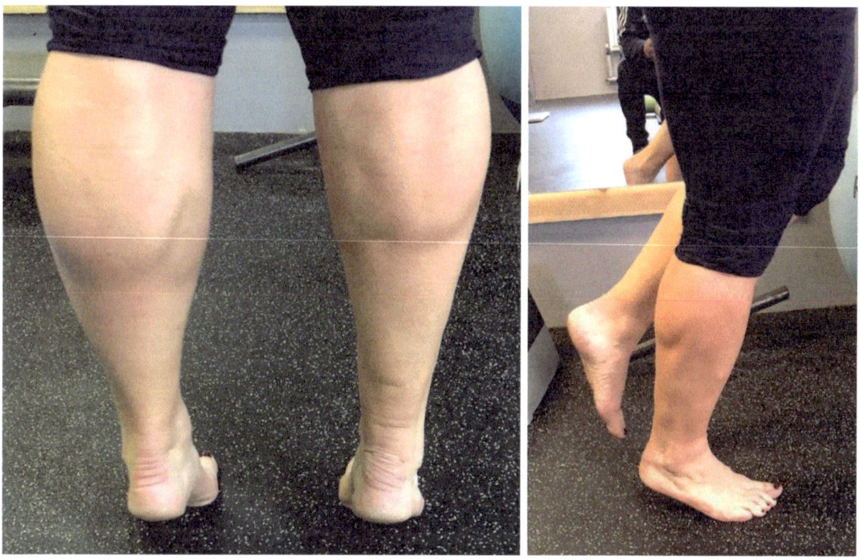

Fig. 14.17 Post-operative recovery—Patient after recovery (6 months post surgery), displaying clear recovery of the triceps surae function (A) and ability to perform single-foot heel rise

The results of ETFHL performed for CATR showed good results and remarkable functional rehabilitation, with all patients being able to resume their previous activities. These results are comparable to open classic techniques, so ETFHL can become standard treatment for CATR due to the less morbidity and risk of skin complications. Nevertheless, further studies are necessary to validate this assumption. ETFHL is a demanding technique, and therefore might not be suitable for the novice ankle arthroscopy surgeon.

Open Technique of Flexor Hallucis Longus to the Calcaneus—Surgical Technique

The open technique of FHL tendon transfer is more commonly performed and is described here. A single incision technique is used. The patient is positioned prone and a thigh tourniquet is applied. The incision is placed in the midline on the posterior aspect. The soft tissues are handled with care to avoid wound healing issues. The Sural nerve that is on the lateral aspect distally but can be more medial proximally, should be protected. The Achilles tendon is identified and the diseased segment is excised (Fig. 14.18). The next step is to divide the fascia overlying FHL muscle belly (Fig. 14.19). The FHL tendon is dissected carefully in the medial

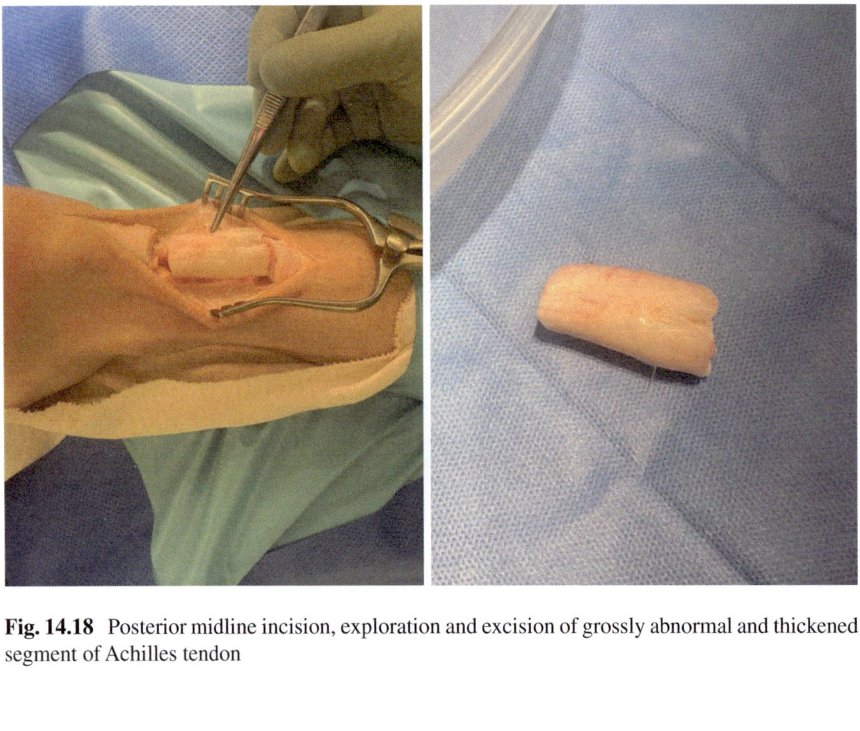

Fig. 14.18 Posterior midline incision, exploration and excision of grossly abnormal and thickened segment of Achilles tendon

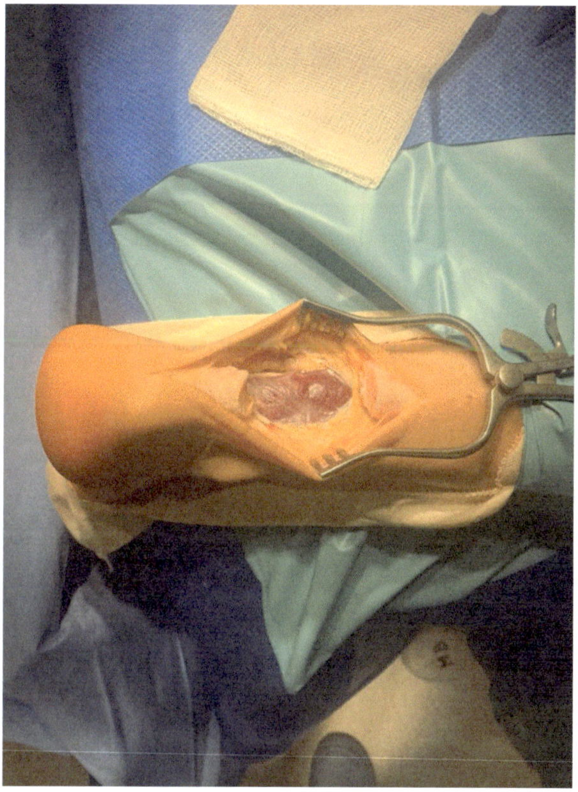

Fig. 14.19 Division of fascia overlying FHL muscle belly

calcaneal tunnel protecting the tibial nerve that is close to this tendon on the medial aspect (Fig. 14.20). The FHL muscle belly is tensioned & retracted with a retractor and the FHL tendon is divided (Fig. 14.21). A length of about 2 cm of the divided tendon is sufficient.

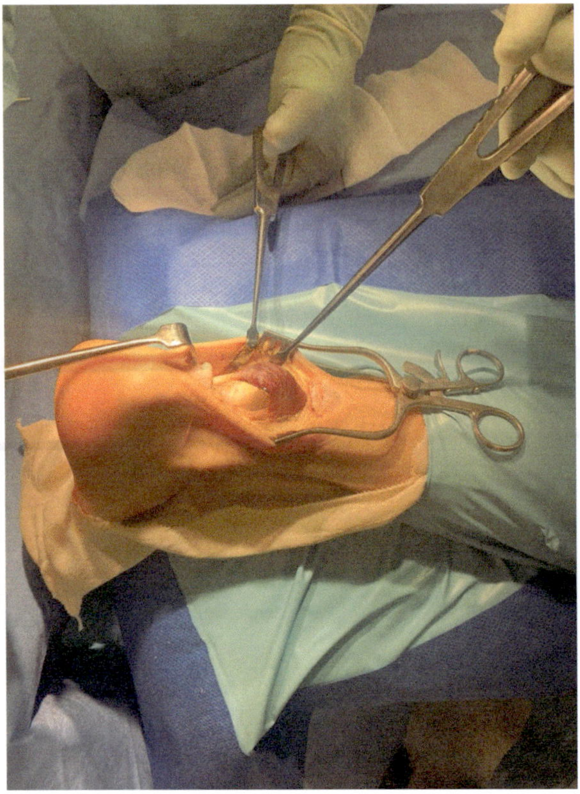

Fig. 14.20 Careful dissection of FHL tendon protecting the tibial nerve

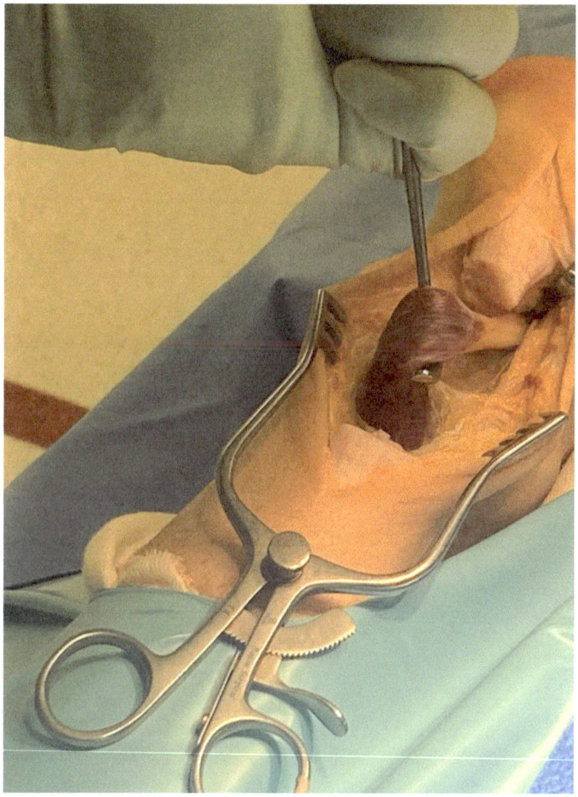

Fig. 14.21 FHL muscle belly is retracted to provide adequate length of FHL tendon prior to it's division

The FHL tendon graft is then whipstitched using a thick (Number 2) looped fiber wire (Fig. 14.22). The thickness of the tendon graft is measured (usually 5–6 mm) (Fig. 14.23). A guidewire is used in the calcaneus that comes out of skin on the plantar aspect of the foot (Fig. 14.24). It is better to make a small incision in the skin where the wire comes out as patients sometimes report pain in this region of heel.

The calcaneal tunnel is then drilled over the guidewire for at least 2 cm (the length of the FHL tendon) (Fig. 14.25). The thickness of the drill should be based upon the bone consistency. In soft bone it is better to avoid over drilling and the same size drill as the FHL tendon should be used. In hard, sclerotic bone on the other hand, 1–1.5 mm over drilling might be required. It is advisable to drill gradually in the increments of 0.5 mm so that the tendon transfer fits snugly in the tunnel.

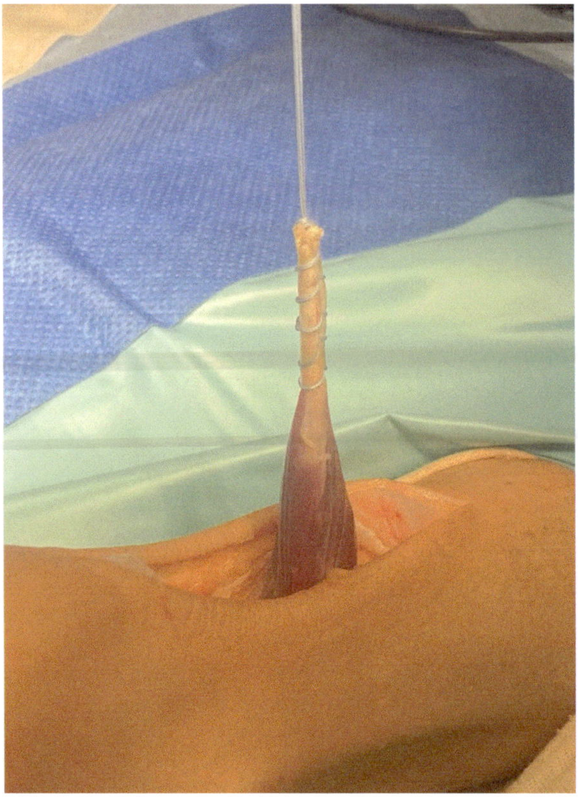

Fig. 14.22 Preparation of the FHL tendon graft using looped Fiber wire

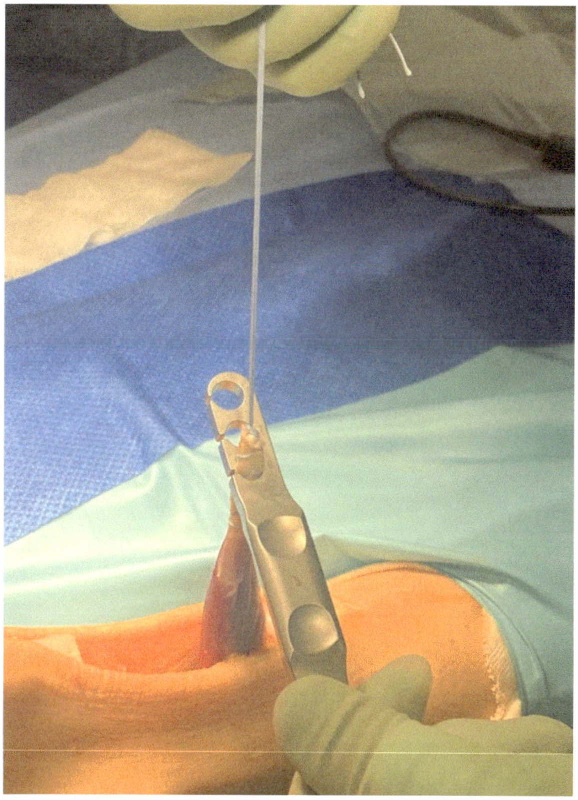

Fig. 14.23 Measurement of thickness of FHL tendon graft

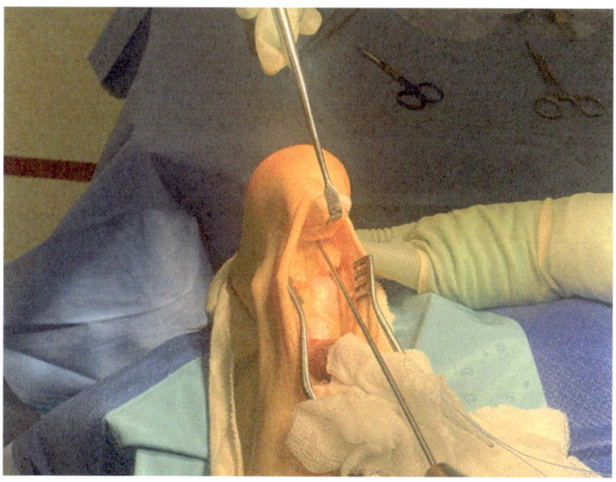

Fig. 14.24 Insertion of guide wire in calcaneum just below the insertion of Achilles

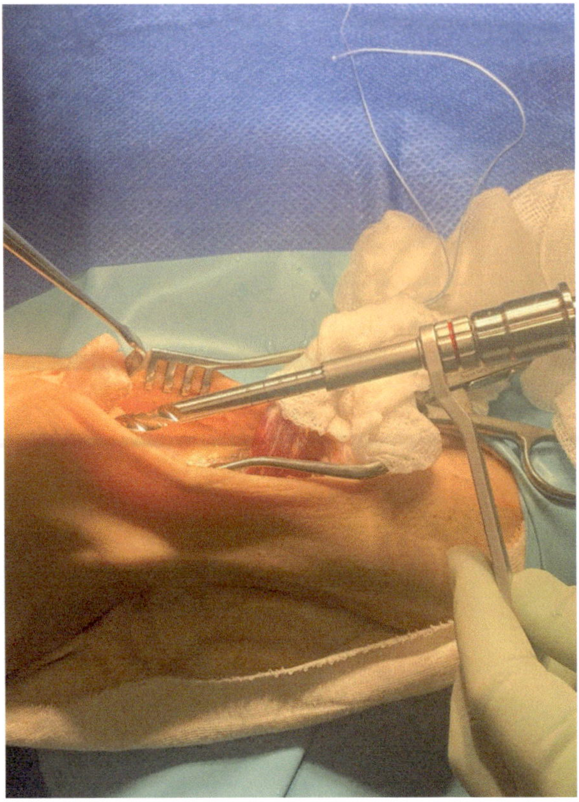

Fig. 14.25 Drilling of calcaneal tunnel over the guide wire

The FHL tendon graft is then passed in the tunnel using an eyed or looped wire (Fig. 14.26). The assistant provides traction to keep the FHL tendon graft under tension and the tendon transfer is then secured with an interference screw usually of the same thickness as the tendon graft (Fig. 14.27). Once the FHL tendon graft is fixed with the screw, the foot is moved to confirm the integrity of the tendon transfer. The distal end of the divided Achilles is then repaired to the FHL tendon using fiber wire to provide extra stability (Fig. 14.28).

The wound is closed in layers and a dorsal slab is applied with the foot in an anti-gravity position.

Post-operative plan: The wound is inspected at 2 weeks and the plaster splint is replaced with a boot with a wedge allowing full weight bearing in the boot. The boot is removed after 6 weeks and physiotherapy is started. It is important to provide thromboprophylaxis for 4–6 weeks after surgery to reduce the risk of clot.

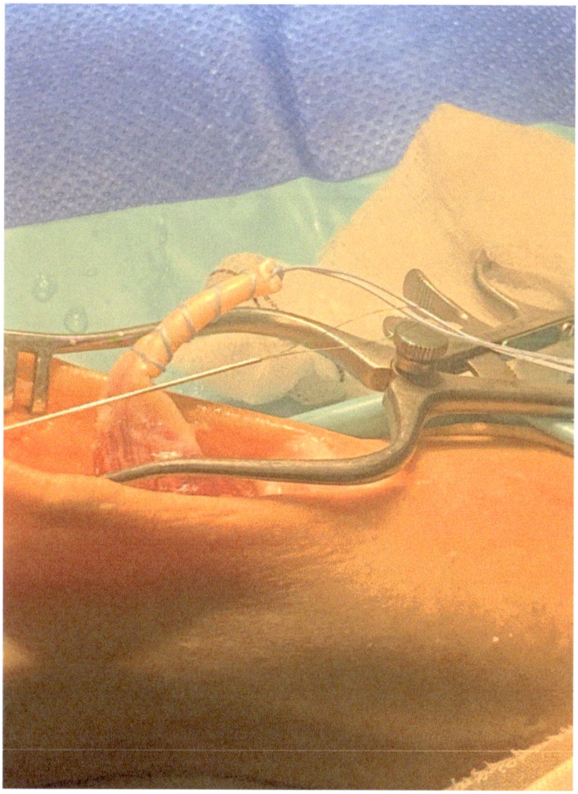

Fig. 14.26 Use of wire with a loop to position the FHL tendon graft in the calcaneal tunnel

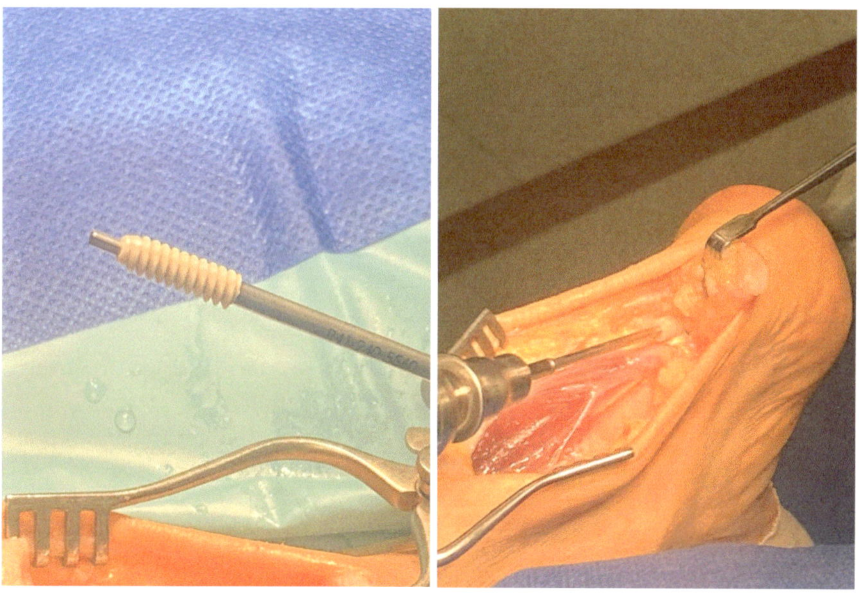

Fig. 14.27 Use of interference screw to secure the FHL tendon graft under tension

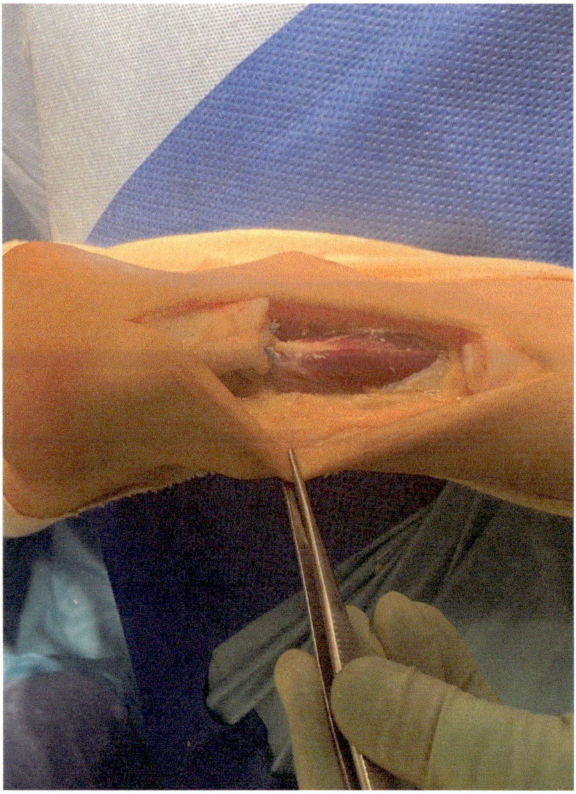

Fig. 14.28 Repair of distal Achilles stump with FHL tendon graft to enhance stability of tendon transfer

Proximal Medial Gastrocnemius Release (PMGR)—Surgical Technique

The indications of PMGR are refractory plantar fasciitis [23] or chronic non insertional Achilles tendinopathy with marked tightness of Gastrocnemius [24]. The patient position is prone (Fig. 14.29). It can be performed under local or general anaesthetic, with or without tourniquet. If performed under local anaesthetic without tourniquet, it is better to use the local anaesthetic with adrenaline.

A small transverse incision is made about 2 cm distal to the popliteal crease or dimple medial to the midline (Fig. 14.30). After clearing the fat, the glistening

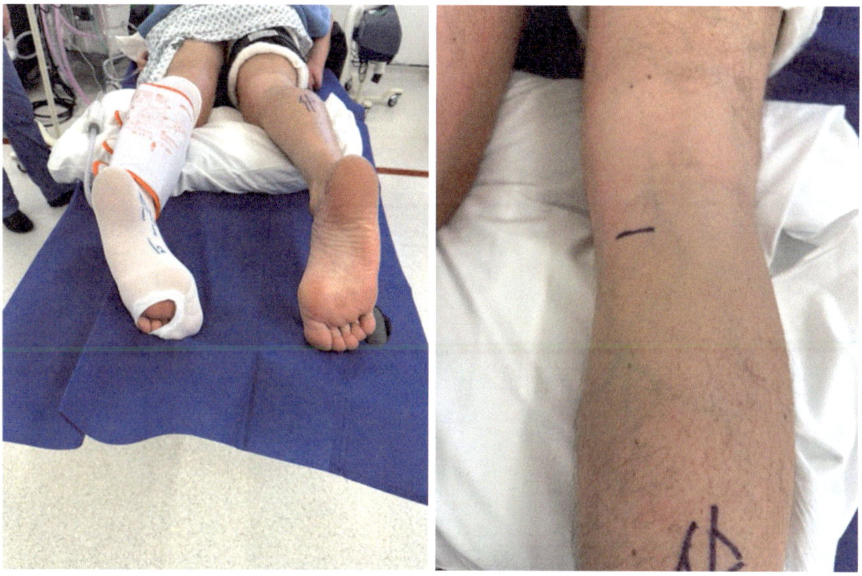

Fig. 14.29 Patient positioning and marking of the skin incision for PMGR

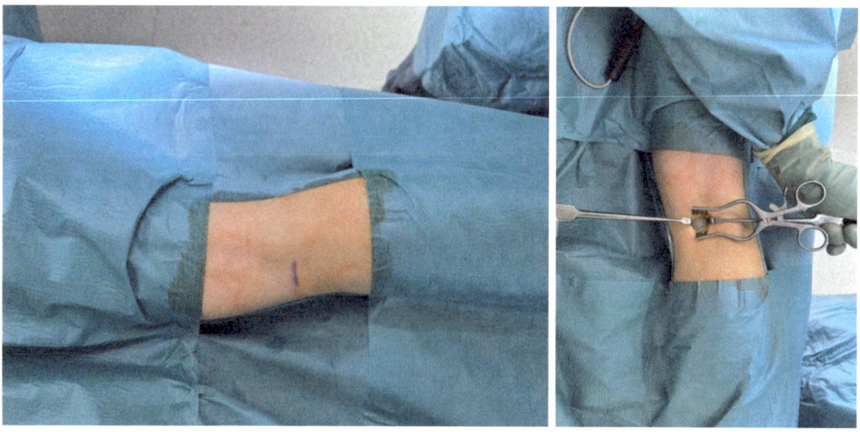

Fig. 14.30 Skin incision for PMGR

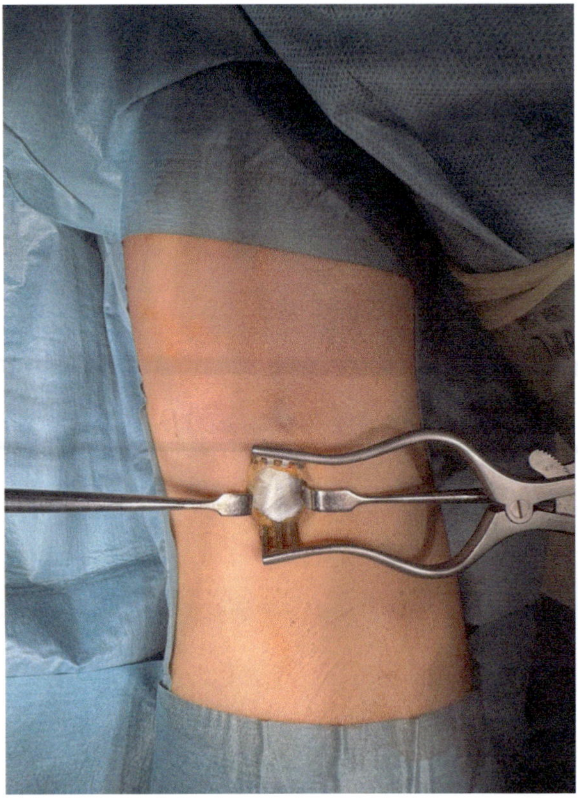

Fig. 14.31 Exposure of glistening fascia overlying medial gastrocnemius

fascia overlying the medial gastrocnemius is identified (Fig. 14.31). There is usually a subtle distinction in the consistency of the fascia overlying the medial head of gastrocnemius (thicker) as compared to that overlying the lateral head of gastrocnemius (thinner).

The fascia is divided to reveal the gastrocnemius muscle underneath. It is easy to miss the medial margin of the fascia and one must ensure with retraction that the fascia overlying the medial gastrocnemius has been divided completely (Fig. 14.32). This is confirmed by movements of the knee or ankle where one can see change in the gap between proximal and distal ends of the divided fascial layers with movements.

Post-operative plan: A small dressing is applied. There is no need for boots or plaster. Full weight bearing mobilisation along with an active range of movement exercises are encouraged immediately post-surgery. Thromboprophylaxis should be considered specially in patients with risk factors for clot.

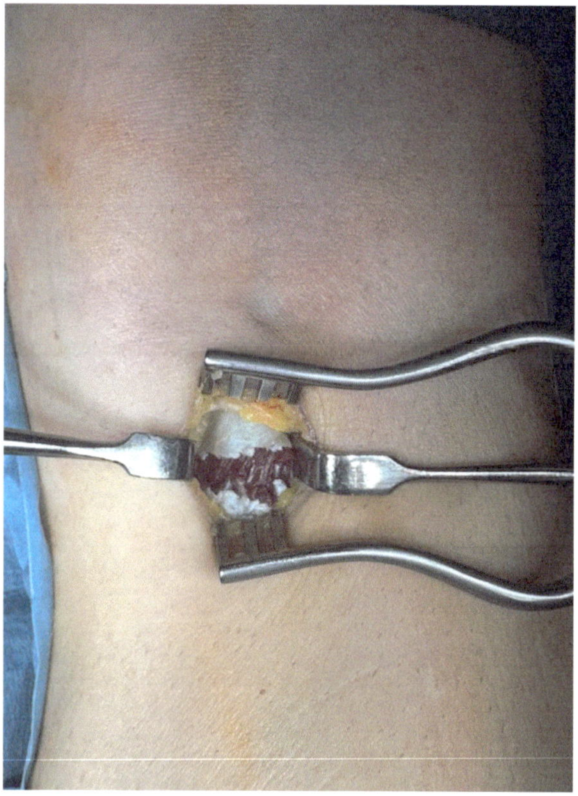

Fig. 14.32 Complete division of the fascia revealing medial gastrocnemius muscle

References

1. Pavone V, Vescio A, Mobilia G, et al. Conservative treatment of chronic Achilles tendinopathy: a systematic review. J Funct Morphol Kinesiol. 2019;4 https://doi.org/10.3390/jfmk4030046.
2. Li H-Y, Hua Y-H. Achilles tendinopathy: current concepts about the basic science and clinical treatments. Biomed Res Int. 2016;2016:6492597. https://doi.org/10.1155/2016/6492597.
3. Vallance P, Hasani F, Crowley L, Malliaras P. Self-reported pain with single leg heel raise or single leg hop offer distinct information as measures of severity in men with midportion and insertional Achilles tendinopathy: an observational cross-sectional study. Phys Ther Sport Off J Assoc Chart Physiother Sport Med. 2021;47:23–31. https://doi.org/10.1016/j.ptsp.2020.10.009.
4. Olewnik Ł, Wysiadecki G, Podgórski M, et al. The Plantaris muscle tendon and its relationship with the Achilles tendinopathy. Biomed Res Int. 2018;2018:9623579. https://doi.org/10.1155/2018/9623579.
5. Lohrer H, David S, Nauck T. Surgical treatment for achilles tendinopathy—a systematic review. BMC Musculoskelet Disord. 2016;17:207. https://doi.org/10.1186/s12891-016-1061-4.
6. Chimenti RL, Cychosz CC, Hall MM, Phisitkul P. Current concepts review update: insertional Achilles tendinopathy. Foot Ankle Int. 2017;38:1160–9. https://doi.org/10.1177/1071100717723127.

7. van Dijk CN, van Sterkenburg MN, Wiegerinck JI, et al. Terminology for Achilles tendon related disorders. Knee Surg Sports Traumatol Arthrosc. 2011;19:835–41. https://doi.org/10.1007/s00167-010-1374-z.
8. Zhi X, Liu X, Han J, et al. Nonoperative treatment of insertional Achilles tendinopathy: a systematic review. J Orthop Surg Res. 2021;16:233. https://doi.org/10.1186/s13018-021-02370-0.
9. Kunkle BF, Baxter NA, Caughman AM, et al. Risk factors for failure of conservative management of insertional Achilles tendinosis. Foot Ankle Spec. 2023;16:370–6. https://doi.org/10.1177/19386400221090358.
10. Lugani G, Santandrea A, Mercurio D, et al. Treatment of Achilles insertional tendinopathy: our surgical procedure and medium-term results. Acta Biomed. 2023;94:e2023053. https://doi.org/10.23750/abm.v94i2.13834.
11. Gatz M, Spang C, Alfredson H. Partial Achilles tendon rupture-a neglected entity: a narrative literature review on diagnostics and treatment options. J Clin Med. 2020;9 https://doi.org/10.3390/jcm9103380.
12. Singh MS, Harna B, Singh S, Vishwakarma G. Evaluation of Flexor hallucis tendon transfer in chronic insertional Achilles tendinopathy in over 50-year-old population using validated ankle scores. Foot (Edinb). 2023;54:101969. https://doi.org/10.1016/j.foot.2023.101969.
13. Peterson KS, Hentges MJ, Catanzariti AR, et al. Surgical considerations for the neglected or chronic Achilles tendon rupture: a combined technique for reconstruction. J foot ankle Surg Off Publ Am Coll Foot Ankle Surg. 2014;53:664–71. https://doi.org/10.1053/j.jfas.2013.10.001.
14. Bevilacqua NJ. Treatment of the neglected Achilles tendon rupture. Clin Podiatr Med Surg. 2012;29:291–9. viii. https://doi.org/10.1016/j.cpm.2012.01.004.
15. Oksanen MM, Haapasalo HH, Elo PP, Laine H-J. Hypertrophy of the flexor hallucis longus muscle after tendon transfer in patients with chronic Achilles tendon rupture. Foot ankle Surg Off J Eur Soc Foot Ankle Surg. 2014;20:253–7. https://doi.org/10.1016/j.fas.2014.06.003.
16. Hahn F, Meyer P, Maiwald C, et al. Treatment of chronic achilles tendinopathy and ruptures with flexor hallucis tendon transfer: clinical outcome and MRI findings. Foot Ankle Int. 2008;29:794–802. https://doi.org/10.3113/FAI.2008.0794.
17. Baumfeld D, Baumfeld T, Figueiredo AR, et al. Endoscopic flexor halluces longus transfer for chronic Achilles tendon rupture—technique description and early post-operative results. Muscles Ligaments Tendons J. 2017;7:341–6. https://doi.org/10.11138/mltj/2017.7.2.341.
18. Gonçalves S, Caetano R, Corte-Real N. Salvage flexor Hallucis longus transfer for a failed Achilles repair: endoscopic technique. Arthrosc Tech. 2015;4:e411–6. https://doi.org/10.1016/j.eats.2015.03.017.
19. Vega J, Vilá J, Batista J, et al. Endoscopic flexor Hallucis longus transfer for chronic noninsertional Achilles tendon rupture. Foot Ankle Int. 2018;39:1464–72. https://doi.org/10.1177/1071100718793172.
20. Maffulli N, Gougoulias N. Letter regarding: endoscopic flexor Hallucis longus transfer for chronic noninsertional Achilles tendon rupture. Foot Ankle Int. 2019;40:121.
21. Karousou E, Ronga M, Vigetti D, et al. Collagens, proteoglycans, MMP-2, MMP-9 and TIMPs in human achilles tendon rupture. Clin Orthop Relat Res. 2008;466:1577–82. https://doi.org/10.1007/s11999-008-0255-y.
22. Martin RL, Manning CM, Carcia CR, Conti SF. An outcome study of chronic Achilles tendinosis after excision of the Achilles tendon and flexor hallucis longus tendon transfer. Foot Ankle Int. 2005;26:691–7. https://doi.org/10.1177/107110070502600905.
23. Arshad Z, Aslam A, Razzaq MA, Bhatia M. Gastrocnemius release in the management of chronic plantar fasciitis: a systematic review. Foot Ankle Int. 2022;43(4):568–75. https://doi.org/10.1177/10711007211052290. Epub 2021 Nov 12
24. Arshad Z, Al Shdefat S, Iqbal AM, Bhatia M. Gastrocnemius release is an effective management option for Achilles tendinopathy: a systematic review. Knee Surg Sports Traumatol Arthrosc. 2022;30(12):4189–97. https://doi.org/10.1007/s00167-022-07039-7. Epub 2022 Jul 11

Chapter 15
Lateral Ligament Reconstruction & Peroneal Tendon Surgery

Jesús Vilá Rico

Lateral Ligament Reconstruction Surgery

Introduction

Ankle sprains are among the most common reasons for consultation in hospital emergencies. The lateral ligament complex is affected 77% of the time, in which the most frequent mechanism of injury is plantar inversion and flexion, forcing the anterior talofibular ligament to act as the main stabilizer of the ankle [1].

Initial evaluation and treatment are crucial to avoid complications, errors in diagnosis and the progression to chronic ankle instability.

Most acute ankle sprains can be treated successfully with conservative measures, including rest, icing, anti-inflammatory drugs, bracing, progressive weight bearing, and physical therapy, especially functional rehabilitation methods such as range-of-motion exercises, peroneal and ankle dorsiflexion strengthening, Achilles tendon stretching, and proprioception training in conjunction with proper ankle immobilization devices.

Approximately 20–40% of patients develop chronic lateral ankle instability (CLAI) [2, 3]. Eighty percent of ankle osteoarthritis cases are posttraumatic, with the initial cause typically being ankle fractures, followed by ankle instability [4].

In recent years, issues related to the treatment of CLAI and certain aspects related to ankle instability have generated considerable controversy.

J. V. Rico (✉)
University Hospital, Madrid, Spain

Quironsalud Ruber Hospitals, Madrid, Spain

Complutense University of Madrid, Madrid, Spain

M. Bhatia (ed.), *Surgical Techniques of the Foot and Ankle*,
https://doi.org/10.1007/978-3-031-93742-2_15

Anatomical Tips

The ankle is a highly congruent synovial, hinge-type joint in which the talus fits perfectly into the mortise formed by the tibial plateau and the tibial and fibular malleoli. This anatomical configuration allows movement through only one axis, the bimalleolar axis, through which dorsiflexion and plantar flexion are produced. The normal range of motion is 13–33° for dorsiflexion and 23–56° for plantar flexion [5].

The lateral joint capsule of the ankle is supported by the anterior talofibular ligament (ATFL), the posterior talofibular ligament (PTFL), and the calcaneofibular ligament (CFL). These structures, together with the superior and inferior retinacula and the medial collateral ligament, are important static stabilizers of the ankle.

The lateral collateral ligament (LCL) is the most commonly injured ligamentous structure of the lower limb due to inversion sprain. It consists of the ATFL, the CFL, and the PTFL [5].

When the foot is in a neutral position, the ATFL and CFL form a 105° angle on the sagittal plane and a 90–100° angle on the frontal plane. These ligaments are not completely independent since some fibres form an arch between the CFL and the inferior part of the ATFL [6].

Tension among these ligaments changes during flexion and extension: in plantar flexion, the lower bands of the ATFL and CFL remain relaxed, whereas the upper ATFL band becomes taut. During dorsiflexion, the upper band relaxes, and the lower bands of the ATFL and CFL bands become taut [5].

Anterior Talofibular Ligament (ATFL)

The ATFL is the anterior component of the LCL and the first ligament to be injured in an ankle inversion sprain. This ligament is responsible for controlling the anterior tilt of the talus. According to early descriptions made by Testut [7], the ATFL is flat and quadrilateral; it is also relatively thin and the weakest lateral ligamentous structure (Fig. 15.1).

The ATFL inserts into the anterior edge of the lateral malleolus of the fibula and courses towards the lateral side of the talus; it then immediately inserts under a triangular area, the identification of which is extremely important in anatomical reconstruction or capsular augmentation procedures for managing chronic ankle instabilities [8].

The ligament is approximately 15–20 mm long, 6–10 mm wide, and 2 mm thick [9].

Recent studies have shown that the ATFL is always formed by two bands and have suggested that single-band ligaments are pathological structures in which the superior band has been reabsorbed after injury [10]. This could be because the ATFL's superior fascicle is an intra-articular ligament [11] and thus has difficulty healing, therefore explaining why the percentages of chronic pain after an ankle sprain are so high following conservative treatment.

Calcaneofibular Ligament (CFL)

Unlike the ATFL, which acts only on the transverse tarsal joint (TTJ), the CFL is extracapsular and plays an important role in the stability of both the TTJ and the subtalar joint (STJ). Morphologically, it has a thick and cord-like shape. It inserts into the anterior side of the cortex of the lateral malleolus, immediately below and very close to the insertion point of the ATFL, to which it is usually joined by arciform fibres [7].

It measures approximately 4–8 mm in diameter, 20 mm in length and 4–5.5 mm in width [12] (Fig. 15.1).

It follows an oblique course towards the posterior and distal directions, at the end of which it inserts into the lateral side of the calcaneus, 15 mm or 20 mm dorsally and posteriorly in relation to the lateral tubercle of this osseous structure, at which point its medial surface becomes involved with the lateral talocalcaneal ligament. Immediately above the anterior edge of the ligament and separated by thin, fatty tissue, which sometimes goes unnoticed, we find the talocalcaneal ligament, which separates the CFL from the STJ [9].

The CFL is a very strong ligament, and when it is relaxed, ankle movements allow the ankle valgus position and ankle eversion. In some situations of varus stress, the CFL is tensioned and may become injured if the ankle is not moving during flexion–extension.

This ligament is the second structure to become injured during an ankle sprain, with an incidence of approximately 20%. When the CFL is injured, the ATFL is usually injured as well [13].

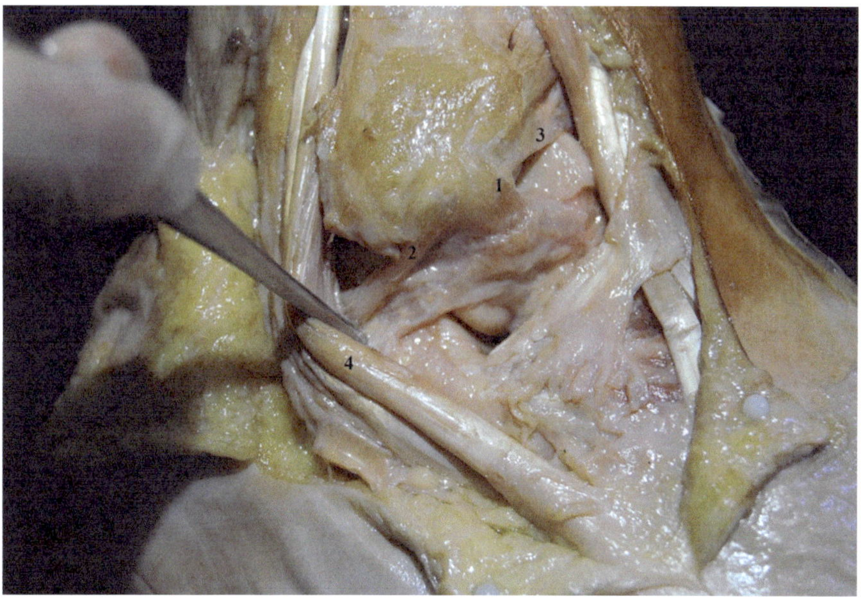

Fig. 15.1 Anatomy of the lateral complex. 1 ATFL. 2 CFL. 3. AITFL. 4 Peroneal tendons

Posterior Talofibular Ligament (PTFL)

Testut described the PTFL as a flat ligament that occupies the posterior region of the joint. Anatomic dissections and arthroscopic visualizations reveal that it has a semicord-like shape and is the strongest and most resilient of the 3 ligaments [7].

The PTFL is shaped like a trapezoid and measures 30 mm in length, 5 mm in width, and 5–8 mm in thickness [14]. This ligament is rarely injured, except in cases of peritalar ankle fracture or dislocation. Rasmussen and Tovborg–Jensen [15] reported that the PTFL plays a minor role in ankle stability if the rest of the lateral structures are intact.

Arciform Fibres

These fibres are an expansion of the regular, collagenous, and elastic dense connective tissues, taking the shape of a triangle or a semicircle, with an anteroinferior base that connects the inferior band of the ATFL with the interosseous talocalcaneal ligament (ITCL) and the CFL continuously (Fig. 15.1). These structures were clearly described by Kelikian and Sarrafian [16] in 2011 and were confirmed by Golanó et al. [8]; however, they have attracted attention again in recent years because of the critical role they play in endoscopic repairs of the ATFL [9] and have been jointly named the lateral fibulotalocalcaneal ligament complex of the ankle.

Assessment of Chronic Instability

Ankle instability can be grouped into two main types: mechanical instability, which is related to anatomic abnormalities of the ankle, usually due to ligament laxity; and functional instability, related to posture defects or tendon and muscle adjustment, usually due to a proprioceptive deficit [17].

When determining the method for treating CLAI, it is essential to assess subtalar stability, hindfoot malalignments in valgus and especially in varus, and the pathology of the peroneal tendons.

Why Perform Anatomical Techniques?

There is some consensus that surgical treatment for CLAI should be considered if rehabilitative treatment has not been successful after 6 months or if the patient has a long history of feeling instability or failure in the ankle that prevents him or her from performing his or her daily activities or sports.

Traditionally, two large groups of surgical techniques have been used: "anatomical techniques", in which the tissue is directly repaired in situ or replaced with allografts or autografts in its original anatomical position; that is, the reconstruction of the layout of the ligament by means of bone tunnels in the correct position; the other group is called "non anatomical techniques".

For many years, non anatomical techniques have involved the use of a hemitendon from the peroneus brevis (PB) and the conductance of tenorrhaphy or fibular tunnels to provide stability to the ankle.

In a systematic review, Noailles [18] reported a greater incidence of ankle osteoarthritis with non anatomical techniques than with direct repair. In addition, he questioned the use of the PB because of its important role in stabilizing tibiotalar inversion. Vuurberg [19] also reported better functional results with anatomical techniques than with non anatomical techniques.

Should We Correct Hindfoot Varus Malalignment in the Context of CLAI?

Surgical treatments for CLAI remain a challenge for orthopaedic surgeons and a subject of debate.

A correct clinical assessment is essential, with special attention given to hindfoot varus malalignments. In 2007, Vienne [20] introduced the concept of static and dynamic correction of ankle instability in cases of varus deformities of the hindfoot, which would imply correction of the varus by means of a lateral calcaneal sliding osteotomy. In 2018, Krause [21] concluded that young patients needed correction of the varus associated with treatment of CLAI; in line with this conclusion, Lintz [22] and the international weight-bearing CT study group identified a greater risk of ankle instability associated with varus malalignment in a study carried out in 2019. In 2023, Yoshimoto [23] reported worse functional results in the presence of varus deformity.

Although treatment must be individualized, for all these reasons, the scientific literature supports combination treatments for this group of patients, given the rise of minimally invaSsive techniques for performing calcaneal osteotomy.

Technique Recommended by the Authors

In these cases, we recommend lateral sliding calcaneal osteotomy with a translation of approximately 10 mm, essentially producing a Dwyer effect by creating a wedge with a lateral base of approximately 10 mm. We prefer fixation with two cannulated headless screws. This should be the first stage of treatment (Fig. 15.2).

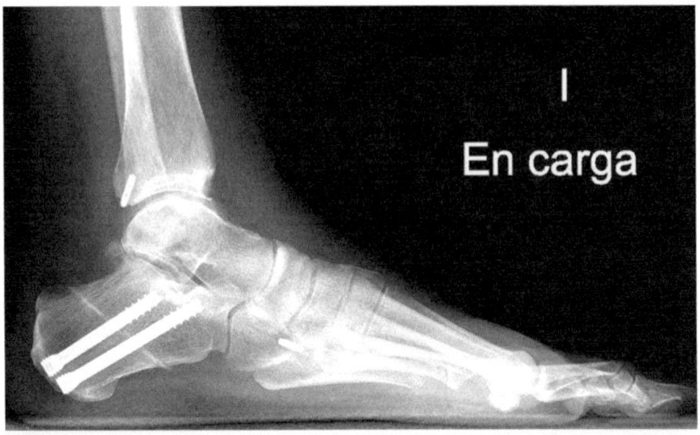

Fig. 15.2 Lateral displacement calcaneal osteotomy in varus malalignment in CLAI. The osteotomy is fixed with two cannulated headless screws

Arthroscopic or Open Treatment in Chronic Lateral Instability?

The popularity of arthroscopic procedures is indisputable. In the last 15 years, we have witnessed the development of numerous arthroscopic techniques for treating CLAI. The availability of specific implants and knotless systems has contributed greatly to all of this.

Initially, the first systematic reviews reported similar results between arthroscopic and open techniques in terms of assessment scales such as the American Orthopaedic Foot & Ankle Society (AOFAS) scale, the Karlsson scale and the visual analogue scale (VAS) without statistically significant differences, although they noted less postoperative pain and average stay and fewer soft tissue complications following arthroscopic techniques [24–27].

In a meta-analysis, Brown [23] reported similar results from arthroscopic techniques according to the AOFAS and Karlsson scales.

Although some systematic reviews have described a relatively high rate of complications with arthroscopic techniques, it is necessary to clarify that these studies included percutaneous techniques with high rates of nerve injury [28, 29]. However, the latest systematic reviews have revealed a lower rate of soft tissue and surgical wound complications [30]. The most frequent complications of both arthroscopic and open techniques include neurological lesions, surgical or portal wound problems, deep vein thrombosis and the recurrence of instability.

In recent studies, the results of arthroscopic techniques seemed to be superior to those of open techniques. In a systematic review and meta-analysis, Xiaosong [31] concluded that arthroscopic repair had better results than open surgery, improving postoperative pain due to its minimally invasive nature, whereas the rates of complications, including nerve injuries, persistent pain, deep vein thrombosis, surgical wound complications and recurrence of instability, were similar between the two. The author concluded that the clinical results according to different scales were superior with arthroscopic techniques.

In 2020, Moorthy [32] concluded that arthroscopic techniques have become the method of choice in the treatment of CLAI and allow the diagnosis and treatment of associated injuries. Similar to open techniques, arthroscopic techniques are simple and reproducible, while also imparting fewer skin complications.

Attia [33] reported that although arthroscopic techniques are more demanding from a technical perspective, compared with open techniques, the AOFAS scale score, the VAS pain score and the time to full weight bearing are superior; however, the surgical time, rate of complications and the results of the anterior drawer and varus stress tests are excellent and statistically comparable. Woo [34] found that compared with the open techniques, arthroscopic techniques yield superior results in terms of the VAS and AOFAS scale scores at 6 and 12 months after surgery.

In short, for the repair and reconstruction of the lateral ligament complex, compared with non anatomical techniques, anatomical techniques yield similar clinical results and tend to achieve a lower rate of complications as well as less postoperative pain and a shorter average hospital stay.

The second argument in favour of arthroscopic techniques is related to their use in the assessment and treatment of associated injuries. The incidence of associated injuries in CLAI ranges from 70% to 100% [35–38] . There is consensus that CLAI should be treated simultaneously with osteochondral lesions [39] using any of the spinal stimulation techniques available.

Direct Repair of ATFL

Direct arthroscopic repair of the ATFL yields excellent results, and multiple techniques involving one or two knotless implants with bone augmentation have been described. Conte-Real [30] and Acevedo [40] initially described an "all-inside" technique with a knotless implant and a third accessory portal; this technique was later modified by Vega [41]. As initially described by Conte-Real [30] in 2009, many neurological lesions of the sural nerve were found due to the use of a mixed technique with a percutaneous approach for suture recovery and plicating the lateral retinaculum of the extensors, similar to the Bröstrom technique as modified by Gould.

The main indication for this technique is rupture of the upper fascicle of the ATFL at the point of insertion into the fibula while the remaining ligament demonstrates good tissue quality (Fig. 15.3).

The technique can be performed through a modified single anterolateral portal or an accessory portal. The use of a single portal reduces the risk of injury to the dorsal cutaneous intermediate branch of the superficial peroneal nerve [37].

Vega [42] advocated the use of synthetic augmentation with high-strength sutures, achieving excellent results. Ulku [43] reported results comparable to those of the open Broström method with this technique, finding it to be an arthroscopically safe procedure. In an interesting systematic review of different augmentation techniques published in 2021, Lan [44] concluded that the best results were obtained when the ATFL remnant had been previously repaired either through an open or arthroscopic procedure and did not advise the use of isolated augmentation, as this could yield the worst results. Wittig [45] and Mercer [46] recently reported that augmentation allows use of an accelerated rehabilitation protocol without compromising ankle stability.

Recommended Technique

We recommend drawing anatomical reliefs and working with a modified lateral portal to avoid injury to the intermediate cutaneous branch of the superficial peroneal nerve. We suggest performing arthroscopic repair with two 2.5- or 2.9-mm knotless biodegradable implants and a direct suture passage system, taking the utmost care to avoid injuring the remnant ligament. The repair should be fixed in dorsal flexion and slight eversion. If the quality of the remnant ATFL is inadequate, one would have to opt for augmentation with synthetic fibres or reconvert the technique to reconstruction (Figs. 15.3, 15.4 and 15.5). We published excellent results with this technique using a single modified anterolateral portal and two anchors in a series of 100 patients in 2023 [47].

Synthetic fibre augmentation could be useful in patients with high functional demand or who participate in intense sports activities.

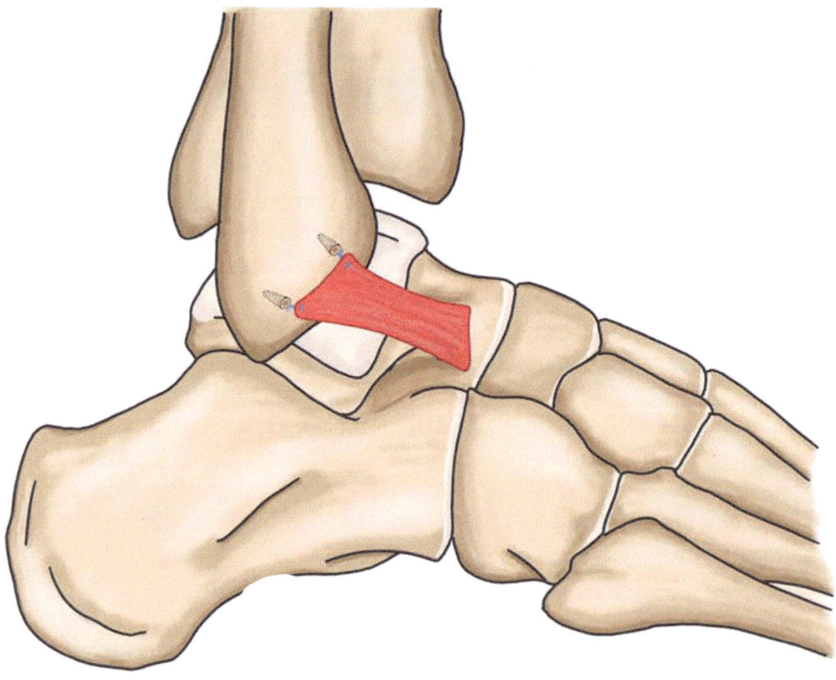

Fig. 15.3 Direct ATFL repair

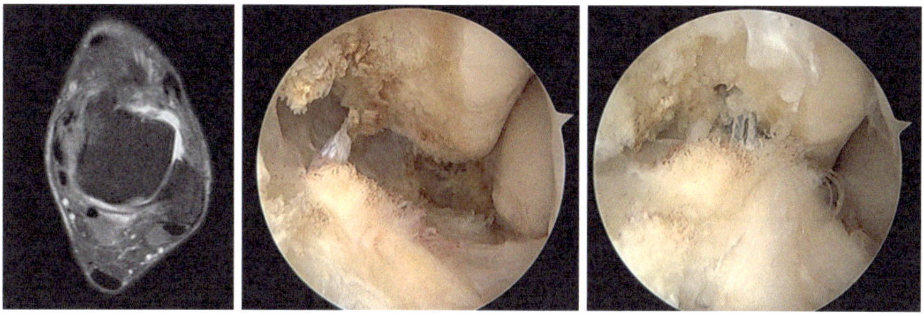

Fig. 15.4 Rupture of the ATFL and arthroscopic "all inside" repair with two anchors. 1 MRI. 2. Arthroscopic view. 3. "All inside" direct repair

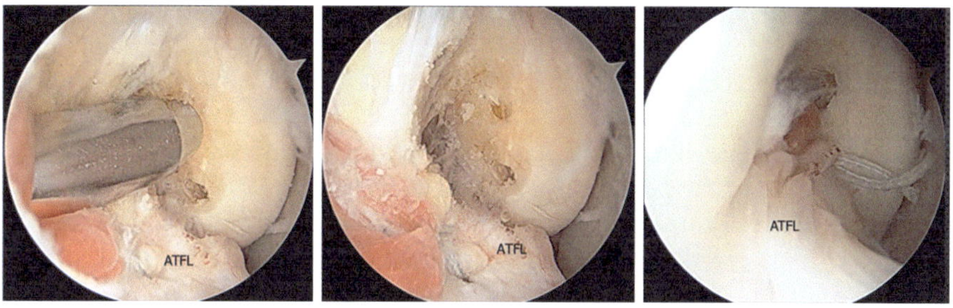

Fig. 15.5 Rupture of the ATFL and arthroscopic "all inside" repair with two anchors using a single modified anterolateral approach. See the correct position of the anchors

Arthroscopic Reconstruction ATFL

Open reconstruction techniques with ATFL grafts were described by Jeys [48] and Coughlin [49] in the early 2000s. Subsequently, different arthroscopic techniques have been described [50, 51] that allow the restoration of joint stability with a low rate of complications; briefly, these are the technique of choice in cases of poor tissue quality; when the ATFL tear is in the talar insertion or in the middle part of the ligament; revision surgery; patients with high functional demand; hypermobility; and high body mass index (BMI).

Arthroscopic reconstructions are highly demanding techniques from a technical perspective, although the development of biotenodesis-type implants and dynamic cortical anchoring systems has greatly facilitated their performance and allowed the creation of blind tunnels, reducing neurovascular complications. A wide variety of techniques and the use of grafts have been described, each with potential advantages and disadvantages [31].

In a systematic review, Brambilla [52] investigated the best graft for lateral ankle reconstruction but did not find studies of sufficient quality in the literature to support the use of either allografts or autografts. The conclusions of that meta-analysis showed similar results in terms of stability between the two grafts, although allografts had the advantages of shortening the surgical time and fundamentally avoiding morbidity in the donor area.

In two meta-analyses that included 12 and 6 English-language papers, Lu [53] and Li [54], respectively, reported excellent results with arthroscopic reconstruction techniques, indicating that they are excellent methods of stabilization with few complications and no problems related to the allograft.

There are few biomechanical studies on this topic. Clanton [55] performed a study using a semitendinous graft, and the maximum load at failure was not significantly different from that of an intact ATFL. The mean stiffness of the reconstructed graft was also not significantly different from that of the intact ATFL, and so the author concluded that anatomical graft reconstruction results in a strength and stiffness similar to that of the intact ligament in a cadaveric model at time zero. Similarly, Mellado [56, 57] published a comparative biomechanical study in cadavers between direct repair and reconstruction with grafts, observing good results with both techniques and finding only significantly better internal rotation in the axial plane with reconstruction.

One debated topic in this field is BMI. Many studies have indicated that a high BMI is an indication for performing reconstruction, but there is no consensus on the value at which reconstruction is preferable; Xu [58] and Jung [59], for example, reported a value greater than 25 kg/m^2, while Dierckman [60] reported a value above 30 kg/m^2.

Recommended Technique

We recommend arthroscopic reconstruction with bench allografts of an approximate thickness of 4.5–5.0 mm via the construction of a blind tunnel at the talar insertion point of the ATFL and a complete tunnel in the fibula in the footprint with an orientation of approximately 30° from caudal to cranial and from anterior to posterior. The graft should be fixed with biodegradable screws (Figs. 15.6 and 15.7). It is important to make a small incision at the exit point of the guide wire to avoid injuring the peroneal tendons. The plasty should be fixed in dorsal flexion and slight eversion.

Reconstruction of the CFL

The CFL is a powerful stabilizer of not only the ankle but also the STJ. Approximately 30% of ankle instabilities coexist with instability of the STJ [57, 61].

A recent consensus [62] recommended ATFL and CFL reconstruction in cases of generalized laxity or when the tissue quality is poor. Other indications include doubts about subtalar stability or the presence of a ruptured LCF. For some authors, a BMI greater than 30 kg/m^2 is also an indication for this technique (Fig. 15.9).

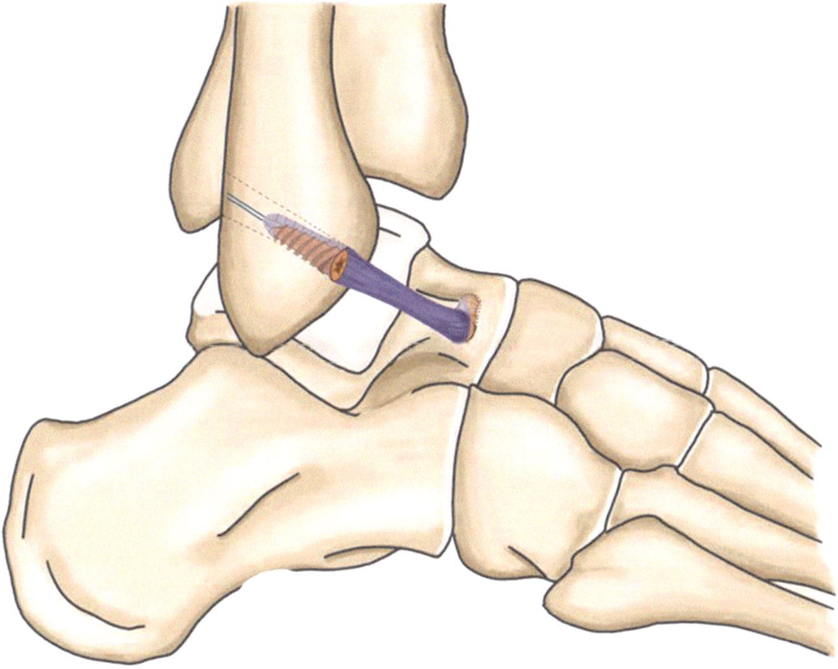

Fig. 15.6 ATFL reconstruction with allograft

Fig. 15.7 Rupture of the ATFL and arthroscopic "all inside" reconstruction with allograft

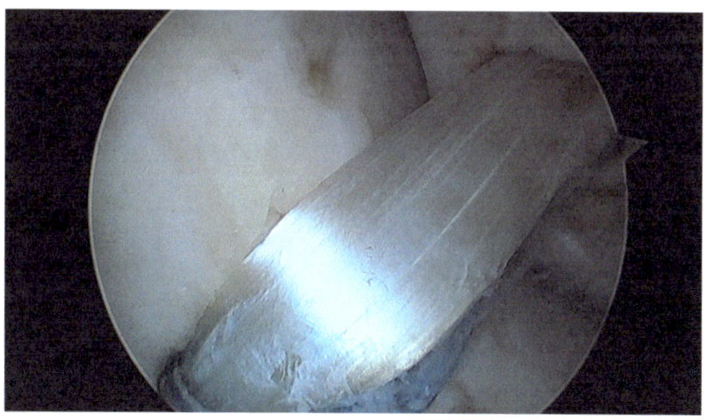

In 2022, Ferkel [63] specified the indications for reconstruction: ligament repair failure; BMI greater than 30 kg/m^2; cases of generalized laxity; high functional demand on the part of the patient (e.g., athletes or workers); poor tissue quality observed intraoperatively; and significant instability with a talar tilt angle greater than 10° different from the tilt angle of the contralateral ankle or an absolute angle greater than 15°. Ferkel concluded that direct arthroscopic repair of the ATFL is an excellent technique in selected cases but that prospective randomized comparative studies are necessary to recommend this technique.

In a systematic review, Lu [53] reported that 80% of athletes rejoined their sports at the same level before the injury following CFL reconstruction. Therefore, he concluded that allograft reconstruction procedures significantly improve functionality and clinical scale scores, with low rate of complications and recurrence of instability.

In a biomechanical study, Hung [64] placed great importance on the CFL as a stabilizer in tibiotalar and subtalar inversion.

Recommended Technique

We recommend arthroscopic reconstruction with bench allografts of an approximate thickness of 4.5–5.0 mm via the creation of a blind tunnel at the site of talar insertion of the ATFL and a blind tunnel in the fibula in the footprint with an orientation of approximately 30° from caudal to cranial and from anterior to posterior. A percutaneous approach should be used to identify the peroneal tubercle and recover the plasty below the peroneal tendons (Fig. 15.8). It is important to make a small incision at the exit point of the guide wire to avoid injuring the peroneal tendons. The ATFL plasty will be fixed in dorsal flexion and slight eversion, and the CFL plasty will be fixed in plantar flexion and slight inversion.

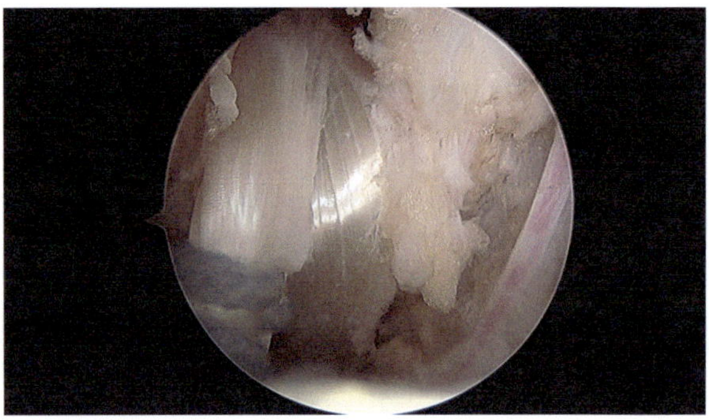

Fig. 15.8 Arthroscopic "all inside" reconstruction of ATFL and CFL with allograft

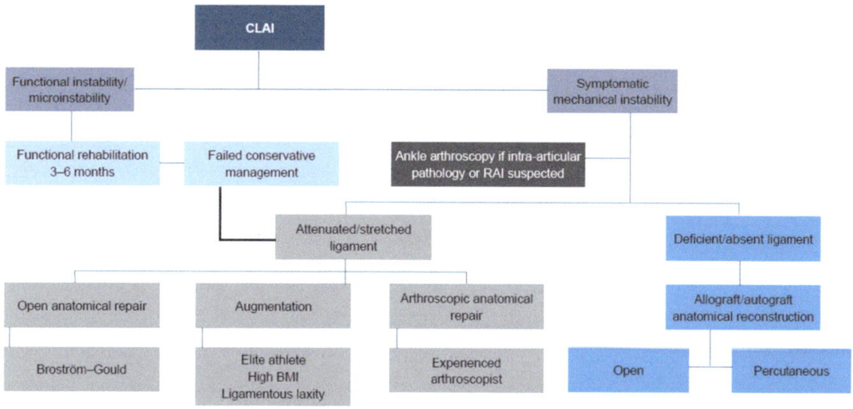

Fig. 15.9 Proposed treatment algorithm

Rotational and Multidirectional Instability

Rotational instability is a relatively novel concept described in 2011 by Buchhorn [65], involving combined injuries of the lateral complex and deltoid ligament (Figs. 15.10 and 15.11) and treatment with an anatomical reconstruction technique for both injuries. Although there is no biomechanical evidence as to why medial injury occurs in patients who have not suffered eversion trauma, the maintenance of stress on the medial complex in lateral instability can likely lead to the development of rotational instability [66]. It is estimated that up to 10–15% of CLAIs can progress to injury to the medial complex, especially its most anterior fibres. Vega [67] described the combination of lateral complex injuries with "book-sheet" injury of the superficial tibiotalar fascicle of the deltoid ligament due to excessive internal rotation in chronic lateral instabilities as well as treatment by direct repair of both injuries. Acevedo [68] and Vega [67] also described safe positions for the anchors in the medial malleolus.

However, the literature remains inconsistent regarding whether the best option for managing cases of long-term instability is direct repair or reconstruction. In view of the works reviewed on this update topic, the reconstruction of ATFL and CFL is probably more effective.

Potential risks of arthroscopic repair of the medial complex include iatrogenic nerve injury, fracture of the medial malleolus, persistent medial instability, or pain in the medial gutter. The procedure is not technically complex but requires experience in arthroscopic ankle techniques [69].

De Cesar [70, 71] described the concept of multidirectional instability and identified the combined instabilities in which CLAI coexists with medial instability, CLAI with syndesmosis instability (frequently in the context of varus malalignment) or medial instability with syndesmosis instability (frequently in the context of valgus malalignment) as well as those in which CLAI, medial instability and chronic instability of the syndesmosis may or may not be associated with subtalar instability.

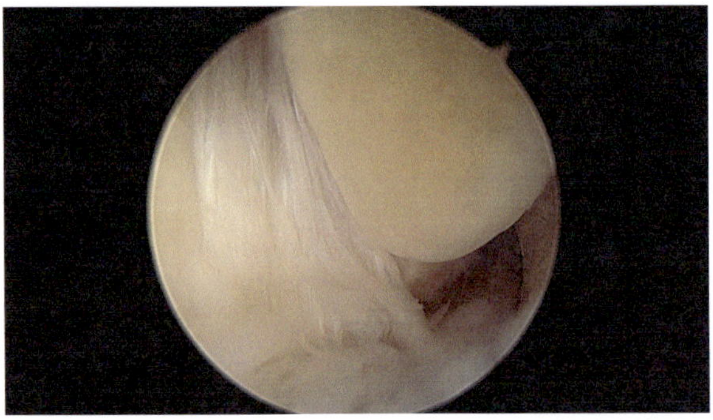

Fig. 15.10 Rupture of the deep deltoid ligament in a rotational instability

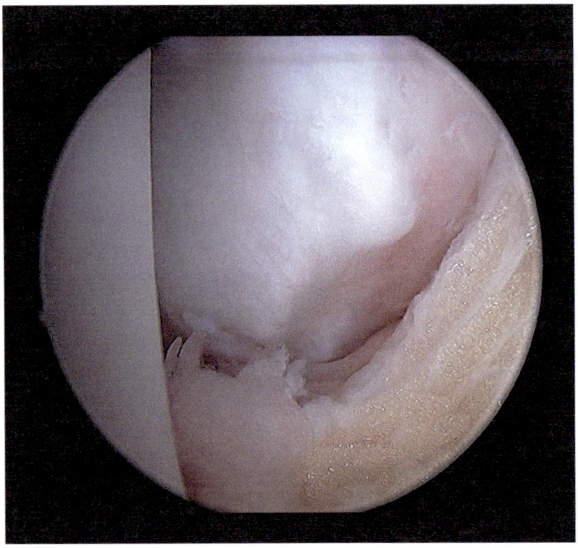

Fig. 15.11 “Open book” rupture of the deep deltoid ligament in a rotational instability with degenerative changes in the medial malleolus

Peroneal Tendon Surgery

Anatomical Tip

The peroneal muscles are located in the lateral compartment of the leg. The PB originates from the distal two thirds of the fibula and the interosseous membrane. The peroneus longus (PL) originates from the proximal two thirds of the fibula to the external malleolus.

The two muscles become tendons before reaching the ankle joint, the PL approximately 4 cm from the tip of the fibula with a long musculotendinous junction, whereas the muscle fibres of the PB reach somewhat more distally, frequently passing beyond the malleolus. Both are innervated by the superficial peroneal nerve. At the level of the lateral malleolus, the PB is located within an osteofibrous tunnel adjacent to and posterior to the fibula and is stabilized inside by the tendon of the PL muscle and the lateral retinaculum. The synovial sheath passes through a fibrous bone tunnel that is stabilized posterolaterally by the superior peroneal retinaculum (SPR) and medially by the posterior talofibular ligament, the calcaneofibular ligament, and the posteroinferior tibiofibular ligament. Anteriorly, it is stabilized by the distal fibula. The SPR is essential for maintaining the stability of the peroneal tendons. This structure originates from the lateral region of the distal fibula. Its insertion point varies, and at least 5 different types have been identified [72]. The most common type (47%) has 2 bands, an upper band that inserts anteriorly into the Achilles tendon sheath and a lower band that inserts into the lateral wall of the calcaneus at the level of the peroneal tubercle.

Both tendons have independent vascularization through the vinculum, a structure that connects each tendon to its tendon sheath and that, in addition to providing vascularization dependent on the posterior peroneal artery, has a controversial role in proprioception that could be related to chronic ankle pain. This vinculum penetrates the posterolateral region of each tendon within the retromalleolar groove and throughout its entire length [73].

Sanmarco, in 2009, described 4 anatomical regions according to the organization of the tendons throughout their courses [74]: the proximal region, from the SPR to the tip of the fibula, in which the tendon of the PB is arranged anterior to the PL; a second region from the inferior peroneal retinaculum (IPR) to the lateral peroneal tubercle of the calcaneus where the PL is inferior to the PB; and 2 areas distal to the lower portion of the IPR, in which the tendon sheath bifurcates into separate sheaths at the level of the peroneal tubercle of the calcaneus towards its insertions at the base of the first and fifth metatarsals.

The os peroneum is an accessory bone found within the PL tendon. It is ossified in approximately 20% of feet. It is located plantar to the cuboid and the calcaneocuboid joint. An accessory muscle can be identified in the lateral compartment, the peroneus quartus, in 13 to 22% of the population [75]. The peroneus quartus usually originates from the PC and inserts into the peroneal tubercle of the calcaneus. Knowledge of these anatomical variants is important for ruling out peroneal impingement syndromes due to space conflicts in the retromalleolar canal.

Tendoscopic Technique

Peroneal tendoscopy is a technique described by Van Dijk and Kort in 1998. Van Dijk [76, 77] conducted a study of the anatomy of the tendons. Since then, this technique has gained great importance and popularity in the treatment of peroneal tendon injury (Fig. 15.12).

Owing to this technique, we can perform not only an anatomical evaluation of the tendons but also a dynamic evaluation of their position and mobility within the sheaths through which they run. Using a minimally invasive approach, we can diagnose and treat tenosynovitis, tendon rupture, dislocations, anatomical variants such as accessory muscles, a low insertion belly of the PB (Fig. 15.13), the presence of a peroneus tertius or quartus, bony prominences or sheath rupture.

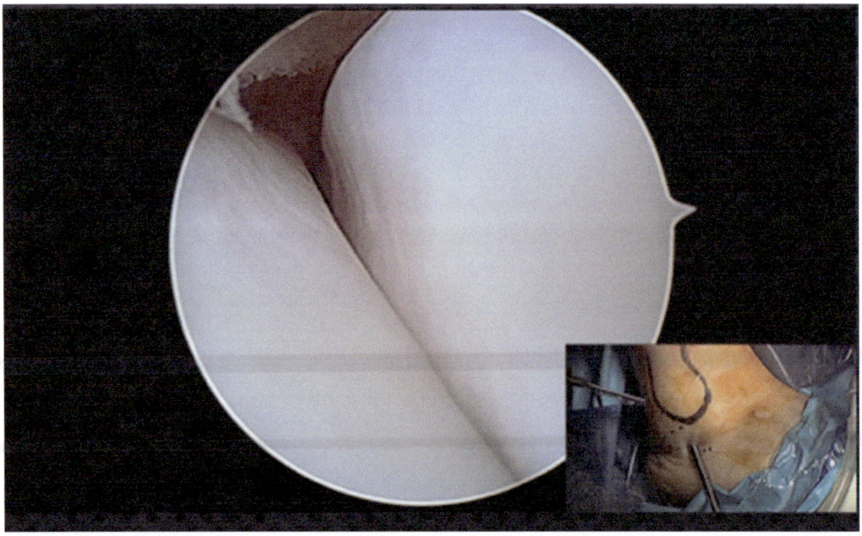

Fig. 15.12 Peroneal tendoscopy. View from the distal portal

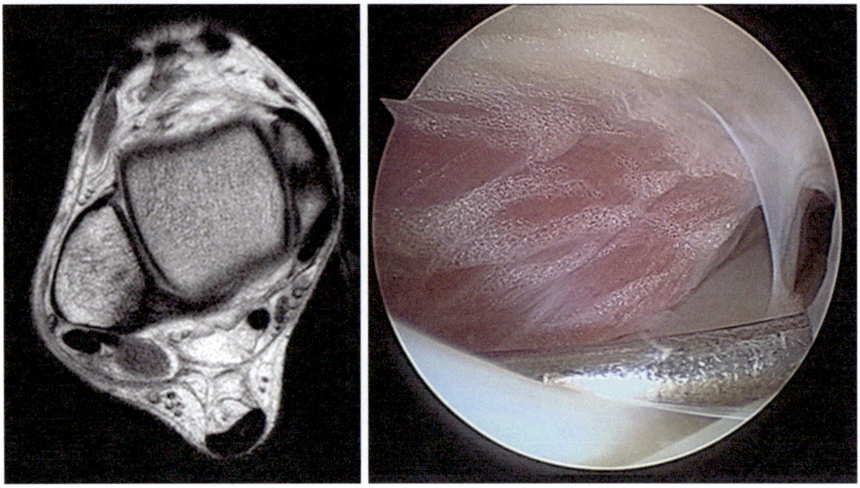

Fig. 15.13 Variant of normality. Low muscle belly of PB

In addition to its minimal invasiveness, tendoscopy has great accessibility, in part owing to the anatomical arrangement of the tendons and the lower risk of neurovascular and soft tissue injury compared with open techniques.

The patient is placed in the lateral decubitus position under regional spinal anesthesia and ischemia. Distal and proximal portals are made along the length of the peroneal tendons 1–1.5 cm distal and 3 cm proximal to the tip of the lateral malleolus, respectively. Accessory portals can be made according to the location and extent of the pathology.

The distal portal is first made with an incision in the skin and in the tendon sheath with a standard 4.0 mm 30° arthroscope. To avoid tearing the sheath and injuring the tendons, we perform this step with the ankle in plantar flexion. Once the distal portal is created, the proximal portal is created under direct visualization.

It is common to identify the presence of synovitis, in which case we perform endoscopic synovectomy prior to exploration of the tendon.

Peroneal Tendon Rupture

Isolated peroneal tendon tears are rare; most are the result of inversion ankle trauma. The prevalence of injury to the PB tendon reported in cadaver studies ranges from 11% to 37%, whereas ruptures of the PL occur less frequently. Dombek et al. [78] described injury to the PB in 88% and the PL in 13% of 40 patients treated surgically for a tendon tear. Among the patients treated with surgery for peroneal tendon rupture, up to 33% also have lateral ankle instability that requires ligament reconstruction, 20% have dislocation, 10% have an insufficient retromalleolar groove, 33% have a low insertion belly of the PB muscle, and 32–82% have cavus varus hindfoot.

PB tears are generally found within the retromalleolar sulcus, indicating that they likely originate from mechanical trauma in this region (Fig. 15.14). Less frequently, ruptures of the PB tendon can occur just proximal to its insertion into the fifth metatarsal via abrupt inversion of the foot. PL tears normally occur at the level of the cuboid, in ossa peroneal, in the peroneal tubercle, or at the tip of the lateral malleolus. Like Krause and Brodskym [79] proposed, in partial longitudinal tears (those involving less than 50% of the cross-section of the tendon) (Fig. 15.15), we recommend tendoscopic debridement and tubulization, whereas for those tears that affect more than 50% of the tendon, the treatment of choice is tendon suture with or without the deepening of the retromalleolar sulcus.

When repair requires more than 2 or 3 sutures, we believe that performing selective open repair is more appropriate.

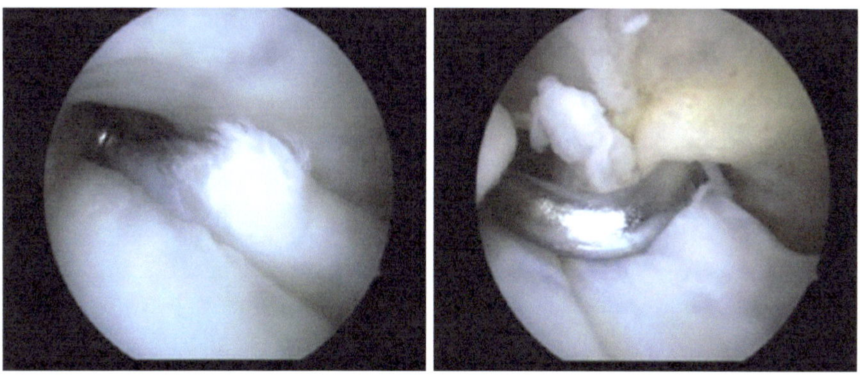

Fig. 15.14 Peroneus brevis tear

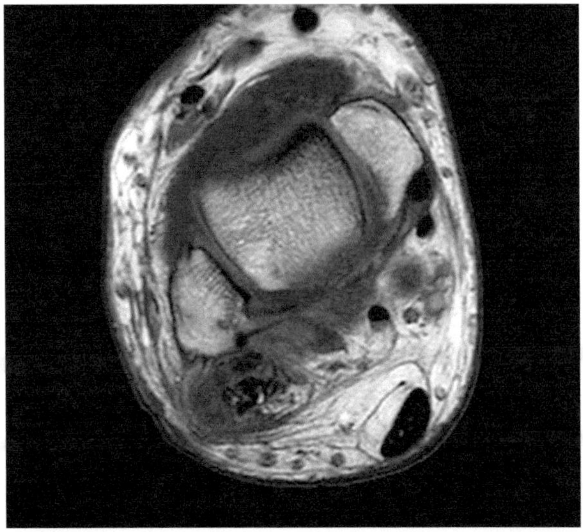

Fig. 15.15 MRI showing an extensile peroneal tendons rupture

Peroneal Tendon Dislocation

Monteggia [80] was the first author to describe instability of the peroneal tendons in a classical ballet dancer in 1803. This condition is estimated to occur in between 0.3–0.5% of ankle injuries. In general, dislocation of the peroneal tendons is secondary to a traumatic history, with the foot in dorsiflexion, abduction and inversion, producing a sudden contraction of the peroneal muscles. The patient presents with pain in the posterolateral region of the ankle and sometimes experiences instability on irregular surfaces and protrusion of the lateral malleolus.

Two main factors can contribute to tendon dislocation: lateral ankle instability and hindfoot varus malalignment, both of which should be evaluated and treated if they coexist. Certain anatomical variants can predispose the patient to instability or subluxation, including the shape and depth of the retromalleolar groove and the presence or absence of the fibrocartilage groove. In Edwards' classic corpse work [81] involving 178 feet, 82% presented with concave retromalleolar grooves, 11% with flat grooves and 7% with convex grooves.

The width of the sulcus when present is 6 mm on average (range 5–10 mm) and relatively shallow, occasionally reaching 3 mm in depth. An inadequate retromalleolar groove, laxity of the SPR due to calcaneal valgus or neuromuscular diseases, and a congenital absence of the SPR may contribute to the mechanisms of dislocation.

In 1976, Eckert and Davis [82] classified peroneal tendon dislocations on the basis of the detachment of the SPR from the periosteum and/or the fibrous canal.

Later, Oden [83] modified this classification by adding a fourth grade. Grade 1, or subluxation (51%), occurs when the SPR is detached from the peroneal malleolus (Fig. 15.16), allowing the tendons to move anteriorly. In Grade 2 patients (33%), the annulus fibrosus is disinserted along with the SPR (Fig. 15.17). Grade

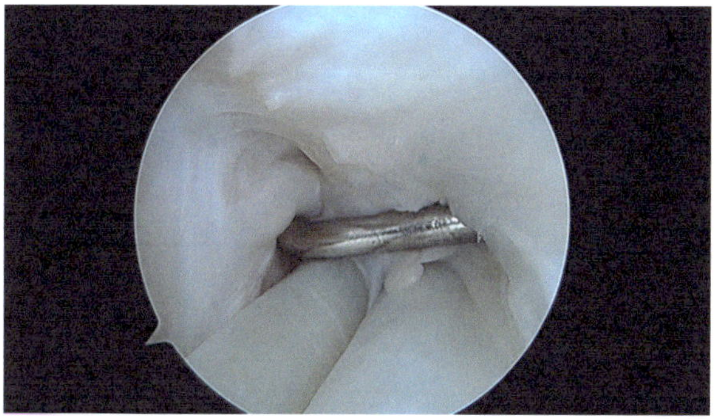

Fig. 15.16 Rupture SPR. Extrasheath dislocation grade 1

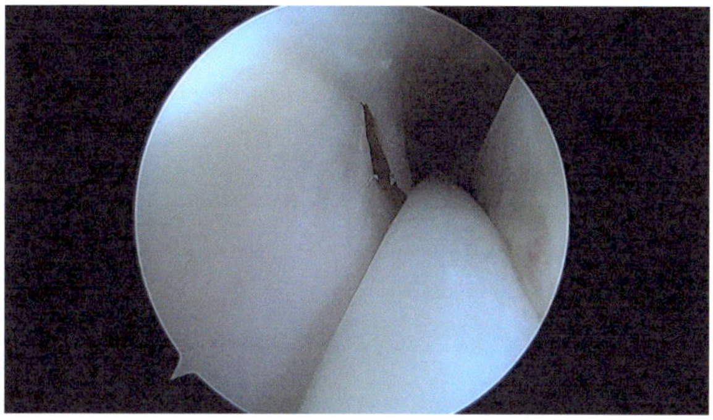

Fig. 15.17 Extrasheath dislocation grade 2, the annulus fibrosus is disinserted along with the SPR

3 (13%) occurs when a small bone fragment of the peroneal malleolus is avulsed with the SPR and the annulus fibrosus (radiologically described as the "fleck sign"). Grade 4, the least frequent grade, is defined as a break or complete avulsion of the posterior insertion of the SPR running through the superficial and lateral tendons.

Recently, Raikin et al. [84] described a new type of dislocation of the peroneal tendons in which the SPR is intact and defined it as an intrasheath dislocation (Fig. 15.18).

He classified this dislocation into two subgroups: type A, in which there is no tendon rupture and the tendons change their relative positions along certain locations (the PL runs below the PB), and type B, in which the PL tendon is dislocated through a longitudinal tear in the PB tendon, losing its position in the retromalleolar groove.

The failure of conservative treatment is very high. It can be an option for cases of acute dislocation.

Surgical treatment offers excellent results, mainly in cases of acute dislocation, and is the only option in cases of recurrent dislocation. It is indicated in young patients who play sports at high levels and who therefore require a rapid return to their activity.

Surgery prevents conditions such as tenosynovitis and longitudinal tears, which are frequently associated with instability of the peroneal tendons.

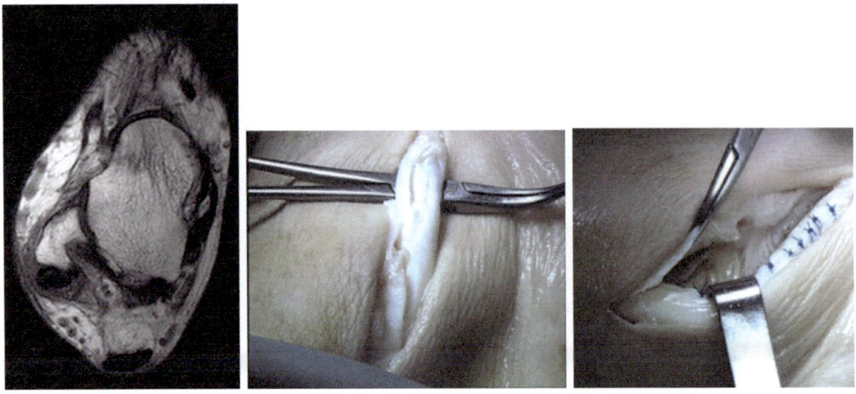

Fig. 15.18 Intrasheath dislocation subgroup B, there is a PB rupture. An open repair

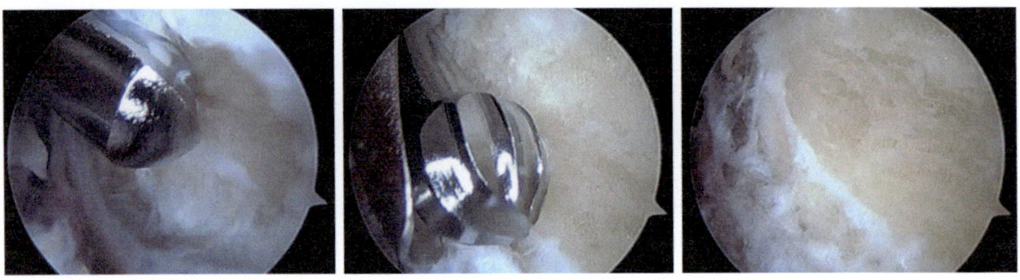

Fig. 15.19 Endoscopic deepening of the retromalleolar groove using a shaver and a small bur of 4.5 mm

In cases of grade 1 and 2 extrasheath dislocation and type A intrasheath dislocation, we recommend techniques for deepening [85] the retromalleolar groove (Fig. 15.19), particularly tendoscopic techniques when used as an isolated procedure. The use of reconstruction techniques for grade 1 and 2 dislocations of the SPR remains disputed (Fig. 15.20). In grade 3 dislocations, the treatment of choice is reconstruction of the retinaculum, often with the use of bone anchors, with the goal of consolidating the avulsed fragment. In grade 4 dislocations, reconstruction or deepening techniques are often insufficient and reinforcement is required. Finally, in intrasheath type B dislocations, the treatment of choice is repair of the longitudinal rupture of the PB as well as deepening of the sulcus.

In 2006, Lui [86] described endoscopic reconstruction of the peroneal retinaculum. Eckert and Davis [82] reported excellent results with this technique with a 5% reluxation rate. Adachi [87] subsequently published a series of 20 patients without any cases of reluxation.

Deepening of the retromalleolar sulcus is undoubtedly the most commonly performed technique tendoscopically. With a vaporizer or synoviotome, the periosteum is debrided, and a 4.0 or 4.5 mm spherical bur is used to deepen the retromalleolar groove. The advantages of the tendoscopic technique are unquestionable; in

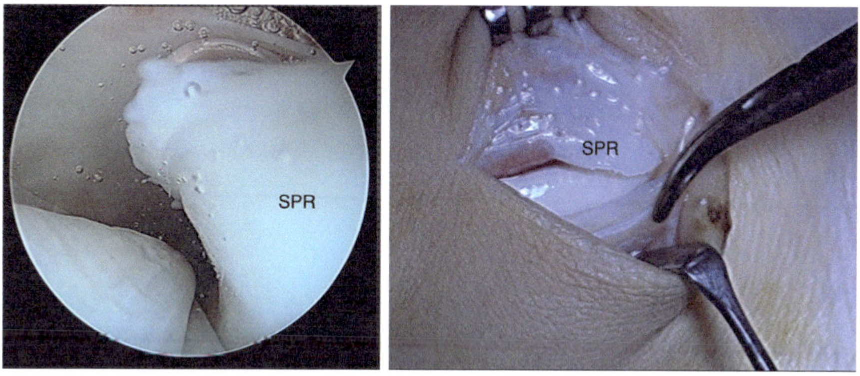

Fig. 15.20 Rupture SPR. Mini open approach and repair with knotless anchors

addition to its minimal invasiveness and low numbers of neurovascular complications and morbidities, it allows early return to sports activities, a dynamic evaluation of the tendons and a ruling out of the presence of associated tendon ruptures. It is also the treatment of choice in cases of type A intrasheath dislocation [88].

References

1. Hølmer P, Søndergaard L, Konradsen L, Nielsen PT, Jørgensen LN. Epidemiology of sprains in the late-ral ankle and foot. Foot Ankle Int. 1994;15:72–4. https://doi.org/10.1177/107110079401500204.2.
2. Maffulli N, Ferran NA. Management of acute and chronic ankle instability. J Am Acad Orthop Surg. 2008;16:608–15.
3. Giannini S, Ruffilli A, Pagliazzi G, Mazzotti A, Evangelisti G, Buda R, et al. Treatment algorithm for chronic lateral ankle instability. Muscles Ligaments Tendons J. 2014;4:455–60.
4. Valderrabano V, Horisberger M, Russell I, Dougall H, Hintermann B. Etiology of ankle osteoarthritis. Clin Orthop Relat Res. 2009;467(7):1800–6.
5. Dalmau-Pastor M, Guelfi M, Malagelada F, Mirapeix R, Vega J. Anatomy of the ankle joint and hindfoot. Springer; 2020. p. 3–9.
6. Espinosa N, Smerek JP, Myerson MS. Acute and chronic syndesmosis injuries: pathomechanisms, diagnosis and management. Foot Ankle Clin. 2006;11(3):639–57.
7. Testut L, Latarjet A. Tratado de anatomía humana, vol. 1. Salvat; 1975.
8. Golanó PD-PM, Vega J, Batista JP. The ankle in football. D'Hooghe PPRN KG, editor. Springer; 2014.
9. Golano P, Vega J, Leeuw P, Malagelada F, Manzanares Céspedes M-C, Götzens V, et al. Anatomy of the ankle ligaments: a pictorial essay. Knee Surg Sports Traumatol Arthrosc. 2010;18:557–69.
10. Vega J, Malagelada F, Manzanares Cespedes MC, Dalmau-Pastor M. The lateral fibulotalocalcaneal ligament complex: an ankle stabilizing isometric structure. Knee Surg Sports Traumatol Arthrosc. 2020;28(1):8–17.
11. Dalmau-Pastor M, Malagelada F, Kerkhoffs GM, Karlsson J, Guelfi M, Vega J. Redefining anterior ankle arthroscopic anatomy: medial and lateral ankle collateral ligaments are vis-

ible through dorsiflexion and non-distraction anterior ankle arthroscopy. Knee Surg Sports Traumatol Arthrosc. 2020;28(1):18–23.
12. Milner CE, Soames RW. Anatomy of the collateral ligaments of the human ankle joint. Foot Ankle Int. 1998;19(11):757–60.
13. Michels F, Matricali G, Vereecke E, Dewilde M, Vanrietvelde F, Stockmans F. The intrinsic subtalar ligaments have a consistent presence, location and morphology. Foot Ankle Surg. 2021;27(1):101–9.
14. Dalmau-Pastor M, Yasui Y, Calder JD, Karlsson J, Kerkhoffs GM, Kennedy JG. Anatomy of the inferior extensor retinaculum and its role in lateral ankle ligament reconstruction: a pictorial essay. Knee Surg Sports Traumatol Arthrosc. 2016;24(4):957–62.
15. Rasmussen O, Tovborg-Jensen I. Anterolateral rotational instability in the ankle joint. An experimental study of anterolateral rotational instability, talar tilt, and anterior drawer sign in relation to injuries to the lateral ligaments. Acta Orthop Scand. 1981;52(1):99–102.
16. Kelikian AS, Sarrafian SK. Sarrafian's anatomy of the foot and ankle: descriptive, topographic, functional. Lippincott Williams & Wilkins; 2011.
17. Sarcon AK, Heyrani N, Giza E, Kreulen C. Lateral ankle sprain and chronic ankle instability. Foot Ankle Orthop. 2019;4(2):2473011419846938.
18. Noailles T, Lopes R, Padiolleau G, Gouin F, Brilhault J. Non-anatomical or direct anatomical repair of chronic lateral instability of the ankle: a systematic review of the literature after at least 10 years of follow-up. Foot Ankle Surg. 2018;24:80–5.
19. Vuurberg G, Pereira H, Blankevoort L, van Dijk CN. Anatomic stabilization techniques provide superior results in terms of functional outcome in patients suffering from chronic ankle instability compared to non-anatomic techniques. Knee Surg Sports Traumatol Arthrosc. 2018;26(7):2183–95. https://doi.org/10.1007/s00167-017-4730-4.
20. Vienne P, Schöniger R, Helmy N, Espinosa N. Hindfoot instability in cavovarus deformity: static and dynamic balancing. Foot Ankle Int. 2007;28(1):96–102. https://doi.org/10.3113/FAI.2007.0018.
21. Krause F, Seidel A. Malalignment and lateral ankle instability: causes of failure from the varus tibia to the cavovarus foot. Foot Ankle Clin. 2018;23(4):593–603. https://doi.org/10.1016/j.fcl.2018.07.005.
22. Lintz F, Bernasconi A, Baschet L, Fernando C, Mehdi N. Weight Bearing CT International Study Group, de Cesar Neto C, Relationship between chronic lateral ankle instability and hindfoot varus using weight-bearing cone beam computed tomography. Foot Ankle Int. 2019;40(10):1175–81. https://doi.org/10.1177/1071100719858309.
23. Yoshimoto K, Noguchi M, Maruki H, Tominaga A, Okazaki K. Hindfoot alignment and ankle stability following arthroscopic lateral ankle ligament repair. Foot Ankle Int. 2023;44(9):872–8. https://doi.org/10.1177/10711007231181123.
24. Yeo ED, Lee KT, Sung IH, Lee SG, Lee YK. Comparison of all-inside arthroscopic and open techniques for the modified Brostrom procedure for ankle instability. Foot Ankle Int. 2016;37(10):1037–45.
25. Li H, Hua Y, Li H, Ma K, Li S, Chen S. Activity level and function 2 years after anterior talofibular ligament repair: a comparison between arthroscopic repair and open repair procedures. Am J Sports Med. 2017;45(9):2044–51.
26. Rigby RB, Cottom JM. A comparison of the "all-inside" arthroscopic Brostrom procedure with the traditional open modified Brostrom-Gould technique: a review of 62 patients. Foot Ankle Surg. 2019;25(1):31–6.
27. Yasui Y, Murawski CD, Wollstein A, Takao M, Kennedy JG. Operative treatment of lateral ankle instability. JBJS Rev. 2016;4(5):e6. https://doi.org/10.2106/JBJS.RVW.15.00074.
28. Brown AJ, Shimozono Y, Hurley ET, Kennedy JG. Arthroscopic versus open repair of lateral ankle ligament for chronic lateral ankle instability: a meta-analysis. Knee Surg Sports Traumatol Arthrosc. 2020;28(5):1611–8. https://doi.org/10.1007/s00167-018-5100-6.
29. Guelfi M, Zamperetti M, Pantalone A, Usuelli FG, Salini V, Martin OX. Open and arthroscopic lateral ligament repair for treatment of chronic ankle instability: a systematic review. Foot Ankle Surg. 2018;24(1):11–8. https://doi.org/10.1016/j.fas.2016.05.315.

30. Corte-Real NM, Moreira RM. Arthroscopic repair of chronic lateral ankle instability. Foot Ankle Int. 2009;30:213–7.
31. Xiaosong Z, Lv Z, Zhang C, Kong C, Wei S, Feng X. Does arthroscopic repair show superiority over open repair of lateral ankle ligament for chronic lateral ankle instability: a systematic review and meta-analysis. J Orthop Surg Res. 2020;15:355. https://doi.org/10.1186/s13018-020-01886-1.
32. Moorthy V, Sayampanathan AA, Meng Yeo NE, Tay KS. Clinical outcomes of open versus arthroscopic Broström procedure for lateral ankle instability: a meta-analysis. J Foot Ankle Surg. 2021;60(3):577–84. https://doi.org/10.1053/j.jfas.2020.10.001.
33. Attia AK, Taha T, Mahmoud K, Hunt KJ, Labib SA, d'Hooghe P. Broström surgery for chronic lateral ankle instability: a systematic review and meta-analysis of comparative studies. Orthop J Sports Med. 2021;21(7):23259671211015207. https://doi.org/10.1177/23259671211015207.
34. Woo BJ, Lai MC, Koo K. Arthroscopic versus open Brostrom Gould repair for chronic ankle instability. Foot Ankle Int. 2020;41(6):647–53. https://doi.org/10.1177/107110072.
35. Lee J, Hamilton G, Ford L. Associated intra-articular ankle pathologies in patients with chronic lateral ankle instability: arthroscopic findings at the time of lateral ankle reconstruction. Foot Ankle Spec. 2011;4:284–9.
36. Hintermann B, Boss A, Schafer D. Arthroscopic findings in patients with chronic ankle instability. Am J Sports Med. 2002;30:402–9.
37. Ferkel RD, Chams RN. Chronic lateral instability: arthroscopic findings and longer-term results. Foot Ankle Int. 2007;28:24–31.
38. Arroyo-Hernández M, Mellado-Romero M, Páramo-Díaz P, García-Lamas L, Vilà-Rico J. Chronic ankle instability: arthroscopic anatomical repair. Rev Esp Cir Ortop Traumatol. 2017;61:104–10. https://doi.org/10.1016/j.recot.2016.10.003.15.
39. Zengerink M, Struijs PAA, Tol JL. Treatment of osteochondral lesions of the talus: a systematic review. Knee Surg Sports Traumatol Arthrosc. 2010;18:238. https://doi.org/10.1007/s00167-009-0942-6.
40. Acevedo JI, Mangone P. Arthroscopic Brostrom technique. Foot Ankle Int. 2015;36:465–73.
41. Vega J, Golanó P, Pellegrino A, Rabat E, Peña F. All-inside arthroscopic lateral collateral ligament repair for ankle instability with a knotless suture anchor technique. Foot Ankle Int. 2013;34:1701–9.
42. Vega J, Montesinos E, Malagelada F, et al. Arthroscopic allinside anterior talo-fibular ligament repair with suture augmentation gives excellent results in case of poor ligament tissue remnant quality. Knee Surg Sports Traumatol Arthrosc. 2020;28(1):100–7.
43. Ulku TK, Kocaoglu B, Tok O, Irgit K, Nalbantoglu U. Arthroscopic suture-tape internal bracing is safe as arthroscopic modified Broström repair in the treatment of chronic ankle instability. Knee Surg Sports Traumatol Arthrosc. 2020;28(1):227–32. https://doi.org/10.1007/s00167-019-05552-w.
44. Lan R, Piatt ET, Bolia IK, Haratian A, Hasan L, Peterson AP, et al. Suture tape augmentation in lateral ankle ligament surgery: current concepts review. Foot Ankle Orthop. 2021;6(4):1–15. https://doi.org/10.1177/24730114211045978.
45. Wittig U, Hohenberger G, Ornig M, Schuh R, Reinbacher P, Leithner A, et al. Improved outcome and earlier return to activity after suture tape augmentation versus Broström repair for chronic lateral ankle instability—a systematic review? Arthroscopy. 2022;38(2):597–608.
46. Mercer NP, Kanakamedala AC, Azam MT, Hurley ET, Samsonov AP, Walls RJ, et al. Clinical outcomes after suture tape augmentation for ankle instability: a systematic review. Orthop J Sports Med. 2020;10(5) https://doi.org/10.1177/23259671221095791.
47. Mortada-Mahmoud A, Fernández-Rojas E, Iglesias-Durán E, Sánchez-Morata E, Vilá-Rico J. Results of anatomical arthroscopic repair of anterior Talofibular ligament in chronic lateral ankle instability patients. Foot Ankle. 2023;44(12):1219–28. https://doi.org/10.1177/10711007231185062.
48. Jeys LM, Harris NJ. Ankle stabilization with hamstring autograft new technique using interference screws. Foot Ankle Int. 2003;24(9):677–9.

49. Coughlin MJ, Schenck RC, Grebing BR. Comprehensive reconstruction of the lateral ankle for chronic instability using free gracilis graft. Foot Ankle Int. 2004;25(4):231–41.
50. Vilá-Rico J, Cabestany-Castellà JM, Cabestany-Perich B, Núñez-Samper C, Ojeda-Thies C. All-inside arthroscopic allograft reconstruction of the anterior Talo-fibular ligament using an Accesory Transfibular portal. Foot Ankle Surg. 2017;pii: S1268-7731(17):31369–3. https://doi.org/10.1016/j.fas.2017.12.008.
51. Allegra F, El Boustany S, Cerza F, Spiezia F, Maffulli N. Arthroscopic anterior talofibular ligament reconstructin in chronic ankle instability. Two years results. Injury. 2020;51(Suppl 3):S56–62. https://doi.org/10.1016/j.injury.2020.03.054.
52. Brambilla L, Bianchi A, Malerba F, Loppini M, Martinelli N. Lateral ankle ligament anatomic reconstruction for chronic ankle instability: allograft or autograft? A systematic review. Foot Ankle Surg. 2020;26(1):85–93. https://doi.org/10.1016/j.fas.2018.11.014.
53. Lu A, Wang X, Huang D, Tu Y, Chen L, Huang J, et al. The effectiveness of lateral ankle ligament reconstruction when treating chronic ankle instability: a systematic review and meta-analysis. Injury. 2020;51(8):1726–32. https://doi.org/10.1016/j.injury.2020.05.031.
54. Li H, Song Y, Li H, Hua Y. Outcomes after anatomic lateral ankle ligament reconstruction using allograft tendon for chronic ankle instability: a systematic review and meta-analysis. J Foot Ankle Surg. 2020;59:117–24. https://doi.org/10.1053/j.jfas.2019.07.008.
55. Clanton TO, Viens NA, Campbell KJ, Laprade RF, Wij-dicks CA. Anterior talofibular ligament ruptures, part2: biomechanical comparison of anterior talofibularligament reconstruction using semitendinosus allograftswith the intact ligament. Am J Sports Med. 2014;42:412–6. https://doi.org/10.1177/0363546513509963.16.
56. Mellado-Romero MA, Guerra-Pinto F, Guimarães-Consciência J, Sánchez-Morata EJ, Vacas-Sánchez E, Arroyo-Hernández M, et al. Estudio biomecánico de la reconstrucción ligamentosa anatómico con autoinjerto en la inestabilidad lateral de tobillo. Rev Esp Cir Ortop Traumatol. 2021;65(2):124–31. https://doi.org/10.1016/j.recot.2020.06.010.
57. Mellado-Romero MÁ, Guerra-Pinto F, Ojeda-Thies C, Arroyo-Hernández M, Abarquero-Diezhandino A, Ramos-Pascua L, et al. Comparison of direct repair versus anatomic graft reconstruction of the anterior talofibular ligament: a biomechanical cadaveric study. J Foot Ankle Surg. 2023;S1067-2516(23):00195–3. https://doi.org/10.1053/j.jfas.2023.08.008.
58. Xu X, Hu M, Liu J, Zhu Y, Wang B. Minimally invasive reconstruction of the lateral ankle ligaments using semitendinosus autograft or tendon allograft. Foot Ankle Int. 2014;35:1015–21.
59. Jung HG, Shin MH, Park JT, Eom JS, Lee DO, Lee SH. Anatomical reconstruction of lateral ankle ligaments using free tendon allografts and biotenodesis screws. Foot Ankle Int. 2015;36:1064–71.
60. Dierckman BD, Ferkel RD. Anatomic reconstruction with a semitendinosus allograft for chronic lateral ankle instability. Am J Sports Med. 2015;43:1941–50.
61. Iglesias-Durán E, Guerra-Pinto F, Ojeda-Thies C, Vilá-Rico J. Reconstruction of the interosseous talocalcaneal ligament using allograft for subtalar joint stabilization is effective. Knee Surg Sports Traumatol Arthrosc. 2023;31(12):6080–7. https://doi.org/10.1007/s00167-023-07622-6.
62. Michels F, Pereira H, Calder J, Matricali G, Glazebrook M, Guillo S, et al. Searching for consensus in the approach to patients with chronic lateral ankle instability: ask the expert. Knee Surg Sports Traumatol Arthrosc. 2018;26:2095–102.
63. Ferkel E, Nguyen S, Kwong C. Chronic lateral ankle instability: surgical management. Clin Sports Med. 2020;39:829–43. https://doi.org/10.1016/j.csm.2020.07.004.
64. Hunt KJ, Pereira H, Kelley J, Anderson N, Fuld R, Baldini T, Kumparatana P, D'Hooghe P. The role of Calcaneofibular ligament injury in ankle instability: implications for surgical management. Am J Sports Med. 2019;47(2):431–7. https://doi.org/10.1177/0363546518815160.
65. Buchhorn T, Sabeti-Aschraf M, Dlaska CE, Wenzel F, Graf A. Combined medial and lateral anatomic ligament reconstruction for chronic rotational instability of the ankle. Foot Ankle Int. 2011;32(12):1122–6.

66. Aicale R, Maffulli. Rotational ankle instability: a current concept review. NJ Orthop Surg (Hong Kong). 2023;31(2):10225536231182347. https://doi.org/10.1177/10225536231182347.
67. Vega J, Allmendinger J, Malagelada F, Guelfi M, Dalmau-Pastor M. Combined arthroscopic all-inside repair of lateral and medial ankle ligaments is an effective treatment for rotational ankle instability. Knee Surg Sports Traumatol Arthrosc. 2020;28(1):132–40.
68. Acevedo JI, Kreulen C, Cedeno AA, Baumfeld D, Nery C, Mangone PG. Technique for arthroscopic deltoid ligament repair with description of safe zones. Foot Ankle Int. 2020;41(5):605–11. Mansur NSB, Lemos AVKC, Baumfeld DS, Baumfeld TS, do Prado MP, Raduan FC, Nery CAS. Medial and lateral combined ligament arthroscopic repair for multidirectional ankle instability. Foot Ankle Orthop. 2021;6(1):1–8. https://doi.org/10.1177/2473011420986150
69. Li CCH, Lui TH. Arthroscopic deltoid ligament reconstruction in rotational ankle instability. Arthrosc Tech. 2023;12(7):e1179–84. https://doi.org/10.1016/j.eats.2023.03.007.
70. de Cesar NC, Valderrabano V, Mansur NSB. Multidirectional chronic ankle instability: what is it? Foot Ankle Clin. 2023;28(2):405–26. https://doi.org/10.1016/j.fcl.2023.01.012.
71. de Cesar NC, Femino JE. State of the art in treatment of chronic medial ankle instability. Foot Ankle Clin. 2021;26(2):329–44.
72. Davis WH, Sobel M, Deland J, Bohne WH, Patel MB. The superior peroneal retinaculum: an anatomic study. Foot Ankle Int. 1994;15:271–5.
73. Sobel M, Geppert MJ, Hannafin JA, Bohne WH, Arnoczky SP. Microvascular anatomy of the peroneal tendons. Foot Ankle. 1992;13:469–72.
74. Sammarco VJ. Peroneal tendoscopy: indications and techniques. Sports Med Arthrosc. 2009;17:94–9.
75. Sobel M, Levy ME, Bohne WH. Congenital variations of the peroneus quartus: an anatomic study. Foot Ankle. 1990;11:81–9.
76. Van Dijk CN, Kort N. Tendoscopy of the peroneal tendons. Arthroscopy. 1998;14:471–8.
77. Van Dijk CN. Hindfoot endoscopy. Foot Ankle Clin. 2006;11:391–414.
78. Dombek MF, Orsini R, Mendicino RW, Saltrick K. Peroneus brevis tendon tears. Clin Podiatr Med Surg. 2001;18:409–27.
79. Krause JO, Brodskym JW. Peroneus brevis tendon tears: pathophysiology, surgical reconstruction, and clinical results. Foot Ankle Int. 1998;19:271–9.
80. Monteggia GB. Instituzioni Chirurgiche, Part III. Milan: Stamperia Pirottae Maspero; 1803. p. 336–41.
81. Edwards ME. The relations of the peroneal tendons to the fibula, calcaneus and cuboideum. Am J Anat. 1928;42:213–53.
82. Eckert WR, Davis EA Jr. Acute rupture of the peroneal retinaculum. J Bone Joint Surg Am. 1976;58:670–2.
83. Oden RR. Tendon injuries about the ankle resulting from skiing. Clin Orthop Relat Res. 1987:63–9.
84. Raikin SM, Elias I, Nazarian LN. Intrasheath subluxation of the peroneal tendons. J Bone Joint Surg Am. 2008;90:992–9.
85. Leeuw PAJ, van Dijk CN, Golano P. A 3-portal endoscopic groove deepening technique for recurrent peroneal tendon dislocation. Tech Foot Ankle Surg. 2008;7:250–6.
86. Lui TH. Endoscopic peroneal retinaculum reconstruction. Knee Surg Sports Traumatol Arthrosc. 2006;14:478–81.
87. Adachi N, Fukuhara K, Tanaka H, Nakasa T, Ochi M. Superior retinaculoplasty for recurrent dislocation of peroneal tendons. Foot Ankle Int. 2006;27:1074–8.
88. Bravo Giménez B, Mellado Romero MA, Martín López CM, Cano Egea JM, Llanos Alcázar LF, Vilà y Rico J. Tendoscopia de los peroneos; nuestra experiencia. Rev Esp Cir Ortop Traumatol. 2013;57:268–75. ISSN 1888-4415.

Chapter 16
Surgical Techniques in Charcot Neuroarthropathy Reconstruction

Raju Ahluwalia, Thomas Hester, and Ines Reichert

This chapter focuses on the surgical management of Charcot neuroarthropathy (CN), examining the advantages and disadvantages of surgical intervention. In the Diabetic Charcot Foot, a combination of Neuropathy/Vasculopathy/Diabetes leads to common deformity patterns, including AVN with fragmentation of the talus or dislocation (see Figs. 16.1 and 16.2). Patients requiring reconstruction are either those who have acute CN where total contact casting is failing or those where chronic deformities have developed, and the foot is at risk of ulceration and infection or has developed these complications already. Surgical relevant factors are an alteration of the position of neurovascular bundle, development of vascular insufficiency and tendons, and an assessment of bone stock as there are usually multiple geographical and bone defects.

The broad aims of Charcot foot reconstruction surgery are outlined below:

1. A foot with no ulcers
2. A foot which fits into specialised custom-adapted footwear
3. A foot which permits weight bearing ambulation
4. A foot without collapse or recurrent instability
5. A plantigrade foot with no bony prominences and ideally with a medial longitudinal arch
6. A limb which is not painful or a burden to the patient

There are multiple ways to undertake Charcot neuroarthropathy reconstruction; operative planning depends on several factors, including the severity and location of the deformity, the presence of infection or osteomyelitis, bone quality, soft tissue condition, vascular sufficiency and the patient's overall health. Each surgical

R. Ahluwalia (✉) · T. Hester · I. Reichert
King's College Hospital NHS Foundation Trust, London, UK
e-mail: Venu.Kavarthapu@nhs.net; Thomashester@nhs.net; Ines.reichert@kcl.ac.uk

M. Bhatia (ed.), *Surgical Techniques of the Foot and Ankle*,
https://doi.org/10.1007/978-3-031-93742-2_16

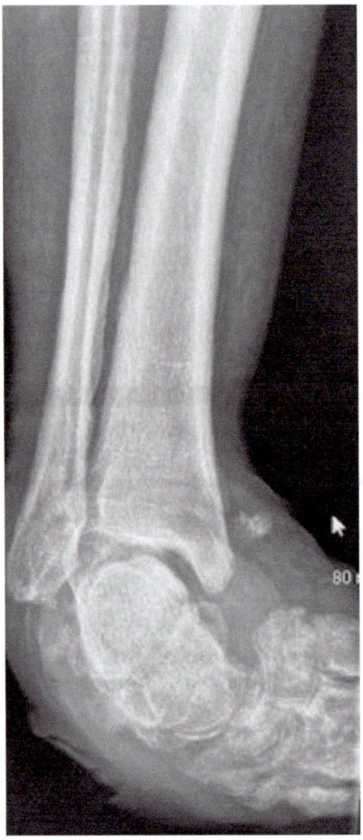

Fig. 16.1 Hind foot Eichholtz stage 3, with Fig destruction and hind foot instability and bone loss

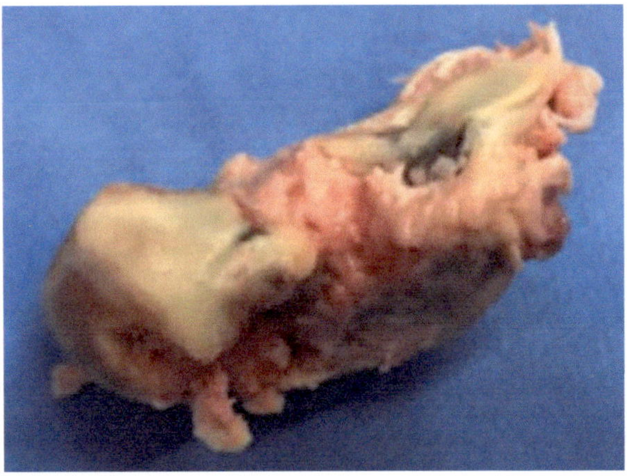

Fig. 16.2 Talus from an acute Charcot stage 1 Eichholtz, excised as part of reconstruction as avascular

approach has its advantages and limitations, and the choice should be individualised. Table 16.1 provides an overview. There are some key considerations in the type of surgery to be offered and include the following:

(a) **Patient factors**: Age, comorbidities (e.g., diabetes), and activity level.
(b) **Infection control**: Active infection necessitates careful debridement and consideration of external fixation or provisional internal fixation.

Table 16.1 The forms of Charcot reconstruction surgery

Surgical method	Best suited for	Surgical techniques	Advantages	Disadvantages
Internal fixation	Patients with adequate bone quality and no active infection Stable soft tissue condition	Beaming (intramedullary screws): Used to stabilise medial and lateral columns in midfoot Charcot deformities Tibiotalocalcaneal (TTC) fusion with hindfoot nailing: Ideal for hindfoot and ankle deformities Plates and screws: For multi-segmental reconstruction and joint fusion	Provides immediate stability and rigid fixation Less cumbersome compared to external fixation Faster recovery and earlier weight-bearing in many cases	High risk of hardware failure in poor bone quality Inappropriate for active infections or soft tissue compromise
External fixation	Patients with severe deformities, poor bone quality, or active infection Complex cases where soft tissue or vascular compromise is a concern	Circular external fixators (e.g., Ilizarov, Taylor Spatial Frame): Used for gradual deformity correction and stabilisation Cobination fixator: Combine circular and mono-lateral fixation for specific application	Ideal for patients with compromised soft tissue or ongoing infection Allows gradual deformity correction and offloading of pressure points Limb salvage is possible in many high-risk cases	Requires long treatment times with meticulous pin site care Patient compliance is critical; some find external frames cumbersome Higher complication rates (e.g., pin tract infections)
Hybrid fixation	Patients who would benefit from the advantages of both internal and external fixation Complex deformities requiring stabilisation and infection control	Combines internal fixation (e.g., beaming or screws) with external fixation for additional stability	Offers rigid internal stabilisation with the ability to manage infection externally Lower hardware stress and failure rates compared to internal fixation alone	Technically demanding and associated with high complication rates Long treatment durations
Amputation	Patients with non-salvageable limbs due to severe infection, osteomyelitis, or poor vascular status Cases where limb salvage would result in prolonged recovery with limited functionality		Quicker recovery and improved mobility with a well-fitted prosthesis Reduces the risk of ongoing infection or recurrent deformity	Loss of the limb Requires adjustment to prosthesis and lifestyle changes

(c) **Vascular Insufficiency:** Peripheral vascular disease below the knee is common in the Charcot foot and is seen in up to 60% of patients affecting mostly the peroneal and posterior tibial vessels.
(d) **Pathoanatomical challenges:**

    (a) **Bone quality**: there may be defects secondary to severe bone resorption or fragmentation.
    (b) **Distortion of anatomy:** including tendon and neurovascular bundle subluxation.

(e) **Surgeon expertise**: Experience with advanced techniques like circular fixators or hybrid constructs is crucial for success.

Outcomes are dependent on medical care and Multi-Disciplinary-Team (MDT) practices for optimisation of patients and control of factors such as the HBA1C, known to be a key risk factor for soft tissue complications following surgery. Furthermore, many patients will also require re-vascularisation, as poor blood supply will limit healing, and as our own evidence suggests, reduces survivorship of a reconstruction. Therefore, MDT working is key for successful Charcot foot reconstruction surgery.

Common Surgical Principles in Charcot Reconstruction

(a) **Infection Control:**

The starting point for all surgical techniques is to clear infection, as definitive fixation cannot be performed in an infected environment, especially when using internal fixation. The authors follow RED, AMBER & GREEN debridement steps [1] (see Fig. 16.3). This has paved the way for 2-stage reconstructions clearing infection in the first stage. Recent evidence suggests that even in the presence of open wounds

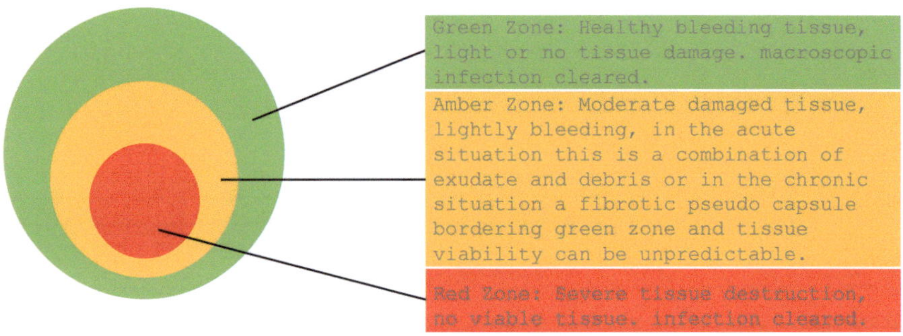

Fig. 16.3 Diagram illustrating three concentric zones representing tissue health. The outermost green zone indicates healthy bleeding tissue with light or no damage and cleared infection. The middle amber zone signifies moderate damage with light bleeding, involving exudate and debris in acute situations or a fibrotic pseudo capsule in chronic cases. The innermost red zone represents severe tissue destruction with no viable tissue, though infection is cleared

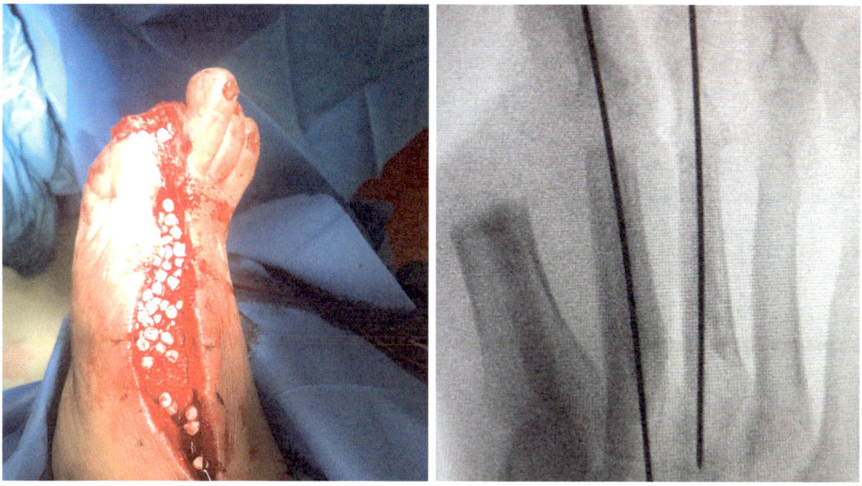

Fig. 16.4 Local antibiotic delivery methods in the form of topical treatments and/or injectable bone void fillers help to minimize resection and consequent dead space. The left panel displays a close-up of a surgical procedure on a foot, with visible white antibiotic pellets of calcium sulphate. on the right we highlight the internal structure and alignment of bones and the injection of local antibiotic carrier within the intramedullary canal. This facilitates local bone ingrowth, and increases local antibiotic levels to reduce the need for systematic antibiotics

due to deformity or ulcers; 2-stage reconstruction offers high rates of successful limb salvage. If there is a suspicion of active or semi-active infection it may be worthwhile to consider a needle biopsy of the site after an appropriate pause of antibiotics to obtain samples prior to surgery for microbiology. During surgery it is routine to sample multiple sites, at least five, using fresh instruments for each sample, for relevant microbiology and before intraoperative antibiotics are given.

Simpson and colleagues [2] concluded that in chronic osteomyelitis, wide resection with clearance margin of 5 mm or more results in no recurrence. However, this view is being recently challenged and the current recommendation is to excise the bone *adequately* and not necessarily widely. Local antibiotic delivery methods have also helped to minimize resection and consequent dead space (see Fig. 16.4) [3].

(b) **Dead space management**

Infection control or reconstruction surgery leads to dead space; active management includes the application of negative pressure wound therapy (NPWT) or local antibiotic delivery systems which are attractive dead-space or void fillers achieving concentrations of 100–1000 times the MIC for bacteria before a biofilm may develop (with agitation). Current management of bone voids includes either shortening osteotomies or the application of bi-composite carriers that can possibly remodel into osseous tissue or bone graft substitutes. There is a role for antibiotic carriers in selected cases and their use is to be determined as long-term data is still not known. Whilst their exact mechanism of action is not fully understood they may suppress the reactivation of further infection or prevent the generation of biofilm especially on newly implanted hardware.

(c) **Deformity Correction**

Combined deformity correction of ankle, and midfoot deformities are not uncommon but can be challenging. Pinzur identified two types of hind foot deformity: a valgus and a varus type [4]. The varus type is less common and results in a clubfoot type deformity with ulceration on the lateral side. The authors reported patients with a valgus deformity pattern were most likely to achieve a favourable clinical outcome, and those with a varus deformity pattern were least likely to achieve a favourable clinical outcome [5]. Deformities can be corrected either gradually or acutely e.g. hindfoot varus deformity is acutely corrected by a lateral shift calcaneal osteotomy or wedge resection using a supra-malleolar osteotomy.

Midfoot deformities can be combined with hindfoot deformities; they are centred around the Lisfranc joints, the medial column and involve divergent or escape of the metatarsals from the hindfoot. They present with a rocker bottom deformity, and the anatomy is distorted through the tarsometatarsal and/or midtarsal joints. This is often associated with forefoot abduction and pronation. Ulcers develop over the bony prominences, often medially due to the extruded medial cuneiform or laterally due to extrusion of the cuboid. Several classifications exist, including the Schon classification based anatomic location and severity, and a new surgical classification, that describes three patterns [6]:

(I) rocker bottom and forefoot abduction
(II) dorsal subluxation/dislocation
(III) forefoot adduction.

Deformities can be characterised utilising CT scans and the bone losses and the dislocations e.g. dorsal subluxation of the tarsus around the Chopart joint. The reader will need weight-bearing X-rays, CT, or MRI to assess the extent of bone destruction, deformity, and soft tissue involvement; utilisation of 3D models to understand spatial deformities (see Fig. 16.5); and MRI scans to assess the neurovascular bundles and the tendons especially the long tendons e.g. we have noted the inferior displacement of the tibialis posterior and the neurovascular bundle in *pes planus* deformities.

Many cases require correction of the hindfoot and midfoot to create a stable plantigrade tripod. This can be achieved using wedge tarsectomy and/or anatomical correction through a subtalar fusion, and reduction of the medial column to the hindfoot and then the middle and lateral columns. The key is to correct or approximate the following angles to normality as shown in Table 16.2. Today, computer-aided planning supports anatomical deformity correction to recreate the anatomical tripod and may offer better longer-term results because internal fixation (implants) or external fixation (wire frame application) are placed in their optimal position s. Early evidence suggests that achieving anatomical reduction offers better results.

(d) **Surgical Timing**

Charcot neuroarthropathy (CN) is traditionally staged using the Eichenholtz classification based on radiographic presentation, which describes the pathophysiological progression of the disease cessation. Treatment should always consider off-loading in a total contact cast and if this fails surgical stabilisation to prevent ulceration or disruption of the osseous anatomy has become important; this can be

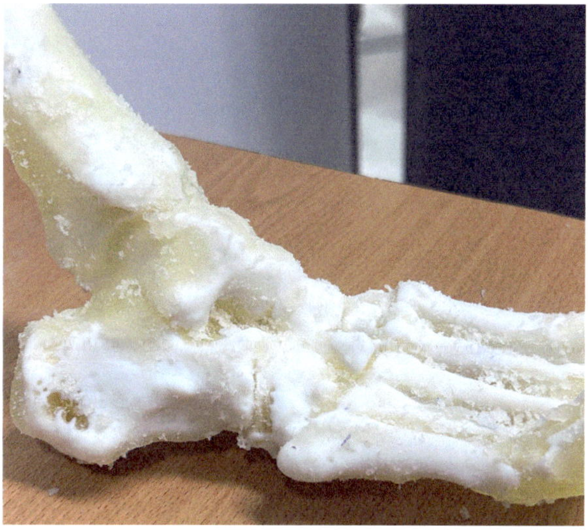

Fig. 16.5 3D model of charcot deformity to help showcase the bones and structure and deformity pattern to better understand the correction required

Table 16.2 Radiographic angles used in charcot deformity correction

Radiographic Angle or measurement	Normal range	Notes
Calcaneal pitch	18° +/− 5°	A line along the inferior surface of the calcaneus connecting the most inferior point of the calcaneal tuberosity with the most distal inferior point of the calcaneus at the calcaneo-cuboid joint
Meary's angle	0–4°	The angle between the long axis of the talus and the long axis of the first metatarsal)
Anterior-posterior talo-calcaneal or kite angle	15°-35°	This is the angle between the longitudinal axes of the talar, and anterior talocalcaneal joints (Kite angle. It decreases in varus feet it increases in hindfoot valgus)
Lateral talo-calcaneal angle	35–50°	An angle formed by a line along the long axis of the talus and another line along the long axis of the calcaneus on a standard weight bearing lateral radiograph of the foot
Cuboid height	1.2 cm	Defined as a perpendicular distance from the plantar aspect of the cuboid to a line drawn from the plantar surface of the calcaneal tuberosity to the plantar aspect of the 5th metatarsal head. Mean normal value is about 1.2 cm above that line. It is a quantitative radiographic measurement of the relationship of the inferior cuboid to the plantar osseous plane of the lateral column of the foot

achieved by surgical stabilisation, open reduction and wires, or percutaneous wire fixation and in select cases internal fixation. Traditionally, reconstructive surgery is avoided in Eichenholtz Stage 1/2, but the recent trend has become more supportive of corrective surgery in the inflammatory phase, utilising modern understanding of fixation requirements in this group of patients. Recent series have shown satisfactory results for hind– and midfoot correction and there is debate if this should be undertaken in 1-stage or 2-stages (in the mid foot). Two stages may be considered more appropriate when infection or ulceration co-exist [7]. All patients should undergo a vascular assessment including formal studies and the results should be discussed with the vascular team prior orthopaedic Charcot reconstruction. As required recommendations may be gleaned for optimal surgical incisions in the presence of vascular insufficiencies. The surgeon needs to be mindful of the effect of deformity correction on a tenuous vasculature. Furthermore, vascular reconstruction may be indicated prior to bone and joint reconstruction.

(e) **Contained and Uncontained Bone Void Defects**

CN leads to both bone loss destruction and uncontained osseous defects. Stable constructs require bony apposition, if this is not possible and stable apposition is required bone void fillers or autologous bone graft can be used in contained defects. Uncontained defects pose significant challenges. Currently, bone voids if contained are filled with bone substitutes releasing antibiotics or bone graft soaked in antibiotics; if uncontained common strategies are significant shortening or autologous bone graft (this can be taken from the foot, e.g. fibula, or where shortening. Utilisation of vascularised bone grafts can be difficult as most patients have peripheral vascular disease (PVD). One newer solution is the use of 3D printed cages, which may integrate into the body, transforming the uncontained into a contained void to be filled with bone graft and bone substitute (see Fig. 16.6). However, the largest reported series cautioned that neuropathy is a relative contraindication as is active infection to these implants [8].

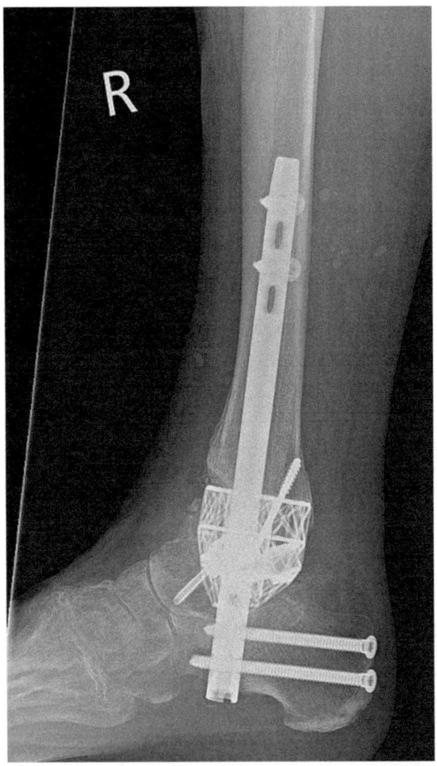

Fig. 16.6 Lateral radiographic of cage fixation in the hind foot for bone loss in a non-diabetes related complication These implants may represent the future but should be used with caution and in specialist centres where other options have been utilised or deemed inappropriate as the literature currently predicts higher failure rates in the presence of neuropathy. Further research is required

General Surgical Processes

Charcot reconstruction is complex surgery, pre-operative preparation requires MDT review and assessment of all medical co-morbidities and optimisation. Once this has been completed surgical planning is undertaken and the key steps are outlined in Table 16.3.

Table 16.3 Critical steps in Charcot reconstruction

Stage	Description
Preoperative assessment	Management of infection is paramount; bone biopsies are ideally required if a history of an ulcer or infection is noted. This can guide local and systemic antibiotics, following surgery. In the elective setting vascular studies to identify arterial disease is essential and guide the utilisation of tourniquets and incision placement and patients may require revascularisation. Surgeons should be aware on the flow to the planter arches, this will help plan incisions in the foot. Identifying all callous and ulcers is important in infection control. Furthermore, many patients will require optimisation of HBA1C and other factors to reduce the risk of systemic complications
Anaesthesia, positioning, and fluoroscopic guidance	Most procedure are performed under general or regional anaesthesia. The patient is positioned supine or lateral with a bump under the contralateral hip, allowing access to the posterior aspect of the hindfoot and ankle. A bolster to raise the affected leg will allow intraoperative imaging to confirm proper alignment in the coronal, sagittal, and axial planes
Preoperative Planning, Imaging & Hardware Selection	Use weight-bearing X-rays, CT, or MRI to assess the extent of bone destruction, deformity, and soft tissue involvement. Utilisation of 3D imaging and models to plan osteotomies is key to understanding the correction. Intraoperatively one can consider further marginal biopsies, to understand clearance and guide the duration and type of post operative antimicrobial therapy. Hardware considerations will be discussed within each type of fixation, but currently there are several implants specifically designed for Charcot reconstruction
Incision and Joint Preparation	The approach is defined by the deformity—longitudinal incisions or extensile approaches are used from either side of the foot and extend proximally to the distal tibia, however arthroscopic or minimally invasive surgical preparation of anatomically well aligned joints is becoming commoner but needs to ensure resection of cartilage and debridement. This is best utilised when infection is not suspected. Excision of articular cartilage from the tibiotalar and subtalar joints to expose bleeding cancellous bone. Remove all non-viable bone and soft tissue, including any sequestrum, this is key as a red, amber, green technique yields the best results. Most surgeons will use curettes, burrs, or osteotomes to prepare the fusion surfaces. Some are wary of burrs and saws due to thermal damage, but little evidence supports this
Alignment and Correction	Surgery aims to achieve a plantigrade position by reducing acute correction with osteotomies e.g. King's cut to correct sagittal plane deformity, multiplanar osteotomies including wedge excision, can correct mid and hind foot mal alignment. An anatomical reduction will aid metalwork placement. After multi-planar deformity correction (e.g., varus, valgus, equinus) temporary Kirschner wires or external fixation are used to stabilise the foot ad then definitive fixation this followed by implantation of hardware. In general shortening will improve soft tissue closure, one should be aware of the changes to neurovascular structures and the authors advice marking out the blood flow to the foot at the time of surgery with a duplex is helpful (see fig)
Closure	Irrigate the surgical site thoroughly, and close the incision in layers, taking care to avoid excessive tension on the soft tissues

Current Evidence and Application of Surgical Fixation Techniques

Following deformity correction, definite fixation is undertaken and there are three different options (Internal, external fixation and hybrid fixation which is a composite of the other two), finally surgery may be staged for infection clearance. Deformity correction and definitive fixation may be combined in a single stage process mostly employed for the closed ulcer and infection-free scenario, or more commonly in the presence of infection and possibly vascular insufficiency a two- or multiple stage procedure is utilised. An overview of the common methods of fixation has been given in Table 16.1.

Internal Fixation in Charcot Reconstruction

Internal fixation is effective in patients with good bone quality and no infection. Fusion rates are generally high, but hardware failure is a concern. There are three predominant methods utilised: the hind foot nail, beams and plates and screws utilising the principles of *long-segment rigid fixation.*

Rigid Long Segment Fixation

This method involves stabilising and fusing multiple joint segments to restore alignment, ensure rigidity, and provide a plantigrade and functional foot. It is particularly useful for addressing extensive instability or deformities affecting multiple bones and joints in the midfoot, hindfoot, and ankle. Long-segment constructs reduce mechanical stress on individual fixation points, minimising the risk of hardware failure which is common with standard fixation techniques. The key indications for Long-Segment Rigid Fixation are outlined below and the key principles are outlined in Table 16.4.

- Severe Charcot deformities involving multiple joints.
- Advanced midfoot collapse with arch failure.
- Combined midfoot and hindfoot deformities.
- Recurrent deformities after previous surgeries.
- Poor bone quality or bone fragmentation requiring stabilisation across larger areas.

Internal fixation and its various methods rely on prolonged periods of immobilisation in a splint or total contact cast applied to protect the surgical reconstruction. Patients may be non-weight-bearing for 8–12 weeks, progressing to partial or full weight-bearing once there is evidence of bone healing on imaging. Regular X-rays or CT scans to monitor the fusion progress are obtained for up to 1-year.

Table 16.4 Explanation of concepts in rigid fixation

Long Segment Fixation Principles	Description
Stability across multiple segments	By spanning several joints (e.g., tarsometatarsal, midfoot, hindfoot, or ankle), the fixation provides structural support and prevents recurrent collapse Typically achieved with intramedullary screws, plates, or hindfoot nails, ensuring long-term stability
Rigid constructs	Large-diameter screws or rods are used to provide strong internal support, especially in areas of poor bone quality or significant deformity
Deformity correction	Simultaneously addresses multi-planar deformities, including sagittal, coronal, and rotational misalignments
Bone fusion	Focuses on achieving arthrodesis (fusion) of affected joints to stabilise the foot and ankle permanently Bone grafts or substitutes may be used to fill voids caused by osteolysis or resection of non-viable bone
Offloading and weight distribution	Ensures even weight distribution across the foot to minimise ulceration risk and avoid excessive pressure on vulnerable areas

A systematic review analysing various surgical reconstruction methods for Charcot neuroarthropathy reported that current surgical options, including internal fixation techniques like beaming, could offer limb salvage with a low amputation risk in a highly selected population. The overall bone fusion rate was reported at 86.1%, with a post-reconstruction amputation rate of 5.5%. However, complications were noted in 36% of individuals, highlighting the complex nature of these procedures [9].

Types of Internal Fixation in Charcot Reconstruction

We now take an in-depth look at the 3 main internal fixation techniques (see Table 16.1); these techniques can be used in combination. A combination of long-segment fixation in the hindfoot and beams in the midfoot allows for a comprehensive reconstruction of complex Charcot deformities.

1. **IM Nailing or tibio-talocalcaneal (TTC) arthrodesis using hindfoot intramedullary nailing.**

The approach corrects deformities, provides stability, and facilitates weight-bearing in patients with Charcot foot. Several studies support the effectiveness of TTC arthrodesis by hindfoot nailing in diabetic patients with Charcot foot joints. The procedure was associated with improved quality of life, with improved stability and decreased ulcer recurrence suggesting its viability as a treatment option. Fusion rates are reported to range from 75–90%, and PROMs score improve; but complications such as infection and hardware failure remain a challenge [9].

Surgical Steps for Hindfoot Nailing in Charcot Reconstruction

1. **Preoperative Planning, Imaging & Hardware Selection**:

There are two types of hind foot nail—straight and angled, the latter is used when a talus is present, as the calcaneum does not naturally sit underneath the tibia. Longer nails are thought to introduce more stability and depending on the patient's anatomy should be isthmic fitting, to prevent failure. A key paper describes the increased risk of failure being associated with a lack of isthmus fit. Additional screw or plate fixation for rotation stability can increase mechanical stability and reduce failure rates. Therefore, pre-selecting implants with appropriate lengths and diameters, according to patient anatomy, is important and can reduce the risk of failure.

2. **Anaesthesia, Positioning, and Fluoroscopic Guidance**

The procedure is performed under general or regional anaesthesia. The patient is positioned supine or lateral with a bump under the contralateral hip, allowing access to the posterior aspect of the hindfoot and ankle. A bolster to raise the affected leg will allow intraoperative imaging to confirm proper alignment in the coronal, sagittal, and axial planes.

3. **Incision and Joint Preparation**

The approach is defined by the deformity—longitudinal incision centred over the calcaneus and extending proximally to the distal tibia, however arthroscopic or minimally invasive surgical preparation of anatomically well-aligned joints is becoming more common requiring resection of cartilage and debridement and may be applied in the Charcot joint as well. The remaining articular cartilage should be excised from the tibiotalar and subtalar joints to expose bleeding cancellous bone. All non-viable bone and soft tissue must be removed, including any sequestrum or infected areas, following the red, amber, green technique yielding the best results. Most surgeons will use curettes, burrs, or osteotomes to prepare the fusion surfaces.

4. **Alignment and Correction**

A plantigrade position is achieved by reducing the hindfoot into proper alignment, and by utilising osteotomes e.g. King's cut to correct sagittal plane deformity and allow correct positioning of the IM nail thus preventing excessive shortening. Anatomical reduction of bone will aid metal work placement. After multiplanar deformity correction (e.g., varus, valgus, equinus) temporary Kirschner wires or external fixation methods are used to stabilise the foot. In general shortening will improve soft tissue closure.

5. **Hindfoot Nail Insertion and application of local antibiotics or bone graft**

The first step is guidewire placement through the plantar aspect of the calcaneus, across the subtalar joint, and into the distal tibia, verified under fluoroscopy. Following this, remaining over the guidewire to create a canal for the nail, ensuring proper alignment and avoiding cortical breaches. Reaming is performed until there is audible cortical chatter, as it is important to insert the largest diameter nail for stability.

Table 16.5 Tips and tricks in the application of a IM nail

Category	Tip
Implants	Nail size: Ensuring isthmic nail fit. Supplementary hindfoot miss a nail screw or hydroxyapatite coated screws, provide additional construct stability
Soft tissue management	Shortening and debulking of prominences will help in wound closure and management and does not stretch the arterial tree and cause vascular insufficiency
Bone Cuts & Osteotomy	Using the king's sliding cut and retaining the medial malleolus and the fibula as anti-rotational support for the nail. A talectomy does not affect union rates, a straight nail will be more amenable to a talectomy as a curved hind foot nail is designed to be used with a talus

Venting holes can be added to the tibial cortex for the insertion of local antibiotics at the time of insertion of the nail (see below). The nail is inserted and locked, proximally and distally with screws to prevent rotation and increase rigidity of fixation. If there are significant bone voids or areas at risk for non-union, autograft, allograft, or bone substitutes to promote fusion e.g. Osmycin (see section below) is placed to fill the void areas. Table 16.5, highlights these key steps in the application of an IM nail.

Midfoot Beaming

Beams or large diameter screws have become part of the modern armoury of internal fixation in the last two decades. The use of beams for long-segment fixation in Charcot neuroarthropathy is an increasingly utilised surgical approach for stabilising and reconstructing severe midfoot deformities. Biomechanically beams work like IM nails, the working length is the distance between the locking screws closest to the fusion site either side of the fusion area (see Fig. 16.7). The longer the working length, the more motion results at the fusion site, and the shorter the working length the stiffer the device becomes. In Charcot midfoot reconstruction the working length is reduced e.g. all joints need to fuse along the beam by preparing all joints and utilisation of the beam for compression, A plate may be used alone or in addition to a beam and these screws reduce the beam working length further. In general beam fixation involves:

(a) ***Large-diameter screws or rigid beams*** (often titanium or stainless-steel screws) are used to stabilise the medial and lateral arches of the foot. They may be cannulated or solid, partially threaded (for compression), or fully threaded (for placement).
(b) ***Spanning screws*** may pass from the talus through the midfoot and into the forefoot, correcting deformities and bridging collapsed midfoot joints e.g. collapse or instability of the tarsometatarsal joints, causing a "rocker-bottom" foot.
(c) ***No active infection***: Beaming is generally used when there is no ongoing infection or active soft tissue issues.

Grant et al. evaluated the "beaming" technique applied to the medial and lateral longitudinal columns in 71 Charcot foot deformities [10]. They reported significant

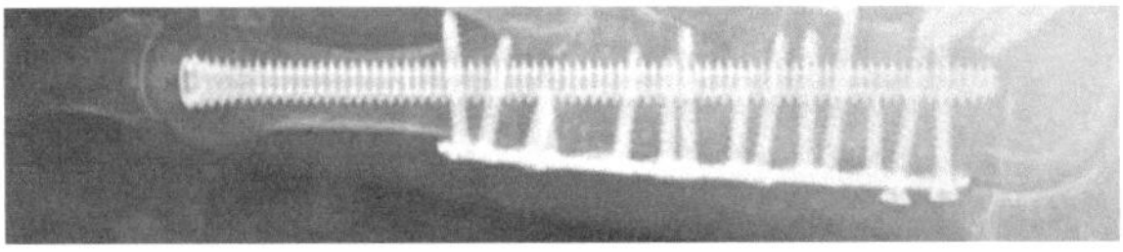

Fig. 16.7 Application of a medial beam and a neutralisation plate, the effect of the plate and screws is to reduce the beam working length to improve construct stability to allow healing

improvements in radiographic alignment postoperatively, indicating the effectiveness of this method in correcting deformities. However, complications such as pin tract infections, broken pins, osteomyelitis, transfer lesions, and ulcerations were noted, underscoring the need for careful patient management. A study by Wiewiorski et al. assessed clinical outcomes and complications, they found the technique allowed for the restoration of an ulcer-free, plantigrade foot in most patients [11]. Nevertheless, the complication rate remained notable, emphasizing the importance of meticulous surgical technique and postoperative care.

Even so, beaming alone is associated with a higher-than-expected risk of complication or failure; subtalar stabilisation can support the creation of a tripod and additional plating to stabilise the construct may prevent beam failure, as it reduces the working length of the beam (see Fig.) [12]. Multiple divergent screws/beams may also create secondary rotational stability. Tarsectomy undertaken with flat cuts may allow column fixation with screws *vs.* anatomical reconstruction allows for conventional bony apposition, beaming and neutralisation plating. Understanding of deformity patterns and instability will support usage of considered bone preparation and fixation techniques, MIS techniques may offer improved outcomes, but further research is necessary to establish long-term efficacy and safety profiles. Recent advancements in minimally invasive surgical (MIS) techniques have introduced percutaneous deformity correction combined with intramedullary beaming. This approach aims to reduce soft tissue dissection and associated complications. Early reports suggest that MIS beaming can achieve satisfactory deformity correction with potentially lower complication rates, though a learning curve is associated with the technique. The authors would not recommend MIS in active infection.

Key Surgical Steps for Midfoot Beaming in Charcot Reconstruction

Here is a step-by-step guide on how to perform beaming for Charcot reconstruction, specifically for the midfoot—certain steps have been omitted as they are used in the hind-foot nail:

1. **Preoperative Planning**

It is important to plan the osteotomies, and beam placement with adequate preoperative imaging. Optimal beam positioning means the medial column beam must end in the medial talus. The lateral beams e.g. fourth and fifth ray would enter the cuboid or calcaneum. Therefore, the surgeon will need to choose appropriately sized intramedullary beams (screws) based on the patient's anatomy. These should span the necessary segments of the foot or ankle and be long enough to provide optimal stability. Ideally joints are fused along the path of the beam, however if there are gaps due to bone loss then a plate should be considered for construct stability and reduce the working length of the screw.

2. **Anaesthesia, Positioning and Approach to the Midfoot (Tarsometatarsal) Deformities:**

The procedure is performed under general or regional anaesthesia. Position of the patient is supine on a radiolucent table with the affected foot accessible, often in a leg holder or with the foot slightly elevated for better access. A bolster or wedge is preferred (see figure of operative positioning) as it allows the foot to be optimally placed for anterior-posterior (AP) views and laterals. A medial, dorsal or lateral incision over the affected midfoot is made to expose the tarsometatarsal joints. Beams can be placed inferiorly or superiorly from the forefoot or retrograde from the talus. Joint preparation, debridement are the same as above, careful apposition of allografts may be used to promote fusion and fill any defects.

3. **Insertion of Beams**

Using fluoroscopic guidance, insert a guidewire into the metatarsal head (see Fig. 16.8) The wire should pass through the bone and across the affected joint into the adjacent bone segment, ensuring proper alignment and orientation for the screw.

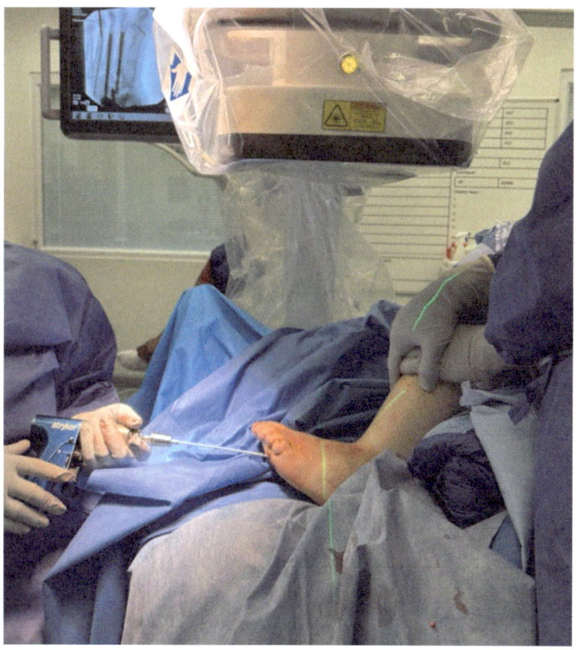

Fig. 16.8 Insertion of beams in theatre with toe is held or placed over a bolster the foot is held dorsiflexed for a planter entry into the metatarsal head

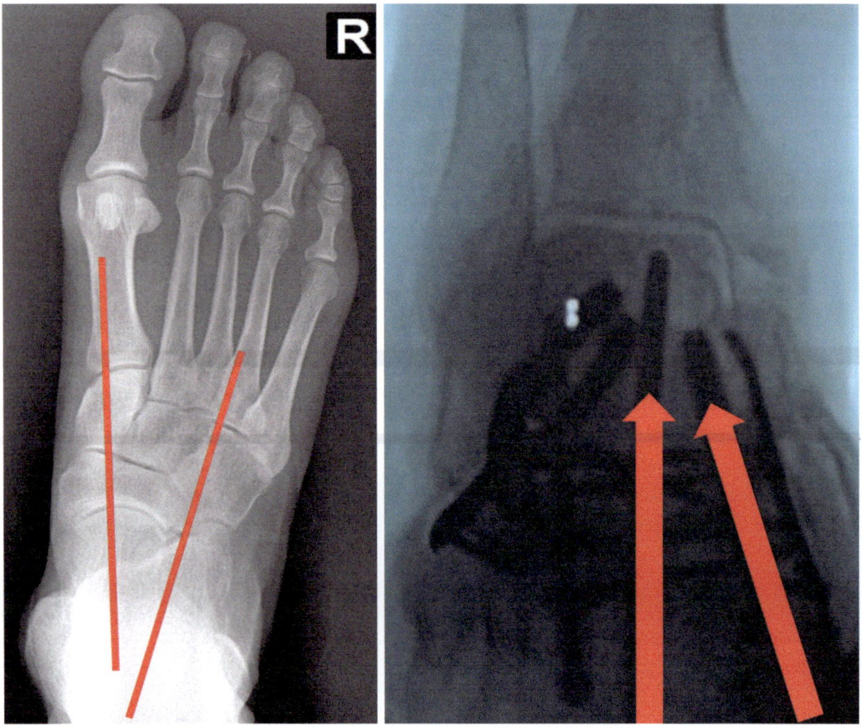

Fig. 16.9 AP radiograph of the foot: Application of medial beams in red line into the first metatarsal from a dorsal approach under image and lateral column. On a AP radiograph of the ankle following the insertion of medial and second ray beam. One can clearly showing the medial beam in the medial half of the talus and the second ray beam into the mid-point of the talus

Verify the position of the guide wire in multiple planes under fluoroscopy (anterior-posterior, lateral). Ream to the appropriate diameter, in some cases the beams may be inserted without reaming especially with a fully threaded beam. Insert the selected intramedullary beam through the prepared canal, spanning the midfoot or hindfoot joints (e.g., through the talus, calcaneus, and tibia for hindfoot beaming). Technique for Medial Column insertion is as follows. The placement following these steps is outlined below in Fig. 16.9.

- Plantar surface—guide wire—free hand/instrumented
- Aim toward the centre of the talus—keep medial
- Aim to keep the beam in the medial half of the talus
- Aim to correct Meary's angle

Technique for Lateral Column Beaming:

- 2nd, 3rd ray beams into the talus—converge; 4th and 5th beams converge into the cuboid as the lateral rays are flatter.

4. **Additional Fixation for a stable construct**

Plate fixation and beams can be combined, or additional screws or plates may be used for supplemental fixation, particularly in areas where there is bone loss. This creates a stable construct and prevents rotational instability or failure where the osteotomies do not oppose, and bony defects exist. External fixation may be used in conjunction with beaming to provide additional stability or to manage deformities that require gradual correction. Midfoot beaming has been shown superior with subtalar (ST) joint fusion in an RCT and is recommended if the ST joint is mobile to create a stable hindfoot [12]. A late complication of this technique may occur if the medial soft tissues are nor repaired and if there is medial ankle instability, which will need to be treated with ankle fusion.

Plate & Screw Fixation

This is the traditional method for midfoot fixation; plate and screw constructs have been primarily employed in Charcot reconstruction. The role of plate fixation is to stabilise bones during realignment or fusion. Today, locking plates are commonly employed due to their rigidity and ability to maintain fixation in compromised bone (e.g., osteoporotic or neuropathic bone in Charcot). Locking plates are used in osteoporotic or neuropathic bone to prevent loss of fixation. Plating is often supplemented by screws, which help compress the fusion site. Low profile titanium plates have improved soft tissue considerations.

Plates are primarily applied to stabilise the medial column, which is critical in maintaining foot stability. Plates can be used in the following modes: bridging fixation where plates may bridge areas of instability or destruction and bypassing weak bone areas to provide strength. They create stable constructs for arthrodesis of joints e.g. the tarsometatarsal (Lisfranc) or ankle joints. Commonly these plates are used with bone grafts (autografts or allografts) to fill defects, stimulate fusion and increase the stability of constructs e.g. with beams or columnar plating to provide three column fixations to the mid- and forefoot and are utilised for stability. The common types of plates are shown in Table 16.6.

Table 16.6 Common plat types and utilisation in Charcot reconstruction

Plate Type	Utilisation
Pre-contoured locking plates	Designed to fit the anatomical curves of the foot and ankle
Straight plates	Used for bridging fixation
Fusion plates	Specifically designed for arthrodesis procedures

Steps in Using Plating for Charcot Reconstruction

1. **Exposure**: The collapsed or deformed area is surgically exposed, requiring extensile approaches, debridement of non-viable bone or tissue is undertaken. Whilst not used by the authors MIS approaches are being developed but subperiosteal plating is considered very difficult due to shifts in anatomic position of bones, tendons and neurovascular bundles
2. **Realignment**: The deformity is corrected using osteotomies, and held with Kirschner wires for reduction, compression screws may be inserted prior to plate application.
3. **Plate application**: Medial or lateral column plates are applied depending on the deformity. Plates can be contoured and locking screws are inserted to secure the plate. They may be combined with compression screws. Patients with multi-segment involvement or combined hindfoot and midfoot deformities have combined application of nails, plates and beams to create stable constructs.

Outcomes of Internal and External Fixation Strategies

Undertaken in the appropriately selected patients, a systematic review reported a fusion rate of 94% in patients treated with external fixation, which was higher compared to 81% in those undergoing internal fixation [9]. The same review found a lower complication rate in the external fixation group (25%) compared to the internal fixation group (41.4%). Post-reconstruction amputation rates were similar between external (5.2%) and internal fixation (4.4%), suggesting comparable limb salvage outcomes. Combined cases of severe mid & hindfoot, may have higher failure rates due to higher technical difficulty e.g. bone stock loss, and deformity (see Fig. 16.10). Patients treated with external fixation began weight-bearing ambulation at an average of 19 weeks postoperatively, slightly longer than the 16 weeks observed in the internal fixation group [9].

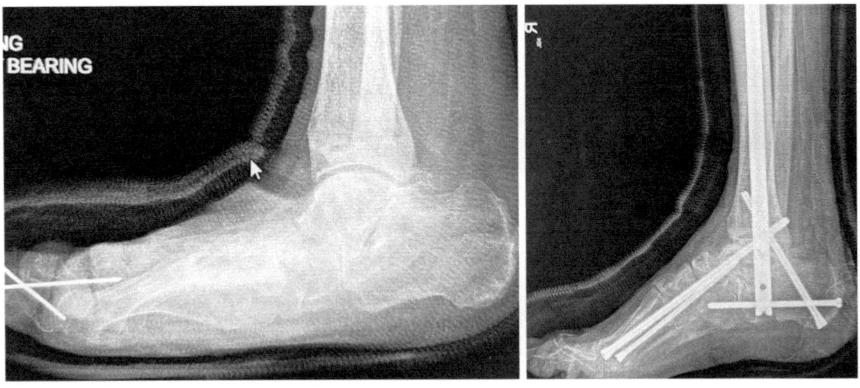

Fig. 16.10 Combined hind and midfoot reconstruction using beams and a hind foot nail with a mis a nail hind foot screw for added stability

External Fixation

External fixator is a generic term covering a range of devices that stabilize the limb skeleton with trans-osseous elements such as half-pins (Schanz screws) and an external frame, the common types are described in table. Circular or ring frames (Ilizarov and/or hexapod frames) can be configured around the deformity; stability may be achieved by adding more pins and wires. (see Table 16.7) The technique is soft tissue friendly, and minimally invasive, and can be combined with internal fixation. Tissues under tension generated by the circular frame also exhibit bactericidal effects *via* activation of biosynthetic processes, which help in the management of osteomyelitis with reduced antibiotic requirements. Another added benefit is considered at the time of frame application when any plantar ulcers are offloaded by correcting alignment and ensuring the foot is plantigrade. Adjunctive plastic surgery techniques (e.g., flap coverage) may be used if required.

Deformity correction can be undertaken acutely intraoperatively for mild deformities and where soft tissues can tolerate the adjustment. Gradual correction is achieved postoperatively by adjusting the frame daily and this is used for severe deformities to minimise soft tissue tension. In cases of non-reconstructable joints (e.g., tibiotalar, subtalar), fusion is achieved through debridement of joint surfaces and compression using the external fixator. Bone grafts or substitutes may be added if there are significant defects. The ideal patients for external fixation are those with:

- Severe deformities unsuitable for internal fixation.
- Poor bone quality or active infection (osteomyelitis).
- Complex soft tissue conditions, such as ulceration or poor wound healing capacity.

Table 16.7 Types of external fixation commonly used in Charcot Reconstruction

Type of External Fixators	Type	Rationale	Description
Circular external fixators	Ilizarov, Taylor Spatial Frame	Used for gradual deformity correction and stabilisation Effective for multi-planar corrections (sagittal, coronal, rotational deformities)	Ring frames can be built to either act as simply holding frames (sometimes called neutral frames) or modular frames capable of deformity correction and compression to promote bone healing. There are well-described safe corridors for the insertion of wires and screws to avoid injury to neurovascular structures
Hybrid external fixators:	Combine circular and mono-lateral components	For targeted support	
Mono-lateral external fixators:	Pin to bar constructs	Primarily used for stabilisation in less complex deformities	Easy to apply and in an emergency set-up. Weight-bearing is generally not possible due to stability concerns

Table 16.8 Indications for external fixation

Ankle and hind foot deformities that are difficult to brace or developing ulceration from the brace/total contact cast
Unstable ankle and subtalar complex with or without fractures, and with poor bone stock and poor soft tissue envelope
Deformity and active ulceration and or deep infection/osteomyelitis
Failure of traditional internal fixation
Poor quality of bone where internal fixation alone is not sufficient
Limbs with suboptimal or compromised vascular status—minimally invasive stabilization with a circular frame minimizes the need for major soft tissue dissection
Part of 2-stage management of deep infection: Circular frame is used as a first-stage treatment to correct the deformity, heal ulcers, and is then converted to internal fixation
Combined treatment: Use of circular frame to complement internal fixation and enhance stability of construct and promote bone healing. This combination allows weight-bearing to some extent in situations where non-weight-bearing is not possible, that is, hyper obese patients

The main drawback of external fixation techniques is the degree of specialist training and equipment required. Frames can be bulky and cumbersome for the patient depending on the type of deformities. Pin site infection is common to all types of external fixators and ring fixators are no exception. Hexapods are advanced ring fixators with dedicated hardware and generally a web-based software that aids gradual deformity correction. They can achieve a plantigrade, ulcer-free, and functional foot and correct deformity and offload pressure directly, from vulnerable areas. The indications of external fixation are outlined below in Table 16.8. External fixation for Charcot reconstruction is a complex procedure to stabilise the foot, correct deformities, and facilitate limb salvage. The specific technique depends on the anatomical location of the deformity and the extent of soft tissue involvement [13]. Below is an overview of how external fixation is typically performed:

Practical Frame Application

Deformity correction may be achieved acutely, with extensile exposures from the apex (convex side) of the deformity. The medial approach is used in *pes planus* deformities to correct the hind foot alignment. The ankle joint is typically exposed from the lateral side by excising or turning down the lateral malleolus. Access to the subtalar joint is available in both approaches. The different types of frame constructs are outlined in the table.

In our institution a hexapod frame is used, however a static frame e.g. Ilizarov frame may be used well for an acute correction. Using the hexapod frame the rings are aligned to the tibia and the struts are aligned to the deformity. In cases where there is hindfoot/ankle involvement, a further proximal tibial ring is applied for stability. Midfoot deformities typically involve rings encircling the

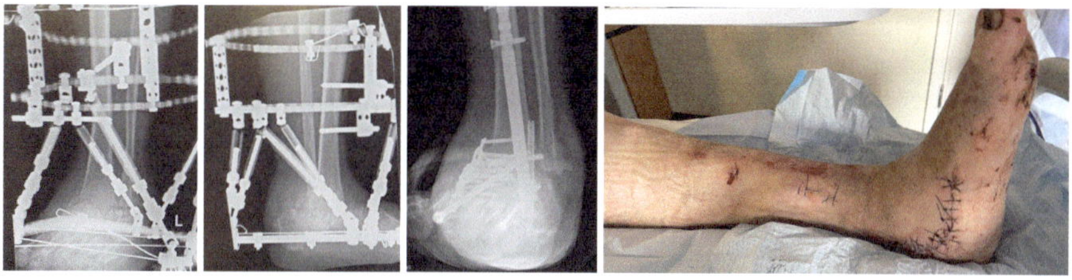

Fig. 16.11 Application of external fixator with struts for 2 stage Charcot reconstruction. Final reconstruction with internal fixation, patient has been ulcer free and WB for 3 yrs, vascular insufficiency was treated prior to 2 stage reconstruction

foot with a U-shaped foot ring. These 2 ring units are connected with 6 struts (see Fig. 16.11). The construct can be made stronger by extending half-pins on the posts above and below the tibial ring. The hexapod is capable of deformity correction, compression, and distraction. Care is taken to avoid neurovascular structures and tension wires to improve stability, the struts or rods connect the rings, allowing multi-planar adjustments. Healing can continue for a couple of years after a ring fixator is used and eventually becomes complete if the alignment is good, the docking site is stable on weight-bearing, and if there is no deep infection.

Complications

Pin site infections and tibial stress fracture through the half-pin track is a well-known complication in diabetic patients. Inserting the half-pins at an angle (30–45°), can reduce this complication, so the two holes of the half-pins are not collinear and act as a single hole on each cortex at different levels. Furthermore, patients require consenting and assessment for suitability, as compliance is very important to allow long treatment times with meticulous pin site care. Patient compliance is critical; some patients find external frames very cumbersome.

Frames for Vascular Insufficiency: Transverse Tibial Bone Transport

TTT harnesses the skeletal system's inherent healing capacity through osteodistraction, governed by two fundamental orthopaedic principles: Wolff's Law and the Law of Tension-Stress [13]. The application of these principles in treating bone non-union by applying gradual and consistent stress on living tissues, thereby stimulating the regeneration of new tissue that is structurally and functionally similar to native tissue [14]. In chronic wound management, TTT applies the same principles to promote localized tissue regeneration while also facilitating revascularization along the entire limb segment, particularly through reconstituting microcirculation in ischemic tissues [15].

Hybrid Fixation Techniques

Combining external and internal fixation methods has been explored to leverage the benefits of both approaches. One study reported a 100% limb salvage rate and a 91.6% fusion rate using a hybrid technique, though the complication rate was higher at 70%. One strategy is to use a circular frame, in the acute stages, to hold the correction whilst utilising beams and IMN for long-term fixation. In this way a patient with an ulcer can be treated with expectant treatment utilising the plastic surgical tree of soft tissue reconstruction.

Revision Surgery Charcot Reconstruction

There is a high overall complication rate of 36%, with an ulceration rate (non-healing or recurrent) of 6.25%; amputation rates are low at 5.5% [9]. Survivorship is currently defined as no amputation, ulceration requiring surgical debridement or revision for any cause, but may not capture all episodes of failure. A patient may ambulate with the help of a CROW-walker for a fibrous non-union or may accept repeated outpatient visits for care of a recurrent or chronic ulceration.

Establishing the cause of CN reconstruction failure is important to determine a treatment strategy; patient factors, implant factors and surgical techniques should be assessed. One study identified peripheral arterial disease, renal disease, delayed postoperative healing, post- operative wound infection, postoperative osteomyelitis, transfer ulceration, new onset of CN in the same foot and post- reconstruction non-union as predictors of post-reconstruction amputation. In addition, there are hardware predictors of failure or success e.g. an intact medial malleolus is protective against non-union and subsequent metalwork failure.

Patient factors include impaired healing due to poorly controlled diabetes, a high BMI, adverse biology, poor soft tissues, wound healing problems, impaired bone stock, and ongoing neurological dysfunction. Patients with Charcot frequently have significant peripheral arterial disease (PAD), and, if untreated, this can lead to failure. After reconstruction, patients have greater activity levels and consequently higher biomechanical requirements and load bearing stress on their metalwork, especially in the presence of bone loss and delayed bone healing.

Implant factors include adverse local tissue reactions, fatigue or implant fracture, and implant loosening at bone implant interfaces. Long segment fixation is championed with rigid fixation and creation of fusion masses that are stable. Therefore,

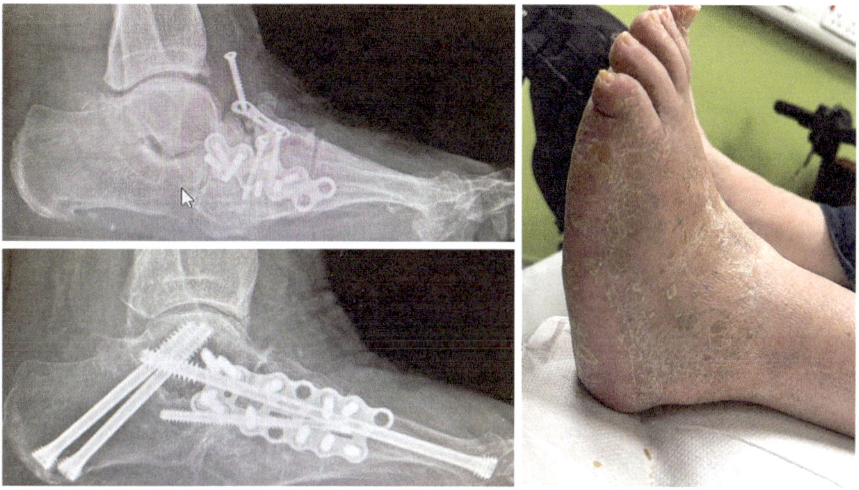

Fig. 16.12 Revision charcot reconstruction surgery, failed midfoot charcot treatment, revised using long-segment fixation

surgical factors such as metalwork position, implantation technique, bone cuts and intra-operative stability are very important. Most implants are not designed to be used with bone loss in mind, hence anatomical positioning and careful creation of stable constructs are recommended.

The key objectives of salvage are infection control, stability and ensuring vascular sufficiency. Early emergent treatment for the great pathologies in diabetes (infection and vascular disease) with local stabilisation to promote healing is at the core of the treatment pathway. A personalised treatment plan, considering compliance, anatomy, vascularity and comorbidities (see Fig. 16.12).

There is a hierarchy of adverse factors to be controlled, with infection needing to be controlled first, whereas instability may be controlled sufficiently with orthotics. Infection control and adequate vascular supply is a prerequisite for wound healing and infection control.

Conclusion

The utilisation of internal fixation (long-segment fixation) in Charcot neuroarthropathy provides a robust surgical option for managing severe deformities and instability. Advances in surgical techniques and materials continue to enhance outcomes, but patient-specific factors and complications remain key considerations.

External fixation is a recognized surgical approach for managing Charcot neuroarthropathy, particularly in cases involving severe deformities, instability, or compromised soft tissue, and may be used in conjunction with other techniques. Ongoing research is required to refine these approaches further and develop evidence-based guidelines for their use.

The key to success is a Multidisciplinary Team management of these patients as their comorbidities limit surgical opportunities and define surgical outcome.

References

1. Ahluwalia R, Vainieri E, Tam J, Sait S, Sinha A, Manu CA, Reichert I, Kavarthapu V, Edmonds M, Vas P. Surgical diabetic foot debridement: improving training and practice utilizing the traffic light principle. Int J Low Extrem Wounds. 2019;18(3):279–86. https://doi.org/10.1177/1534734619853657. Epub 2019 Jun 25
2. Simpson A, Deakin M, Latham J. Chronic osteomyelitis: the effect of the extent of surgical resection on infection-free survival. J Bone Joint Surg Br. 2001;83:403–7.
3. Langit MB, Tay KS, Al-Omar HK, et al. Surgical debridement in long bone chronic osteomyelitis: is wide tumour-like resection necessary? Bone Joint Open. 2023;4:643–51.
4. Pinzur MS. Treatment of ankle and hindfoot charcot arthropathy. Foot Ankle Clin. 2020;25:293–303.
5. Pinzur MS, Schiff AP. Deformity and clinical outcomes following operative correction of Charcot foot: a new classification with implications for treatment. Foot Ankle Int. 2018;39(3):265–70.
6. Kavarthapu V, Vris A. Charcot midfoot reconstruction—surgical technique based on deformity pattern. Ann Joint. 2020;5:28. https://doi.org/10.21037/aoj.2020.02.0.
7. Patel AS, Sivaprakasam M, Reichert ILH, et al. Reconstruction of the 'Foot at Risk' during Acute Charcot Neuroarthropathy. J Foot Ankle Surg (Asia-Pacific). 2023;10(S-1):S15–20.
8. Abar B, Kwon N, Allen NB, Lau T, Johnson LG, Gall K, Adams SB. Outcomes of surgical reconstruction using custom 3D-printed porous titanium implants for critical-sized bone defects of the foot and ankle. Foot Ankle Int. 2022;43(6):750–61.
9. Ha J, Hester T, Foley R, Reichert ILH, Vas PRJ, Ahluwalia R, Kavarthapu V. Charcot foot reconstruction outcomes: a systematic review. J Clin Orthop Trauma. 2020;11(3):357–68. https://doi.org/10.1016/j.jcot.2020.03.025. Epub 2020 Apr 20. PMID: 32405193; PMCID: PMC7211810
10. Richter M, Mittlmeier T, Rammelt S, Agren PH, Hahn S, Eschler A. Intramedullary fixation in severe Charcot osteo-neuroarthropathy with foot deformity results in adequate correction without loss of correction – results from a multi-Centre study. Foot Ankle Surg. 2015;21(4):269–76. https://doi.org/10.1016/j.fas.2015.02.003. Epub 2015 Mar 9
11. Grant WP, Garcia-Lavin S, Sabo R. Beaming the columns for Charcot diabetic foot reconstruction: a retrospective analysis. J Foot Ankle Surg. 2011;50(2):182–9. https://doi.org/10.1053/j.jfas.2010.12.002. Epub 2011 Jan 22
12. Wiewiorski M, Yasui T, Miska M, Frigg A, Valderrabano V. Solid bolt fixation of the medial column in Charcot midfoot arthropathy. J Foot Ankle Surg. 2013;52:88–94.
13. Alammar Y, Sudnitsyn A, Neretin A, et al. Closed arthrodesis in infected neuro- pathic ankles using Ilizarov ring fixation. Bone Joint Lett J. 2020;102-B:470–7.
14. Mittlmeier T, Klaue K, Haar P, et al. Should one consider primary surgical reconstruction in Charcot arthropathy of the feet? Clin Orthop Relat Res. 2010;468:1002–11.
15. Martin B, Chow J. The use of circular frame external fixation in the treatment of ankle/hindfoot Charcot Neuroarthropathy. J Clin Orthop Trauma. 2021;16:269–76.

Chapter 17
Introduction to Minimally Invasive Foot and Ankle Surgery

T. L. Lewis and R. Ray

Introduction to Minimally Invasive Foot and Ankle Surgery

Minimally invasive surgery (MIS), also known as percutaneous surgery, has become increasingly popular for treating a wide range of foot and ankle pathologies including hallux valgus (HV), hallux rigidus, insertional achilles tendinopathy and pes planus amongst others. Minimally invasive surgery requires specific equipment designed for working through small incisions. This includes a high-torque, low-speed burr to perform osteotomies as well as different types of burr design depending on the intended use. The Shannon burr is a cutting burr used to perform osteotomies whilst the wedge burr is used to remove bony prominences (Fig. 17.1). Irrigation is important to reduce the risk of thermal injury to bone which may lead to complications such as non-union or skin damage.

Minimally invasive surgery offers several key benefits compared to open procedures. These advantages primarily stem from the reduced surgical trauma associated with MIS techniques:

- smaller incisions and less scarring
- reduced soft tissue disruption
- reduced postoperative pain and faster recovery

Despite being less invasive, studies suggest that MIS techniques can achieve similar clinical and radiographic outcomes to open procedures for a wide range of foot deformities and pathologies [1].

T. L. Lewis · R. Ray (✉)
King's Foot and Ankle Unit, King's College Hospital NHS Foundation Trust, London, UK
e-mail: robbie.ray2@nhs.net

M. Bhatia (ed.), *Surgical Techniques of the Foot and Ankle*,
https://doi.org/10.1007/978-3-031-93742-2_17

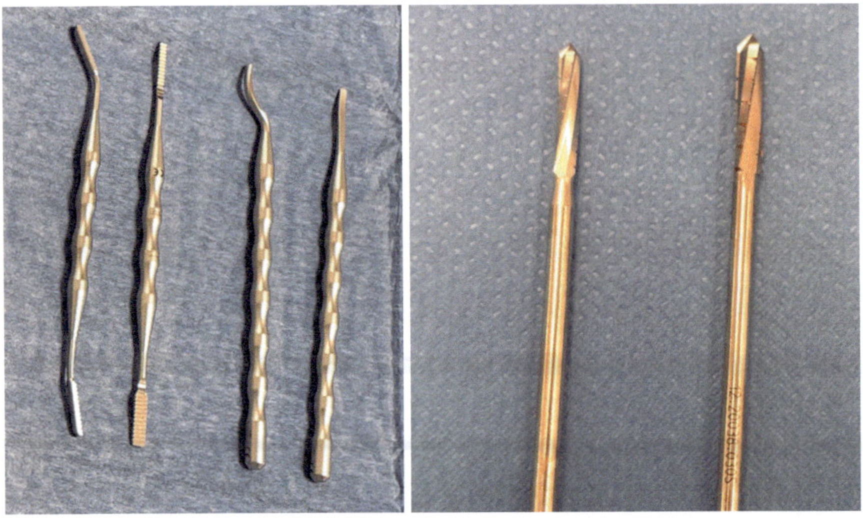

Fig. 17.1 Left: Instruments required for MIS including periosteal elevators and rasps. Right: Common burrs used for MIS (shannon cutting burr and wedge resection burr)

This chapter will explore the surgical techniques for five common pathologies that are amenable to treatment with minimally invasive techniques; hallux valgus, hallux rigidus, lesser toe deformity, calcaneal osteotomy and insertional achilles tendinopathy.

Setup and Positioning

Optimal patient positioning is crucial for successful minimally invasive surgery (MIS), ensuring both surgeon ergonomics and optimal access to the surgical field. For forefoot procedures a supine position is preferred with the patient positioned with their feet extending off the end of the operating table, allowing for natural plantarflexion at the ankle [14]. This facilitates obtaining a true anteroposterior view of the foot during intraoperative fluoroscopy (Fig. 17.2). A true lateral view can usually be achieved through ankle supination or, in cases of limited ankle flexibility, by externally rotating and flexing the knee. The use of a leg support to elevate the non-operative leg can create additional space for the surgeon and imaging.

For hindfoot procedures, a lateral position is preferred with the use of an additional leg support. The lateral position allows assessment of both AP/lateral as well as axial hindfoot views as needed.

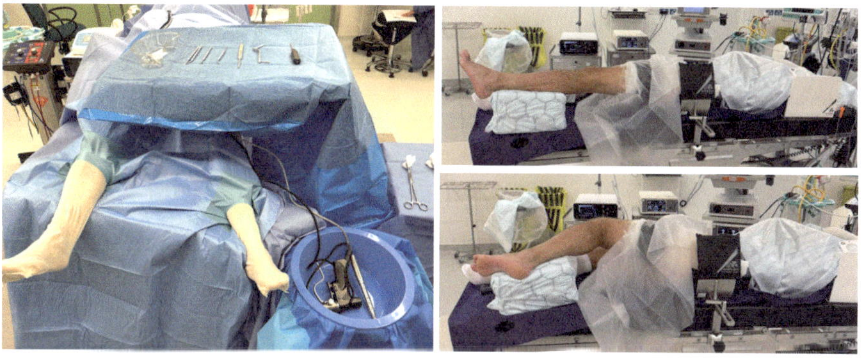

Fig. 17.2 Photo of positioning for forefoot (left) and hindfoot (right)

Hallux Valgus

One of the main uses for minimally invasive techniques is addressing hallux valgus deformity. This procedure can be used to correct mild to severe hallux valgus deformity[12, 13, 16].

Patient Positioning: The patient is placed in a supine position on the operating table, with the feet extending off the end of the table. Antibiotics and tranexamic acid are administered. A thigh tourniquet is typically used, inflated to 300 mmHg to provide a bloodless surgical field.

Incisions: Four small (<3 mm) percutaneous incisions are The first incision is made just proximal to the medial eminence at the flare of the first MT neck. Three further incisions are made; one at the level of the MTPJ, one for the Akin osteotomy site, and the final incision at the level of the TMTJ. All incisions are made using a beaver blade and careful dissection to the bone to reduce risk of neurovascular injury.

Transverse Osteotomy: Under fluoroscopic guidance, a percutaneous transverse osteotomy is performed at the neck of the first metatarsal, just proximal to the capsule, using a 2 × 20-mm Shannon burr. The osteotomy is made in two halves, dorsal and plantar, using a combination of rotating and translating movements with the burr (Fig. 17.3).

Metatarsal Head Correction: After the osteotomy, a 3D Reduction manoeuvre is performed using a reduction tool to correct the intermetatarsal angle, hallux valgus angle and pronation. Once the head position has been confirmed, two guide wires are inserted from the proximal aspect of the first metatarsal into the metatarsal head. The optimal configuration is one bicortical wire and one intramedullary wire [15]. It is important to ensure there is a bony bridge between the screws to reduce the risk of lateral wall fracture. It is important to ensure that the wire is only passed through the lateral cortex once as 'pepper potting' the lateral cortex increases the risk of fracture and subsequent loss of position (Fig. 17.4).

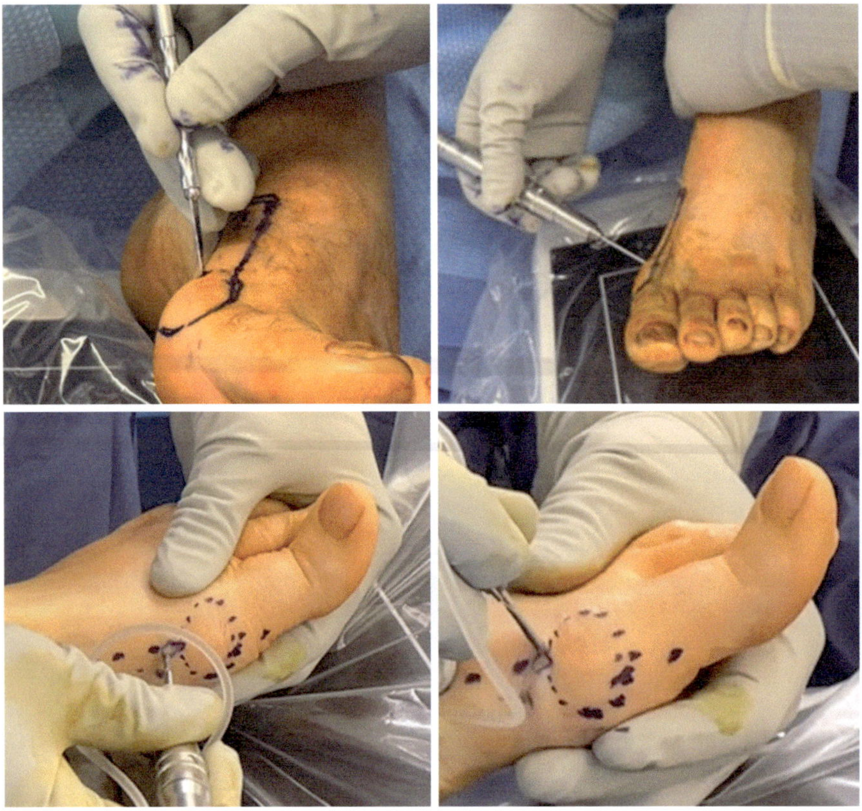

Fig. 17.3 Percutaneous distal first metatarsal transverse osteotomy

Screw fixation: These wires are overdrilled and then the osteotomy is fixed with two cannulated 4 mm compression screws with oblique chamfered heads (Fig. 17.5). Care needs to be taken to maintain the metatarsal head position when the screws enter the head as occasionally this can lead to distraction or loss of position [11].

Medial eminence resection: Using a 2-mm shannon burr, the medial eminence is resected. The medial ledge edge can either be compressed into the osteotomy or removed [3]. Additional prominent bone on the dorsal and medial side of the metatarsal head can be resected using a wedge burr. Copious irrigation will remove any residual bone swarf that can lead to irritation if not removed.

Akin osteotomy: A percutaneous Akin osteotomy is performed to address any residual HVA deformity. This medial closing wedge osteotomy at the base of the proximal phalanx using a 2 × 10 mm burr which is then fixed with a 3-mm compression screw. If required, a limited lateral release, involving the division of the lateral aspect of the plantar first metatarsophalangeal joint capsule and the distal

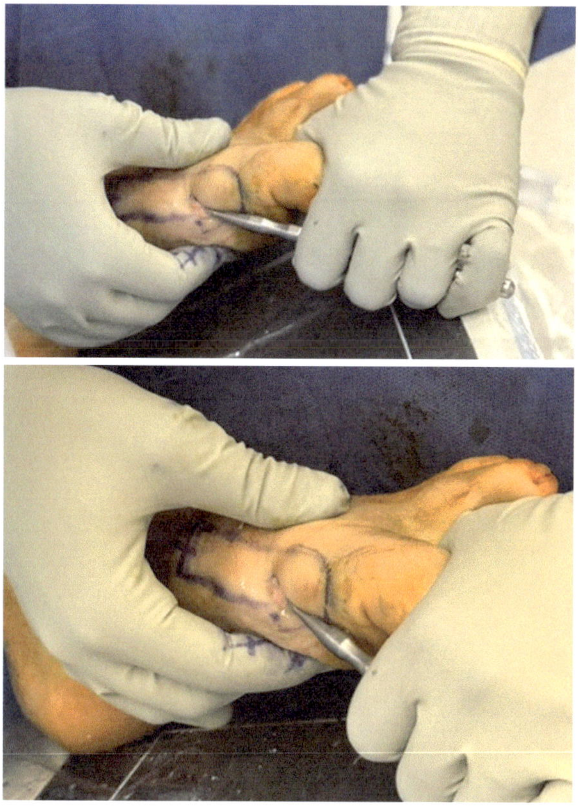

Fig. 17.4 Demonstration of three-dimensional reduction maneuver to correct coronal and frontal plane deformity of hallux valgus

attachment of the adductor hallucis tendon, may be performed to address any residual tightness and optimize joint alignment [8].

Wound Closure and Dressing: The small incisions are closed with simple absorbable sutures such as 4/0 vicryl or 4/0 monocryl. A sterile dressing is applied to the surgical site and a flat surgical shoe is applied.

Postoperative Care: Patients are allowed immediate full weight-bearing postoperatively in a surgical shoe. High elevation is key to reduce swelling and patients can transition into sneakers at 2 weeks following surgery. Active and passive hallux range-of-motion exercises are initiated at 2 weeks postoperatively to prevent stiffness. Patients are advised to wear adhesive tape to maintain hallux position for the duration of 6 weeks [21].

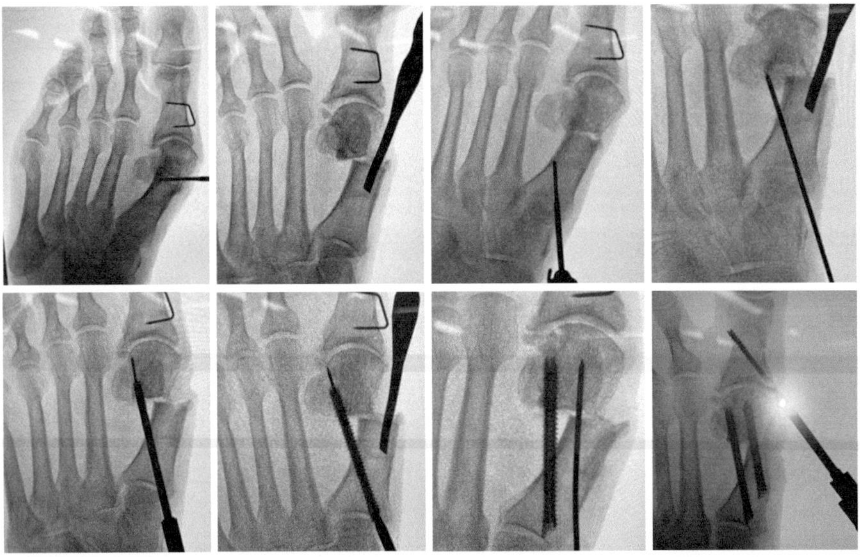

Fig. 17.5 Intraoperative fluoroscopy demonstrating the key steps of percutaneous surgery. Left to right: percutaneous transverse osteotomy, three-dimensional reduction maneuver, entry point for proximal wire, proximal wire ensuring bicortical fixation in metatarsal head, drill to ensure no distraction of head, proximal screw insertion whilst maintaining reduction, second wire and screw insertion and finally, percutaneous akin osteotomy

Hallux Rigidus

Hallux rigidus is a degenerative condition affecting the first metatarsophalangeal joint, leading to progressive stiffness, pain, and loss of motion [5]. It is a form of osteoarthritis characterized by cartilage wear, osteophyte formation, and eventual joint fusion. Treatment options range from conservative measures such as orthotics, NSAIDs, and activity modification to surgical interventions. Surgical approaches may include minimally invasive cheilectomy [2, 24] and arthroscopy [22] or arthrodesis for more advanced cases, aimed at relieving pain and restoring function (Fig. 17.6) [4].

Pre-operative Assessment

Radiographic Evaluation: Weight-bearing radiographs are used to assess the severity of Hallux Rigidus using the Coughlin and Shurnas classification. Patients with a grade of <3 are potentially candidates for joint-preservation procedures such as cheilectomy.

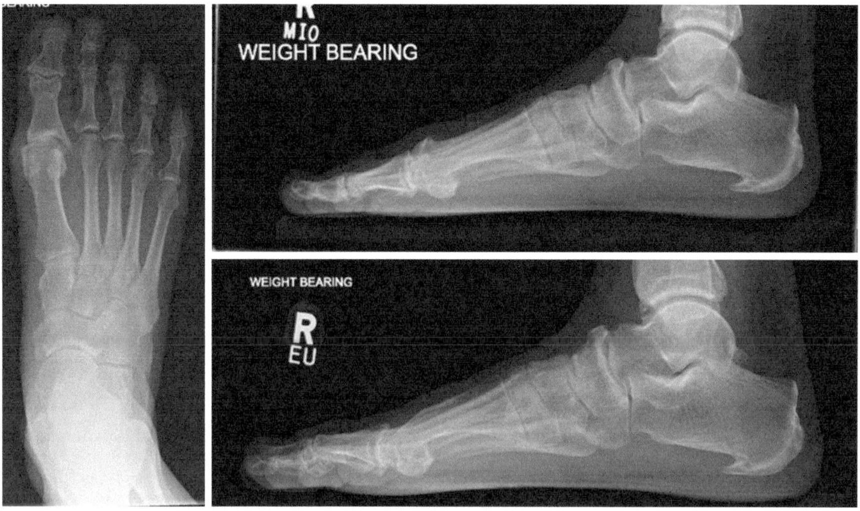

Fig. 17.6 Pre and post operative lateral radiographs demonstrating resection of the dorsal osteophyte through a percutaneous approach

Range of Motion: Assess the range of motion of the first metatarsophalangeal joint (MTPJ), particularly dorsiflexion. Surgery is not recommended for patients with more than 20° of dorsiflexion.

Interphalangeal (IP) Joint Assessment: Evaluate the IP joint for hyper-dorsiflexion. Patients with a hyperextensible IP joint may tolerate stiffness at the MTPJ better, potentially making an isolated cheilectomy sufficient.

Surgical Technique

Patient Positioning: The patient is placed in a supine position on the operating table, with the feet extending off the end of the table similar to the setup for hallux valgus. Antibiotics and tranexamic acid are administered. A thigh tourniquet is typically used, inflated to 300 mmHg to provide a bloodless surgical field. It is important to place the arthroscopy stack at the end of the bed in order to optimize the ergonomics of arthroscopy for the surgeon.

Incisions: A dorsomedial skin incision is made 2–3 cm proximal to the first MTPJ. This location allows for capsular release and osteophyte clearance from lateral to medial. A second incision is made dorsolateral proximal to the MTPJ (Fig. 17.7).

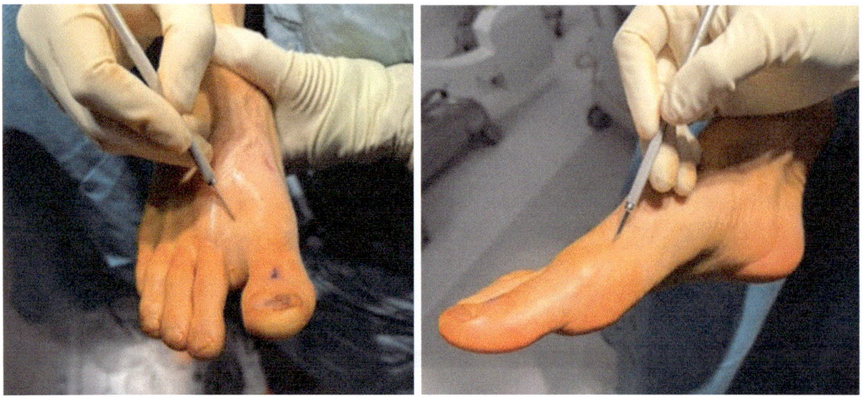

Fig. 17.7 Photographs demonstrating skin incisions for minimally invasive dorsal cheilectomy

Creation of Safe Plane and Capsular Release

It is important to establish a safe plane down to the capsule without injuring the dorsomedial cutaneous nerve at the level of the first metatarsal neck [23]. A minimally invasive periosteal elevator is recommended, keeping the blade in line with the incision to minimize nerve damage. Elevate the periosteum distally to reach the dorsomedial capsule. Puncture the proximal dorsomedial capsule with the elevator and direct it intra-capsularly towards the lateral joint aspect, releasing the capsule from lateral to medial. Ensure complete release of the dorsal capsule from its attachment to the metatarsal head as this will protect EHL from the burr.

Osteophyte Resection: Utilize a wedge burr (minimum size 2.9 mm) for osteophyte resection. The conical shape of the wedge burr facilitates both cutting and grinding, allowing for efficient removal of bone.

The primary burr sweep should create a plane between the osteophyte and the metatarsal head, cutting from lateral to medial, (an inside out technique). Using the dorsal surface of the metatarsal as a guide for the burr can help to create a flat cut. Aim to remove approximately 20–30% of the joint. Care needs to be taken to avoid damaging the joint with the burr. Distract the first MTPJ during the osteotomy to prevent burr injury to the base of the proximal phalanx (Fig. 17.8).

Removal of Dorsal Fragment and Irrigation: After completing the osteotomy, gently place your index and middle fingers over the dorsal fragment on either side of the extensor hallucis longus tendon to stabilize it. The fragment can either be removed or burred away using upward pressure on the burr to thin and resect the dorsal fragment. Copious irrigation with a 20 ml syringe and 18G blunt needle is crucial for removing bone paste and debris whilst a rasp can be used to assist with fragment removal, pulling the dorsal sliver towards the portal. Alternatively a straight mosquito artery clip can then be used to remove any remaining dorsal cortex fragment.

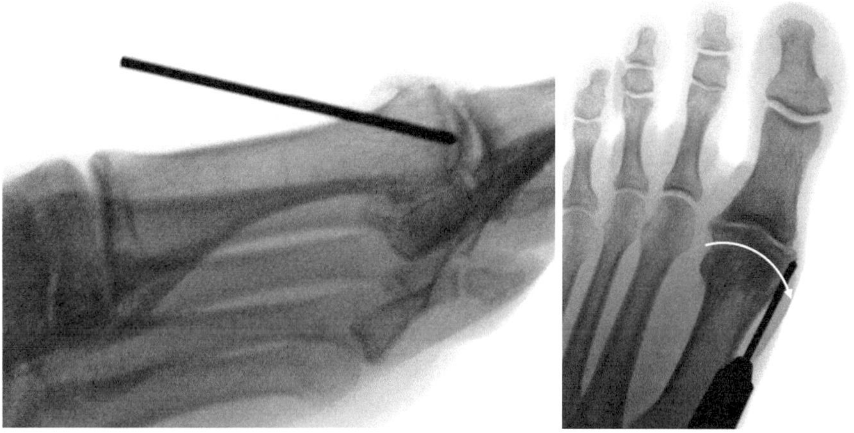

Fig. 17.8 Intraoperative fluoroscopy demonstrating burr position and direction of movement for a percutaneous dorsal cheilectomy aiming to remove the dorsal third of the first MTPJ head

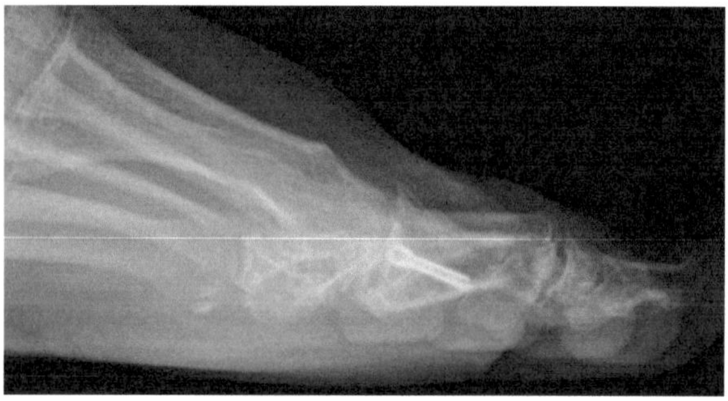

Fig. 17.9 Lateral radiograph demonstrating a percutaneous dorsal cheilectomy and Moberg osteotomy

Moberg-Akin Osteotomy: A Moberg-Akin osteotomy is performed to help improve dorsiflexion and ROM of the first MTPJ. The Moberg osteotomy is performed using a 2 mm × 12 mm Shannon burr. Care is taken to carefully resect all of the dorsal cortex followed by the plantar lateral and plantar medial corners while leaving the central plantar cortex intact. The osteotomy is closed whilst a 1.1 mm cannulated screw guidewire is inserted from the medial base of the proximal phalanx. The wire is aimed slightly more dorsally to facilitate closure of the osteotomy when the screw is tightened. The guidewire is advanced through the far cortex while digital pressure is used to hold the osteotomy closed. The near cortex is overdrilled, but not the far cortex, to utilise a glide-hole technique and help with closure when the screw is tightened. A 2.9 mm screw is then inserted to fix the osteotomy (Fig. 17.9).

First Metatarsal Joint Arthroscopy: There is some discussion regarding the value of performing first MTPJ arthroscopic assistance to ensure thorough debris clearance and visualization of the joint. This can involve irrigation with large volumes of saline (3–6 liters) and inspection of the joint surfaces and remaining cartilage.

Wound Closure: Inspect the wound for any burr or thermal damage, excising the skin edges if necessary. Close the wounds with either a 4/0 monocryl or 3/0 vicryl subcuticular suture. Dress the foot with gauze, wool, and crepe, and place it in a flat surgical shoe.

Postoperative Management

Patients are allowed to weight-bear as tolerated in a postoperative shoe and elevate the foot for the first 2 weeks to minimize swelling and then encouraged to perform gentle range of motion exercises once the wound has healed. Patients can gradually transition to supportive footwear and increase activity as tolerated.

Operative Guide: Management of Lesser Toe Deformity Using Percutaneous Techniques

Percutaneous or minimally invasive surgery techniques for managing lesser toe deformities (hammer toe, mallet toe, and claw toe) provide effective solutions for deformity correction whilst reducing soft tissue dissection and scarring [20, 22, 25]. Deformity correction can be achieved through a combination of osteotomies, fusions and tendon/soft tissue releases.

Preoperative Planning

Radiographic assessment: Weight-bearing X-rays of the foot to assess deformity severity, joint congruity, and presence of any arthritic changes can be used to guide surgical decision making.

Physical examination: Determine the flexibility of the deformity to guide surgical planning (flexible deformities may be treatable with soft tissue procedures alone; rigid deformities typically required arthrodesis).

A number of MIS surgical procedures can be utilized to correct the hammer toe deformity, either in isolation or in combination [20].

- PIPJ FDB release
- Proximal phalangeal (P1) basal osteotomy
- PIPJ/DIPJ fusion with intramedullary screw
- Distal metaphyseal metatarsal osteotomy (DMMO)
- MTPJ soft tissue procedures (capsular release, tenotomy, and tendon lengthening)

The procedure choice or combination will depend on the flexibility of the PIPJ deformity and the stability of the MTPJ.

Patient Positioning

Similar to other forefoot deformity correction procedures using minimally invasive surgery, the patient is positioned supine on the operating table with a bump under the ipsilateral hip to elevate the operative foot and allow access for imaging. Antibiotics and tranexamic acid are administered. A thigh tourniquet is typically used, inflated to 300 mmHg.

PIPJ FDB Release

A small incision is made with a beaver blade at the level of the PIPJ. The blade is swept along the inferior aspect of the proximal phalanx to detach the FDB tendon.

Proximal phalangeal (P1) basal osteotomy: A 2 mm incision is made using a beaver blade at the dorsomedial aspect of the base of the proximal phalanx. An irrigated 2.0 × 8 mm burr set at low speed and high torque is used and positioned on the dorsomedial cortex at the metaphyseal flare of the base of the proximal phalanx just medial to the extensor digitorum longus (EDL) tendon. The position is confirmed on the image intensifier. The burr is then inserted through the dorsomedial cortex as far as the plantar lateral cortex without perforating the lateral cortex. It is important to keep the dorsolateral cortex intact. The burr is then passed through the plantar lateral cortex before completing the osteotomy through the plantar cortex. It is important that the plantar lateral cortex is osteotomised as this tends to be thicker and without division the osteotomy cannot close down. To achieve this the burr is swept medially, taking care to avoid over penetration, which would risk damage to the tendon and neurovascular structures. Finally the burr is rotated medially to complete the osteotomy of the medial cortex The direction of the osteotomy can be adjusted as required in order to correct any coronal or sagittal plane deformity (Fig. 17.10) [19].

PIPJ/DIPJ fusion with intramedullary screw: Use a small skin incision at the PIP or DIP joint and introduce the wedge burr under fluoroscopy. The burr can be used to excise the joint by grinding the cartilage into bone swarf which can be removed with copious irrigation. A 2 mm k-wire or the 2 mm shannon burr can be used to create an entry path for the intramedullary screw. For a PIPJ fusion, the screw should be anchored in the subchondral bone of the DIPJ to reduce risk of losing position.

Distal Metaphyseal Metatarsal osteotomy (DMMO)

This procedure can be used to shorten the lesser metatarsals and allow a subluxed or dislocated MTPJ to reduce. A small incision is made at the lateral aspect of the neck of M2/M3/M4. The periosteum surrounding the bone at the site of the planned

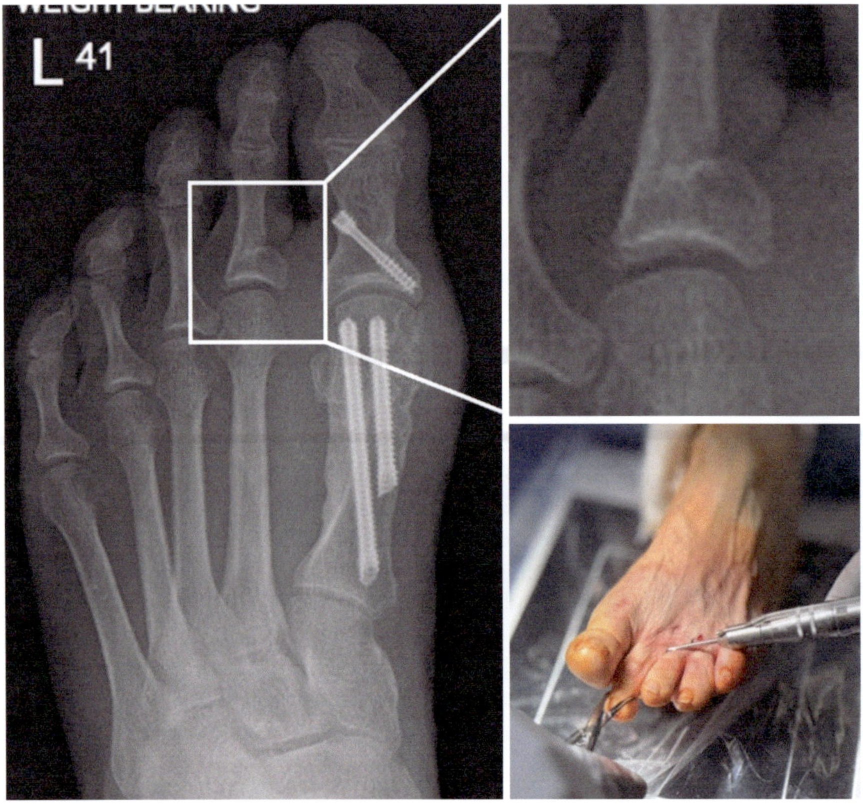

Fig. 17.10 Percutaneous proximal phalanx P1 osteotomy demonstrating a medial closing wedge to correct lesser toe deformity

osteotomy is then detached using an elevator. An extraarticular osteotomy is performed using a 2.0 × 12.0 mm shannon burr slightly more proximally than the Weil osteotomy and begins 2–3 mm from the articular surface in the neck area. The surgeon initially makes a 45° cut to shorten and elevate the MT head. By rotating the burr, a clear osteotomy can be performed and confirmed using imaging (Figs. 17.11 and 17.12).

Closure and Postoperative Management: Close the small stab incisions with Steri-Strips or absorbable sutures. Taping is important for 6 weeks following surgery to ensure the deformity correction is maintained and reduce the risk of floating toes. Apply a bulky, non-compressive dressing with gauze to protect the wounds. Patients are allowed to fully weight-bearing in a post-operative shoe for 2 weeks.

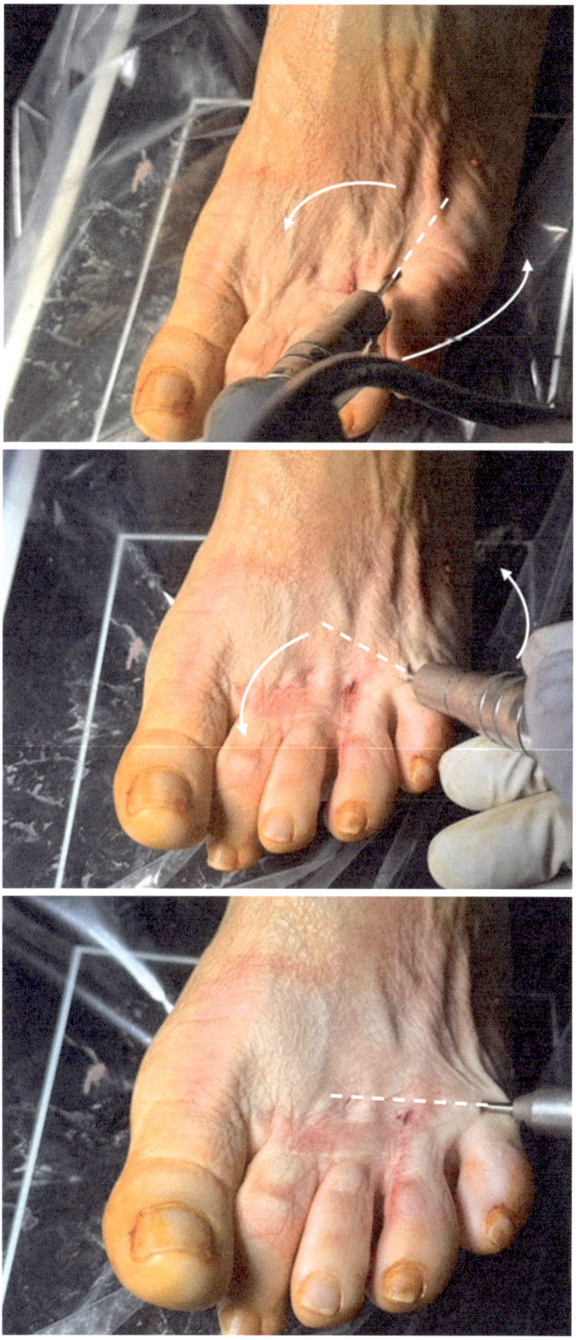

Fig. 17.11 Sequence of hand positions to perform DMMO's. Left to right: Starting oblique neck cut. Hand moving from in line with metatarsal to across metatarsal finishing at 90° to metatarsal to create chevron osteotomy

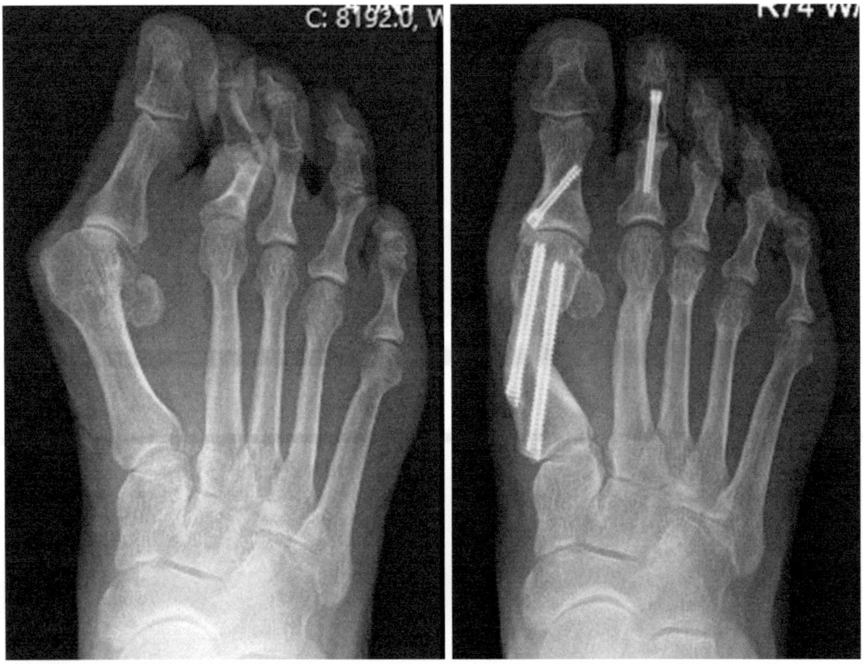

Fig. 17.12 Pre and postoperative radiographs demonstrating percutaneous hallux valgus correction and associated DMMO's of 2/3/4 metatarsals

Minimally Invasive calcaneal Osteotomy

Minimally invasive calcaneal osteotomy is a procedure performed to correct hindfoot malalignment, typically varus or valgus deformities [6]. This guide details the intraoperative steps for performing a minimally invasive medializing (for valgus deformity) or lateralizing (for varus deformity) calcaneal osteotomy. This is typically performed as part of a wider hindfoot reconstruction and this guide focuses on the calcaneal osteotomy alone.

Positioning: All hindfoot minimally invasive procedures are performed with the patient in the lateral position with a bolster to ensure that the hindfoot is parallel to the floor. A tourniquet is used alongside tranexamic acid and intravenous antibiotics.

Incision: Palpate and mark the posterior superior corner of the calcaneus, along with the planned osteotomy site (typically 1–2 cm posterior to the subtalar joint line).

Use fluoroscopy to confirm appropriate placement of the osteotomy plane, usually perpendicular to the axis of the calcaneus. It can also be helpful to mark out the planned location of the hindfoot screws. A small incision (3–4 mm) on the lateral aspect of the heel, posterior to the peroneal tendons and above the sural nerve.

Bluntly dissect through soft tissues down to the bone.

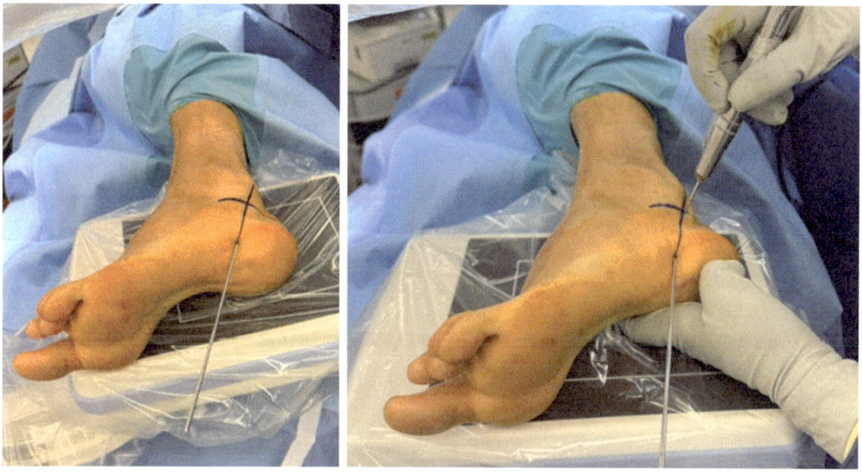

Fig. 17.13 Guidewire inserted subcutaneously under fluoroscopic guidance at the desired angle for the osteotomy (usually perpendicular to the calcaneus) in order to protect the subtalar joint (left). This is used as a guide for the burr (right)

Guidewire Placement: Insert a guidewire under fluoroscopic guidance at the desired angle for the osteotomy (usually perpendicular to the calcaneus). This will protect the subtalar joint (Fig. 17.13).

Osteotomy: A periosteal elevator is used to clear the soft tissues around the planned osteotomy. Using a 2.0 × 30.0 mm shannon burr, make the calcaneal osteotomy along the guidewire, maintaining the plane perpendicular to the calcaneal axis. Due to the length of the cutting flutes, it may be necessary to cut the near cortex first and then proceed to use this as a guide for the distal cortex. Care must be taken to avoid bending the burr as this can lead to the burr breaking. Fluoroscopy can be used to confirm the osteotomy completion (Fig. 17.14).

Mobilizing the Calcaneus

In order to mobilise the calcaneus, a laminar spreader can be inserted through the incision and used to mobilize the osteotomized calcaneal fragment. In order to shift the calcaneus, an elevator can be inserted through the incision and used to lever the fragment either medially or laterally as needed. Confirm the amount of correction via fluoroscopy by checking the position of the calcaneal tuberosity in relation to the talus and ankle axis.

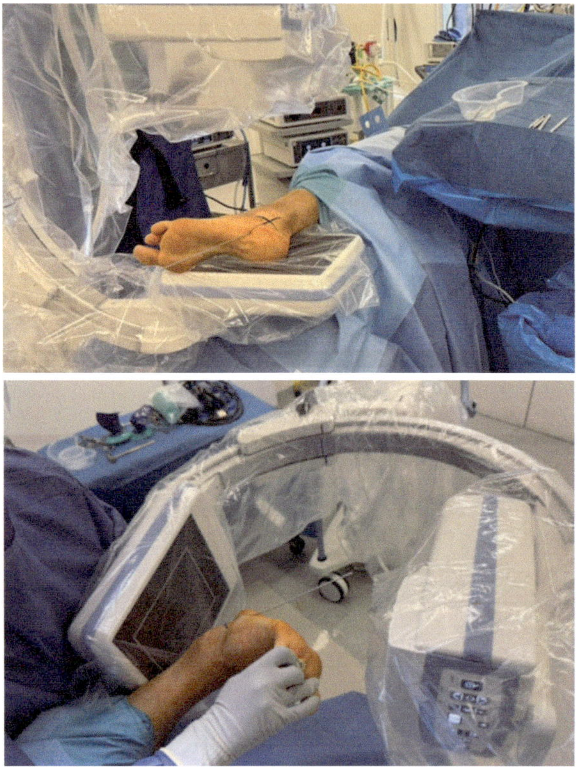

Fig. 17.14 Guidewire placement for fixation can be checked on a true lateral and then by rotating the c-arm to parallel to the floor, an axial calcaneal view can be achieved without adjusting the leg

Fixation

Once the desired position is achieved, insert one or two K-wires across the osteotomy site to temporarily stabilize the fragment.

Using fluoroscopy, insert one or two cannulated screws from posterior to anterior, ensuring purchase across both the superior and inferior aspects of the osteotomy.

Confirm the screw placement and alignment on both lateral and axial fluoroscopy views (Fig. 17.15).

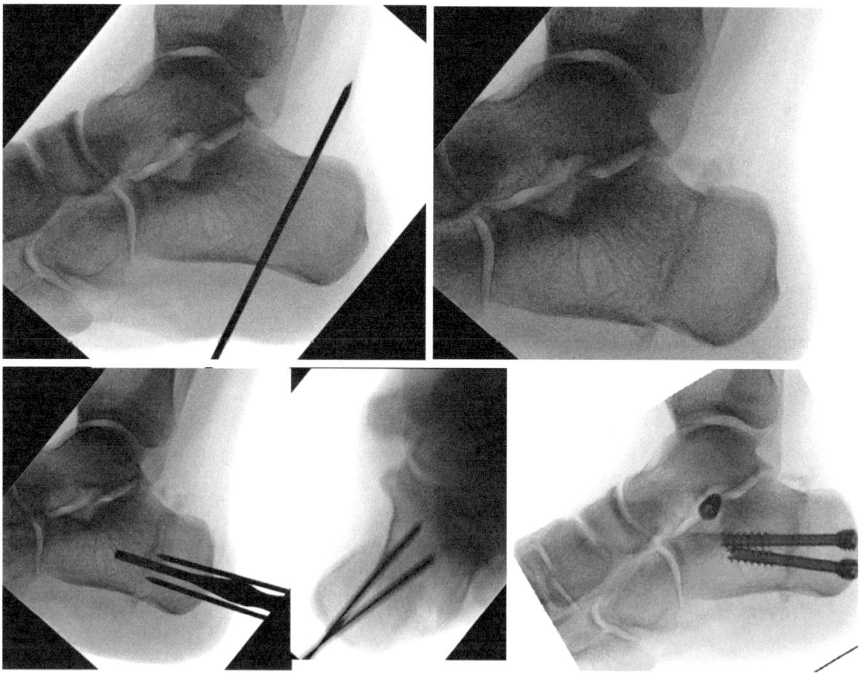

Fig. 17.15 Top row demonstrates intraoperative fluoroscopy demonstrating guidewire placement, and MIS calcaneal osteotomy. The bottom row demonstrate a medial calcaneal shift, axial view and fixation using partially threaded cannulated screws

Wound Closure

The small lateral and posterior heel wounds can be closed using a 4/0 monocryl or 3/0 vicryl rapide. Patients are typically placed in a non-weight bearing in a below knee backslab.

Postoperative Protocol

This depends on the concurrent pathology being treated alongside the calcaneal osteotomy.

Percutaneous Zadek Osteotomy for Insertional Achilles Tendinopathy

The Zadek osteotomy, or dorsal closing wedge calcaneal osteotomy, is primarily used to treat insertional achilles tendinopathy [7, 17, 18]. The procedure involves removing a wedge of bone from the posterior aspect of the calcaneus to reduce the prominence of the heel spur and relieve tension on the tendon. This guide details the steps for performing this procedure using a percutaneous technique, which minimizes soft tissue damage, promotes faster recovery, and reduces complications.

Positioning: This operation is performed with the patient in the lateral position with a bolster to ensure that the hindfoot is parallel to the floor. A tourniquet is used alongside tranexamic acid and intravenous antibiotics.

Incision: Palpate and mark the planned osteotomy site (typically 1–2 cm posterior to the subtalar joint line). Use fluoroscopy to confirm appropriate placement of the dorsal closing wedge apex and osteotomy plan [9]. It can also be helpful to mark out the planned location of the hindfoot screws with the insertion distal to the bone spur. A small incision (3–4 mm) on the lateral aspect of the heel, posterior to the peroneal tendons and above the sural nerve. Bluntly dissect through soft tissues down to the bone and free the soft tissues over the osteotomy site using an elevator.

Guidewire Placement: Insert two guidewires under fluoroscopic guidance at the desired angle for the osteotomy in order to create space for the dorsal closing wedge osteotomy .

Osteotomy: Using a 3.0 × 30.0 mm shannon burr, make the calcaneal osteotomy along the guidewires. Due to the length of the cutting flutes, it may be necessary to cut the near cortex first and then proceed to use this as a guide for the distal cortex. It is important to maintain the plantar cortex integrity. Multiple bony passess will be needed to clear enough bone [10]. Aim for a width of ~1 cm at the dorsal aspect of the closing wedge. Failure to remove enough bone may reduce the effectiveness of the operation. Fluoroscopy can be used to confirm the osteotomy completion. Irrigation is needed to ensure all bone swarf is removed.

Mobilizing the Calcaneus

In order to close the calcaneus dorsal closing wedge osteotomy, the foot is dorsiflexed. The tension of the achilles will lead to closure of the osteotomy. Confirm the osteotomy is closing appropriately via fluoroscopy (Fig. 17.16).

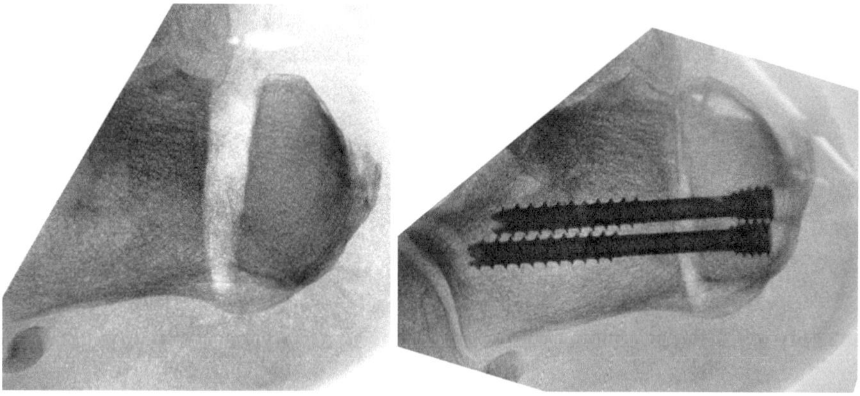

Fig. 17.16 Intraoperative fluoroscopy demonstrating the calcaneal dorsal closing wedge Zadek osteotomy with subsequent closure and fixation using partially threaded cannulated screws

Fixation

Once the desired position is achieved, insert two K-wires across the osteotomy site to temporarily stabilize the osteotomy. Using fluoroscopy, insert two cannulated screws from posterior to anterior, with the insertion point below the insertion of the Achilles tendon. Confirm the screw placement and alignment on both lateral and axial fluoroscopy views.

Wound Closure and Postoperative Protocol

The small lateral and posterior heel wounds can be closed using a 4/0 monocryl or 4/0 vicryl rapide. Patients are typically placed non-weight bearing in a below knee backslab for 2 weeks before being allowed to fully weight bear in a boot from weeks 2–6.

Conclusion

Minimally invasive foot and ankle surgery may potentially offer significant advantages in treating a range of foot and ankle pathologies while minimizing soft tissue trauma potentially reducing recovery time. This chapter has outlined key MIS techniques for addressing hallux valgus, hallux rigidus, lesser toe deformities, hindfoot malalignment and the Zadek osteotomy. Mastery of MIS techniques will equip surgeons with effective tools for addressing a range of pathologies in addition to standard open procedures.

References

1. Alimy A-R, Polzer H, Ocokoljic A, et al. Does minimally invasive surgery provide better clinical or radiographic outcomes than open surgery in the treatment of hallux Valgus deformity? A systematic review and meta-analysis. Clin Orthop Relat Res. 2023;481:1143–55.
2. Esser K, Butler JJ, Roof M, et al. Outcomes following minimally invasive dorsal cheilectomy for hallux rigidus: a systematic review. World J Orthop. 2024;15:585–92.
3. Ferreira GF, Nunes GA, Mattos E, Dinato MC, et al. Technique tip: medial prominence bone spur resection in the third-generation percutaneous Chevron-Akin Osteotomy Technique (PECA) for hallux valgus correction. Foot Ankle Surg. 2022;28:460–3.
4. Ferreira GF, Pedroso JP, Nunes GA, et al. Treatment of hallux rigidus with percutaneous metatarsophalangeal arthrodesis: a case series with a minimum follow-up of 2 years. Arch Orthop Trauma Surg. 2023; https://doi.org/10.1007/s00402-023-04948-1.
5. Gauthier C, Lewis T, O'Keefe J, et al. Minimally invasive Dorsal cheilectomy and Hallux metatarsophalangeal joint arthroscopy for the treatment of Hallux Rigidus. Foot Ankle Surg. 2024; https://doi.org/10.1016/j.fas.2024.02.011.
6. Gutteck N, Zeh A, Wohlrab D, Delank K-S. Comparative results of percutaneous calcaneal osteotomy in correction of Hindfoot deformities. Foot Ankle Int. 2019;40:276–81.
7. Hall S, Schipper O, Kaplan JRM, et al. Outcomes after percutaneous zadek osteotomy for insertional Achilles tendinopathy. Foot Ankle Int. 2024;45:931–9.
8. Izzo A, Vallefuoco S, Basso MA, et al. Role of lateral soft tissue release in percutaneous hallux valgus surgery: a systematic review and meta-analysis of the literature. Arch Orthop Trauma Surg. 2022; https://doi.org/10.1007/s00402-022-04693-x.
9. Kaplan JRM, Hall S, Schipper ON, et al. Percutaneous Zadek osteotomy for insertional Achilles tendinopathy and Haglund deformity: a technique tip. Foot Ankle Int. 2023;44:931–5.
10. Karaismailoglu B, Nassour N, Duggan J, et al. Effect of sequential burr passes on osteotomy magnitude and calcaneal morphology in minimally invasive Zadek osteotomy. Foot Ankle Surg. 2023; https://doi.org/10.1016/j.fas.2023.10.009.
11. Lewis TL, Ray R, Miller G, Gordon DJ. Third-generation minimally invasive Chevron and akin osteotomies (MICA) in Hallux Valgus surgery: two-year follow-up of 292 cases. J Bone Joint Surg Am. 2021a;103:1203–11.
12. Lewis TL, Ray R, Robinson P, et al. Percutaneous Chevron and Akin (PECA) osteotomies for severe hallux valgus deformity with mean 3-year follow-up. Foot Ankle Int. 2021b;42:1231–40.
13. Lewis TL, Ray R, Gordon DJ. Minimally invasive surgery for severe hallux valgus in 106 feet. Foot Ankle Surg. 2022;28:503–9.
14. Lewis TL, Alkhalfan Y, Ferreira GF, et al. Optimizing the operating room setup for minimally invasive forefoot surgery: technical tip. Foot Ankle Orthop. 2023;8:24730114231198235.
15. Lewis TL, Mansur H, Ferreira GF, et al. Comparative biomechanical study of different screw fixation methods for minimally invasive hallux valgus surgery: a finite element analysis. Foot Ankle Surg. 2024; https://doi.org/10.1016/j.fas.2024.09.001.
16. Lewis TL, Barakat A, Mangwani J, et al. Current concepts of fourth-generation minimally invasive and open hallux valgus surgery. Bone Joint J. 2025;107-B:10–8.
17. Nordio A, Chan JJ, Guzman JZ, et al. Percutaneous Zadek osteotomy for the treatment of insertional Achilles tendinopathy. Foot Ankle Surg. 2020;26:818–21.
18. Poutoglidou F, Drummond I, Patel A, et al. Clinical outcomes and complications of the Zadek calcaneal osteotomy in Insertional Achilles Tendinopathy: a systematic review and meta-analysis. Foot Ankle Surg. 2023;29:298–305.
19. Ray R, Lewis TL, Robinson P, et al. Valgus second toe deformity treated with a percutaneous extracapsular closing-wedge osteotomy of the proximal phalanx. Foot Ankle Int. 2022;43:1157–66.
20. Reaney A, Koç T, Lewis TL, Gordon D. Management of hammer toe deformities using percutaneous surgical techniques. Clin Podiatr Med Surg. 2024; https://doi.org/10.1016/j.cpm.2024.06.001.

21. Robinson PW, Lam P. Percutaneous correction of mild to severe hallux Valgus defomity: the evolution and current concepts of the PECA technique. In: Percutaneous and minimally invasive foot surgery. Cham: Springer International Publishing; 2023. p. 101–23.
22. Schipper ON, Day J, Ray GS, Johnson AH. Percutaneous techniques in orthopedic foot and ankle surgery. Orthop Clin North Am. 2020;51:403–22.
23. Teoh KH, Haanaes EK, Alshalawi S, et al. Minimally invasive dorsal Cheilectomy of the first metatarsal: a cadaveric study. Foot Ankle Int. 2018a;39:1497–501.
24. Teoh KH, Tan WT, Atiyah Z, et al. Clinical outcomes following minimally invasive dorsal Cheilectomy for Hallux Rigidus. Foot Ankle Int. 2018b;40:195–201.
25. Vernois J, Redfern D, Mifas GS. Lesser toes deformities: a percutaneous approach. Tech Foot Ankle Surg. 2020;19:69–75.

Chapter 18
Ankle Fracture and Syndesmotic Fixation Techniques

Nikolaos Gougoulias and Anthony Sakellariou

Introduction

The term "ankle fractures" refers to a variety of osseous and soft tissue injuries involving the anatomic region of the tibial and fibular malleoli, and the tibiotalar (ankle) joint, and which are usually the result of rotational injuries in combination with axial loading [1, 2].

In the past these have been described as "malleolar fractures" and were considered as "simple" injuries to treat, usually operated on by the less experienced. Management of these common injuries has received considerable attention by the orthopaedic and traumatology community in the last 15 years, as has the realisation that these injuries are a lot more complex than previously thought [3]. A study from a major trauma centre in the United Kingdom revealed some very interesting results. The malreduction rate of operatively treated ankle fractures was as high as 44% and the major complication rate was 11% in 2015. "System change", introducing specialist foot and ankle trauma operating lists, resulted in dramatic reduction of malreductions to 2.4% and complications to 1% 2 years later [4].

Thus, several dogmata [5] were revisited and research (basic science, cadaveric, and clinical) introduced new insights into the understanding of ankle fractures. The complexity of these injuries lies within the complexity of ankle joint anatomy that involves three bones (tibia, fibula, talus), and multiple ligamentous stabilizing structures.

Stability is the key issue in guiding the decision making regarding nonoperative vs operative management [3, 6–8]. Stable fractures can be safely treated

N. Gougoulias
General Hospital of Katerini, Katerini, Greece
e-mail: talus@doctors.org.uk

A. Sakellariou (✉)
Frimley Health NHS Foundation Trust, Frimley Park Hospital, Frimley, UK

M. Bhatia (ed.), *Surgical Techniques of the Foot and Ankle*,
https://doi.org/10.1007/978-3-031-93742-2_18

nonoperatively, allowing early weight bearing, whilst weight bearing anteroposterior ankle radiographs have been shown to be very helpful for the initial assessment of stability of isolated distal fibula fractures [3, 9]. CT scans are essential for preoperative planning of unstable fractures, allowing diagnosis of all elements of the injury (including assessment of morphology of bony fragments, but also of the alignment/displacement of the distal tibiofibular syndesmosis) [1, 2].

Surgical fixation, indicated for unstable fractures, aims to restore the normal anatomy and stability, allowing joint mobilisation and early weight bearing [10].

In this chapter we present the key elements of applied anatomy and biomechanics that are associated with ankle fractures, propose indications for operative management and describe the relevant surgical techniques.

Applied Clinical Anatomy and Biomechanics

The ankle joint complex, consisting of bones (lower tibia, fibula, talus), and soft tissue structures (deltoid ligament, syndesmotic ligaments, interosseous membrane), should be considered a "ring" (Fig. 18.1), in relation to injury. If it breaks in one place it remains stable, if it breaks in two or more it becomes unstable [1, 2]. Furthermore, every osseous injury has a soft tissue equivalent: (Fig. 18.1).

Osseous injury	Soft tissue injury
Medial malleolus (MM)	Deltoid ligament
Posterior malleolus (PM)	PiTFL
"Anterior malleolus" (AM)	AiTFL
Fibula Wagstaffe fracture	AiTFL

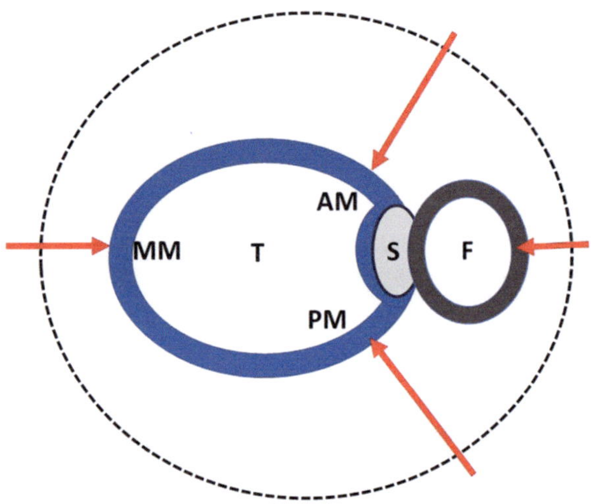

Fig. 18.1 The ankle can be considered a ring (dotted circular line). Tibia (T), and fibula (F), are connected through the syndesmotic ligaments (S). Rotational forces may cause injury (red arrows) to the fibula, the tibia [medial malleolus (MM), "posterior malleolus" (PM), "anterior malleolus" (AM), and/or the syndesmotic ligaments (S)]

It is thought that these rotational injuries follow a sequence of events depending on the position of the foot (supinated or pronated) at the time of the injury, whilst the tibia and the rest of the body, rotates externally. This is the basis of the Lauge-Hansen classification [11]. Although this is an out-dated and un-validated classification, it is still valuable as it encourages clinicians to think about and analyze the mechanism of injury which, in turn, helps predict the osseous and, most importantly—soft tissue injuries [12–14]. Analysis of what may be damaged will allow appropriate decision making to guide treatment, depending on whether the bone and soft tissue components of the injury have resulted in conversion of the stable "ankle ring" into an unstable structure.

Supination external rotation (SER) injuries start on the lateral side, resulting in partial AiTFL damage (stage 1), short oblique trans-syndesmotic fibula fracture (Weber B-type—stage 2). The more severe injuries may progress to a PM fracture and/or PiTFL injury (stage 3) and, finally, a MM fracture or deltoid ligament injury (stage 4) (Fig. 18.2). SER4 injuries can be subdivided into those causing "partial rupture", possibly only affecting the superficial deltoid (SDL), and those causing

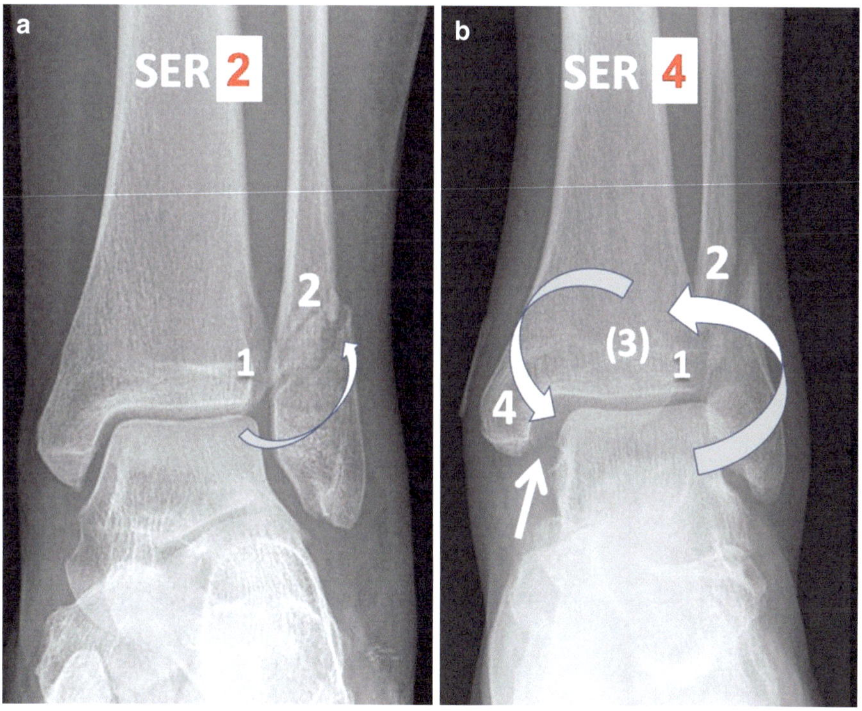

Fig. 18.2 Supination external rotation (SER) injuries may only cause injury to the lateral side (eg anterior syndesmosis (1) and fibula fracture (2), and the ankle remains stable (**a**). More severe injuries may continue damaging structures posteriorly [posterior malleolus or posterior inferior tibiofibular ligament (3)], and medially [medial malleolus or deltoid ligament (4)], producing unstable fracture patterns (**b**)

"complete" rupture, possibly affecting the deep deltoid (DDL), too [3]. Thus, some SER injuries (stages 1 & 2) may leave the medial side intact, or may not cause complete rupture of medial structures.

Pronation external rotation (PER) injuries, start on the medial side (DL injury or MM fracture—stage 1), then result in injury to the anterior syndesmosis (AiTFL—stage 2), then forces drive "upwards" damaging the central syndesmosis and the interosseous membrane resulting in a supra-syndesmotic fibula fracture (Weber C type—stage 3) whilst sometimes, in more severe injuries, forces will also cause a PM fracture—stage 4 (Fig. 18.3).

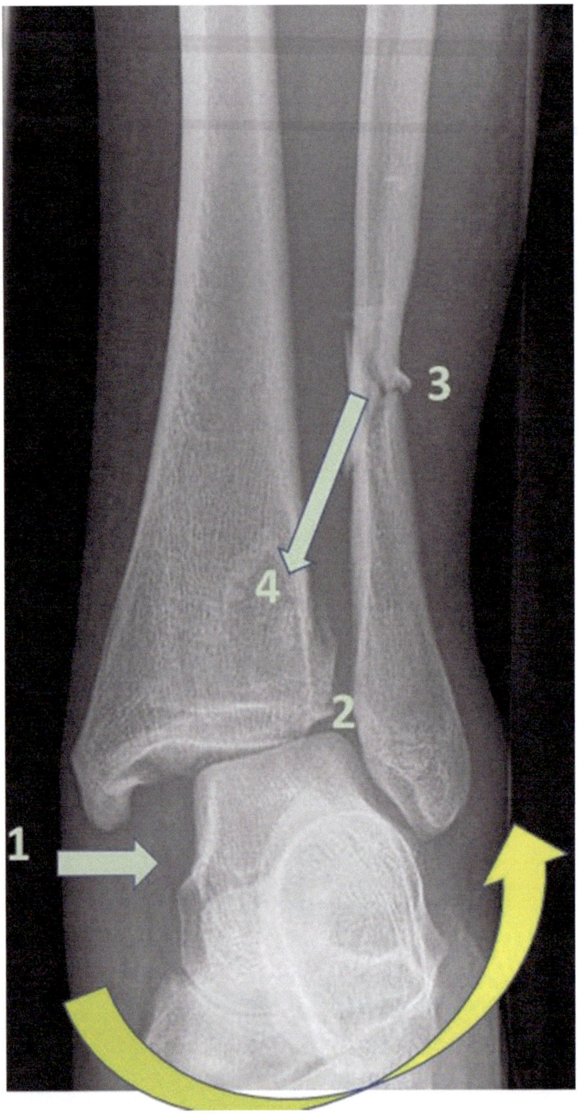

Fig. 18.3 Pronation external rotation (PER) injuries, start damaging structures medially (1), then causing syndesmosis disruption (2), followed by a suprasyndesmotic fibula fracture (3), and may finally extend posteriorly causing a posterior malleolus fracture (4)

The following questions can serve as a guide when treating an ankle fracture:

- Which bones are broken?
  - What is the level of fibula fracture (intra-, or supra-syndesmotic)?
  - Is there a medial malleolus (MM) fracture?
    - What is the morphology of the MM fracture?
  - Is there a posterior malleolus fracture? What type? Best to see the CT-based classifications [15–17].
  - Is there an anterolateral distal tibia (Chaput) avulsion fracture [18]?
  - In the presence of posterior or anterior distal tibia fracture, is the syndesmosis displaced?
- Which ligaments are injured [13]?
  - In the absence of MM fracture, is there widening of the medial clear space, indicating deltoid injury?
  - Is the syndesmosis intact?

The benefits of fixation, regardless of fracture size, arise from restoration of function of the posterior inferior tibiofibular ligament (PiTFL) and include restoration of joint congruity and stability of the syndesmosis without the potential need for trans-syndesmotic screws or suture buttons [12, 14, 19, 20]. A number of studies have supported the trend towards fixation of posterior malleolar fractures regardless of size. Cadaveric studies have shown that fixation of fragments <25% result in improvement in joint pressure distribution and neutralisation of rotational forces to the ankle joint [21], whilst a retrospective review of ankle fractures comparing those with a posterior malleolar component which were fixed and those not fixed, revealed better patient reported outcome scores in the cohort that were fixed [22].

The deltoid ligament is a multifascicular complex consisting of superficial and deep layers. The superficial layer is composed of the tibiospring, tibionavicular, superficial posterior tibiotalar, and tibiocalcaneal ligaments, and crosses the tibiotalar and subtalar joints. The deep layer includes the deep anterior tibiotalar and posterior tibiotalar ligaments and only crosses the ankle joint (Fig. 18.4). Functionally, the superficial layer resists valgus stress, the deep layer acts against lateral talar displacement, and both layers prevent talar external rotation [23]. Additionally, recent cadaveric studies indicate that the deltoid ligament is an indirect stabilizer of the syndesmosis.

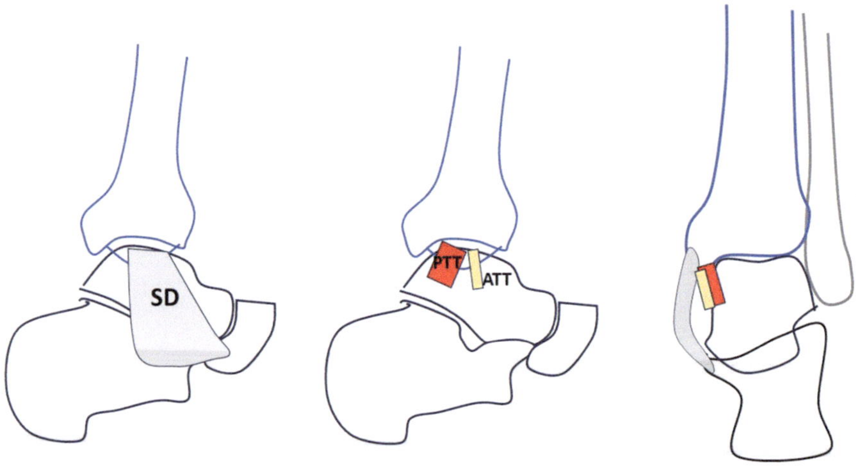

Fig. 18.4 The deltoid ligament consists of two components. The superficial (SD) attaching distal to the talus, and the deep one, attaching onto the talus, consisting of two ligaments, the anterior tibiotalar (ATT) and the posterior tibiotalar (PTT) ligament, of which the latter is the strongest

Treatment Strategy of Ankle fractures

Emergency management for unstable ankle fractures and fracture dislocations consists of the following:

- Reduce
  - Manipulation & splint
  - Spanning external fixation
- Scan
- Plan

Emergency Treatment

Unstable fractures ("ankle ring" broken in two places) require surgical repair. Before that however, closed reduction of displaced fractures, or fracture-dislocations of the ankle is mandatory, to avoid excess swelling and skin necrosis (especially on the medial side) (Fig. 18.5). It is advisable that, for grossly deformed ankles, the reduction is performed prior to radiographic examination, to protect neurovascular structures. The deformity should be documented, preferably by medical photography.

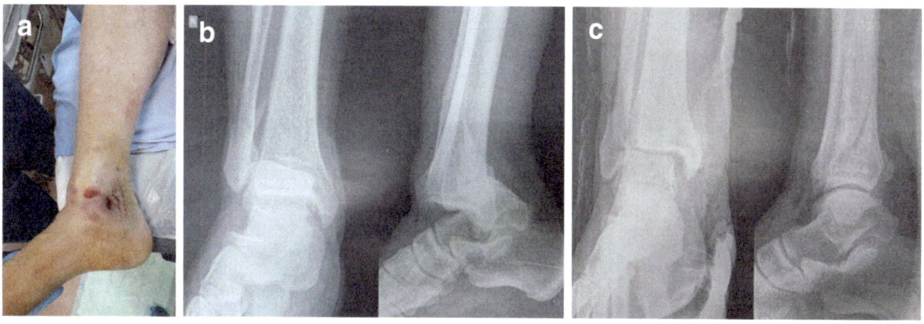

Fig. 18.5 Gross deformity at the ankle, with medial soft tissue swelling, and ecchymosis (**a**), is indicative of fracture dislocation (**b**). Reduction has to be performed (**c**), as soon as possible

Fracture dislocations should "ring a bell", indicating higher energy injuries, with significant damage of osseous and soft tissue structures, and risk for potential complications.

In those cases where satisfactory ankle joint congruity/reduction cannot be restored by manipulation and, depending on the skin condition, one should proceed to spanning external fixation so as to acheive joint re-alignment and to allow the soft tissue envelope to recover (Fig. 18.6).

Planning and Performing Definitive Surgery

Once unstable ankle fractures are reduced and placed in a below knee back slab or, after spanning external fixation, a CT scan should be obtained to identify all components of the injury and allow for surgical planning (Fig. 18.7).

Surgeons treating ankle fractures should have relevant expertise and be familiar with various surgical approaches around the ankle.

A CT scan will reveal the morphology of posterior fragments (posteromedial, and/or posterolateral), anterior fragmentation in the region of the anterolateral tibia ("Chaput fracture"; Fig. 18.8), or fibula ("Wagstaffe fracture"; Fig. 18.9), and consequently, accurate assessment of the distal tibiofibular syndesmosis. Additionally, only the size of posterior malleolar fragments can be reliably assessed with plain x/rays, leading to under-estimation of comminution and surgically relevant information is missed. An early CT scan will mitigate against missing such important information.

Any posterior fragments should be fixed from posterior to anterior (Fig. 18.10). Anterior to posterior percutaneous screw fixation is not recommended as accurate reduction of the fracture is usually not feasible. Fixation in this way is biomechanically irrational (fixing the tibia -"big fragment"- to the small posterior fragment) and percutaneous fixation can put the anterior neurovascular structures at risk.

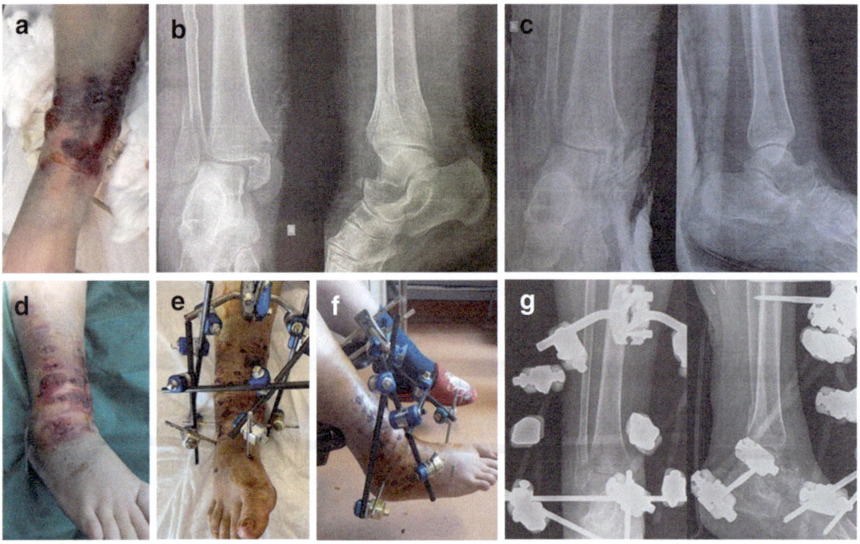

Fig. 18.6 A 59 years old lady presented with significant soft tissue swelling, ecchymosis and blisters (**a**, **d**), following a displaced, unstable ankle fracture (**b**). Manipulation and attempt for closed reduction was not successful (c), due to fracture instability. An ankle spanning "A" frame was applied (**e**, **f**), to achieve ankle joint congruency (**g**), maintain reduction, and allow soft tissues to recover

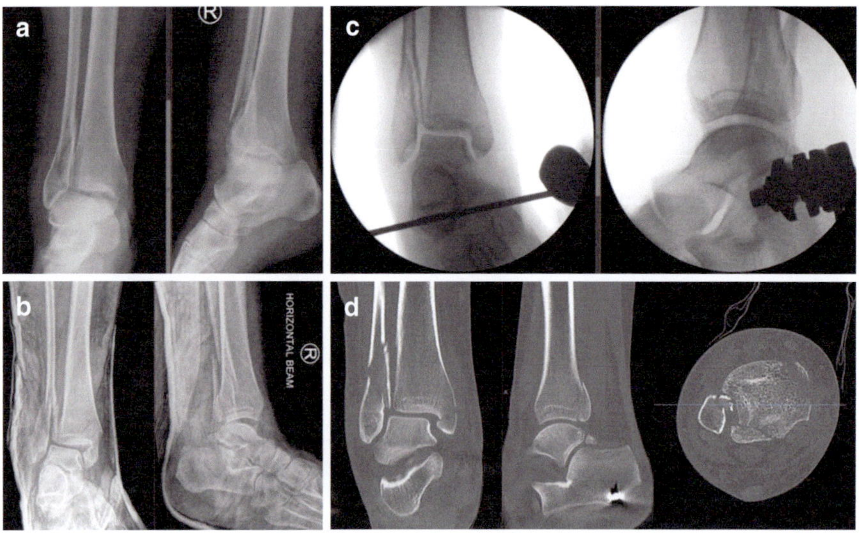

Fig. 18.7 The "Span, Scan and Plan" concept applies on unstable ankle fractures. An unstable ankle fracture (**a**, **b**), was reduced and stabilised on the day of injury, using ankle spanning external fixation (**c**). CT scan imaging is required for preoperative planning, before internal fixation

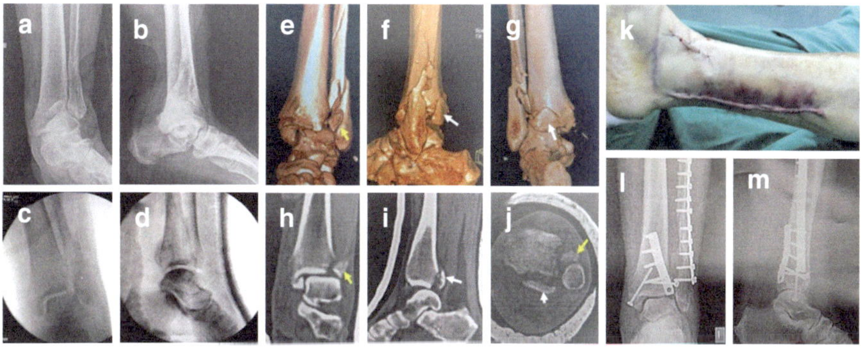

Fig. 18.8 Ankle fracture dislocation (**a**, **b**) in a 79 years old patient, required manipulation under anaesthetic for reduction (**c**, **d**). CT scan imaging (e-j) allowed for accurate assessment of all fractures, including fractures of the posterior (white arrows) and anterior malleoli (yellow arrows). The latter is the so called Chaput fracture. Preoperative planning indicated the need for open reduction internal fixation using posterolateral (posterior malleolus and fibula fractures), anterolateral (for Chaput fracture) and medial (for medial malleolus fracture) approaches (**k**–**m**)

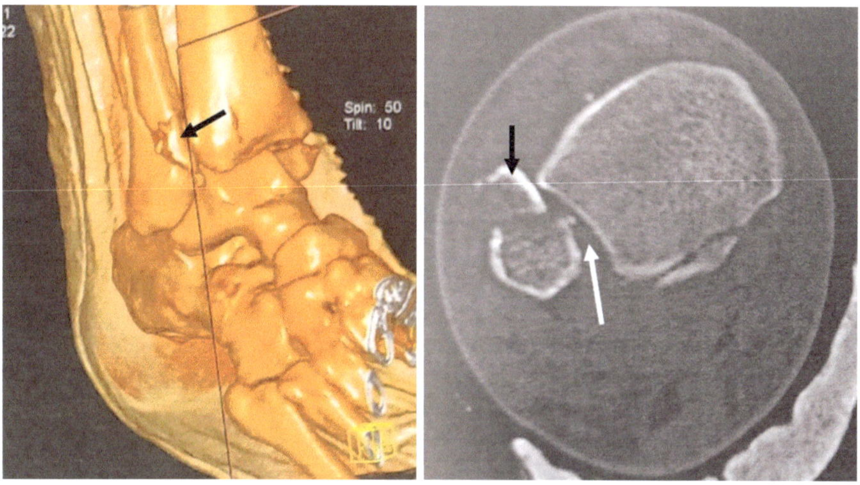

Fig. 18.9 Images show the, so called, Wagstaffe fracture of the distal fibula (black arrows). These are avulsion injuries of the anterior inferior tibiofibular ligament (AiTFL), causing syndesmosis instability and displacement of the fibula within the incisura (white arrow)

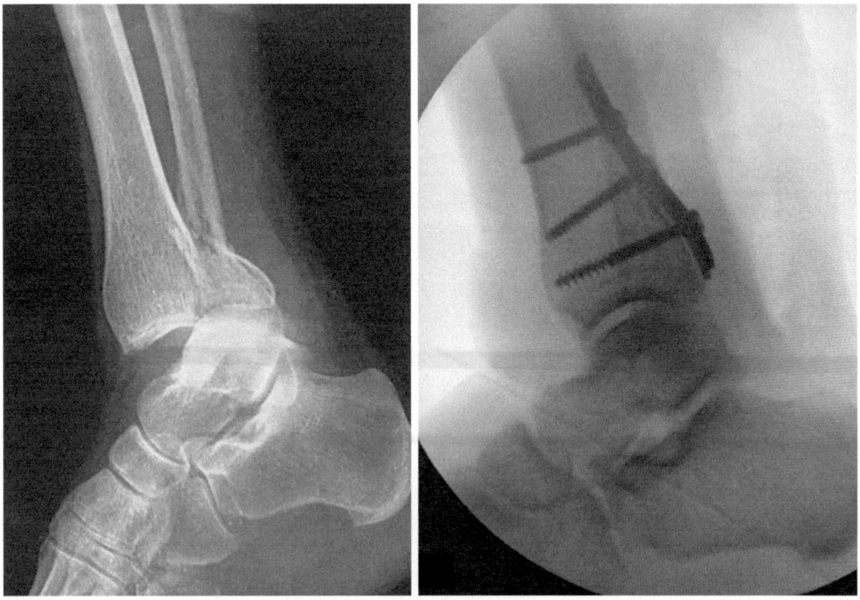

Fig. 18.10 Posterior buttress plating of posterior malleolus fracture

Fibula displacement within the incisura is often associated with avulsion of small bony fragments from the posterior and anterior rim of the distal tibia (Fig. 18.11). Reduction and fixation of (even small) fragments onto the tibia is recommended for tibiofibular syndesmosis reduction, as this allows healing in anatomic alignment, thereby making the use of syndesmosis screws or suture button devices unnecessary. Small fragments can be fixed with partially threaded screws and/or buttress plating (Fig. 18.11).

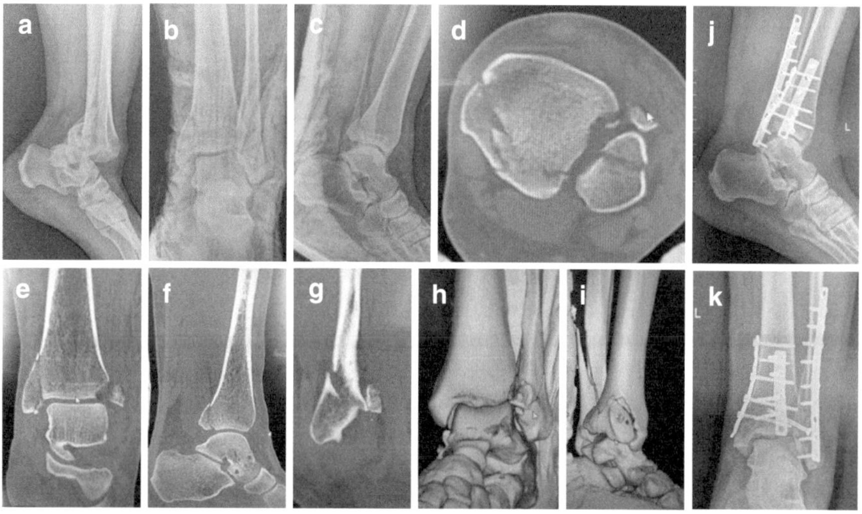

Fig. 18.11 Fracture dislocation of the ankle (**a**), was reduced (**b**, **c**), and CT imaging was obtained (d-i), including 3-D reconstruction (**h**, **i**). Imaging revealed a complex fracture pattern, including posterior malleolus fracture, with posteromedial extension (2B according to Mason), Chaput ("anterior malleolus") fracture, and a multifragmentary fibula fracture. Open reduction internal fixation was performed, using three surgical approaches: Posterolateral for posterolateral malleolar fragment and fibula fixation using plates, anterolateral for fixation of the Chaput fracture using a partially threaded screw, and medial posteromedial for fixing the posteromedial malleolar fragment, using plate

In cases of ligamentous avulsions or, in the presence of very small undisplaced fractures attached to the syndesmotic ligaments, indirect fixation using syndesmotic screws can be performed (Fig. 18.12).

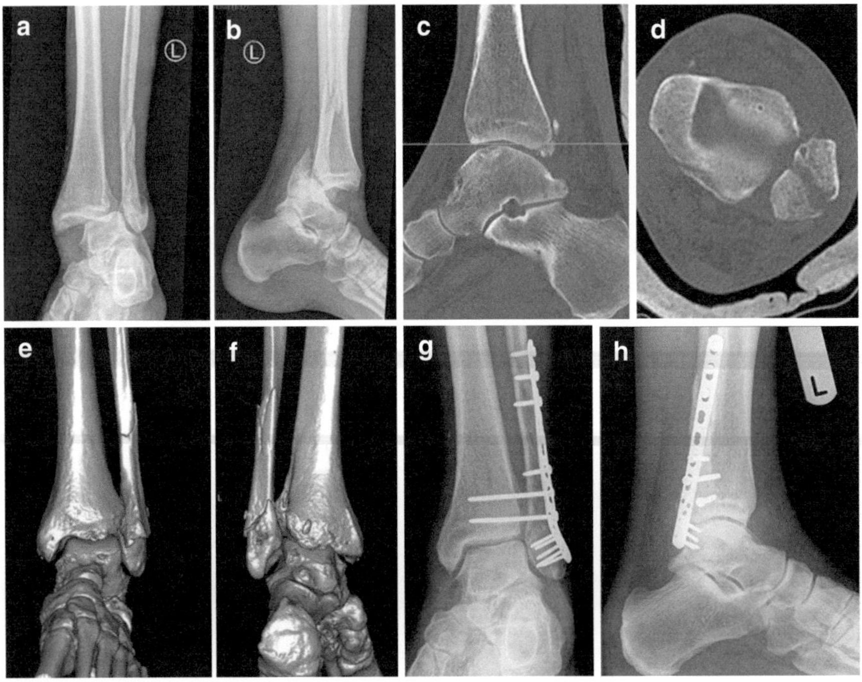

Fig. 18.12 Fracture dislocation of the ankle, with a suprasyndesmotic fibula fracture (**a**, **b**), possibly a result of pronation external rotation type injury. CT imaging (c,d,e,f) revealed small posterior malleolus avulsion and syndesmosis injury. Length of fibula was restored and fixed with an anatomic locking plate, whilst the syndesmosis was stabilised with two syndemsosis screws, also -indirectly- fixing the posterior malleolus avulsion injury

Surgical Techniques

Direct Lateral Approach for Fibula Fixation

Widely used for fixation of fibula fractures. Simple dissection for distal fractures (e.g. Weber B, trans-syndesmotic). Care should be taken to avoid damaging branches of the superficial peroneal nerve and the peroneal tendons distally. More proximal fractures (eg. Weber C - suprasyndesmotic) require more invasive dissection separating the peroneal muscles and care so as not to injure the common peroneal nerve.

Typical short oblique distal fibula fractures are fixed using one lag screw (anterior to posterior) to compress the oblique fracture and a lateral neutralisation (1/3 tubular) plate (Fig. 18.13). Long oblique fractures in good quality bone can be fixed with two compression screws (without the need of plate), as neutralisation of torsional forces are controlled by the second screw (Fig. 18.14). In osteoporotic or comminuted fractures, 'bridge plating' using locking screws may be preferred, often supplemented by fibula pro tibia fixation. Supra-syndesmotic (e.g. Weber C)

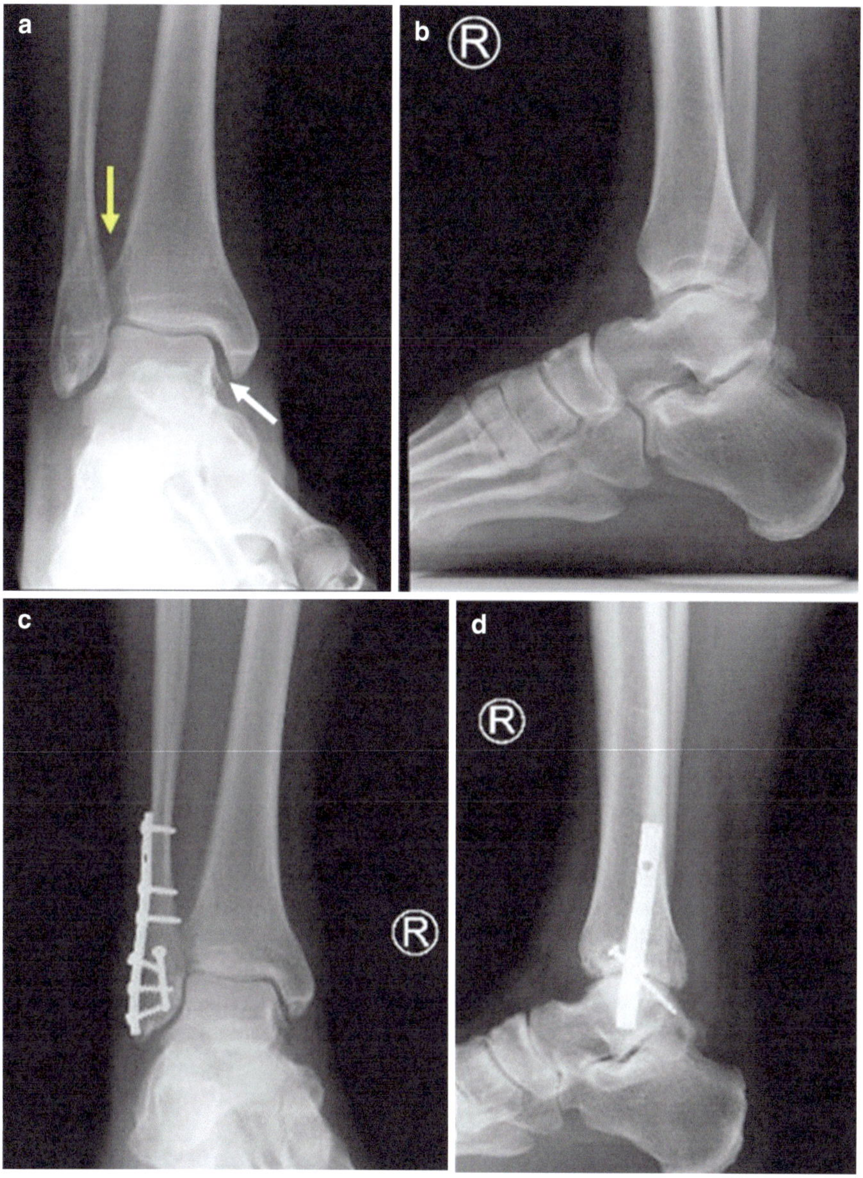

Fig. 18.13 Unstable supination external rotation fracture (**a**, **b**), with widening of the syndesmosis (yellow arrow) and medial clear space (white arrow), on weight bearing ankle radiograph (**a**). Operative management was indicated. The fibula fracture was reduced and fixed with a lag screw, and a neutralisation 1/3 tubular plate was applied (**c**, **d**)

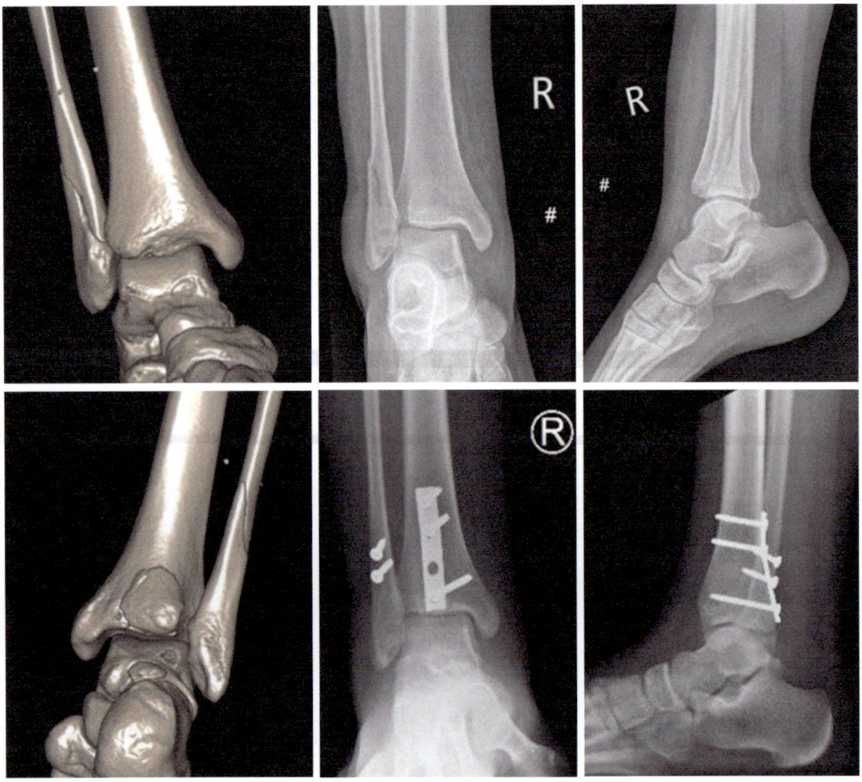

Fig. 18.14 Long oblique fractures in good quality bone (eg. young athletic patients), can be fixed with two compression (lag) screws, rather than one screw combined with neutralisation plate, to avoid potential soft tissue irritation by the fibula plate

fractures often require stronger plates (e.g. DCP) to resist torsional forces as fracture patterns in high fibula fractures do not usually allow interfragmentary screw compression. Instead, with thicker DCP-type plates, compression can be applied in transverse fractures, and bridging fixation in comminuted fractures.

Posterolateral Approach for "Posterior Malleolus" (PM) and Fibula Fixation

Typically performed to fix posterolateral tibia ("posterior malleolus") fractures. It is performed with the patient in the prone, recovery [24], or lateral decubitus [25] positions (Fig. 18.15). A longitudinal incision is performed, midway between the posterior edge of the fibula and the lateral edge of the Achilles tendon. Peroneal tendons are dissected and their fascia is longitudinally incised, whilst taking care to avoid damaging the sural nerve (Fig. 18.16). The incision is extended distally to the

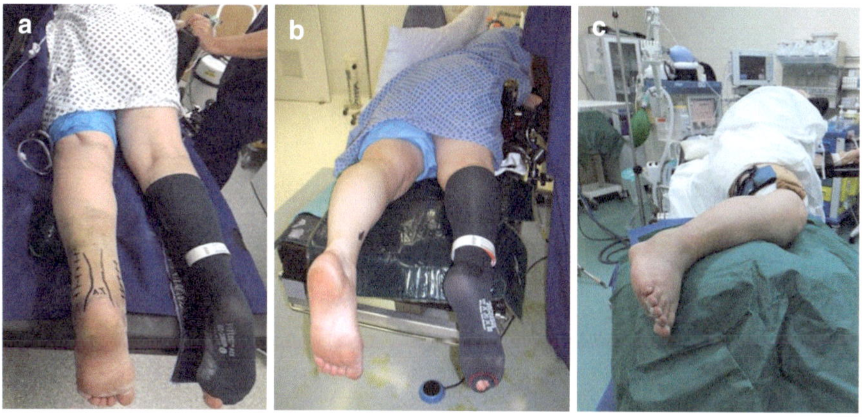

Fig. 18.15 Patients can be positioned prone (**a**), in recovery (**b**), or lateral decubitus positions, for posterior malleolus fracture fixation

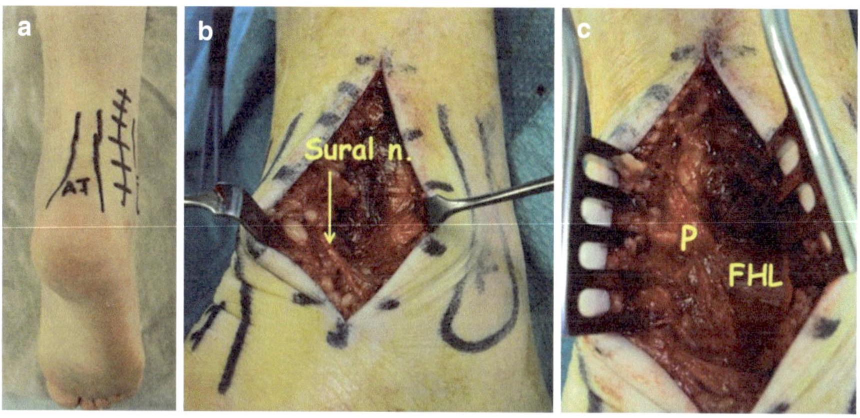

Fig. 18.16 The patient was placed prone on the operating table, and a longitudinal incision half-way between the lateral edge of the Achilles tendon and the posterior margin of the fibula (**a**). Care is taken to identify and avoid damaging the sural nerve (**b**). The peroneal muscles (P) are reflected laterally (towards the Achilles tendon), and flexor hallucis muscle (FHL) is identified, covering the posterior aspect of the distal tibia (**c**)

level of the tip of the fibula, and proximally, depending on the configuration of the fibula fracture, should this be fixed through the same approach. Distal extension however, carries the risk of damaging the peroneal artery and angiosome causing skin necrosis. Peroneal tendons and muscles are retracted laterally and the muscle belly of flexor hallucis longus (FHL) is identified, overlying the distal tibia. The FHL muscle is retracted medially using a Hohman retractor against the medial edge of the tibia, giving good access to the posterolateral tibia (Fig. 18.17). The (lateral) PM fragment is usually fixed first (Fig. 18.10), unless there is also a posteromedial fracture fragment as well, when the latter is reduced and fixed first This is feasible

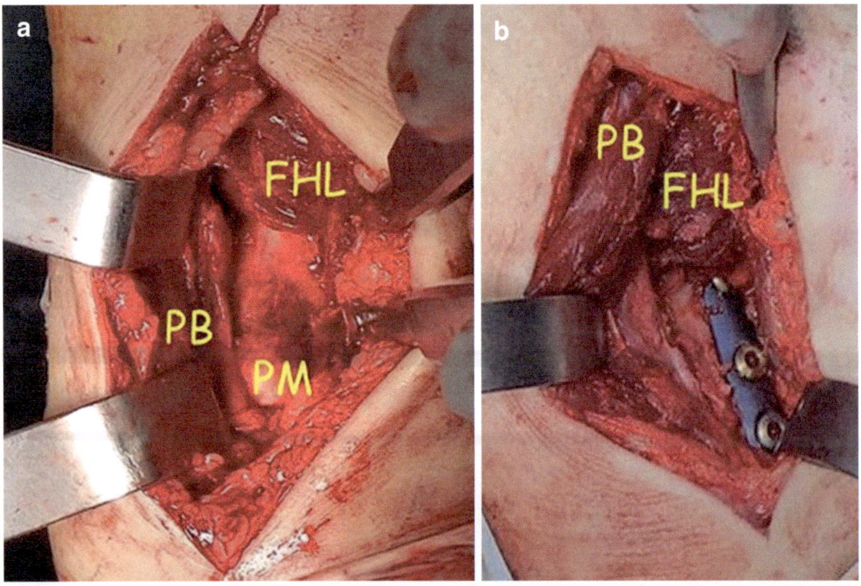

Fig. 18.17 Retraction of peroneus brevis (PB) muscle laterally, and flexor hallucis longus (FHL) muscle medially, to posterior malleolus (PM) is identified (**a**). Fixation of the PM fracture is performed, applying a posterior plate (**b**)

by applying a 4- or 5-hole 1/3 tubular plate, slightly pre-bent to match the curvature of the posterior aspect of the distal tibia. Alternatively, specialised posterior malleolar plates can be used. One cortical screw is used first, through the plate, proximal to the fracture line, to "push" the plate onto the bone, so as to buttress and reduce the fracture (Fig. 18.10).

Exposure of the distal fibula is possible through the same approach, often by reflecting the peroneal tendons medially (Fig. 18.18). Fixation of the distal fibula fractures is usually performed using a posteriorly applied antiglide plate (Figs. 18.18, 18.19 and 18.20). For more proximal fibula fractures (eg. suprasyndemsotic, Weber C), the same approach may be used (extended proximally) (Fig. 18.21) or, a separate lateral incision may be used.

This is the authors' preferred approach to fix posterolateral distal tibia combined with distal fibula fractures [1, 2].

Posteromedial and Modified Posteromedial Approaches

Depending on fracture configuration (eg in Mason 2B type fractures) the posteromedial approach may be preferred to fix the PM fracture(s) (Fig. 18.22). The tendons (tibialis posterior, flexor digitorum longus, tibial artery and nerve, flexor hallucis longus, running behind the medial malleolus in that order), are retracted in

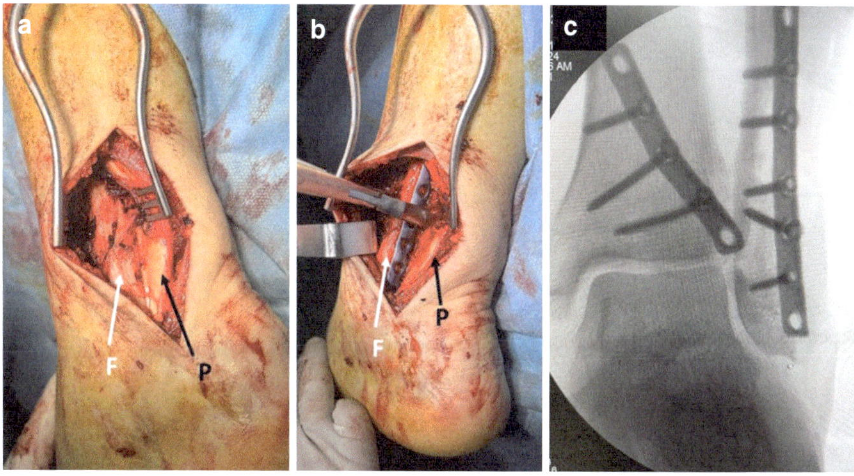

Fig. 18.18 Peroneal muscles and tendons (P) are retracted medially and the fibula (F) is exposed (**a**). The fibular fracture is exposed and reduced and a posterior antiglide plate is applied (**b**), and fixation is performed (**c**)

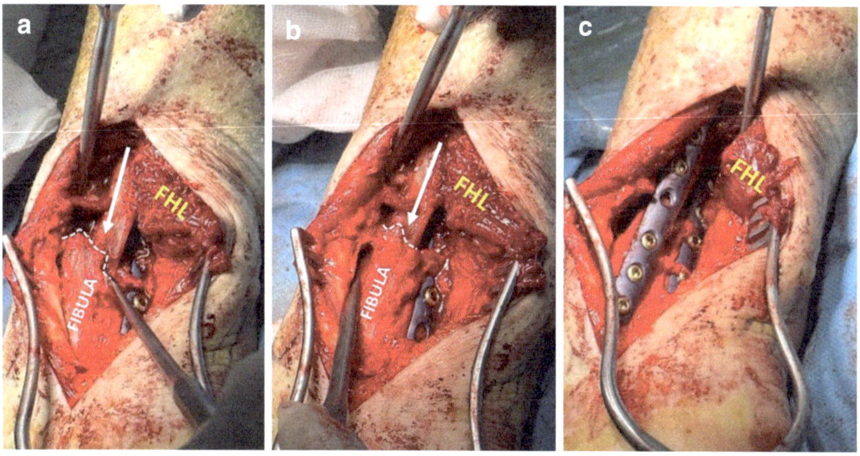

Fig. 18.19 After posterior malleolus fixation, the fibular fracture is exposed (**a**), reduced (**b**), and fixed (**c**). Flexor hallucis longus (FHL) muscle is retracted medially, to allow exposure if the posterior aspect of the distal tibia

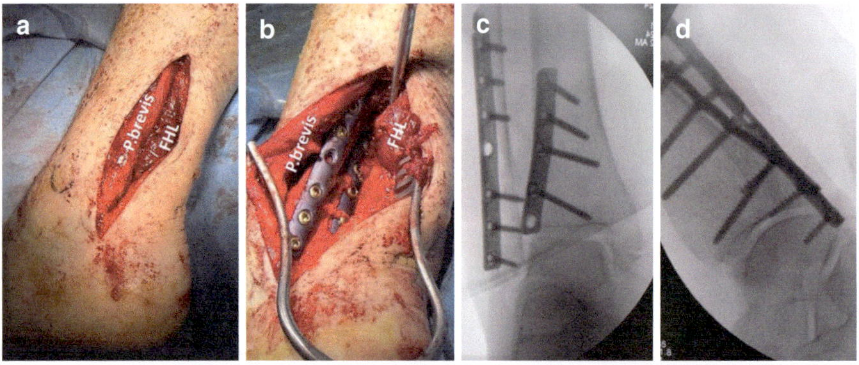

Fig. 18.20 Peroneus brevis (PB) and flexor hallucis longus (FHL) muscles are identified under the skin incision (**a**). Retraction of the muscles allows exposure of the posterior malleolus and fibula fractures (**b**), that are fixed sequentially, usually in that order, using posterior plates (**c**, **d**)

Fig. 18.21 A suprasyndesmotic fibula fracture (**a**) was fixed using a DCP plate, extending the posterolateral approach, proximally (**b**)

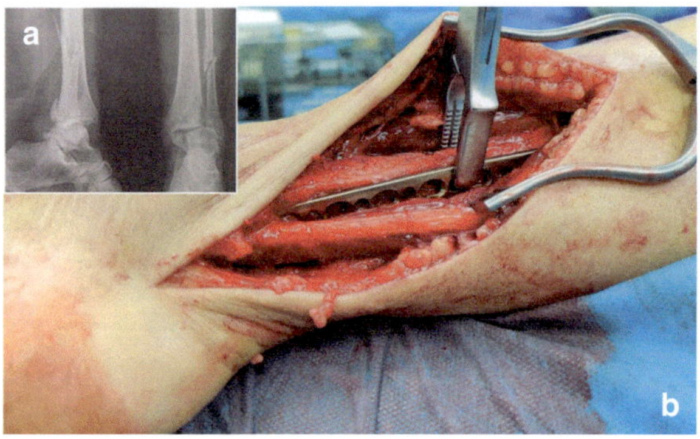

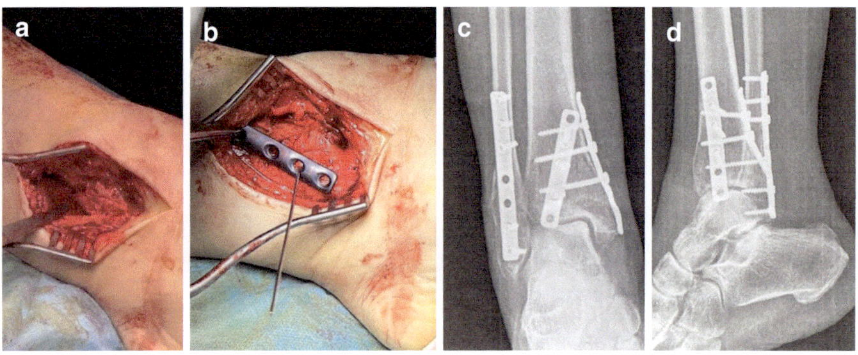

Fig. 18.22 Posteromedial approach (**a**), to fix the posteromedial fragment. The fracture was reduced by applying an 1/3 tubular plate (**b**), after the posterior and lateral malleolus fractures were fixed (**c**, **d**)

a posterolateral direction, to expose the posterior aspect of the tibia. Plate and/or screws are used to fix the fractures, starting with the posteromedial fragment first, followed by the posterolateral fragment. In such cases a direct lateral approach is used for distal fibula fracture fixation [26].

Syndesmosis Fixation

Syndesmosis fixation is controversial in various aspects. There are probably more questions than answers, as listed below:

1. When is it required and how is syndesmosis rupture confirmed intra-operatively?
2. How to assess accurate reduction?
3. Screws or suture-button devices (eg. tightrope)?
4. What is the preferred ankle position during fixation of the syndesmosis?
5. Screw(s): 3 or 4 cortices?
6. Small (3.5 mm) fragment or bigger (4.5 mm) screws?
7. Does it matter if screws break?
8. Remove syndesmosis screws (and when), or not?

There is lack of consensus regarding the above-mentioned issues, due to the lack of strong scientific evidence (mostly associated with level IV and/or under-powered studies). It seems that routine syndesmosis screws removal is not required, and patients should be treated on an "as needed" basis [27]. Given these controversies, and the fact that syndesmosis malreduction can be as common as approx. 50% [19], it is recommended that surgeons should not rely on syndesmosis fixation to compensate for inadequately fixed fractures.

We can provide some guidelines based on the available evidence, personal experience and application of some of the concepts mentioned earlier. The surgeon should always bear in mind that the ankle behaves like a ring regarding stability and every osseous injury has a soft tissue equivalent, and by fixing (even small) fragments, ligaments are re-attached to bone. Thus, once (all) bony fragments are fixed (fibula—including Wagstaffe fragment if present, PM and anterior Chaput fragments), the ankle should be stable and no syndesmosis screws are needed (Figs. 18.11, 18.23, 18.24 and 18.25).

However sometimes, small avulsion injuries (such as Mason type 1), or PiTFL injuries, require indirect stabilisation using syndesmosis screws.

The "hook test" (Fig. 18.26) (probably not as useful as previously thought) and external rotation stress testing using fluoroscopy, are performed to confirm stability (once all fractures have been fixed). Widening of syndesmosis and/or medial clear space are indicative of syndesmosis instability (Fig. 18.27). The authors want to emphasize that if instability persists despite fracture(s) fixation, the surgeon should question whether anatomic reduction and fixation has been achieved (eg. has the fibula been fixed to correct length and/or rotation?) and that all fragments have been

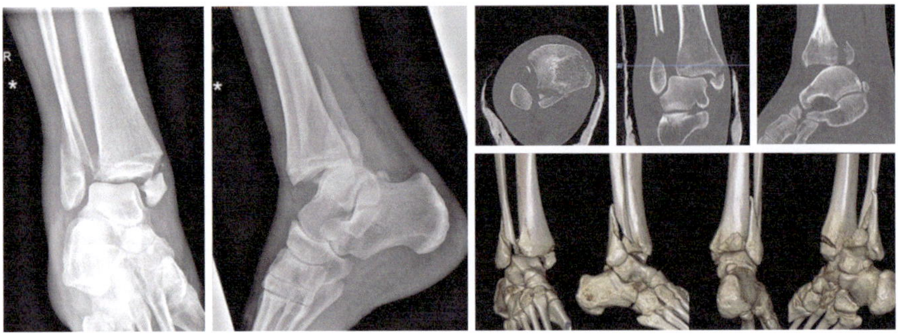

Fig. 18.23 An unstable ankle fracture, involving the posterior malleolus and the syndesmosis is shown

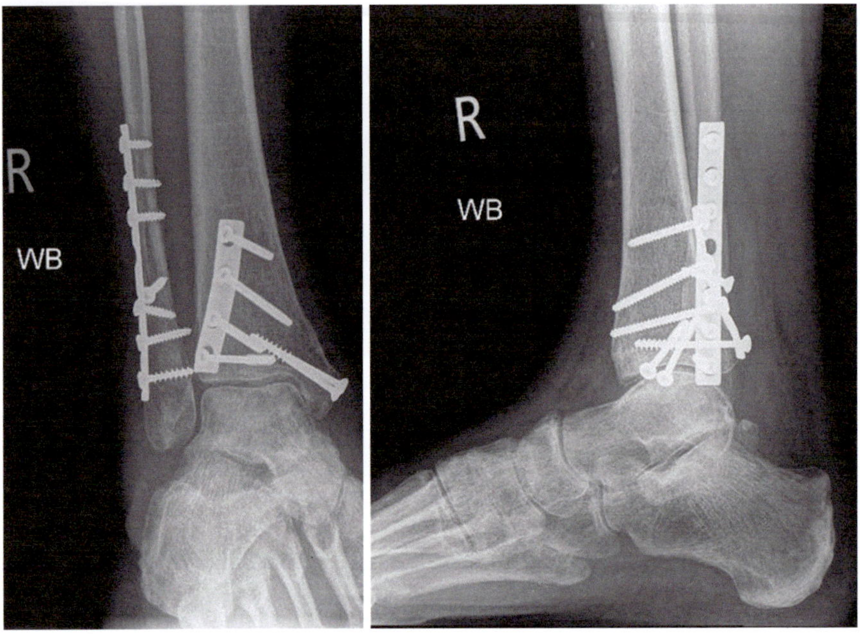

Fig. 18.24 Fracture shown in Fig. 18.23, was fixed anatomically

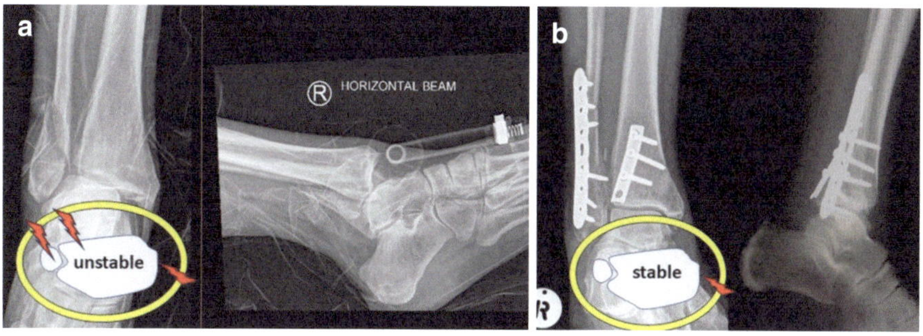

Fig. 18.25 Unstable ankle fracture involving the fibula, posterior malleolus, and the deltoid ligament (**a**). Fixation of the osseous injuries, resulted in stabilisation of the "ankle ring" stable. Fixation of the posterior malleolus reduced and stabilised the syndesmosis (**b**). The medial soft tissue (deltoid ligament) injury, was not directly repaired. However, the ankle ring was stable, to allow soft tissue injuries to heal over time

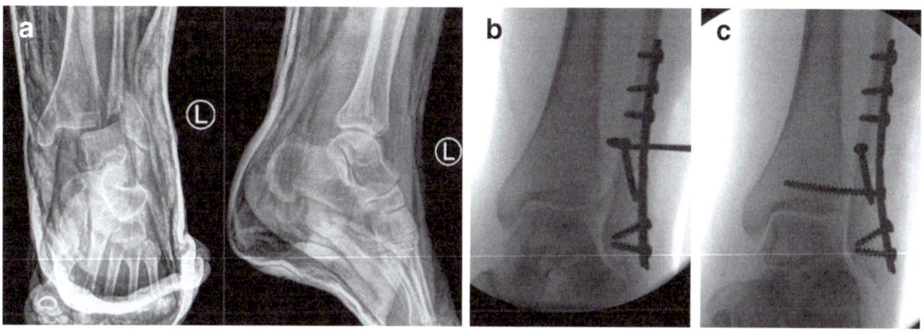

Fig. 18.26 Unstable ankle fracture (**a**), requiring operative treatment. The "hook test" performed intraoperatively (lateral translation of the fibula), revealed syndesmosis widening (**b**), indicating the need for syndesmosis screw fixation (**c**)

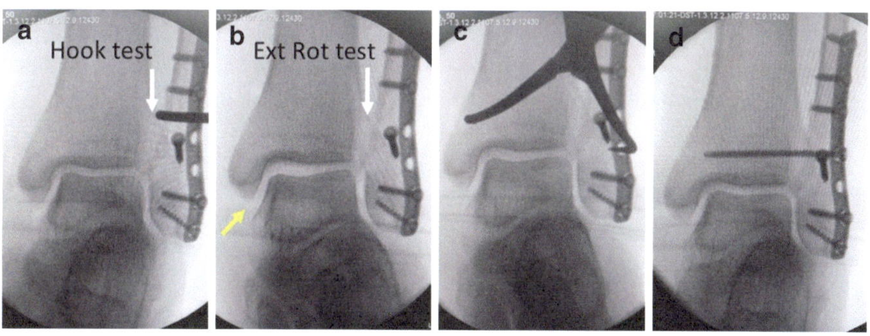

Fig. 18.27 In this case, the "hook test" revealed no instability (**a**). After applying external rotation of the foot, syndesmosis (white arrow) and medial clear space (yellow arrow) widening were evident (**b**). Syndesmosis reduction (**c**) and screw fixation (**d**), were performed

fixed (eg. has an anterior Chaput type fracture, also called "anterior malleolus" in the literature, been overlooked or ignored?). In those cases, supplementary syndesmosis fixation may be required.

It is important to understand that the hook test, if used, only tests for coronal plane stability whereas, one should also consider (and test for) sagittal (antreroposterior) plane instability (which is common). Also, if there is a high, comminuted fibula fracture (Weber C-type) that has not been, or can't be adequately stabilised/fixed, then vertical instability is present. Understanding the types of syndesmotic instability that can be present has important implications for what type of syndesmosis stabilisation can be used. If there is coronal plane instability, then either 1–2 screws can be used (correctly sited) or 1 suture button (also correctly sited). If however, there is sagittal plane instability then, although 1–2 screws can be used, 1 suture button is insufficient; it has to be two suture buttons sited divergently. Finally, with vertical instability (present with shortened, comminuted high Weber C-type fractures), suture buttons should not be used at all, as they do not provide any degree of vertical stability.

Deltoid Ligament (To Repair or Not)

Deltoid damage can be one of the components of the injury. If the fracture is unstable and surgical fixation of the bony elements of the injury is performed, the issue of deltoid repair is controversial. One can argue that anatomic fixation of bony injuries and syndesmosis fixation (if required) will turn the unstable ankle injury into a stable one. In such cases the "ankle ring" remains 'broken' only on the medial side (deltoid ligament). Thus, it is stable, and the deltoid could be left to heal without surgical repair, provided there is no talar tilt on intraoperative stress testing of the ankle (Figs. 18.25, 18.27 and 18.28). Some surgeons choose, however, to regularly explore and repair the superficial deltoid ligament. There is currently no strong scientific evidence in favour of, or against deltoid repair, although there is some evidence that deltoid repair may yield better results [28]. In the authors' opinion intraoperative testing using the external rotation test after fixation of the osseous injuries is important, in order to detect those cases where superficial ligament repair is needed.

If the external rotation stress test, performed after fibula and syndesmosis fixation reveals talar tilt and/or medial clear space widening, this may be because the superficial deltoid (also called "tibiospring") ligament is completely avulsed. As this ligament attaches distally to the talus, it follows the rest of the foot when manipulated in external rotation, leading to talar tilt and medial clear space widening (Fig. 18.29). In such cases it may be beneficial to perform a direct superficial deltoid ligament repair (Figs. 18.30 and 18.31) so as to prevent later medial arch collapse. It is also essential to carefully study the preoperative imaging (including CT scan), as a "fleck sign" indicating deltoid avulsion may be detected (Figs. 18.31, 18.32, 18.33, 18.34 and 18.35).

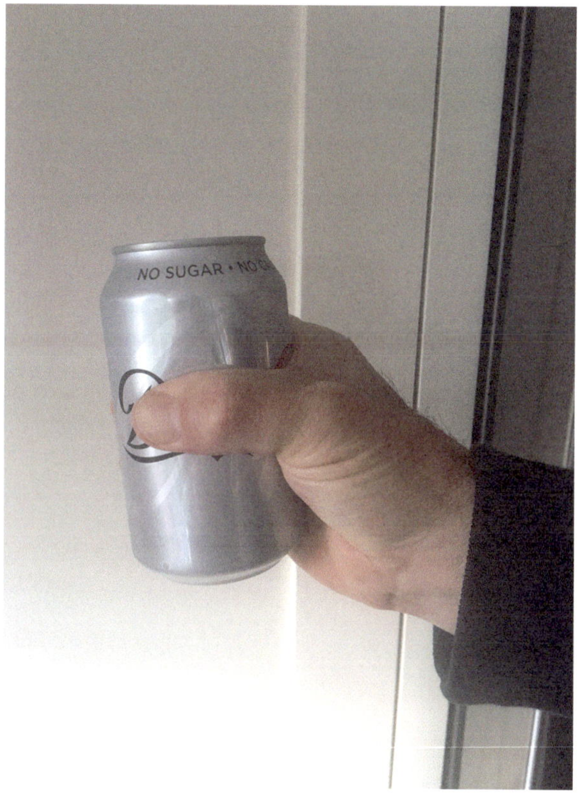

Fig. 18.28 The pressure applied to the "syndesmosis" clamp should be similar to the digital pressure that might be used to just indent an un-opened can of carbonated beverage

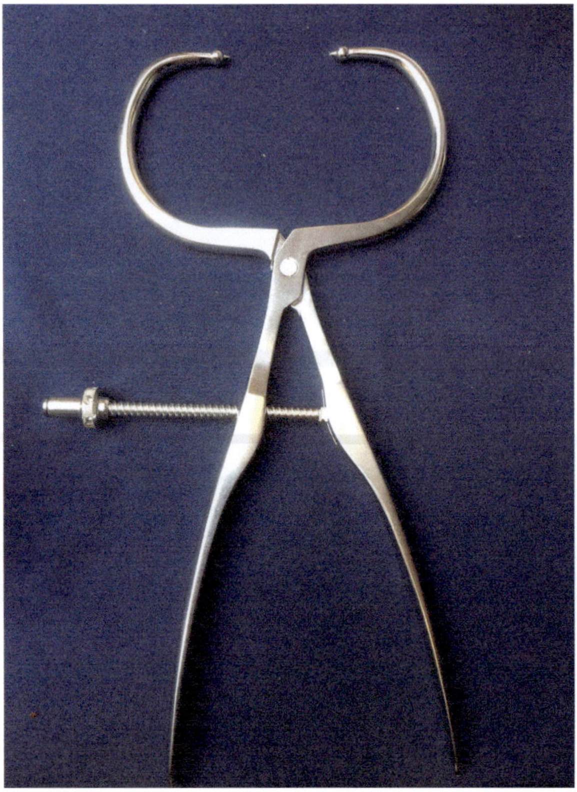

Fig. 18.29 Example of instrument / clamp, used to reduce the distal tibiofibular syndesmosis

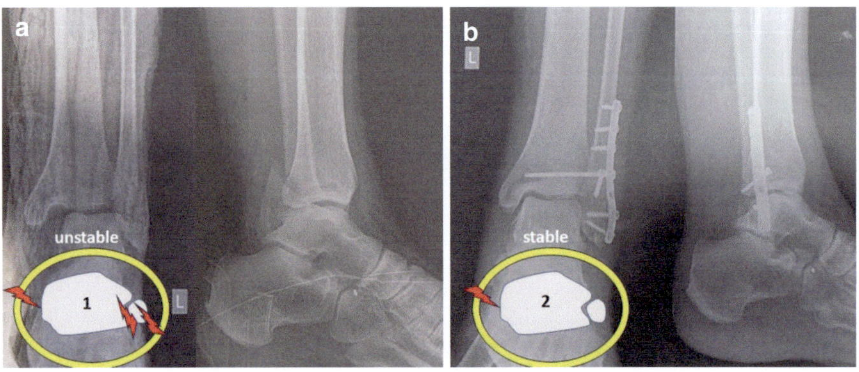

Fig. 18.30 An unstable ankle fracture is shown (**a**). Radiographs show an intrasyndesmotic fibula fracture (Weber B), with medial clear space and syndesmosis widening, indicative for deltoid ligament and syndesmosis injury. Thus the "ankle ring" is broken in three places as shown in diagram 1. Fixation of the fibula and the syndesmosis (**b**), leaves the "ankle ring" broken only in one place (deltoid ligament injury), thus, stable (diagram 2). Repair of the deltoid ligament is optional

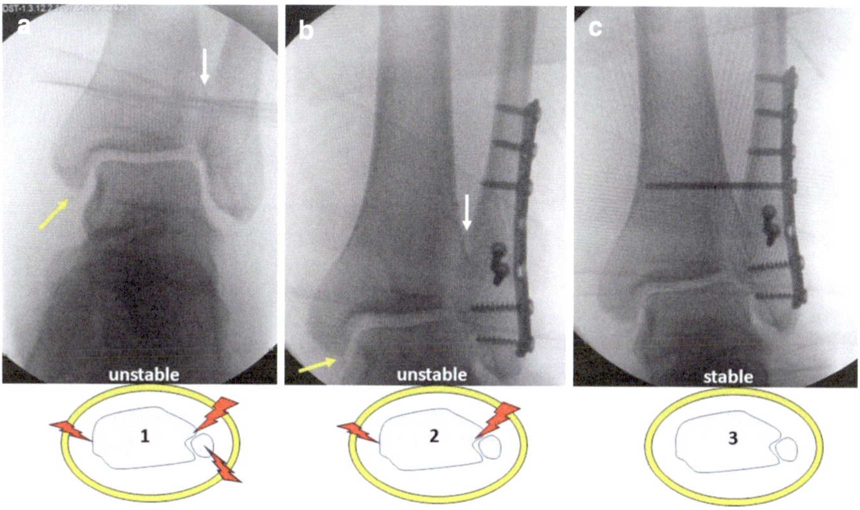

Fig. 18.31 Supination external rotation (SER) type 4 (unstable) fracture (**a**) with syndesmosis widening (white arrows) and medial clear space widening with evidence of "fleck sign" (yellow arrows), indicating deltoid ligament avulsion. Fibula fixation (**b**), was not sufficient to restore ankle stability. Diagrams 1 and 2 show that the "ankle ring" is broken in three and two places, respectively. Thus, the ankle is unstable in both conditions (**a**, **b**). Syndesmosis fixation and direct repair of superficial deltoid ligament, avulsed off the medial malleolus in this case (using trans-osseous sutures), was performed (**c**). "Ankle ring" is now stable structure, as all lesions were repaired (diagram 3)

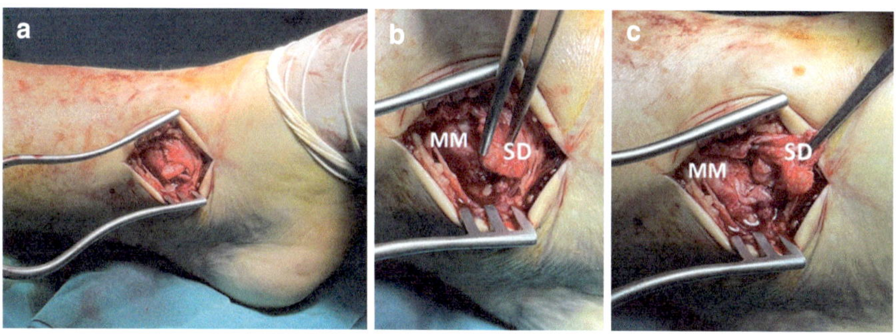

Fig. 18.32 Pictures (**a**–**c**) show avulsion of the superficial deltoid (SD) ligament, from the medial malleolus (MM)

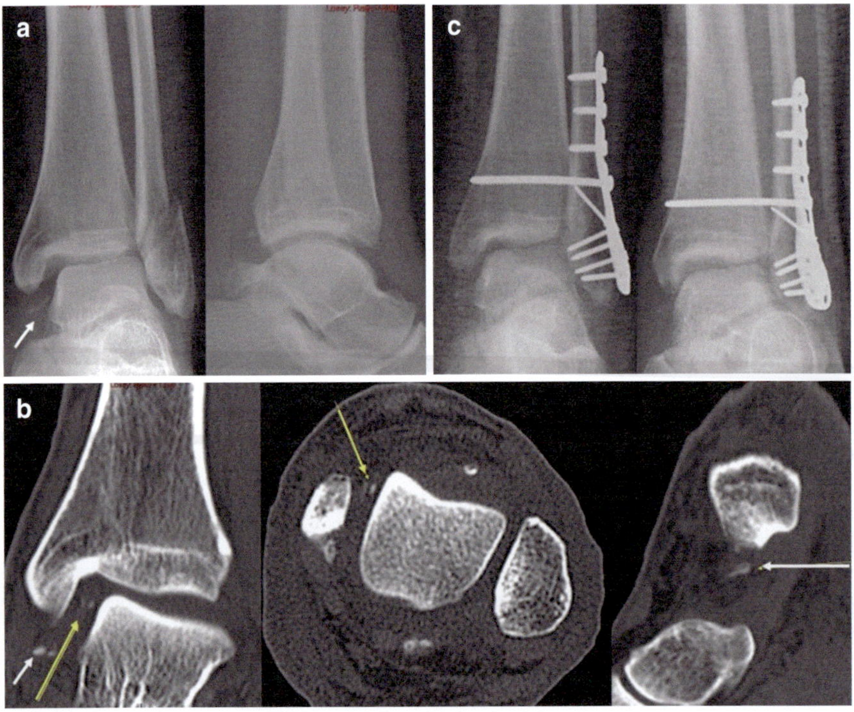

Fig. 18.33 Unstable SER4 fracture is shown (**a**). There is positive "fleck sign" (white arrows) (**a**, **b**), and loose fragments within the medial gutter (yellow arrows) (**b**). The fibula fracture and syndesmosis were fixed (**c**), however, the deltoid ligament avulsion was not taken into consideration, thus, leaving residual talar tilt (**c**). Ideally superficial deltoid ligament repair should have been performed

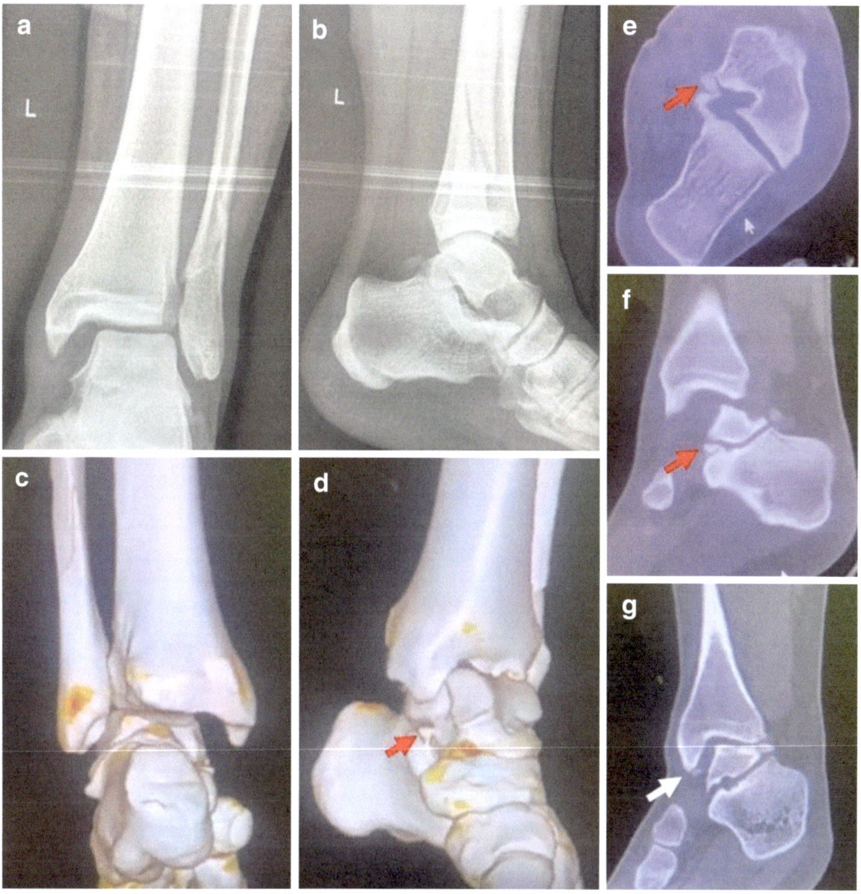

Fig. 18.34 A 29 years old man landed on his left foot playing football, sustaining a pronation external rotation injury. Radiographs (**a**, **b**) revealed a suprasyndesmotic fibula fracture with syndesmosis and medial clear space widening. Computed tomography (**c**–**g**) revealed an avulsion injury of the sustenaculum tali (red arrows; **d**–**f**) indicative of superficial deltoid and possibly spring ligament injury and "fleck sign" in the region of the medial malleolus (white arrow; g), indicative of potential deep deltoid ligament injury

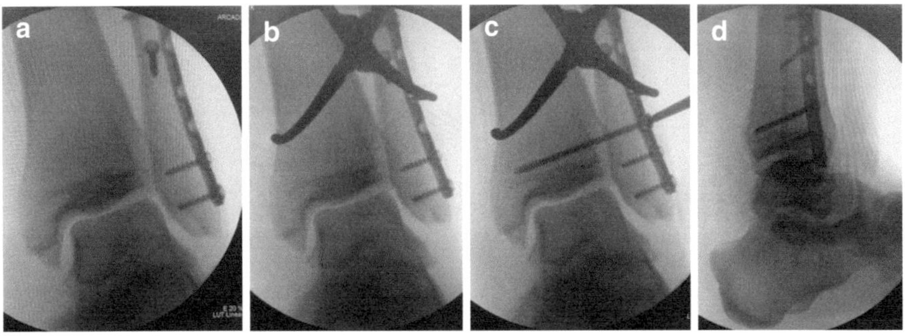

Fig. 18.35 The fracture presented in Fig. 18.34 was deemed unstable and operative fixation was performed. With the patient in supine position the distal fibula was exposed (direct lateral approach) and fixed with a lag screw and 1/3 tubular neutralisation plate (**a**). Large reduction forceps were applied to reduce the syndesmosis (**b**), and syndesmosis fixation through the plate was performed (**c**, **d**)

Peructaneous Fixation

Percutaneous fixation of (selected) ankle fractures is an attractive option offering ankle stability and allowing early mobilisation with minimal surgical trauma. This is of importance particularly in geriatric patients and/or in those with bad soft tissue condition (Figs. 18.36 and 18.37). The authors do not advocate routine use of percutaneous fixation for all ankle fractures, as anatomic reduction may not always be possible, especially in relation to the medial malleolus. An alternative to the use of large cannulated screws in the fibula, is the fibular nail.

Some geriatric and/or diabetic patients may also be candidates for stabilisation using a retrograde hindfoot nail (Fig. 18.38) in order to avoid complications and allow immediate and unrestricted weight bearing [29].

In either case (fibular nail or large percutaneous screws), after 2 weeks of restricted weight-bearing in a backslab, weight-bearing as tolerated in a below knee cast should be encouraged in these elderly patients.

Arthroscopically Assisted Ankle fracture Fixation

There is a new trend in using arthroscopy during ankle fracture fixation. Currently, there is no high quality evidence to support routine use of arthroscopy in ankle fracture fixation. Theoretically, accuracy of joint congruity and intra-articular (e.g. osteochondral) lesions can be assessed and treated. The clinical benefits however, are yet to be confirmed. The authors believe that arthroscopy has its place, in order, for example, to assess syndesmosis integrity and/or reduction (Figs. 18.39, 18.40, 18.41, 18.42, 18.43 and 18.44), and potentially also medial collateral ligamentous injuries (eg. assessing the anterior portion of the deep deltoid ligament).

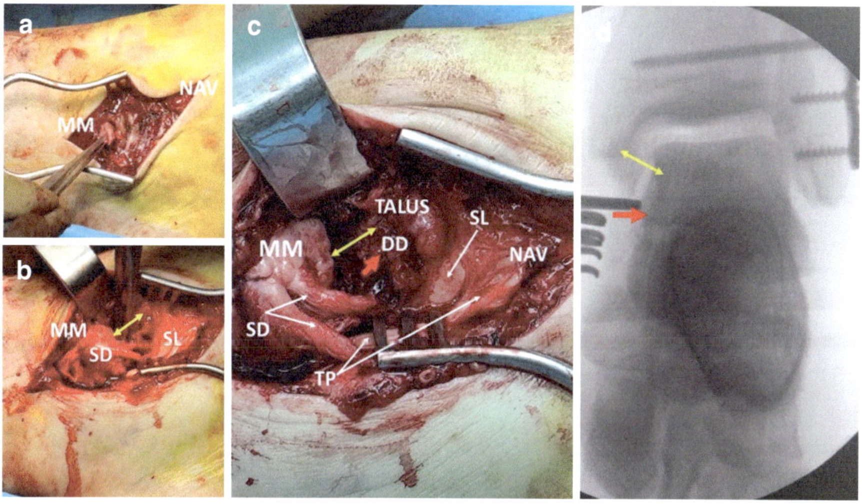

Fig. 18.36 Following fixation of the fibula fracture and the syndesmosis (presented in Figs. 18.32 and 18.33), the medial side was exposed through a curved incision (**a**) extending from the medial malleolus (MM) to the naviculum (NAV). After blunt dissection, injuries were confirmed. The superficial deltoid (SD) was ruptured distally and the proximal stump was attached to the medial malleolus (MM). The spring ligament (SL) was identified distally (**b**). The tibialis posterior (TP) tendon sheath was incised, to allow exploration of TP, SL and the sustenaculum tali. There was evidence of injury to the SL, attached on to the sustenaculum tali, that was avulsed, but the fragment was not displaced and stable. Slight abduction of the foot, resulted in widening of the space between talus and medial malleolus (yellow, double arrow), and showed clearly that there was also injury to the deep deltoid (DD) ligament, that was avulsed from the medial malleolus, still attached onto the talus (**c**, **d**)

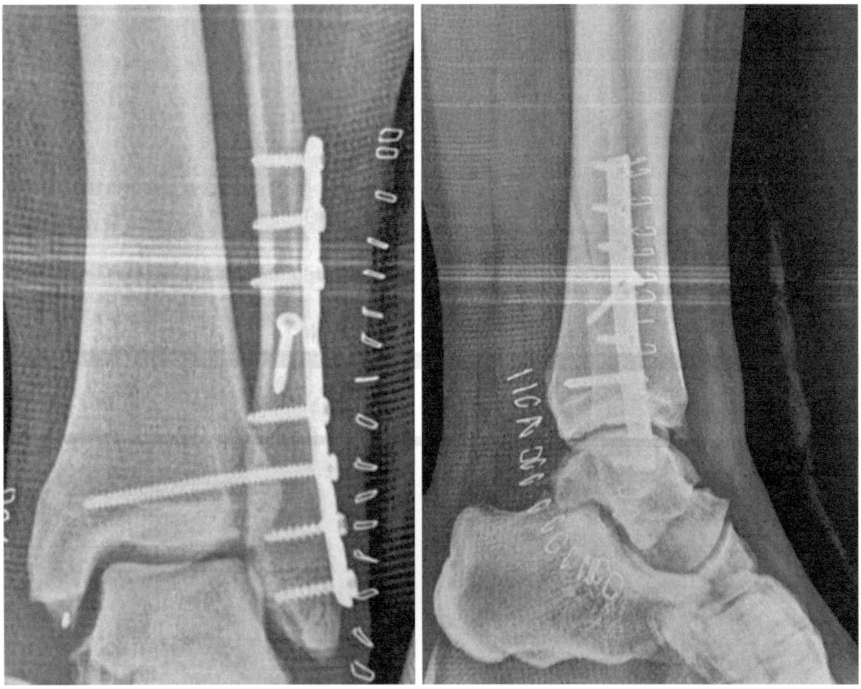

Fig. 18.37 Immediate postoperative radiographs of the fracture presented in Figs. 18.34, 18.35 and 18.36. The deep deltoid ligament was repaired onto the medial malleolus using a suture anchor. The superficial deltoid ligament was reattached onto the spring ligament using sutures

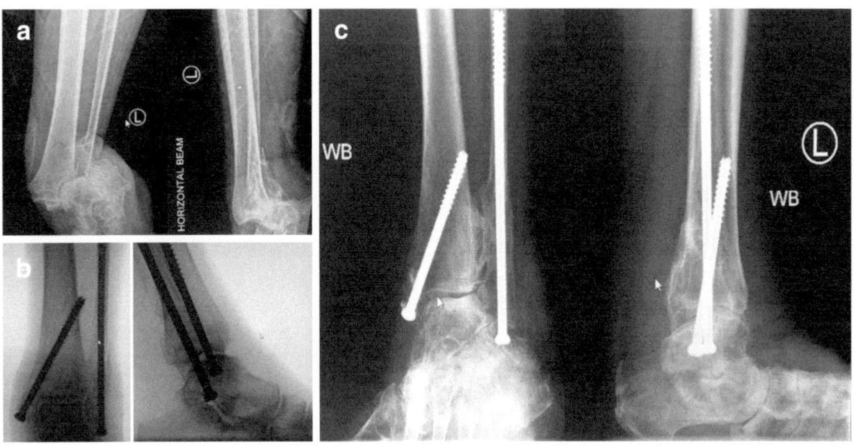

Fig. 18.38 Pronation abduction ankle fracture dislocation in a geriatric patient (**a**), was associated with significant soft tissue swelling and fracture blisters. Percutaneous fixation using cannulated 6.5 mm screws was performed (**b**, **c**)

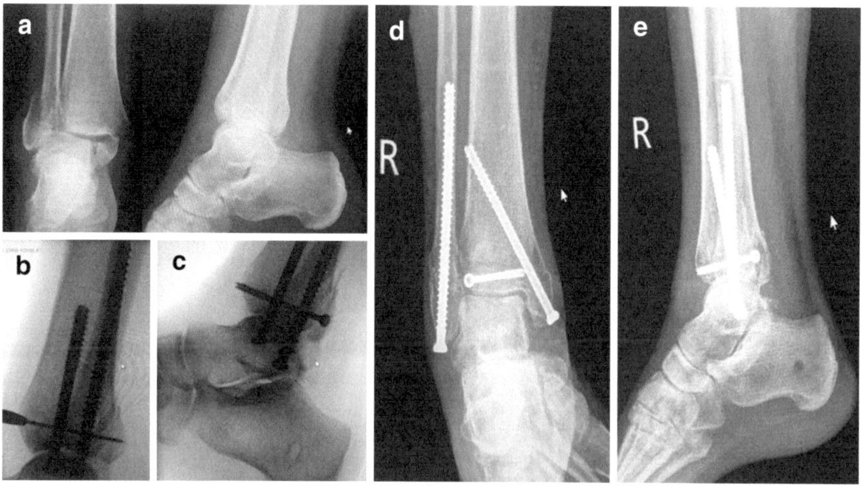

Fig. 18.39 A geriatric patient with bad soft tissue envelope presented with a supination external rotation ankle fracture also involving the posterior malleolus (**a**). Although the authors routinely recommend direct fixation of the posterior malleolus fracture through posterior approaches, in this case, percutaneous fixation was the preferred treatment option. After fixation of the fibula and medial malleolus using 6.5 mm cannulated screws (**b**), the posterior malleolus was fixed, to stabilize the syndesmosis, and thus, the "ankle ring". The guide wire for a cannulated 4.0 mm screw was inserted from anterior to posterior direction (**b**), whilst the screw was inserted percutaneously from posterior to anterior to reduce and compress the posterior malleolus fragment (**c**). Postoperative radiographs at 4 weeks show healing of fractures in optimal alignment (**d**, **e**)

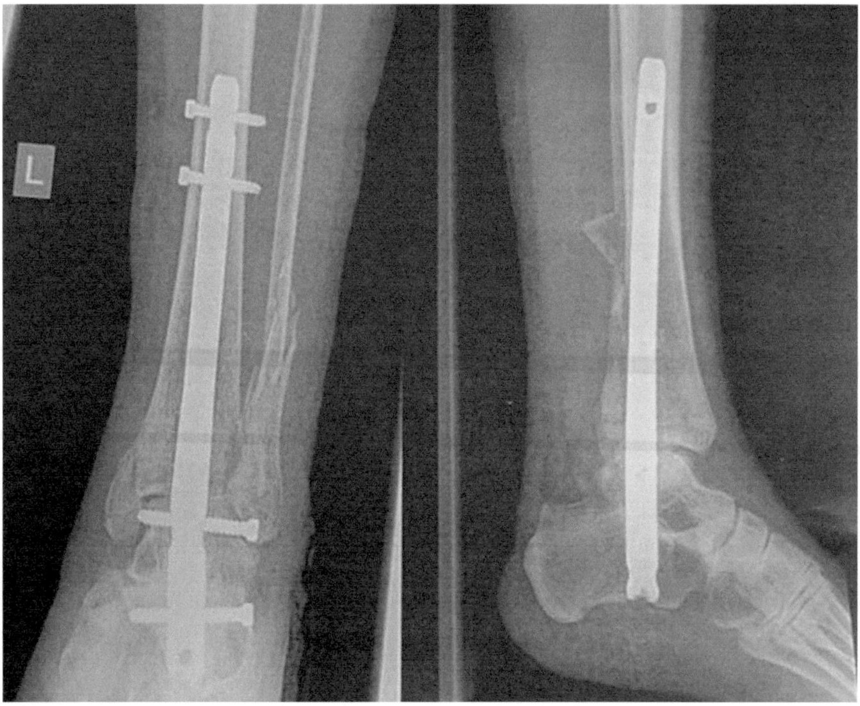

Fig. 18.40 An unstable ankle fracture in a 74 years old patient with uncontrolled ("complicated") diabetes and peripheral neuropathy, was stabilised with retrograde hindfoot nail

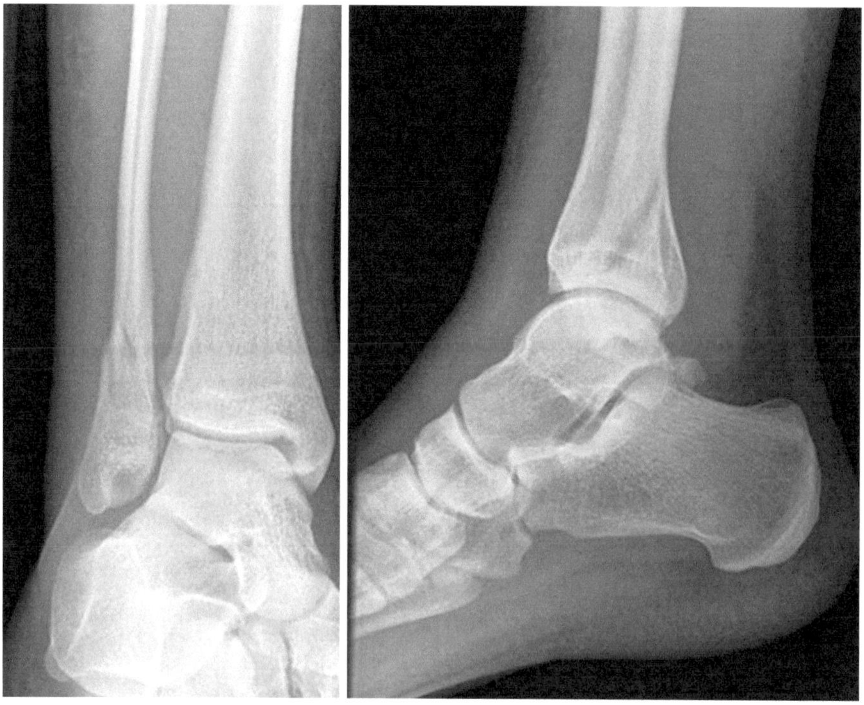

Fig. 18.41 A supination external rotation fracture (**a**) in a 17 years old male patient, was deemed stable and was initially treated nonoperatively

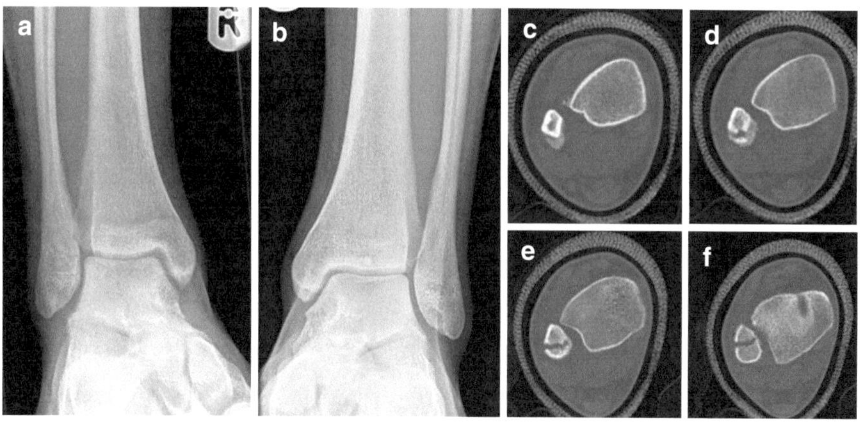

Fig. 18.42 A few weeks later, weight bearing radiographs were obtained, with evidence of syndesmosis widening (**a**) compared to the contralateral (healthy) side (**b**). CT scan confirmed syndesmosis malalignment, whilst there were already signs of fracture healing in the 17 years old patient (**c**–**f**)

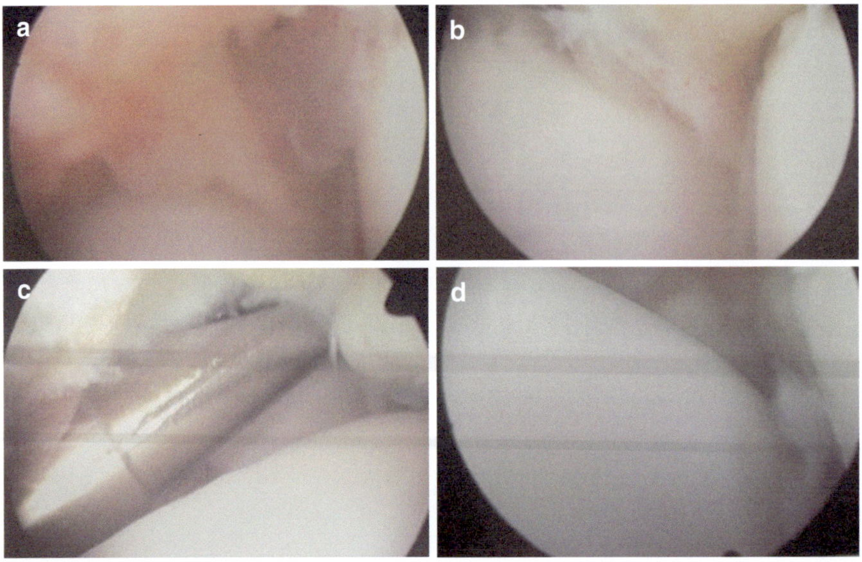

Fig. 18.43 The injury presented in Figs. 18.41 and 18.42 was assessed arthroscopically. Syndesmosis synovitis (**a**), was debrided (**b–d**)

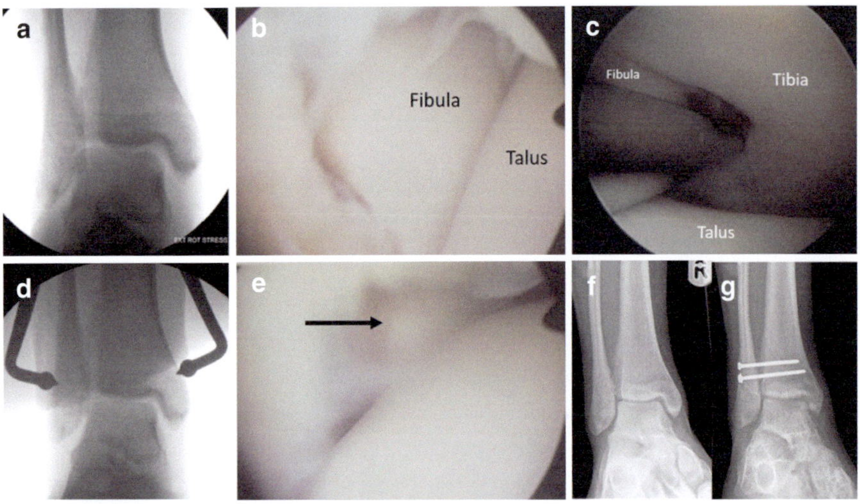

Fig. 18.44 External rotation testing of the ankle injury presented in Figs. 18.41 and 18.42, revealed syndesmosis widening (**a**). Arthroscopy showed anterior translation of the fibula (**b**), and instability of the syndesmosis (**c**), while external rotation was performed. Reduction of the syndesmosis using large reduction forceps was confirmed using fluoroscopy (**d**) and arthroscopy (**e**). The preoperatively unstable syndesmosis (**f**), was fixed with two syndesmosis screws (**g**). No plate was applied as the fracture had clinically united

Summary

- Ankle fractures are stable or unstableStable fractures can safely be treated nonoperatively
- Weight bearing radiographs can aid decision making
- Recognize all elements of the injury (osseous and soft tissue)
- Reduce dislocated joints
- Spanning external fixation if non-reducible, and/or soft tissues in bad condition
- CT scan reveals all elements of the injury and affects preoperative planning
- Be aware of posterior and anterolateral avulsion injuries
- Detect syndesmosis malalignment / instability (external rotation test)
- Fixation of posterior malleolus and anterolateral avulsion fractures (Chaput and Wagstaffe) restores syndesmotic stability.
- Posterolateral and/or posteromedial surgical approaches are increasingly used.
- Residual talar tilt on external rotation testing, after fracture and syndesmosis stabilisation is indicative of superficial deltoid ligament injury, that may require operative repair

References

1. Gougoulias N, Sakellariou A. Ankle Fractures. In: Bentley G, editor. European surgical Orthopaedics and traumatology: the EFORT textbook. Berlin: Springer; 2014. p. 3735–65.
2. Lampridis V, Gougoulias N, Sakellariou A. Stability in ankle fractures: diagnosis and treatment. EFORT Open Rev. 2018;3(5):294–303. https://doi.org/10.1302/2058-5241.3.170057.
3. Gougoulias N, Sakellariou A. When is a simple fracture of the lateral malleolus not so simple? How to assess stability, which ones to fix and the role of the deltoid ligament. Bone Joint J. 2017;99-B(7):851–5. https://doi.org/10.1302/0301-620X.99B7.BJJ-2016-1087.
4. Whitehouse S, Mason LW, Jayatilaka L, Molloy AP. Fixation of ankle fractures – a major trauma centre's experience in improving quality. Ann R Coll Surg Engl. 2019;101(6):387–90. https://doi.org/10.1308/rcsann.2018.0098.
5. Nelson MC, Jensen NK. The treatment of trimalleolar fractures of the ankle. Surg Gynec Obst. 1940;71:509–14.
6. Gougoulias N, Khanna A, Sakellariou A, Maffulli N. Supination-external rotation ankle fractures: stability a key issue. Clin Orthop Relat Res. 2010;468(1):243–51. https://doi.org/10.1007/s11999-009-0988-2.
7. Michelson J, Solocoff D, Waldman B, Kendell K, Ahn U, Ankle fractures. The Lauge-Hansen classification revisited. Clin Orthop Relat Res. 1997;345:198–205.
8. Michelson JD, Magid D, McHale K. Clinical utility of a stability-based ankle fracture classification system. J Orthop Trauma. 2007;21:307–15.
9. Dawe EJ, Shafafy R, Quayle J, Gougoulias N, Wee A, Sakellariou A. The effect of different methods of stability assessment on fixation rate and complications in supination external rotation (SER) 2/4 ankle fractures. Foot Ankle Surg. 2015;21(2):86–90. https://doi.org/10.1016/j.fas.2014.09.010.
10. Baumbach SF, Rellensmann K, Spindler FT, Böcker W, Barg AD, Mittlmeier T, Ochman S, Rammelt S, Polzer H. Immediate weight bearing without immobilization for operatively treated ankle fractures is safe – a systematic review. Foot Ankle Surg. 2023;29(4):306–16. https://doi.org/10.1016/j.fas.2023.04.006.

11. Lauge-Hansen N. Fractures of the ankle. III. Generic roentgenologic diagnosis of fractures of the ankle. Am J Roentgenol. 1954;71:456–71.
12. Gardner MJ, Demetrakopoulos D, Briggs SM, Helfet DL, Lorich DG. The ability of the Lauge-Hansen classification to predict ligament injury and mechanism in ankle fractures: an MRI study. J Orthop Trauma. 2006a;20(4):267–72.
13. Rammelt S, Boszczyk A. Ligament ruptures in Ankle Fractures-Was Lauge-Hansen right? Foot Ankle Clin. 2023;28(2):445–61. https://doi.org/10.1016/j.fcl.2023.01.007.
14. Gardner MJ, Brodsky A, Briggs SM, Nielson JH, Lorich DG. Fixation of posterior malleolar fractures provides greater syndesmotic stability. Clin Orthop. 2006b;447:165–71.
15. Mason LW, Marlow WJ, Widnall J, Molloy AP. Pathoanatomy and associated injuries of posterior malleolus fracture of the Ankle. Foot Ankle Int. 2017; https://doi.org/10.1177/1071100717719533. [Epub ahead of print]
16. Bartoníček J, Rammelt S, Tuček M. Posterior malleolar fractures: changing concepts and recent developments. Foot Ankle Clin. 2017;22(1):125–45. https://doi.org/10.1016/j.fcl.2016.09.009.
17. Rammelt S, Bartoníček J. Posterior malleolar fractures: a critical analysis review. JBJS Rev. 2020;8(8):e19.00207. https://doi.org/10.2106/JBJS.RVW.19.00207.
18. Kroker L, Neumann AP, Beyer F, Rammelt S. Ankle fractures involving the anterolateral distal tibia: medium-term clinical results of 50 cases. Eur J Trauma Emerg Surg. 2023;49(2):941–9. https://doi.org/10.1007/s00068-022-02161-0.
19. Miller AN, Carroll EA, Parker RJ, Helfet DL, Lorich DG. Posterior malleolar stabilization of syndesmotic injuries is equivalent to screw fixation. Clin Orthop Relat Res. 2010;468(4):1129–35. https://doi.org/10.1007/s11999-009-1111-4.
20. Solan MC, Sakellariou A. Posterior malleolus fractures: worth fixing. Bone Joint J. 2017;99-B(11):1413–9. https://doi.org/10.1302/0301-620X.99B11.BJJ-2017-1072.
21. Evers J, Fischer M, Zderic I, Wähnert D, Richards RG, Gueorguiev B, Raschke MJ, Ochman S. The role of a small posterior malleolar fragment in trimalleolar fractures: a biomechanical study. Bone Joint J. 2018;100-B(1):95–100.
22. Jeyaseelan L, Bua N, Parker L, Sohrabi C, Trockels A, Vris A, Heidari N, Malagelada F. Outcomes of posterior malleolar fixation in ankle fractures in a major trauma Centre. Injury. 2020;S0020-1383(20):31034–2.
23. Kelikian AS, Sarrafian SK. Sarrafian's anatomy of the foot and Ankle: descriptive, topographical, functional. 3rd ed. Philadelphia: JB Lippincott Williams & Wilkins; 2011. p. 176–95, 537–41.
24. Gougoulias N, Dawe EJ, Sakellariou A. The recovery position for posterior surgery of the ankle and hindfoot. Bone Joint J. 2013;95-B(10):1317–9. https://doi.org/10.1302/0301-620X.95B10.32527.
25. Gougoulias N, Christidis P, Christidis G, Markopoulos P, Biniaris G. Posterior malleolus fracture fixation in lateral decubitus position: surgical technique and results in 60 patients. J Foot Ankle Surg. 2024;63(6):742–6. https://doi.org/10.1053/j.jfas.2024.07.012.
26. Philpott MDG, Jayatilaka MLT, Millward G, Molloy A, Mason L. Posterior approaches to the ankle – an analysis of 3 approaches for access to the posterior malleolar fracture. Foot (Edinb). 2020;45:101725. https://doi.org/10.1016/j.foot.2020.101725.
27. Acevedo D, Suarez A, Kaur K, Checkley T, Jimenez P, MacMahon A, Vulcano E, Aiyer AA. Syndesmotic screws, unscrew them, or leave them? A systematic review and meta-analysis of randomized controlled trials. J Orthop. 2024;54:136–42. https://doi.org/10.1016/j.jor.2024.03.012.
28. Sogard O, McDonald J, Waters ME, Lee W. The clinical outcome comparison between trans-syndesmotic fixation and anatomic deltoid ligament repair in unstable ankle fractures with medial clear space widening: a systematic review and meta-analysis. Foot Ankle Surg. 2024;S1268-7731(24):00187–5. https://doi.org/10.1016/j.fas.2024.08.008.
29. Gougoulias N, Oshba H, Dimitroulias A, Sakellariou A, Wee A. Ankle fractures in diabetic patients. EFORT Open Rev. 2020;5(8):457–63. https://doi.org/10.1302/2058-5241.5.200025.

Chapter 19
Surgery for Malunited Ankle, Talus and Calcaneal Fractures

Stefan Rammelt and Choon Chiet Hong

Introduction

Malunion of the ankle and hindfoot after fractures of the ankle, talus and calcaneus is not uncommon and can lead to significant sequelae such as deformity, pain and severe disability [1–11]. Malunion predominantly affects articular congruency and anatomical axis of the joints leading to eccentric loading, altered peak stresses on the articular surfaces and impingement pain [1–20]. If left alone, this abnormal loading of the joint surfaces will add to the primary cartilage injury already triggered by the initial trauma mechanism resulting in progressive development of post-traumatic osteoarthritis. [1–19] The majority of these malunion cases are caused by missed, neglected or underestimated fractures and ligamentous injuries, inadequate reduction and/or fixation of fracture dislocations, and secondary displacement due to inadequate after treatment [1–3]. Patient-related factors include noncompliance, poor bone quality, systemic diseases like diabetes and rheumatoid arthritis, vascular disease and other conditions that may lead to impaired healing. Besides solid malunions, non-unions, aseptic and septic necrosis may be observed.

In this chapter, we will review malunions of the hindfoot including ankle, talus and calcaneal fractures and discuss the types of deformities and reconstructive options including joint preserving osteotomies and corrective arthrodeses.

S. Rammelt (✉)
University Center for Orthopaedics, Trauma and Plastic Surgery, University Hospital Carl Gustav Carus at the TU Dresden, Dresden, Germany
e-mail: stefan.rammelt@uniklinikum-dresden.de

C. C. Hong
Department of Orthopaedic Surgery, National University Hospital, Singapore, Singapore

M. Bhatia (ed.), *Surgical Techniques of the Foot and Ankle*,
https://doi.org/10.1007/978-3-031-93742-2_19

Patient Assessment

A complete assessment starting with medical history should be routinely performed followed by appropriate clinical examination and radiological imaging modalities. Clinical history should include the patient's primary complaint and functional impairment affecting the ambulatory status, activities of daily living, work and sporting activities. Medical comorbidities such as diabetes, peripheral arterial disease, systemic conditions and risk factors like smoking and substance abuse (alcohol/drugs) must also be evaluated early and optimized medically as these can negatively affect surgical outcomes. Clinical examination should assess the general deformity and malalignment of the whole lower limb, soft tissue conditions such as swelling, previous surgical scars, callosities indicating eccentric loading, chronic wounds or skin defects, neurovascular status, joint range of motion and joint stability (Fig. 19.1). The unaffected contralateral side serves as a template for potential correction. A holistic assessment allows the surgeon to better identify and plan the reconstructive surgery as well as manage the patient's expectation in terms of potential complications and residual deformity that cannot be corrected due to soft tissue contractures and scarring in addition to residual deficits such as stiffness, swelling and pain [1–3, 20–24].

For the ankle and hindfoot, it is imperative to obtain bilateral weight-bearing anteroposterior and lateral radiographs of the foot and ankle [1–3]. In addition, a hindfoot alignment view which demonstrates the heel alignment with respect to the tibial axis with the patient standing such as the Saltzman view is important to show the amount of angular deformity at the hindfoot with associated compensatory deformities [1–4]. The anteroposterior ankle radiograph with the foot in 15 degrees

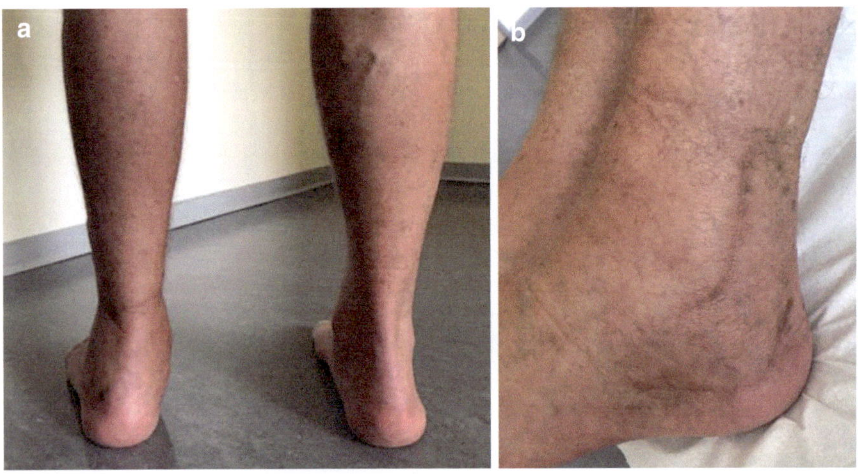

Fig. 19.1 (**a**) Clinical examination is crucial for evaluating visible deformities like valgus deviation, broadening, and loss of height of the hindfoot in case of a malunited left calcaneal fracture. (**b**) The location and condition of pre-existing scars is important for planning corrective surgery

of internal rotation (mortise view) will reveal any malleolar or supramalleolar deformities (Fig. 19.2), talar tilt in case of instability, loss of hindfoot height and fibulocalcaneal abutment resulting from calcaneal malunions. The lateral view radiograph of the foot will provide information such as sagittal talo-metatarsal alignment, presence of anterior ankle impingement, loss of hindfoot height (Böhler's angle) and joint depression in cases of malunited calcaneal fracture with severe loss of hindfoot height while malunited talar neck fracture, cavus or flatfoot deformity can be detected easily. The anteroposterior (dorsoplantar) view radiograph of the foot with the tube tilted 20 degrees towards the toes will demonstrate talar head/neck deformities with associated Chopart joint involvement, forefoot and midfoot abduction or adduction (axial talo-metatarsal malalignment) if present. If there is a clinically apparent limb length discrepancy or proximal deformities at the knee and/or hip, standing long leg alignment radiographs should be acquired from the hip to the heel.

Computed tomography (CT) scanning is extremely useful as it provides a 3-dimensional (3D) illustration of the complex malunion, nonunion and extent of bone loss, presence of subchondral cysts and avascular necrosis, articular alignment with severity of arthritis (Fig. 19.3) [1–3, 20]. Weight-bearing CT scan enhances interpretation of the ankle and hindfoot alignment under physiological loading particularly in case of peritalar instability. Newer tangible 3D printed reconstruction of the deformity can also be produced to help aid preoperative planning for complex deformities in terms of planning the level of osteotomy and optimal implant placement [25]. However, this resource may not be widely available at present and can be costly. Besides, magnetic resonance imaging (MRI) can also be used for evaluation of osteochondral defects, ligamentous and tendon injuries as well as determining

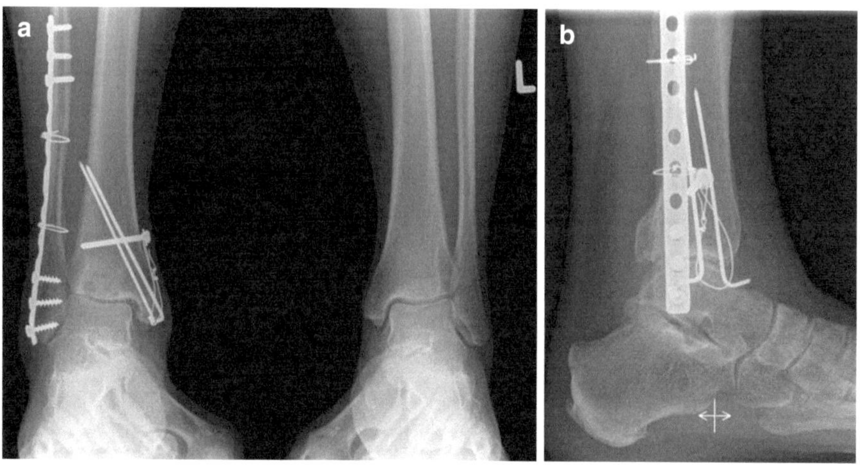

Fig. 19.2 Radiographs should evaluate axial alignment and posttraumatic arthrosis under weight-bearing conditions and include the formerly unaffected side. (**a**) Anteroposterior and (**b**) lateral standing radiographs of a 53-year old female 10 months after ankle fracture-dislocation showing shortening and valgus deviation of the right distal fibula, lateral shift of the talus with slight widening of the tibiofibular and medial clear space

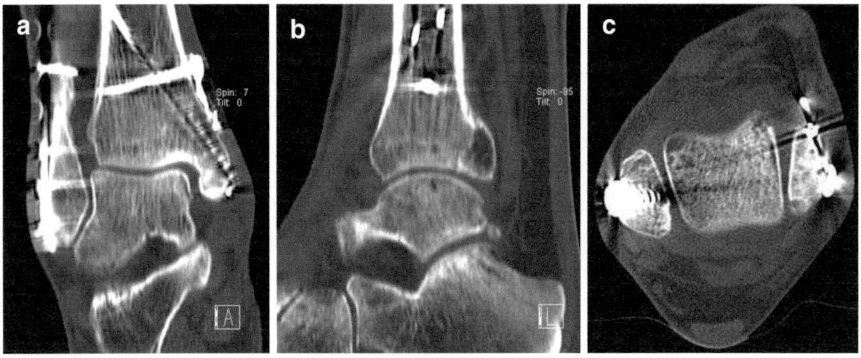

Fig. 19.3 (**a**) Coronal CT image confirming lateral shift of the right talus with slight widening of the tibiofibular and medial clear space. (**b**) Sagittal CT image showing a posterior malleolar fracture left unfixed but without posterior talar shift or step-off in the joint. (**c**) Axial CT image showing external rotation of the distal fibula. (Same patient as in Fig. 19.2)

the presence and extent of AVN within the tibial plafond and talus. Nonetheless, it is in the authors' experience that MRIs produce many false-positive pathologic diagnoses in the foot and ankle and tend to overread cartilage damage and AVN although quantitative T2 mapping sequences for cartilage quality can be useful [1–3, 26].

Malunion of the Ankle

Malreduction of ankle fractures have been reported to affect up to 44% of patients following operative treatment leading to malunions or nonunions [27, 28]. These can be supramalleolar, intra-articular (involving the tibial plafond) or malleolar [27, 28]. This chapter will focus on the latter, which is the most common pathology. Malunion of the malleoli deviates from normal hindfoot alignment resulting in eccentric loading and abnormally high contact stresses on the articular surfaces [1–5, 7, 8, 12–14, 20]. A simple 1 mm lateral translation of the talus reduces the articular contact surface by 42% in a biomechanical model while a deviation of ≥10° from the anatomical axis decreases the tibiotalar contact area significantly [5, 12, 13]. In addition, fibular shortening of ≥2 mm was associated with excessive lateral loading in the ankle joint and development of valgus deformity. [1, 3, 14] Similarly, posterior malleolus malunion with intra-articular step-off of ≥2 mm have also been shown to be an independent risk factor for poor outcomes and development of posttraumatic osteoarthritis regardless of the fragment size [3, 20–22]. Finally, malreduction and malunion has been reported following neglected displaced anterior malleolus (Tillaux-Chaput) fractures. [29, 30] This is consistent with multiple studies demonstrating inferior clinical outcomes following malreduced ankle fractures when compared to those with anatomically reduced fractures during the index surgery. [1–5, 7, 8, 12–14, 20]

The types of deformities in ankle malunions typically follow the initial mechanism of injury according to the location of the malaligned malleoli [3]. The pathoanatomy of malleolar malunion can then be described in analogy to acute ankle fractures (AO/OTA 44) (Fig. 19.4) [3]

1. Lateral malleolus
2. Medial malleolus
3. Posterior malleolus
4. Anterior malleolus

Despite being classified into each malleolus individually, ankle malunion can occur concomitantly affecting 2 or more malleoli including ligamentous instability such as syndesmosis and/or collateral ligaments. One also has to take note that partial impaction of tibial plafond can occur in ankle malunions which is vital to address to prevent posttraumatic arthrosis due to articular incongruency. We discuss 2 common ankle malleolar malunions and treatment options.

Lateral Malleolar Malunion

One of the commonest ankle malunion scenarios involves the lateral malleolus where the typical pathoanatomy often includes an inadequately treated ankle fracture (nonoperatively or surgically) with fibular shortening, external rotation with

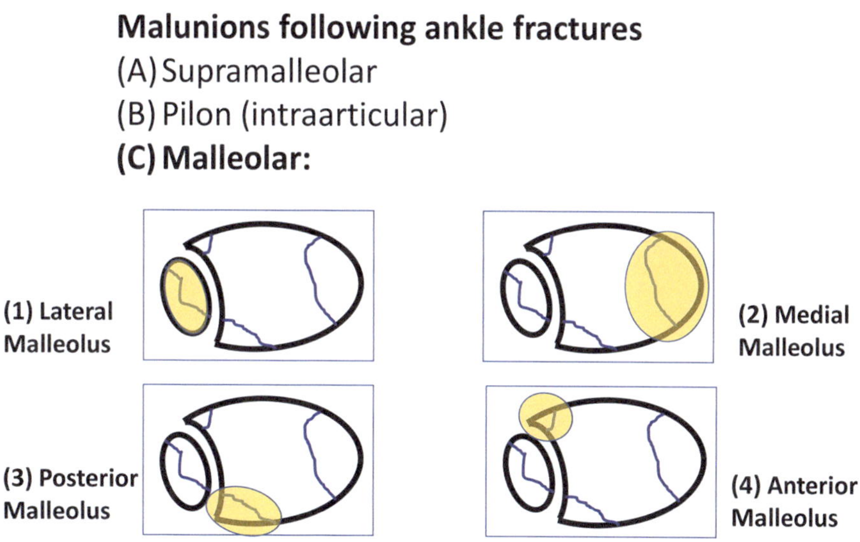

Fig. 19.4 Ankle malunions may be easily characterized like acute fractures with respect to the affected malleoli. Malunions of the tibial pilon (supramalleolar and intraarticular) and talus are of distinct etiologies. (From: Rammelt and Hong [3], with permission)

lateral and posterior displacement of the distal fragment (see Fig. 19.2) [3]. This leads to significantly increased loading of the lateral tibiotalar surfaces due to the lateral shift and rotation of the talus following the displaced distal fragment of the lateral malleolus especially in the presence of medial malleolar malunion, nonunion or deltoid ligament instability (see Fig. 19.3) [13, 31]. In some cases, concomitant malunited posterior malleolus and/or the anterolateral tibial tubercle (anterior malleolus/Chaput fragment) can occur manifesting as syndesmotic instability with widening of the mortise and tibiofibular clear space due to bony displacement and malunion or an isolated syndesmotic instability from ligamentous injury itself [3].

Joint-preserving corrections have a good potential for delaying or halting the progression of posttraumatic arthritis at the ankle despite visible signs of arthrosis at the time of surgery. It should be pursued in active and compliant patients with preserved range of motion, reasonable bone stock and a cartilage cover over about 2/3 of the joint surface.

The most common malunion with shortening of the lateral malleolus typically requires a fibular osteotomy aimed at lengthening the shortened fibula while addressing any associated valgus or rotational deformity (Fig. 19.5). A lateral approach to the fibula is used for this technique with special attention given to protect the superficial peroneal nerve at the proximal portion of the incision. An oblique

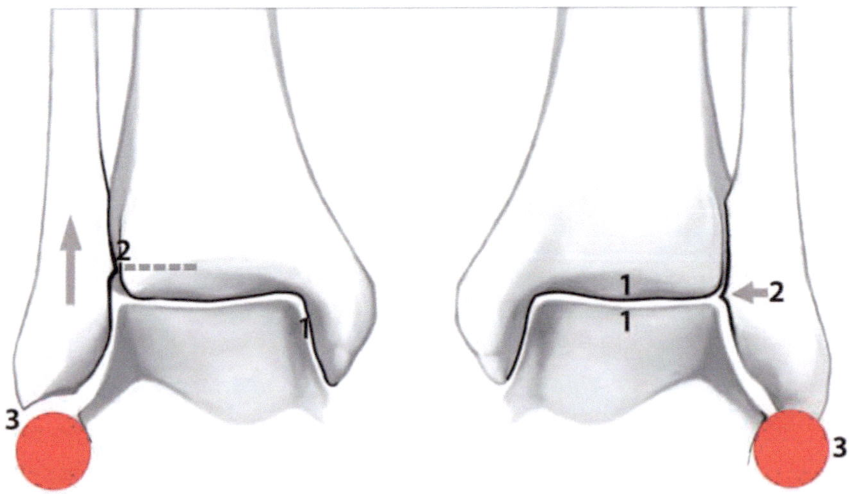

Fig. 19.5 Radiographic landmarks for fibular reduction and correction (Weber indices). (1) Trilateral intervals of the ankle joint should be equal and parallel, the medial clear space should not be wider than the superior clear space. (2) The medial spike of the distal fibula ("Weber's nose") should indicate and continue the level of the tibial subchondral bone ("Menard-Shenton line of the ankle"). (3) The contour of the lateral talar process continues as an unbroken curve to the peroneal recess in the distal fibula ("Weber–Kreis", German for "Weber circle" or "dime sign"). (From: Rammelt S, Zwipp H. Korrektur fehlverheilter Fibulafrakturen. In: Hamel, J, Zwipp H (eds.): Meistertechniken in der operativen Orthopädie und Unfallchirurgie. Sprunggelenk und Rückfuß. Berlin, Springer, 2016, S. 83–92, with permission)

or Z-shaped osteotomy can be utilized for lengthening of up to 5 mm without any need for bone grafting although a transverse osteotomy with corticocancellous bone from the tibia or iliac crest would be more reliable if lengthening >5 mm is required [1, 3, 9, 32]. Following the fibula osteotomy, distraction is usually performed with assistance from a plate where a rigid straight plate is first fixed to the distal fragment of the fibula and lengthened progressively to the desired correction using a lamina spreader or plate tensioner between the proximal part of the plate and a single cortical screw proximal to the plate (Fig. 19.6). The amount of lengthening can be ascertained with the use of an image-intensifier at the ankle mortise to achieve congruency and correction of the deformity. Once the desired length and deformity has been corrected, the plate can be fixed proximally [1, 3, 9, 32, 33]. Typically, the residual valgus deformity will be corrected once the rigid straight plate is fixed and tightened proximally to push the talus medially [1, 3, 9, 32]. Any rotational deformity will also correct as the distal fibula fragment glides distally through the curved lateral facet of the talus with the ankle held in neutral position [1, 3, 9]. On the other hand, if significant rotational deformity correction is needed, it can be adjusted using K wires inserted into the proximal and distal fibula fragment at the exact angle of malrotation as measured on the preoperative CT scan followed by careful derotation during the lengthening process with both K wires being visibly parallel at the end of the corrective manoeuvre [1, 3, 34]. A cadaveric study has shown that this K wire technique to correct for malrotated fibular malunion can be reliably corrected within 1.6° of the values of the normal contralateral ankle as confirmed with CT imaging [34].

Special attention has to be given in situations where the deformity is only partially corrected with residual widened medial clear space following lengthening because debridement and scar tissue removal in the medial gutter is needed to allow the talus to be reduced adequately [3]. In the event of concomitant medial malleolar deformity due to malunion, the medial malleolus has to be osteotomized along the

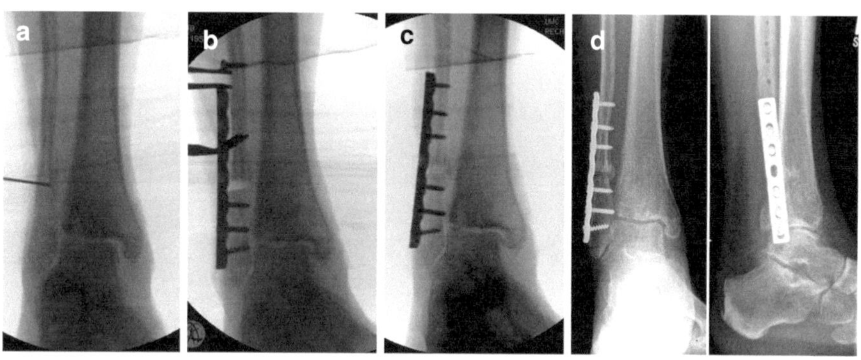

Fig. 19.6 (**a–c**) Fibular lengthening osteotomy in the classic Weber technique. Note the correction of the wide tibiofibular and medial clear space through suprasyndesmal fibular osteotomy. (**d**) Standing radiographs at 3 months showing physiological ankle alignment and osseous consolidation. (Same patient as in Figs. 19.2 and 19.3)

former fracture and released from intervening scar tissue prior to attempting fibular lengthening osteotomy. [3] Any residual deltoid instability can be evaluated and treated simultaneously with transosseous reefing and fixation once the fibular lengthening osteotomy is completed. In cases of fibular nonunion, debridement of fibrous tissue and nonviable bone is absolutely necessary until bleeding bone ends are visible. The resultant gap can always be filled with autologous or allogeneic bone graft followed by plate and screw fixation as described earlier once the deformity is corrected. The tibiofibular syndesmosis typically tightens with fibular lengthening, particularly when the osteotomy is performed on a suprasyndesmal level. Nevertheless, syndesmotic stability should be assessed at the end of the corrective surgery and addressed in case of residual instability. [35]

Posterior Malleolar Malunion

Up to 50% of ankle fractures have posterior malleolar involvement that, if not adequately treated, may lead to malunions or nonunions [20–22]. They can present as isolated malunited posterior tibial fragments or concomitantly with lateral malleolar, medial malleolar or intra-articular malunions of the ankle following the initial pathomechanism of injury [20–22]. Bartoníček and Rammelt Type 1 (shell-like extra incisural avulsions) do not lead to ligamentous instability while even smaller posterolateral fragments (Type 2) may lead to ligamentous instability from rotational injury, fibular malposition or articular incongruity if displaced (Fig. 19.7) [36]. The larger two-part or multifragmentary fractures with medial extension and large triangular fractures from Bartoníček and Rammelt Types 3 and 4 if not treated properly usually result in three-dimensional deformities due to the amalgamation of rotational, abduction and axial compression forces which is associated with pronation injury mechanism [36]. Of note, posterior malleolar malunion is invariably associated with syndesmotic incongruity and instability as it carries the attachment of the posterior inferior tibiofibular ligament (PiTFL) [20, 36].

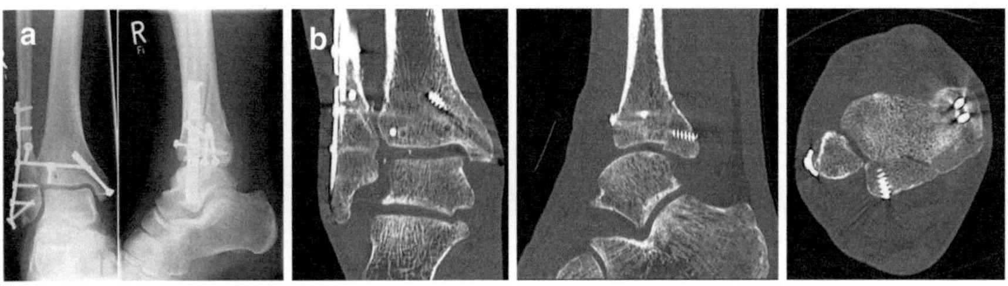

Fig. 19.7 (**a**) Anteroposterior and lateral ankle radiographs of a 46-year old male patient with pain on attempted weight-bearing 3 months after internal fixation of a trimalleolar fracture. Due to overlap of bone contours and implants, there is no visible malunion. (**b**) CT imaging reveals multiple intraarticular loose bodies and a malunited posterior malleolar fracture with articular step-off of 2 mm and lateral shift of 1 mm

The posterior malleolar fragment is commonly malunited in a vertically displaced position with a posterior articular step-off [1, 3]. This may be associated with a shortened, malrotated, anteverted/retroverted and/or valgus malposition of the fibula as illustrated earlier in combination injuries [1, 3]. Corrective osteotomies along the former fracture line may be pursued in cases with a single malunited fragment and a simple intra-articular fracture (Fig. 19.8) [1, 3, 9, 37].

In the authors' preference, the patient is placed prone and a posterolateral approach to the posterior malleolus is utilized. Notably, one has to identify the sural nerve in the subcutaneous plane and keep it gently retracted together with the lesser saphenous vein and within the subcutaneous fat during the dissection to prevent iatrogenic injury. Dissection is extended through the superficial and deep fascia to identify the interval between the flexor hallucis longus and peroneal tendons in order to reach the posterior distal tibia surface. At this stage, the posterior ankle joint capsule can be dissected to visualize the joint while ensuring that the PiTFL remains intact. Using fluoroscopy, the former fracture line is marked with 1 or 2 K-wires and osteotomy is performed with a chisel carefully along this line towards the articular step-off margin. A separate (postero-)medial incision may be necessary in cases with medial extension in malunited Bartoníček and Rammelt Type-3

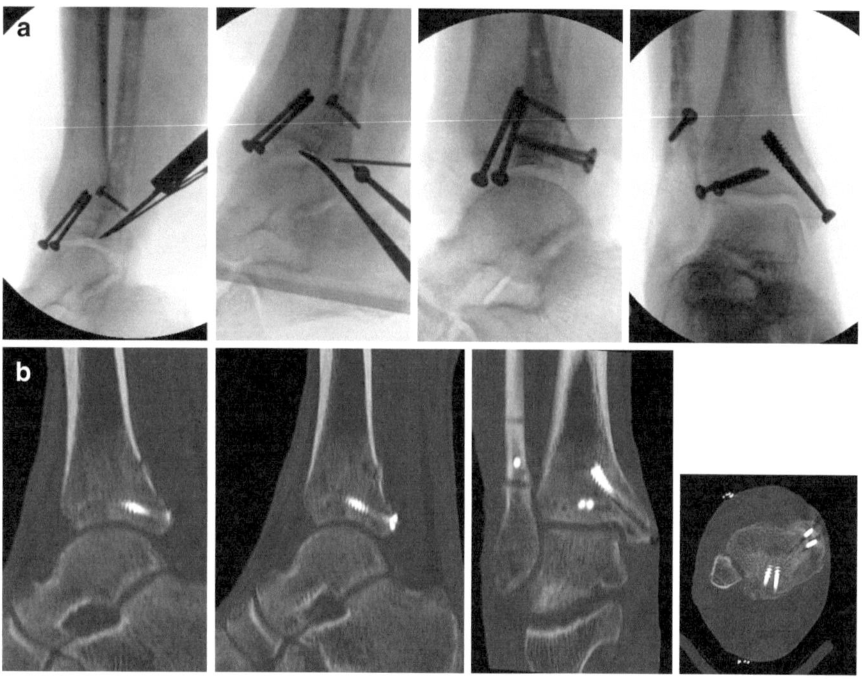

Fig. 19.8 (**a**) Corrective surgery consisted of removal of the loose bodies, partial implant removal, and posterior malleolar osteotomy with the patient in prone position. (**b**) Postoperative CT scanning demonstrates anatomic alignment of the posterior malleolus with restoration of the joint surface and tibial notch (incisura) resulting in a centered position of the distal fibula. (Same patient as in Fig. 19.7)

fractures. A transfibular approach may alternatively be used, particularly when there is a need for fibular osteotomy and/or syndesmosis reconstruction as a part of a more complex deformity correction.

Once the malunited posterior malleolar fragment has been osteotomized, the reduction is typically biplanar where the fragment is brought down so that the articular surface is flush with the anterior articular surface of the tibial plafond and adjusted medially because the posterior malleolar fragment is often displaced laterally due to the pull of the PiTFL. With adequate reduction, fixation can be performed with interfragmentary screws alone or antiglide plating with compression screws through the plate [1, 3, 9, 20, 37, 38]. Once the posterior malleolar malalignment has been corrected anatomically, syndesmosis stability would be restored in most cases without the need for additional tibiofibular stabilization.

Malunion of the Talus

Malunion of the talus is debilitating for patients because they are almost exclusively intraarticular and even minor malalignment can impair the function of peritalar joints that are essential for gait and ambulation [1, 2, 10, 15–19, 39–42]. This is especially true because any axial malalignment of the talar body will certainly lead to a 3D malposition of the hindfoot resulting in deformity and eccentric loading [1, 2, 10, 15–19, 39–42]. Talus fractures can be divided to central and peripheral fractures and therefore malunion of the talus can also be grouped into the same categories. Malunions and nonunions of the central talar fractures are frequently a result of inadequate reduction and fixation or nonoperative treatment of a displaced fracture (Fig. 19.9) while malunion of peripheral talar fractures (i. e. talar head, lateral and posterior process) are often a result of overlooking these intra-articular injuries [1, 2, 10, 15–19, 39–44].

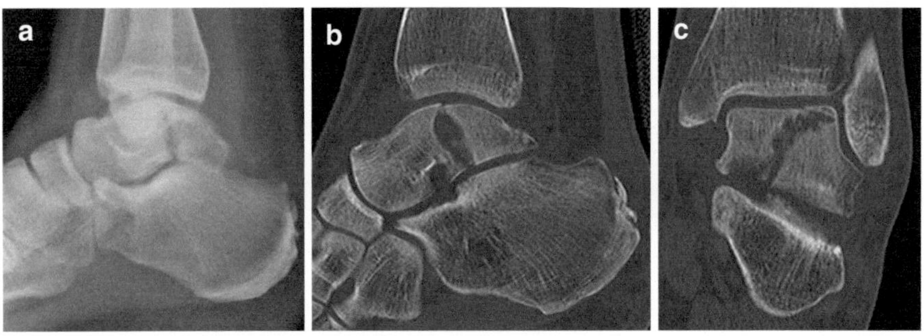

Fig. 19.9 (**a**) Lateral radiograph and (**b**) CT images of a non-union of the left talar body (Type II deformity) with displacement of the articular joint surfaces in a 35-year old female patient, 4 months after an initially overlooked talar body fracture

Specifically related to the talus, one has to take note of a particular complication which is avascular necrosis (AVN) of the talar body. AVN can occur in up to 50% of cases depending on the initial amount of displacement and/or dislocation [1, 2, 10, 39–42, 45]. To some extent, there will always be some areas of reduced blood supply in virtually all cases of displaced talar fractures. Despite that, only total AVN of the talar body is clinically relevant because this will inadvertently lead to collapse of the talar dome while partial AVN of the talar body will typically be progressively replaced by creeping substitution and asymptomatic partial AVN does persists in many cases [1, 2, 10, 39–42, 45]. Additionally, deep seated infection should always be considered as a differential diagnosis because this can occur in 3–8% of open talar fractures. [10, 18, 19, 39, 40, 46]

Reconstruction of a malunited talar fracture depends on several fracture-related factors such as the extent of AVN, severity of posttraumatic osteoarthritis, presence of infection and bone quality as well as patient-related factors including co-morbidities and compliance. A simple classification depicted in Table 19.1 can be used as a guideline for treatment options [2, 15, 19, 42].

Treatment of Type I–III Deformities

Corrective osteotomies for joint preservation aim to correct the deformity and realign the ankle and hindfoot in the absence of severe posttraumatic osteoarthritis without complete AVN of the talar body. Despite that, the decision to reconstruct or fuse one or more peritalar joints is more often than not made intraoperatively when direct visualization and probing of the articular cartilage can be performed (Fig. 19.10a). Hence, the options of joint preservation surgery and/or fusion must always be discussed with the patient and informed decisions made before the

Table 19.1 Classification for post traumatic deformities of the talus with corresponding treatment options [2, 15, 19, 42]

<table>
<tr><th rowspan="2">Type</th><th rowspan="2">Features</th><th colspan="2">Treatment options</th></tr>
<tr><th>Active, reliable patients with no symptomatic arthritis</th><th>Noncompliant patient, presence of multiple co-morbidities and symptomatic arthritis</th></tr>
<tr><td>I</td><td>Malunion and/or joint displacement</td><td rowspan="3">Osteotomy, secondary reconstruction and internal fixation with joint preservation</td><td rowspan="5">Corrective fusion of the affected joint(s)</td></tr>
<tr><td>II</td><td>Nonunion with displacement</td></tr>
<tr><td>III</td><td>Type I/II with partial AVN</td></tr>
<tr><td>IV</td><td>Type I/II with complete AVN</td><td>Necrectomy, (vascularized) bone grafting, corrective fusion</td></tr>
<tr><td>V</td><td>Type I/II with septic AVN</td><td>Radical debridement(s), bone grafting, corrective fusion</td></tr>
</table>

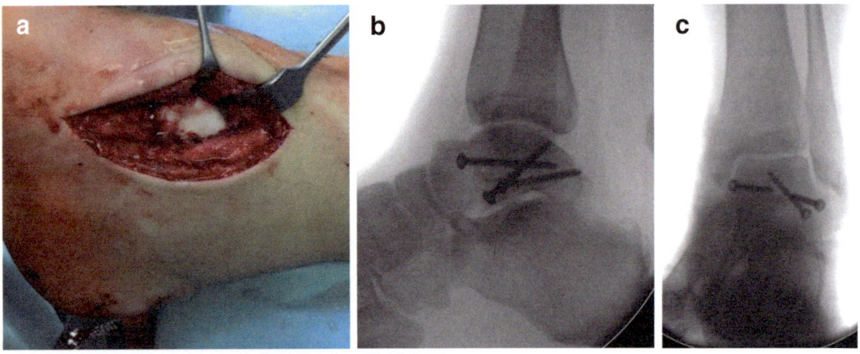

Fig. 19.10 (**a**) Anteromedial approach to the medial talar body showing complete cartilage cover, thus confirming the indication to a joint-preserving procedure for talar non-union. (**b**, **c**) Intraoperative fluoroscopic images following curettage, drilling, bone-grafting of the fibrous non-union and secondary screw fixation. (Same patient as in Fig. 19.9)

surgery. In type IV deformities where there is total AVN and collapse of the talar body, necrotic bone should be excised and debrided followed by autologous bone grafting, realignment and fusion of the affected joints. In the presence of infection such as in Type V deformities, repeated debridement of infected and dead bone should be performed until tissue cultures are negative. Typically, this will result in subtotal talectomy following repeated debridements albeit preservation of the talar head and talonavicular joint is preferred. Following that, a tibiocalcaneal or tibiotalocalcaneal fusion can be performed depending on the residual defect size and bone graft availability. On the other hand, malunions or nonunions of talar process fractures can be easily salvaged by excision of the malunited fragments but if left for a longer period, symptomatic subtalar joint arthritis can occur rapidly leading to a necessary in situ fusion of the subtalar joint.

Surgical approaches for corrective osteotomies of properly selected type I-III talar malunion are typically the same as in acute fractures although it often based on the type of deformity and malunited fracture lines [1, 2, 10, 19, 39–42]. The two most common approaches include the anteromedial and anterolateral windows. The anteromedial approach is commonly used to expose the medial talar neck, head and anterior body. If access to the central and posterior medial talar body is required, a medial malleolar osteotomy can be added. The anterolateral approach over the sinus tarsi allows access to the lateral talar process, lateral talar body and neck including the subtalar joint. If a more extensile exposure of the lateral talar neck and head up to the talonavicuar joint is needed, an oblique Ducroquet-Ollier approach along the relaxed skin tension lines is preferred. As with acute fracture fixation, most deformities require both approaches for optimal surgical correction. Occasionally, malunion affecting the posterior talar process or body will necessitate a posterior approach to be performed either from posterolateral or posteromedial depending on the deformity. In most cases, a posterolateral approach provides adequate access and visualization of the posterior third of the talar body and subtalar joint particularly when a femoral distractor with Schanz pin in the tibia and the calcaneus is used for distraction. Alternatively, a collinear foot distractor placed at the posterolateral distal tibia and the calcaneus can also help to enlarge the surgical window.

One must always take note of the blood supply to the talar body with careful dissection and avoidance of excessive soft tissue stripping particularly around the deltoid ligament, the sinus and canalis tarsi. This is especially important in corrective osteotomies for Type I and III deformities where there is solid malunion requiring osteotomy to be performed exactly along the former fracture line. It is best to carry out the osteotomy step-wise using small osteotomes carefully. On the contrary, Type II deformities typically present with fibrous pseudoarthrosis and sclerotic bone edges needing more tenacious curettage until viable bleeding cancellous bone is seen. Viability of the talus can be assessed with the tourniquet released. Visibly necrotic bone areas can be curetted and drilled to stimulate bone healing and remodelling. Bone grafting can be used to fill up the resultant defect to prevent secondary collapse or axial deviation. Furthermore, fibrous adhesions around the peritalar joints, tight gastrosoleus complex or deep flexors must be released or lengthened to allow the ease of deformity correction. Once the fragments have been mobilized, K-wires are often used as joysticks for reduction and provisional pinning of the reduction. Anatomic reduction is vital to ensure correction of the malalignment and this is easily recognized via the dual window (medial and lateral) approach. Certain parts of the subtalar joint that may not be easily accessible to assess articular congruity after reduction despite distraction may benefit from arthroscopy performed open using a small-diameter arthroscope to directly visualize the articular surfaces. Additionally, fluoroscopy is used to ensure the reduction and overall alignment is optimal (Fig. 19.10b, c).

In malunited fractures of the talar head, there is often involvement of the Chopart (mid-tarsal) joints. Besides the obvious incongruity of the talonavicular joint, any residual incongruity of instability at the calcaneocuboid joint has to be ruled out as well. For correction of the talar head, the anteromedial approach is extended distally to access the talonavicular joint and the Ducroquet-Ollier approach is used to access the talar head from lateral [1]. It is very important to achieve anatomic reduction of the talonavicular joint as it prevents peritalar subluxation by establishing a stable relationship between the medial and lateral columns of the foot.

Once reduction is achieved and held provisionally with K-wires, fixation can be performed with 2.7–3.5 mm screws. Following debridement and bone grafting for a non-union, a mini fragment plate may be preferred as a bridging plate construct in comminuted fractures either applied medially on the compression site to prevent varus collapse or bilaterally in some cases. 3D fluoroscopy may be useful in this situation to visualize the correct placement of implants.

Notably, cartilage lesions from the previous trauma can be found at the ankle, subtalar or talonavicular joints during corrective osteotomies. If the lesions are small and superficial, loose flaps can be fixed or resected. In cases with larger full thickness cartilage lesions, bone marrow stimulation procedure such as curettage to stable rim of cartilage followed by microfracture can be performed to encourage formation of fibrocartilage. In reality, the majority of Type I-III talar malunions and nonunions will present with end-stage arthritic changes (>50% articular surfaces affected) and arthrodesis of the affected joint(s) will be the treatment of choice. This entails correction of the axial malalignment of peritalar joints followed by fusion of these individually affected joints. Total ankle replacement is an alternative treatment option for symptomatic end-stage ankle arthritis if the tibial and talar bone stock is well preserved. Total ankle replacement should be particularly considered for cases where the subtalar joint and talonavicular joints are already arthritic to avoid a pantalar fusion resulting in a stiff ankle/hindfoot complex. The ankle can be replaced concomitantly with the subtalar and/or talonavicular joint fusion as a single procedure or staged as interval procedures.

The treatment of choice for malunion or (more frequently) nonunion of **lateral or posterior process fractures** is typically resection of the unstable fragments and arthrolysis as these loose fragments frequently affect the intact cartilage on the corresponding joint facets of the tibia and/or calcaneus. If joint irritation has already progressed to symptomatic arthritis, in situ fusion of the subtalar joint is performed [41, 43, 44].

It is the authors' experience that partial AVN does not develop or progress after corrective osteotomy of Type I-III deformities (Fig. 19.11). However, development or progression of posttraumatic arthritis maybe observed in a substantial number of patients depending on the initial severity of injury and duration of follow-up [40]. Only about one third of these patients actually require a secondary fusion.

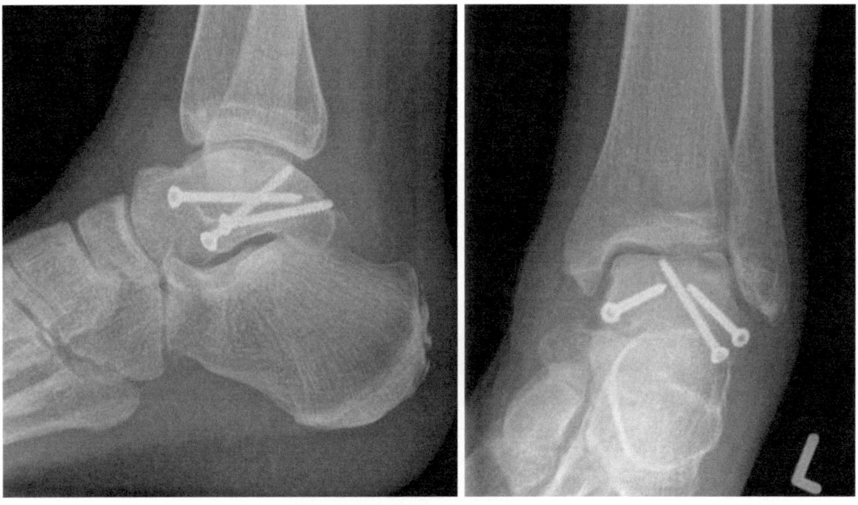

Fig. 19.11 Radiographs at one year after secondary reconstruction of a Type II deformity showing complete osseous union without signs of avascular necrosis or osteoarthritis. (same patient as in Figs. 19.9 and 19.10)

Treatment of Type IV–V Deformities

If AVN extends to the whole talar body, options with joint-preservation are limited. As long as there is no collapse of the joint facets, treatment options for AVN include protection, medication, extracorporeal shock wave therapy, bone marrow aspirate, drilling, and (vascularized) bone grafting, e. g. from the medial femoral condyle [45].

Complete AVN with collapse of the talar dome are mainly salvaged with necrectomy, bone grafting and fusion of the arthritic and incongruent joints (Fig. 19.12). Alternatively, custom 3D prostheses providing either total talar replacement or talar body replacement with preservation of the talar head, may preserve peritalar joint function at least for some time [47]. Talar replacement may also be combined with ankle replacement and / or subtalar fusion [48]. A recent long-term study showed superior long-term results with talar body prosthesis than with tibitalocalcaneal fusion following total talar AVN with collapse [49]. However, the overall experience with these implants is limited and more studies with long-term follow-up are needed [50, 51].

Septic AVN of the talar body as the worst case scenario warrants staged treatment with radical debridements until negative bacteriological specimens are obtained. Besides allograft and autograft bone, customized cages, trabecular metal, or biomaterials like bioglass with antiinfective properties may be used for secondary defect filling. Reconstruction and fusion is then mostly obtained with internal fixation. Fixation methods include ventral or dorsal plates and retrograde intramedullary nailing which may incorporate custom cages [45]. With critical soft tissue conditions and lingering infection, partial or total astragalectomy and tibiocalcaneal fusion may serve as a salvage procedure.

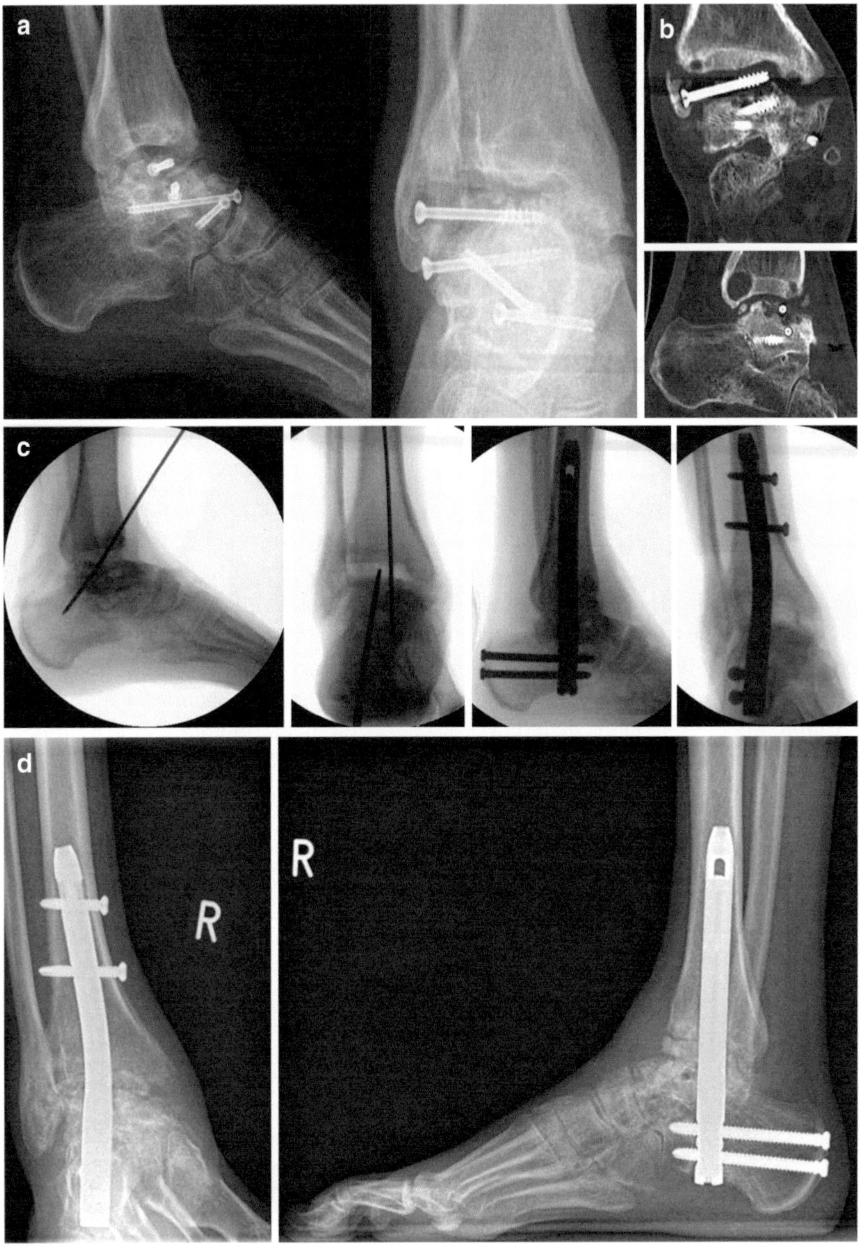

Fig. 19.12 (**a**) Radiographs and (**b**) CT images of a patient with complete avascular necrosis of the right talar body with collapse of the talar dome (Type IV deformity), loss of cartilage over the ankle and subatalar joint and hardware irritation one year following open reduction and screw fixation of a comminuted talar body fracture. The talar head still appears viable. (**c**) Treatment consists of implant removal, necrectomy with debridement of any avital bone, and tibiotalocalcaneal fusion with a curved retrograde nail and corticocancellous bone grafting from the iliac crest. (**d**) Standing radiographs at 6 months show stable fusion and physiological hindfoot alignment

Malunion of the Calcaneus

Calcaneal fractures are the commonest fractures of the hindfoot which can lead to a high level of dysfunction and morbidity [1, 2, 6, 11, 15, 24, 52–55]. Although treatment options have evolved significantly from conservative treatment to open surgical fixation and now minimally invasive via sinus tarsi approach or percutaneous reduction and fixation, malunion of the calcaneus continues to be a problem. This is largely due to conservative management or poor surgical technique with respect to reduction and fixation (Fig. 19.13) of displaced, intra articular fractures, resulting in hindfoot deformity, painful and stiff subtalar joint due to bony and soft tissue impingement with progressive posttraumatic arthrosis [1, 2, 6, 11, 15, 24, 52–55]. The pathomechanism of calcaneus malunion is a direct reflection of its original fracture mechanism where an axial impact to the calcaneus leads to a burst fracture pattern with widening of calcaneus, loss of height, varus or valgus deformity, and

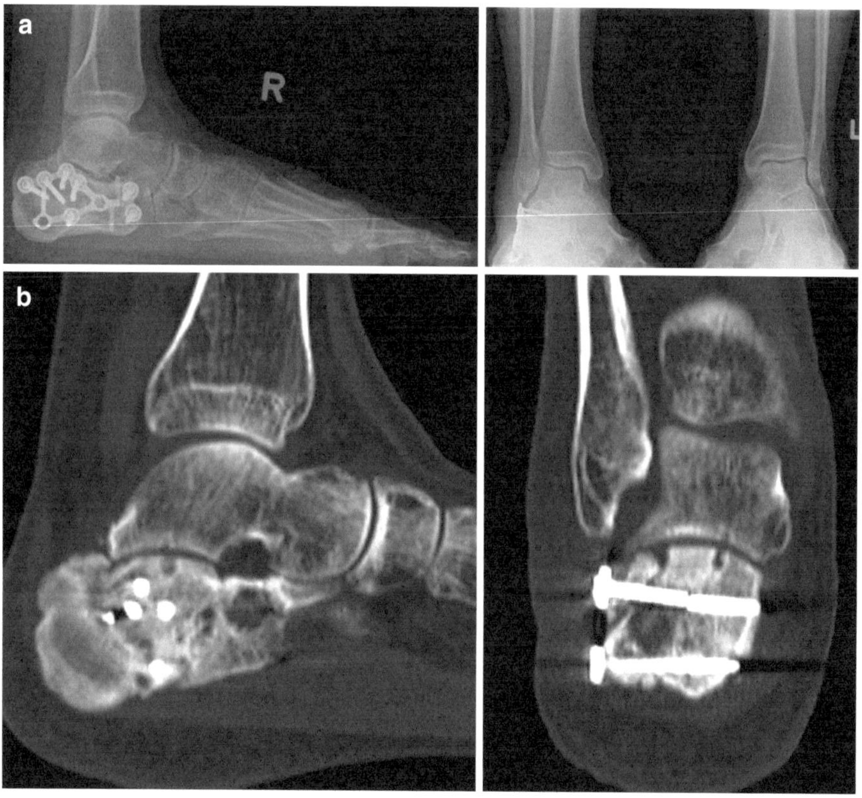

Fig. 19.13 (**a**) Standing lateral and anteroposterior radiographs of a Type III calcaneal malunion with loss of height, broadening and posttraumatic subtalar arthritis. (**b**) CT imaging confirms subtalar arthritis and reveals articular incongruity

articular cartilage damage [1, 2, 6, 11, 15, 24, 52–55]. When treated nonoperatively, the lateral wall displacement or blow out can cause impingement of the peroneal tendons and subfibular space. Due to the impaction of the talus through the calcaneus, the posterior facet of the calcaneus is often fractured severely leading to articular cartilage destruction with plantar displacement as well as shortening of the calcaneus body and subsequent varus deformity of the posterior tuberosity. There is also often decreased talar declination angle due to the depression of the talar body into the center of the fracture creating anterior ankle impingement. Intra-articular incongruity produces subtalar and calcaneocuboid joint arthritis while a missed sustentacular fracture can result in failure of medial support of the talus leading to varus malalignment of the hindfoot.

With severe deformities of the malunited calcaneus, the foot function is frequently affected due to loss of hindfoot motion, impingement pain, deformed heel shape restricting regular footwear and inability to walk on uneven ground. In order to improve the foot function, joint-preserving osteotomies can be utilized in cases of extraarticular malunions or selected intraarticular malunions without severe arthritis [55]. Unfortunately, end-stage arthritis of the subtalar joint develops rapidly with a residual step-off in the subtalar joint and is manifested already during presentation. Therefore, corrective arthrodesis rather than osteotomy is the preferred treatment in most cases.

Analogous to the treatment of malunited talar fractures, treatment of calcaneal malunion is very dependent on the specific complication associated with the particular type of malunion, patients' functional requirements, compliance and comorbidities. Because of this, Stephens and Sanders were the first to develop a classification system for malunion of the calcaneus based on CT scans into 3 categories [11]. Type I involved malunited calcaneus with a large lateral exostosis with subfibular impingement but without subtalar arthritis and malalignment although in some cases, extremely lateral subtalar joint arthritis can be present. This can be treated with a simple exostectomy of the lateral wall exostosis and peroneal tenolysis (originally described by Cotton in 1921) [56]. Type II malunion included additional advanced subtalar arthritis, while Type III malunions included an additional hindfoot varus malalignment of greater than 10°.

Following that, Zwipp and Rammelt developed another classification system in order to address all types of calcaneal malunion and defined 5 types of deformities (Table 19.2) including the quality of bone stock to enable surgical planning. Type 0 encompasses all extra articular and intra articular malunions with viable cartilage in the subtalar joint (including Stephens & Sanders Type I malunions) which can be treated with joint-preserving osteotomy and secondary internal fixation. [2, 15]

The classification by Zwipp and Rammelt provided the ability to add on deformities classically seen in malunions of calcaneus fractures so to provide stepwise surgical options for intervention [2, 15, 24, 54, 55]. Type I malunions with symptomatic subtalar joint arthritis (similar to Stephens & Sanders Type II) can be treated with in situ fusion of the subtalar joint which is often accompanied by lateral wall exostectomy, decompression and tenolysis of the peroneal tendons. Type II deformities

Table 19.2 Zwipp and Rammelt classification of posttraumatic malunion of calcaneus with proposed treatment strategies [2, 15]

Type	Characteristics	Treatment options
0	Extra articular or intra articular malunion without arthritis	Joint-preserving osteotomy
I	Subtalar joint arthritis without deformity	Subtalar joint in situ fusion
II	Additional hindfoot varus/valgus	Subtalar joint bone block fusion (+ osteotomy)
III	Additional loss of height	Subtalar joint distraction bone-block fusion (+ osteotomy)
IV	Additional lateral translation of the tuberosity	Oblique calcaneal osteotomy with subtalar joint fusion
V	Additional talar tilt at the ankle joint	Ankle revision, subtalar joint distraction bone block fusion and osteotomy

with additional varus (similar to Stephens & Sanders Type III) or valgus deformity require corrective subtalar joint fusion with asymmetric joint resection to correct for the varus or valgus malalignment. Minor deformities can be addressed with placement of wedge-shaped bone blocks while marked deformities—particularly those in varus—due to the pull of the deltoid ligament require an additional displacement osteotomy through the tuberosity.

The most common pathology following displaced intra-articular calcaneal fractures is substantial loss of height. These Type III malunions will require a subtalar distraction bone block fusion to restore the calcaneal height and alleviate the anterior ankle impingement (Fig. 19.14). Excessive cranial displacement of the tuberosity or varus (or valgus) malalignment requires an additional vertical osteotomy. [2, 15, 54, 55] Type IV calcaneal malunions are typically a result of fracture dislocation of the calcaneus with lateral, upward and posterior dislocation of almost the entire calcaneal body relative to the talus. The preferred treatment option for this type of deformity is a corrective osteotomy along the former fracture plane and subtalar joint fusion. It is also mandatory to reroute the dislocated peroneal tendons to its original retrofibular position with reconstruction of the superior peroneal retinaculum. Type V deformities are more complex in that the severe depression and deformity of the malunited calcaneus has affected the position of the talus leading to a varus tilt within the ankle mortise. An anteromedial or anterior midline approach to the ankle joint with careful debridement of ingrown fibrous scar tissue is necessary to mobilize the talus followed by realignment of the calcaneus and corrective subtalar joint fusion with additional osteotomy as needed.

This classification (Table 19.2) also provided modifiers in terms of quality of bone stock where solid malunion is termed “A”, nonunion is termed “B” and avascular necrosis is termed “C”. Solid malunion (A) cases can be treated successfully with corrective osteotomies/fusions as described earlier whereas nonunion (B) cases will always require curettage and debridement of the fibrous nonunion supplemented by bone grafting. Avascular necrosis (C) is less frequently seen in calcaneal

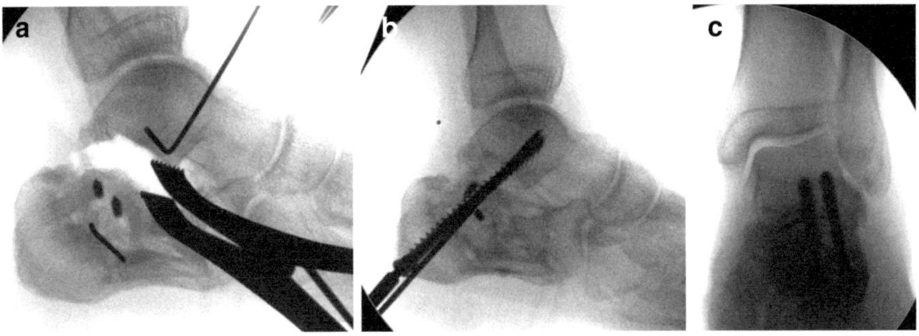

Fig. 19.14 Subtalar distraction bone block fusion of a Type III calcaneal malunion. (**a**) Following hardware removal and joint debridement, a lamina spreader is introduced into the subtalar joint to measure the amount of correction needed. (**b**, **c**) A tricortical bone block from the iliac crest of the required size is introduced into the subtalar joint to restore hindfoot alignment. The arthrodesis is fixed with screws. (Same patient as in Fig. 19.13)

than in talar malunions, but, if present, would necessitate a complete debridement of necrotic bone and soft tissues followed by stepwise realignment with corticocancellous or vascularized bone grafting.

In **Type I malunions** with isolated posttraumatic arthritis of the subtalar joint, in situ fusion can be performed via a sinus tarsi approach or even arthroscopically if there was no previous surgery. In case of remaining surgical hardware, the former extended lateral or posterolateral approach is utilized for implant removal and subtalar fusion. Removal of the lateral plate is followed by lateral wall exostectomy and peroneal tendon decompression with tenolysis. The lateral wall decompression starts posteriorly with an osteotome or oscillating saw aimed medially relative to the longitudinal axis of the calcaneaus in order to remove the subfibular impingement. For this, the peroneal tendons are gently freed from adhesions along the lateral calcaneal wall. Notably, the talofibular joint should be protected with a blunt retractor during this procedure and the resected exostosis should be kept as an autograft for subtalar joint fusion. The subtalar joint is then prepared for fusion by debriding the articular surfaces of remaining cartilage and sclerotic bone followed by perforation of the subchondral bone with small drill bits to improve bony union. Depending on the individual bone quality, cancellous bone grafting should be added generously.

Patients with a **Type II malunion** will also require subtalar joint fusion but with a lateral shift and closing wedge osteotomy for varus malalignment (Dwyer osteotomy) or a medial displacement calcaneal osteotomy for valgus malalignment. The subtalar joint is then fused in a physiological valgus alignment with 2 large (6.5–8 mm) cancellous screws inserted via stab incisions from the posteroinferior calcaneal tuberosity into the talar dome and neck. A less severe deformity can be corrected with wedge-shaped bone blocks inserted into the debrided subtalar joint.

The treatment of choice for **Type III malunions** with additional loss of height is a subtalar distraction bone block fusion preferably using the posterolateral (Gallie) approach with the patient in the prone position [57]. This approach confers good visualization of the fusion site and assessment of the overall hindfoot axis with respect to the lower leg. Most importantly, the incisional wound can be closed without tension even if substantial distraction is needed. Often, 1 or 2 tricortical bone blocks would be harvested from the posterior iliac crest and inserted press fit into the subtalar joint after preparation of the articular surfaces (Fig. 19.15). Minor varus or valgus deformities can be corrected based on adjustments of the shape and size of the bone grafts while more pronounced axial malalignment would necessitate an additional osteotomy.

In analogy to the type II malunions, marked varus deformity (<10°) will require an additional lateralizing closing wedge (Dwyer) osteotomy of the tuberosity. Valgus malalignment can mostly be corrected with wedge-shaped bone blocks introduced from lateral into the subtalar joint, correcting both coronal malalignment and loss of height.

In cases where the calcaneal tuberosity is significantly displaced superiorly, an additional vertical osteotomy would be required for plantar displacement to restore the level arm for Achilles tendon and plantar aponeurosis as well as the longitudinal arch of the foot. Alternatively, an additional closing wedge osteotomy at the calcaneal neck is useful to correct for substantial sagittal plane malalignment and ideally the wedge can be used for bone grafting in the subtalar joint. [54] Fusion of the subtalar joint can be achieved with 2 large 6.5 mm cancellous screws and additional screws may be needed for fixation of the concomitant osteotomy performed.

Type IV malunions (Fig. 19.16) are best treated with a corrective 3D osteotomy along the former fracture which is modified from the technique originally described by Romash [58]. This involves realignment of the entire dislocated calcaneal body through a medial and plantar shift with stable fixation to the sustentaculum fragment which is often the only portion of the calcaneus that is still in the correct position (Fig. 19.17). This maneuver reestablishes the calcaneal

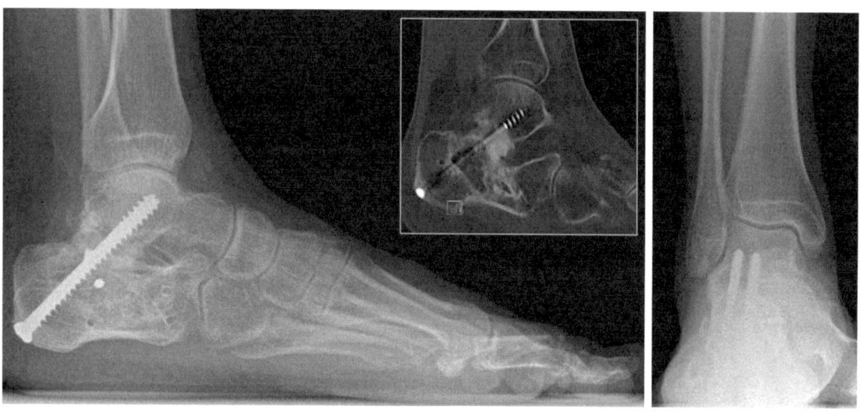

Fig. 19.15 (**a**) Standing radiographs and (**b**) CT imaging at 1 year following corrective surgery demonstrating solid fusion and physiological realignment of the heel. (Same patient as in Figs. 19.13 and 19.14)

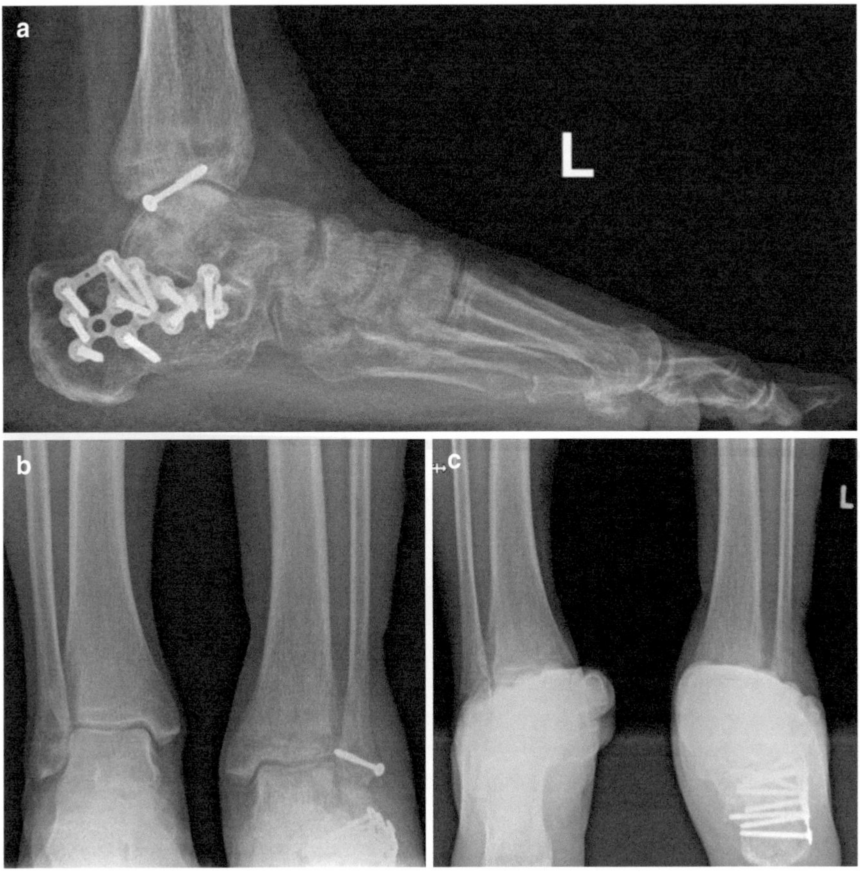

Fig. 19.16 Type IV deformity in a 59-year old male patient after lateral plate fixation of a left calcaneal fracture-dislocation in a still dislocated position. This kind of treatment combines the worst of both operative and nonoperative treatment. (**a**) The lateral weight-bearing radiograph reveals a double contour at the level of the subtalar joint and inclination of the talus due to loss of support of the calcaneus. (**b**) Bilateral anteroposterior ankle radiographs show a massive loss of height and subfibular impingement by the left calcaneal body that is displaced laterally and upward. (**c**) The hindfoot alignment view shows the massive axial deviation of the left calcaneus. (Same patient as in Fig. 19.1)

height, width and axial alignment. The patient is positioned on the uninjured side or supine with a wedge under the ipsilateral hip ("floppy lateral position") allowing bilateral manipulation. The lateral approach starts over the lateral malleolus and is aimed towards the 4th metatarsal base along the lateral utility line [1] and extended over the anterior process to the calcaneocuboid joint as needed. If there is a need to remove a lateral plate, the former extensile lateral approach can be utilized and a full-thickness fasciocutaneous flap is raised as in acute fractures. Care is taken to not injure the chronically dislocated peroneal tendons which lie subcutaneously and have to be gently freed from adhesions and retracted plantarly or dorsally with the flap (Fig. 19.18). The calcaneal body is moved plantarly

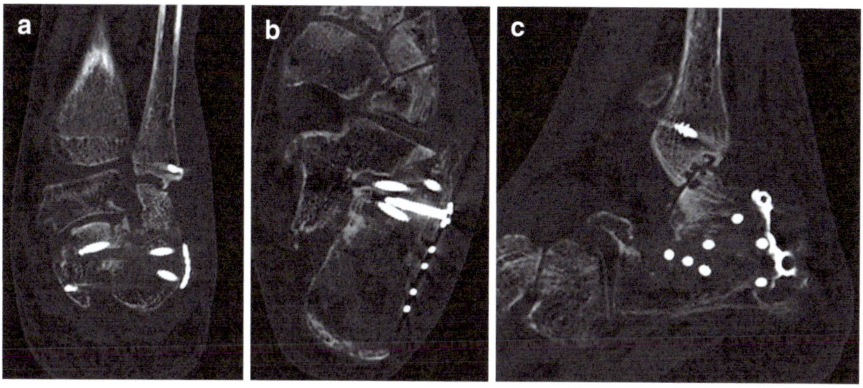

Fig. 19.17 (**a**) Coronal CT image showing the dislocation of the lateral calcaneal body and tuberosity towards the fibula resulting in painful abutment. (**b**) Axial CT image showing the lateral displacement along the former primary fracture line. (**c**) Sagittal CT image showing the fibulocalcaneal abutment with the lateral part of the body / tuberosity appearing intact. (Same patient as in Figs. 19.1 and 19.16)

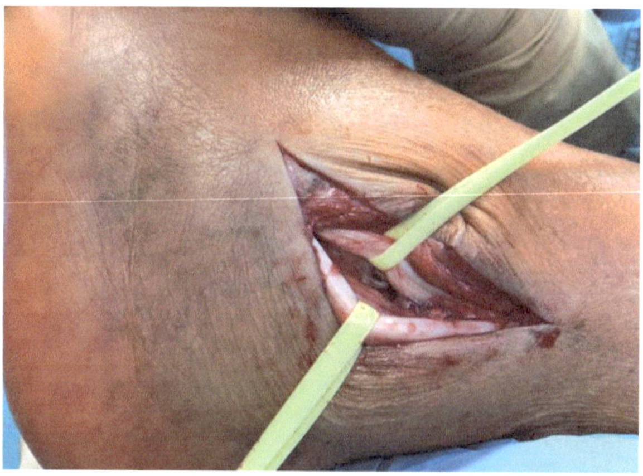

Fig. 19.18 Correction of a malunited calcaneal fracture-dislocation is carried out via anterior and posterior extension of the sinus tarsi approach along the lateral utility line from the posterior tip of the fibula to the calcaneocuboid joint. The chronically displaced peroneal tendons are freed from adhesions in the subcutaneous tissue and gently held away with a soft strap. (Same patient as in Figs. 19.1, 19.16, and 19.17)

in a stepwise manner and away from the tip of the fibula. The subtalar joint is accessed between the fibula and calcaneus, a laminar spreader between the latter is most helpful for that. The large step-off in the articular surface is then easily identified and a K-wire is introduced obliquely along the former fracture. The correct plane is determined with the Harris axial view using fluoroscopy (Fig. 19.19). Once the trajectory of the K-wire is confirmed, osteotomy can be performed with a standard osteotome from superolateral to posteromedial exiting

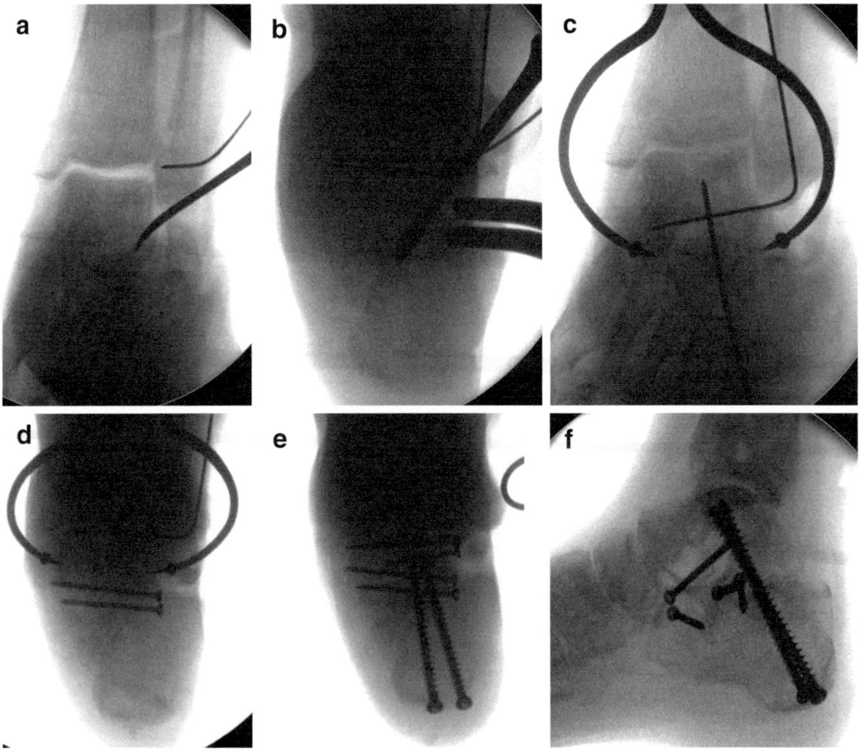

Fig. 19.19 (**a**) The former primary fracture line is accessed and identified through the fibula-calcaneal space. (**b**) The corrective osteotomy is then carried out along the former fracture. (**c**) The tuberosity and lateral body are shifted back plantarly and medially and a curved reduction clamp placed between the sustentaculum tali and the lateral calcaneal wall. (**d**) The main fragments are fixed first with 2–4 compression screws like acute fracture-dislocations. (**e**) Subtalar fusion is completed with 2 axial cancellous screws introduced percutaneously from the tuberosity and bone grafting as needed. (Same patient as in Figs. 19.1, 19.16, 19.17, and 19.18)

below the neurovascular bundle. Occasionally, there could be a wide gap between the sustentaculum and tuberosity fragments leading to an obvious nonunion with fibrous scar tissue intervening between these fragments. In such cases, debridement and curettage of the fibrous tissue and adjacent bone is needed until viable bleeding bone surfaces. Residual cartilage from the subtalar joint surfaces needs to be debrided and prepared for fusion as well.

Upon completion of the osteotomy through the former fracture line or debridement of the fibrous nonunion tissues, the calcaneal body is then shifted plantarly and medially. In some cases, Achilles tendon lengthening (or, rarely, gastrocnemius recession) may be needed to allow easier mobilization and reduction. Typically, soft tissue contractures can limit immediate mobilization of the fragments and therefore, adequate adhesiolysis and periosteal elevation is vital where blunt elevators can be inserted into the osteotomy site for leverage. Next, stepwise distraction using distraction devices such as the femoral distractor placed between the distal tibia and the medial part of the calcaneal tuberosity or a laminar spreader introduced between the superior aspect of the calcaneal body and the tip of the fibula can help to assist correction. A curved reduction clamp is placed between the sustentaculum and the calcaneal body to reduce the main fragments to each other. Once the reduction is satisfactory, provisional K-wires are inserted to hold the fragments in place for verification via orthogonal views (lateral and anteroposterior ankle/hindfoot with Harris axial calcaneal view) from intraoperative fluoroscopy. Residual bony defects in the subthalamic region of the calcaneus are filled with autologous bone graft from the anterior iliac crest. Stable fixation of the main fragments from the lateral calcaneal body to the sustentaculum is essential and achieved with horizontal 3.5–4.5 mm cortical or cancellous lag screws depending on the size of the fragments. Subtalar fusion is typically achieved with 6.5 mm cancellous screws. Once the bony deformity is corrected, peroneal tendons are rerouted back to its original retrofibular position with reconstruction of the superior peroneal retinaculum (Fig. 19.20). Lastly, final fluoroscopic views are taken to verify the correct hindfoot alignment and screw position.

Depending on the elapsed time since the injury, in Type III and IV malunions, anterior ankle impingement may have led to some degree of anterior cartilage damage and osteophyte formation necessitating anterior ankle debridement, arthrolysis, cheilectomy and microfracturing of cartilage defects via an additional anterior approach.

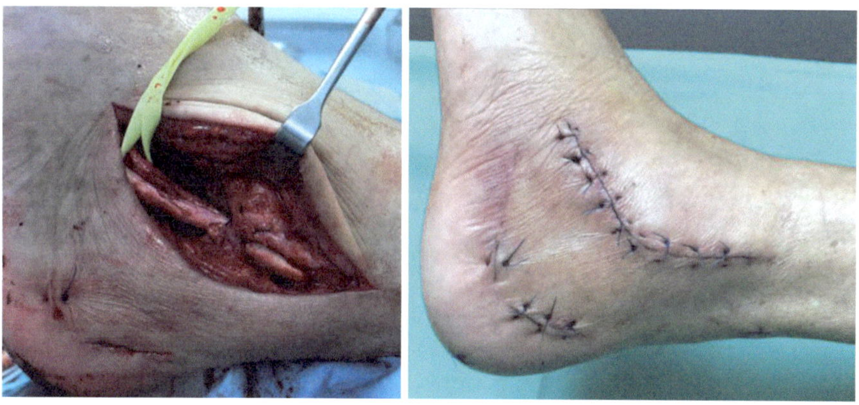

Fig. 19.20 (**a**) After decompression of the lateral wall through correction of the tuberosity, the peroneal tendons are rerouted behind the tip of the fibula and the retinaculum is reconstructed. (**b**) Wound closure is achieved without any tension. In this case, the preexisting plate was removed via a lateral utility approach and 2 small incisions along the former extensile lateral approach. This avoided dissection of the extensile soft tissue flap over the lateral calcaneal wall that was largely intact. (Same patient as in Figs. 19.1, 19.16, 19.17, 19.18, and 19.19)

Type V malunions always require additional access to the ankle usually via the anteromedial or midline approach to the ankle. This is because the talus is tilted in varus within the ankle mortise as a secondary deformity from the severely deformed calcaneus. The most essential step is to ensure adequate clearance of capsular adhesions and fibrous scar tissue in order to mobilize the talar body. The malunited calcaneus is then reduced step-by-step as described earlier according to the individual deformity and the talus is elevated gradually from within the calcaneal body using lateral or bilateral incisions while taking utmost precaution to avoid injury to its blood supply. Once the calcaneus malunion is reduced and the talus is mobilized back into the optimal position, the subtalar joint is fused with 2 large screws as illustrated earlier. Regularly, bone graft may be needed for residual bony defects and the lateral ankle ligaments can be repaired as needed mostly with a modified Brostrøm / Gould augmentation.

Extraarticular malunions and selected intraarticular malunions with preserved cartilage surfaces can be treated with joint-preserving osteotomies and secondary internal fixation and they are collectively termed "**Type 0 malunions**" [2]. In those with extra articular malunions, it is frequently the fracture of the tuberosity just behind the posterior facet of the subtalar joint where it is displaced cranially [52]. This type of deformity can be approached from a small vertical lateral approach at the former fracture plane where the osteotomy is performed. Once mobilized, the tuberosity is shifted plantarly progressively after adhesions and scar tissues have been freed. Achilles tendon lengthening is often required to allow the plantar shift and may be carried out percutaneously. Fixation is achieved with 2 large partially threaded cancellous lag screws.

Rarely, selected cases of simple (2-part) intraarticular calcaneal malunion and/or fracture-dislocations can benefit from joint-preserving corrective osteotomies as long as patients have intact viable cartilage, adequate bone stock and good compliance [55]. Despite that, it is in our experiences that, because of the shearing forces acting on the subtalar joint while walking, the vast majority of intraarticular calcaneal malunions rapidly lead to progressive articular cartilage deterioration and symptomatic arthritis needing subtalar joint fusion at the time of corrective surgery. In the event of corrective osteotomies, the surgical approach is similar to primary fracture fixation where an extensile lateral approach (or, increasingly a less invasive sinus tarsi approach that also allows for good joint visualization) is utilized for the classical joint-depression or tongue type fractures. The approach is also determined by the necessity of removing metal implants from previous surgery. Fibrous scar tissues are released, lateral osteophytes and a prominent lateral wall are removed to enable sufficient visualization and assessment of the status of the articular cartilage surfaces. Next, the osteotomy is performed using small chisels along the former fracture plane gradually. In malunited joint depression type fractures, an osteotomy at the angle of Gissane is required with a second one behind the posterior facet and a third osteotomy below the depressed posterior facet fragment connecting the other initial 2 osteotomy lines [55]. In malunited tongue-type fractures, the osteotomy is continued along the superior aspect of the tuberosity [59]. The depressed posterior articular facet fragment is then derotated and elevated to the posterior facet of the talus that is used as a template for reduction. Provisional K-wires are used to hold that reduction in place and orthogonal views with fluoroscopy are obtained to confirm satisfactory reduction followed by internal fixation using lateral plate and screws. Any residual bony defects at the subthalamic area can be filled with local bone graft from the prominent lateral wall or a corticocancellous bone graft from the anterior iliac crest.

Likewise, malunited calcaneal fracture-dislocations with intact cartilage over the posterior facet of the subtalar joint can be salvaged with the same corrective 3D realignment osteotomy as in Type IV malunions with arthritis as described earlier where the displaced calcaneal body is shifted medially and plantarly to correct the initial displacement [55]. Once satisfactory reduction is achieved, the fixation can be achieved with cancellous screw to the sustentaculum fragment followed by decompression of the peroneal tendons and rerouting of the tendons behind the lateral malleolus and reconstruction of the superior peroneal retinaculum [54, 60].

Postoperative Rehabilitation

Following corrective surgery at the ankle and hindfoot, a well-padded below knee posterior splint is applied with the ankle in neutral for the first few days following surgery until the swelling subsides. Active range of motion for the ankle and partial weight bearing up to 20 kg on 2 crutches in a walker boot is allowed from the 2nd postoperative day. The duration of partial weight bearing is adjusted according to the quality of the bone stock during surgery and extent of bony defects requiring bone graft. Progression to full weight bearing is only allowed after radiographic evidence of fusion, typically at 6–12 weeks postoperatively (Fig. 19.21). An extensive protocol of physical therapy is essential to regain a maximum of foot function (Fig. 19.22).

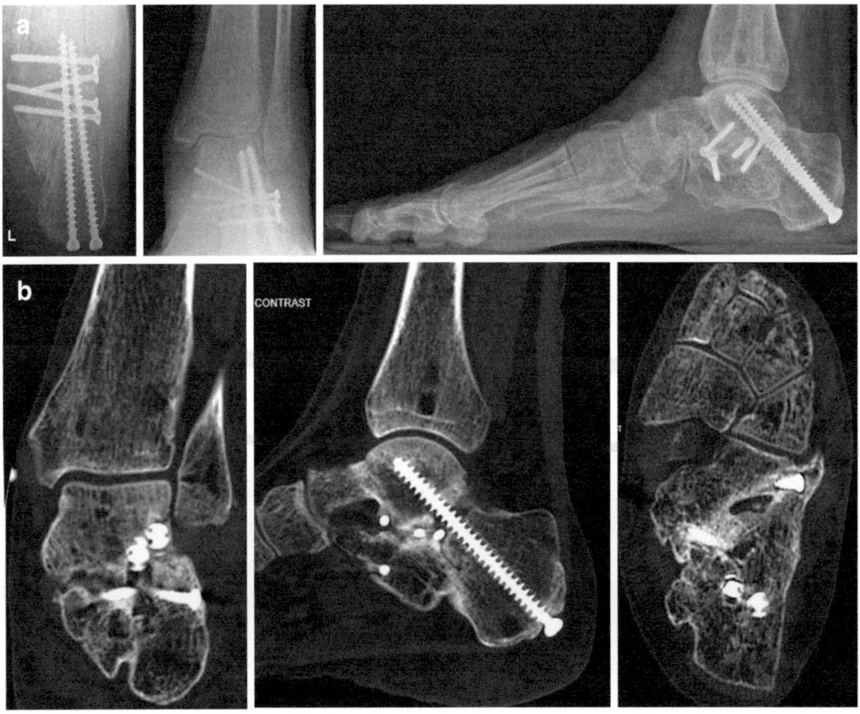

Fig. 19.21 (**a**) Standing radiographs and (**b**) CT scans demonstrating consolidation of the osteotomy and fusion with axial realignment of the foot at 3 months postoperatively. (Same patient as in Figs. 19.1, 19.16, 19.17, 19.18, 19.19, and 19.20)

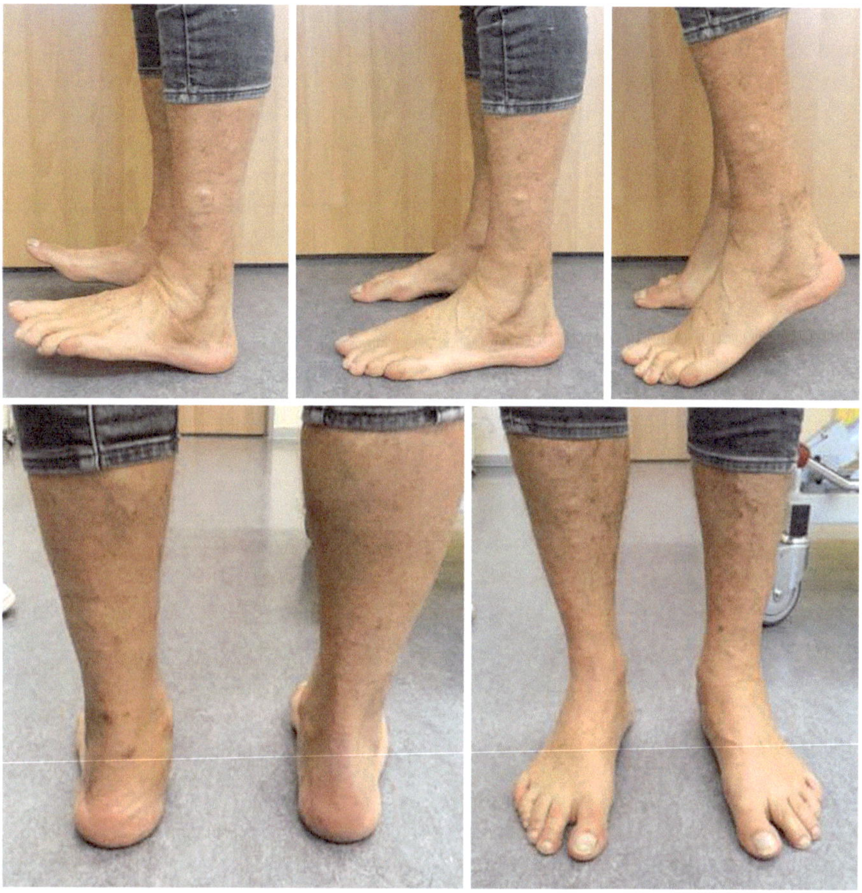

Fig. 19.22 Clinical aspect and sagittal range of motion 4 months following reconstruction of a malunited left calcaneal fracture-dislocation/Type IV deformity. (Same patient as in Figs. 19.1, 19.16, 19.17, 19.18, 19.19, 19.20, and 19.21)

Conclusion

Ankle and hindfoot malunions can lead to severe pain, disability and affect functional status of the afflicted patients. A thorough and complete preoperative assessment of the types of deformity, source(s) of pain generator, adequate imaging of the malunion, presence of posttraumatic arthritis, nonunion, infection or extent of avascular necrosis need to be established prior to any intervention. It is also essential to identify the patient's comorbidities, compliance and expectations in order to provide a holistic treatment plan to address the malunion. Existing classification systems for posttraumatic ankle, talar and calcaneal malunions are robust and easy to use in determining optimal treatment strategies in properly selected patients.

Corrective osteotomy with secondary internal fixation can be performed as a joint-preserving procedure in carefully selected compliant patients with viable articular cartilage surfaces and sufficient bone stock with little or no avascular necrosis. However, the majority of malunion cases with intra articular involvement will present with end-stage posttraumatic arthritis and require corrective fusion where asymmetric joint resection, distraction, additional osteotomies and structural bone grafting are frequently needed for axial realignment of the malunited deformity followed by fusion although fusion is restricted only for the affected joint(s) to minimize loss of motion and function. Bone grafting is almost always necessary for cases of nonunion, sclerotic, necrotic or infected bone following thorough debridement to achieve good structural stability and union. Multiple clinical studies have shown substantial pain and functional improvement with high satisfaction rates after corrective osteotomies and fusions for the posttraumatic ankle and hindfoot malunions.

References

1. Rammelt S, Zwipp H, Hansen ST. Posttraumatic reconstruction of the foot and ankle. In: Browner BD, Jupiter JB, Krettek C, Anderson PA, editors. Skeletal trauma. 6th ed. Philadelphia: Elsevier Saunders; 2019. p. 2641–90.
2. Rammelt S, Zwipp H. Corrective arthrodeses and osteotomies for post-traumatic hindfoot malalignment: indications, techniques, results. Int Orthop. 2013;37(9):1707–17.
3. Rammelt S, Hong CC. Management of nonunions, malunions and late syndesmotic injuries of the ankle. In: Herscovici D, Anglen JO, Early JS, editors. The evaluation and surgical Management of the Ankle. Springer Nature Switzerland: Cham; 2023. p. 271–98.
4. Fischer B, Mason LW. Reconstruction of severe ankle and pilon fracture malunions. Foot Ankle Clin. 2020;25(2):221–37.
5. Giannini S, Faldini C, Acri F, Leonetti D, Luciani D, Nanni M. Surgical treatment of post-traumatic malalignment of the ankle. Injury. 2010;41(11):1208–11.
6. Sangeorzan BJ, Hansen ST Jr. Early and late posttraumatic foot reconstruction. Clin Orthop Relat Res. 1989;243:86–91.
7. Capogna BM, Egol KA. Treatment of nonunions after malleolar fractures. Foot Ankle Clin. 2016;21(1):49–62.
8. Rammelt S, Zwipp H. Intra-articular osteotomy for correction of Malunions and nonunions of the Tibial Pilon. Foot Ankle Clin. 2016;21(1):63–76.
9. Rammelt S, Marti RK, Zwipp H. Gelenkerhaltende Osteotomien fehlverheilter Sprunggelenk- und Pilonfrakturen [Joint-preserving osteotomy of malunited ankle and pilon fractures]. Unfallchirurg. 2013;116(9):789–96.
10. Rammelt S, Zwipp H. Talar neck and body fractures. Injury. 2009;40:120–35.
11. Stephens HM, Sanders R. Calcaneal malunions: results of a prognostic computed tomography classification system. Foot Ankle Int. 1996 Jul;17(7):395–401.
12. Tarr RR, Resnick CT, Wagner KS, Sarmiento A. Changes in tibiotalar joint contact areas following experimentally induced tibial angular deformities. Clin Orthop Relat Res. 1985;199:72–80.
13. Ramsey PL, Hamilton W. Changes in tibiotalar area of contact caused by lateral talar shift. J Bone Joint Surg Am. 1976;58(3):356–7.
14. Thordarson DB, Motamed S, Hedman T, Ebramzadeh E, Bakshian S. The effect of fibular malreduction on contact pressures in an ankle fracture malunion model. J Bone Joint Surg Am. 1997;79(12):1809–15.

15. Zwipp H, Rammelt S. Posttraumatische Korrekturoperationen am Fuss [Posttraumatic deformity correction at the foot]. Zentralbl Chir. 2003;128(3):218–26. German.
16. Daniels TR, Smith JW, Ross TI. Varus malalignment of the talar neck. Its effect on the position of the foot and on subtalar motion. J Bone Joint Surg Am. 1996;78(10):1559–67.
17. Sangeorzan BJ, Wagner UA, Harrington RM, Tencer AF. Contact characteristics of the subtalar joint: the effect of talar neck misalignment. J Orthop Res. 1992;10(4):544–51.
18. Canale ST, Kelly FB Jr. Fractures of the neck of the talus. J Bone Joint Surg Am. 1978;60:143–56.
19. Rammelt S. Secondary correction of talar fractures: asking for trouble? Foot Ankle Int. 2012;33(4):359–62.
20. Rammelt S, Bartoníček J. Posterior malleolar fractures: a critical analysis review. JBJS Rev. 2020;8(8):e19.00207.
21. Drijfhout van Hooff CC, Verhage SM, Hoogendoorn JM. Influence of fragment size and postoperative joint congruency on long-term outcome of posterior malleolar fractures. Foot Ankle Int. 2015;36(6):673–8.
22. Li Y, Chen Y, Liu X, Chen J, Gan T, Zhang H. Patient pain and function after correction of posterior malleolar malunion. Foot Ank le Int. 2021;42(12):1536–46.
23. Hong CC, Roy SP, Nashi N, Tan KJ. Functional outcome and limitation of sporting activities after bimalleolar and trimalleolar ankle fractures. Foot Ankle Int. 2013;34(6):805–10.
24. Rammelt S, Sangeorzan BJ, Swords MP. Calcaneal fractures – should we or should we not operate? Indian J Orthop. 2018;52(3):220–30.
25. Jastifer JR, Gustafson PA. Three-dimensional printing and surgical simulation for preoperative planning of deformity correction in foot and ankle surgery. J Foot Ankle Surg. 2017;56(1):191–5.
26. Schreiner MM, Mlynarik V, Zbýň Š, Szomolanyi P, Apprich S, Windhager R, Trattnig S. New technology in imaging cartilage of the ankle. Cartilage. 2017;8(1):31–41.
27. Roberts V, Mason LW, Harrison E, M olloy AP, Mangwani J. Does functional o utcome depend on the quality of the fracture fixation? Mid to long term outcomes of ankle fractures at two university teaching hospitals. Foot Ankle Surg. 2019;25(4):538–41.
28. Whitehouse S, Mason LW, Jayatilaka L, Molloy AP. Fixation of ankle fractures – a major trauma centre's experience in improving quality. Ann R Coll Surg Engl. 2019 Jul;101(6):387–90.
29. Rammelt S, Bartoníček J, Kroker L. Pathoanatomy of the anterolateral tibial fragment in ankle fractures. J Bone Joint Surg Am. 2022;104(4):353–63.
30. Rammelt S, Walther EJ. Joint-preserving osteotomy of the lateral tibial plafond for posttraumatic osteonecrosis: a prospective cohort study. Foot Ankle Int. 2024 Apr;45(4):328–37.
31. Curtis MJ, Michelson JD, Urquhart MW, Byank RP, Jinnah RH. Tibiotalar contact and fibular malunion in ankle fractures. A cadaver study. Acta Orthop Scand. 1992;63(3):326–9.
32. Zwipp H, Grass R, Rammelt S. Osteotomien—Distaler Unterschenkel und Sprunggelenk. OP-J. 2011;27:260–7.
33. Weber BG. Lengthening osteotomy of the fibula to correct a widened mortice of the ankle after fracture. Int Orthop. 1981;4(4):289–93.
34. Heineck J, Serra A, Haupt C, Rammelt S. Accuracy of corrective osteotomies in fibular malunion: a cadaver model. Foot Ankle Int. 2009;30(8):773–7.
35. Rammelt S, Boszczyk A. Chronic syndesmotic injuries: arthrodesis vs reconstruction. Foot Ankle Clin. 2020;25:631–52.
36. Bartoníček J, Rammelt S, Kostlivý K, Vaněček V, Klika D, Trešl I. Anatomy and classification of the posterior tibial fragment in ankle fractures. Arch Orthop Trauma Surg. 2015 Apr;135(4):505–16.
37. Weber M, Ganz R. Malunion following trimalleolar fracture with posterolateral subluxation of the talus – reconstruction including the posterior malleolus. Foot Ankle Int. 2003;24(4):338–44.
38. O'Connor TJ, Mueller B, Ly TV, Jacobson AR, Nelson ER, Cole PA. "A to P" screw versus posterolateral plate for posterior malleolus fixation in trimalleolar ankle fractures. J Orthop Trauma. 2015 Apr;29(4):e151–6.

39. Zwipp H, Rammelt S. Secondary reconstruction for malunions and nonunions of the talar body. Foot Ankle Clin. 2016 Mar;21(1):95–109.
40. Zwipp H, Gavlik JM, Rammelt S. Secondary anatomic reconstruction of malunited central talus fractures. Unfallchirurg. 2014;117:767–75.
41. Rammelt S, Winkler J, Grass R, Zwipp H. Reconstruction after talar fractures. Foot Ankle Clin. 2006;11:61–84.
42. Rammelt S, Winkler J, Heineck J, Zwipp H. Anatomical reconstruction of malunited talus fractures: a prospective study of 10 patients followed for 4 years. Acta Orthop. 2005;76(4):588–96.
43. Shank JR, Benirschke SK, Swords MP. Treatment of peripheral talus fractures. Foot Ankle Clin. 2017;22(1):181–92.
44. Boack DH, Manegold S. Peripheral talar fractures. Injury. 2004;35(Suppl 2):SB23–35.
45. Kopp L, Rammelt S. Posttraumatic avascular necrosis of the talus: prevention, course, and treatment options. Foot Ankle Clin. 2025;30(1):83–110.
46. Lindvall E, Haidukewych G, DiPasquale T, Herscovici D Jr, Sanders R. Open reduction and stable fixation of isolated, displaced talar neck and body fractures. J Bone Joint Surg Am. 2004;86(10):2229–34.
47. Dimitrov AS, Westover L, Jomha NM. Clinical use of talar prostheses. JBJS Rev. 2021;9(6).
48. Mitra K, Anastasio AT, Wu KA, Abar B, Schweitzer KM, Parekh SG, Easley ME, Adams SB. Outcomes of cobalt-chrome 3D-printed total talus replacement with and without combined total ankle replacement. Foot Ankle Surg. 2025;31(2):126–37.
49. Harnroongroj T, Arunakul M, Reingrittha P, Chuckpaiwong B, Angthong C, Tharmviboonsri T, Lertwattanachai P. Outcomes of Tibiotalocalcaneal arthrodesis vs talar body prosthesis as treatment of collapsed avascular necrosis of the talus: a 10- to 13-year-follow-up retrospective comparative study. Foot Ankle Int. 2024;45(5):435–43.
50. Morita S, Taniguchi A, Miyamoto T, Kurokawa H, Takakura Y, Takakura Y. Tanaka Y the long-term clinical results of total talar replacement at 10 years or more after surgery. J Bone Joint Surg Am. 2022;104(9):790–5.
51. Abar B, Kim MS, Adams SB, Adams WR, Amendola A, Easley ME, Ellington JK, Ford SE, Hanselman AE, Highlander P, Kwon JY, Miller CP, Nunley JA, Parker C, Parekh SG, Schweitzer KM, Shawen SB, Mann T, Kelly C. Initial safety of total talus replacement used to treat talar avascular necrosis. Foot Ankle Int. 2024;45(11):1258–65.
52. Ketz J, Clare M, Sanders R. Corrective osteotomies for malunited extra-articular calcaneal fractures. Foot Ankle Clin. 2016;21(1):135–45.
53. Benirschke SK, Kramer PA. Joint-preserving osteotomies for malaligned intraarticular calcaneal fractures. Foot Ankle Clin. 2016;21(1):111–22.
54. Rammelt S, Marx C. Managing severely malunited calcaneal fractures and fracture-dislocations. Foot Ankle Clin. 2020;25(2):239–56.
55. Rammelt S, Grass R, Zwipp H. Joint-preserving osteotomy for malunited intra-articular calcaneal fractures. J Orthop Trauma. 2013;27(10):e234–8.
56. Cotton F. Old os calcis fractures. Ann Surg. 1921;74:294–303.
57. Gallie WE. Subastragalar arthrodesis in fractures of the os calcis. J Bone Joint Surg. 1943;25:731–6.
58. Romash MM. Reconstructive osteotomy of the calcaneus with subtalar arthrodesis for malunited calcaneal fractures. Clin Orthop Relat Res. 1993;290:157–67.
59. Yu GR, Zhang MZ, Yang YF. Corrective osteotomies for malunited tongue-type calcaneal fractures. Foot Ankle Clin. 2016;21(1):123–34.
60. Rammelt S, Marx C, Swords G, Swords M. Recognition, treatment, and outcome of calcaneal fracture-dislocation. Foot Ankle Int. 2021;42(6):706–13.

Chapter 20
Fixation of Lisfranc Injuries

Togay Koç and Robert Clayton

Introduction

Early and accurate diagnosis of Lisfranc injuries is crucial to prevent long-term functional impairment and the development of post-traumatic arthritis. Due to the variability in presentation, from subtle ligamentous injuries to severe fracture-dislocations, a systematic approach using clinical assessment, imaging modalities and thorough intra-operative assessment of destabilisation within the zone of injury is required.

Clinical Assessment—A Cautionary Note

Often the orthopaedic foot & ankle surgeon is not at the point of presentation or initial care of a Lisfranc injury, particularly those of a more subtle nature. It is therefore, in their best interests, the surgeons' prerogative or even responsibility to educate first contact practitioners to have a high index of suspicion for and not miss Lisfranc injuries. The authors advise and utilise the production of local protocols for

Supplementary Information The online version contains supplementary material available at https://doi.org/10.1007/978-3-031-93742-2_20.

T. Koç
University Hospital Southampton, Southampton, UK

University of Southampton, Southampton, UK
e-mail: togay.koc@doctors.org.uk

R. Clayton (✉)
NHS Fife - Victoria Hospital, Kirkcaldy, Dunfermline, Scotland, UK

M. Bhatia (ed.), *Surgical Techniques of the Foot and Ankle*,
https://doi.org/10.1007/978-3-031-93742-2_20

emergency department and minor injury unit practitioners and doctors to include a thorough clinical assessment of midfoot injuries including an accurate documentation of the mechanism of injury, points of tenderness and the presence/absence of plantar ecchymosis. Earlier detection of these injuries will lead to expedient onward assessment and management.

Weight-Bearing Radiographs

Weight-bearing (WB) radiographs remain the first-line imaging modality for diagnosing Lisfranc injuries. Weight-bearing X-rays are mandatory over non-weight-bearing images in detecting subtle diastasis between the first and second metatarsals, as well as between the medial cuneiform and second metatarsal base. The identification of a diastasis >2 mm is highly specific for a Lisfranc injury, especially when compared to the contralateral foot [1].

The Fleck sign, a small bony fragment between the bases of the first and second metatarsals, is a reliable indicator of ligamentous disruption, particularly of the Lisfranc ligament. Several studies have identified the presence of this sign as a hallmark of midfoot instability, often warranting surgical intervention [2].

CT Scans

CT imaging offers a more detailed view of the osseous architecture and is useful through the spectrum of Lisfranc injury severities from complex, high-energy injuries for the assessment of bone stock to subtle low-energy injuries for subtle displacement. CT scans are superior to radiographs for evaluating the extent of comminuted fractures, small cortical fractures, and joint subluxations/dislocations, providing a 3D reconstruction of the Lisfranc complex. For high-energy injuries, CT can be invaluable in surgical planning, as it delineates the intricate fracture patterns that plain films may miss.

CT has a sensitivity of 83–93% in identifying bony Lisfranc injuries and plays a vital role in cases where plain radiographs show no obvious diastasis but clinical suspicion remains high [3].

MRI

MRI is the imaging modality of choice for diagnosing purely ligamentous Lisfranc injuries, especially when WB X-rays and CT scans are inconclusive. MRI provides excellent visualization of the Lisfranc ligament, which can be torn without bony injury in low-energy trauma [4]. Bone marrow oedema, indicative of subtle ligamentous injury, is also commonly identified in MRI.

The sensitivity of MRI in identifying ligamentous Lisfranc injuries is reported to be 97–100%, making it a highly effective tool when ligamentous instability is suspected, particularly in athletes or individuals with chronic midfoot pain [5].

Examination Under Anaesthesia (EUA)

When imaging is inconclusive, Examination Under Anaesthesia (EUA) remains a gold standard for confirming joint instability, particularly in subtle injuries. Additionally, in all operatively managed Lisfranc injuries, a systematic examination under anaesthesia of each column and/or tarsometatarsal joint is advised to determine which tarsometatarsal joints are unstable and therefore require stabilisation. Intraoperative fluoroscopy can further guide this assessment.

The importance of EUA is underscored by its ability to detect occult instability that may not be visible on imaging, particularly in low-energy injuries where subtle ligamentous damage is the primary pathology [6].

Despite the central role of EUA in the assessment and management of Lisfranc injuries, there is a paucity of literature in regards to its specific techniques, order of joints examined or how to apply its findings to intraoperative decision making and fixation configuration.

Surgical Algorithm

The surgical approach to Lisfranc injuries varies widely, depending on factors such as the energy of the injury, the presence of fractures, and the degree of soft tissue involvement. As early as soft tissue status permits, accurate fixation or fusion of the appropriate joints is critical to restoring normal foot biomechanics and avoiding complications such as ongoing instability, progressive deformity and/or post-traumatic arthritis.

Some surgeons advocate acute reduction and K-wire stabilisation pending definitive stabilisation after resolution of soft tissue swelling. The authors do not advocate routine use of this technique because any incisions made at the primary procedure risk compromising the ideal placement of incisions at the time of definitive fixation.

Patient Positioning

For most Lisfranc fixation operations, the patient is placed in the supine position with a thigh tourniquet to maintain a bloodless field. This position provides access to both the medial and lateral aspects of the foot, facilitating surgical manoeuvres including EUA, reduction, fixation and intraoperative fluoroscopy.

In cases where extensive lateral column work is anticipated, positioning adjustments may be required to ensure proper access for dual incisions and optimal visualization during fluoroscopy.

A sterile triangular bolster under the knee is helpful to position the foot so that the plantar surface is level with the operating table. This allows the image intensifier to be fixed in a position perpendicular to the operating table and a consistent position of the foot to allow reproducible EUA manoeuvres as well as freedom of movement around the food to perform intraoperative manoeuvres. This positioning allows the easy acquisition of Dorsoplantar images with the bolster in place and its removal combined with external rotation of the hip allows the performance of lateral radiographs without the need to move the image intensifier (Fig. 20.1a–g).

EUA Manoeuvres

EUA continues to be an important tool during Lisfranc fixation procedures, particularly to determine which individual Tarsometatarsal joints demonstrate instability as well as to obtain and confirm reduction prior to final fixation.

During EUA, the surgeon assesses stability both generally and specifically.

The overall stability of the midfoot is assessed through a sequence of stress manoeuvres. Accurate and reproducible intraoperative fluoroscopy is critical to this process therefore positioning and image application should be performed meticulously. With the knee bent over the sterile triangular bolster, keeping the plantar surface of the foot on the operating table and the image intensifier orthogonal to the operating table, the hindfoot is stabilised manually. The forefoot can now be manipulated for stress views, the results of which should be documented in both the operative note as well as with image acquisition. Stress radiographs should be obtained with the normal position as well as with the application of an adduction force followed by an abduction force, a supination force and a pronation force independently. Careful attention should be paid at each of these points to all the tarsometatarsal joints for subluxation in the medial-lateral plane as well as for diastasis in the second metatarsal base—medial cuneiform interval. The diastasis may extend into the intercuneiform joints or indeed into the naviculocuneiform joint. In the case of associated fractures of the navicular in particular, the instability can extend into the talonavicular joint (Fig. 20.2a–e, Video 20.1).

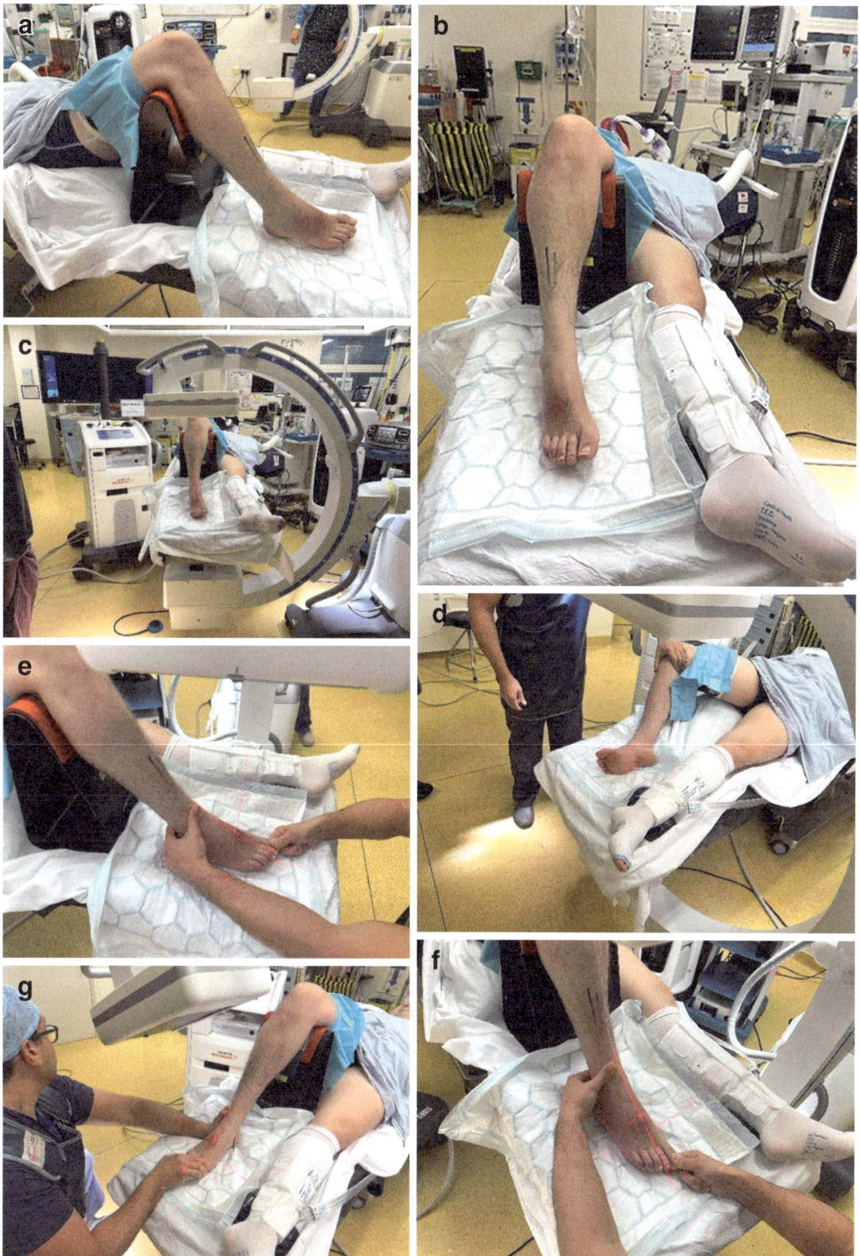

Fig. 20.1 (**a**, **b**) Patient positioning over triangle. (**c**, **d**) Patient/image intensifier positioning for DP & lateral views. (**e**, **f**) Patient positioning for DP & lateral views. (**g**) Patient/image intensifier positioning for oblique view

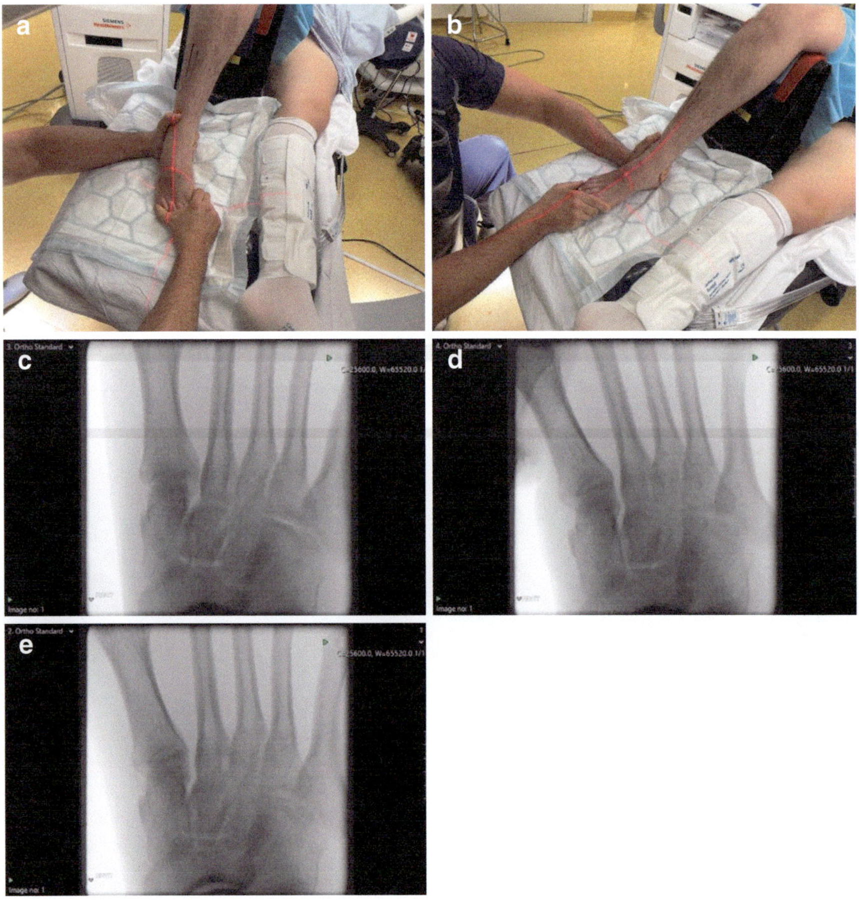

Fig. 20.2 (**a**) Adduction Manoeuvre for EUA. (**b**) Abduction Manoeuvre for EUA. Note the stabilisation counter-manoeuvre of the hindfoot with the non manipulative (left) hand. (**c**) Baseline DP image, (**d**) Adduction EUA DP image, (**e**) Abduction EUA image

Once this series of stress examinations has been performed, it can be repeated with oblique images either through internal rotation of the knee or by rotation of the image intensifier to the appropriate obliquity. Finally, the bolster is removed and the knee is allowed to fall into an externally rotated position to lay the foot with the lateral border on the operating table to assess for instability in the dorsal-plantar plane. After the acquisition of a baseline image, each tarsometatarsal joint can be screened clinically with dorsoplantar pressure at the base of the metatarsal (the "piano key test" or "push-up test") and radiographically by stabilising the Chopart articulation manually and attempting to apply a plantar-dorsal stress to each tarsometatarsal joint observing for dorsal subluxation of the metatarsal base. This movement is akin the Lachmann's test for knee cruciate ligament injury or the metatarsophalangeal joint instability test associated with assessment for plantar plate insufficiency. The obliquity of the imaging acquisition will need to be adjusted to follow the natural curvature of the longitudinal arch of the foot to visualise each joint individually (Fig. 20.3a–f, Video 20.1).

At the conclusion of the EUA, the surgeon will have an understanding of the general stability of the the Lisfranc-tarsometatarsal joints complex which he/she can utilise, combined with their study of the pre-operative imaging to determine which components of the complex require direct visualisation for reduction and fixation and which components of the complex do not require additional iatrogenic insult. Recent studies emphasize the role of intraoperative fluoroscopy during EUA to guide reductions and confirm joint congruity before proceeding with fixation. This allows for precise adjustments to the reduction and helps guide the fixation sequence [7].

Approach and Incisions

Surgical approaches for Lisfranc injuries typically involve one or two incisions to expose both the medial and middle columns. In fewer cases, an approach to the lateral column is required.

The authors' preference is to begin with a dorsal approach which will allow the visualisation of the 2nd metatarsal base—medial cuneiform articulation, 2nd TMTJ in its entirety. The incision is centred along a line following the lateral cortex of the 2nd metatarsal. If stabilisation of the 3rd TMTJ is anticipated, the incision can be placed slightly laterally to allow full access to the 1st web space along with the 2nd and 3rd TMTJs through the one dorsal incision. Radiography may be used to allow the precise localisation of the skin incision which is performed with a surgical blade. Once the superficial nerves have been identified and protected, The Extensor Hallucis Brevis is sought and identified to allow protection of the dorsal neurovascular bundle through its medial retraction. The incision can be extended to observe the intercuneiform joint, lateral border of the 1st TMTJ and medial border of the 3rd TMTJ.

It is important to limit the dissection at this stage to remain extra-articular. If the practitioner begins to incise/excise capsules and therefore ligaments to visualise all TMTJs and the Lisfranc articulation, he/she will potentially further destabilise the injury which he/she will be obliged to stabilise, adding to the severity of the injury as well as the morbidity of the procedure.

Once the dissection to but not through the TMTJ capsules has been completed, the surgeon may now assess stability with additional direct visualisation. Dorsal ligament injuries can be directly seen as long has they have not been incised/excised during the approach. The authors suggest utilising a pointed reduction clamp applied to the 2nd metatarsal just distal to the transverse intermetatarsal joint and/or a threaded K-wire into the 2nd metatarsal base to act as a joystick. Now the 2nd metatarsal base can be manipulated with lateral translation and/or external rotation to observe for Lisfranc joint diastasis as well as dorsal and plantar translation to

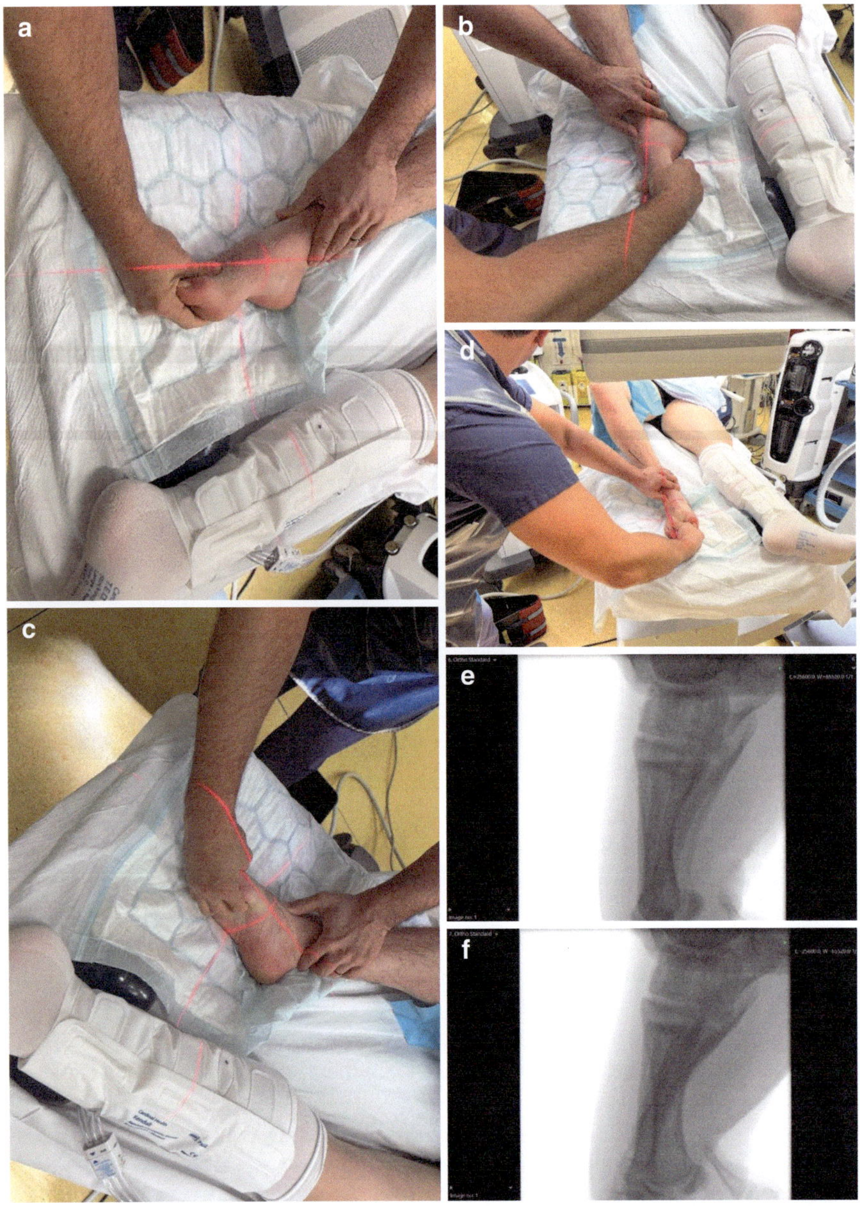

Fig. 20.3 (**a**) Baseline lateral positioning for EUA, (**b**, **c**) "Piano key/Push-up/Lachman test" of TMTJs, note pressure with counter pressure for EUA manoeuvre from fingers under metatarsal heads and thumb dorsally (right hand) and thumb over dorsal midfoot proximal to TMTJs (left hand) to provide counter stabilisation to EUA performed by attempted dorsal/plantar translation of the metatarsal at the TMTJ, (**d**) foot positioning obliquely to follow cascade of TMTJs while "Piano key/Push-up/Lachman test" of TMTJs is repeated. (**e**) Baseline imaging. (**f**) Stress imaging showing 2nd TMTJ dorsal translation under stress

observe for instability of the 2nd TMTJ. Instability can also be checked during these manoeuvres with radiography (Fig. 20.4a, b, Video 20.2).

The corresponding author assesses the proximal extension of instability from the Lisfranc joint (2nd MT base-Medial cuneiform) by inserting a Freer elevator, MacDonald forceps or similar between the medial & middle cuneiforms and applying a rotation under image intensifier guidance to assess for excessive (>2 mm) diastasis of the joint (the Koç twist test). This can be re-assessed subsequent to Lisfranc fixation to determine if additional intercuneiform stabilisation is required (Fig. 20.5a–f).

The surgeon should stabilise the 2nd TMTJ before definitively assessing the stability of the 3rd TMTJ. Particularly in low energy injuries in which the intermetatarsal ligaments between the bases of the 2nd to 5th metatarsals remain intact, it is frequently the case that restoration of stability of the 2nd TMTJ and Lisfranc ligament will reduce and stabilise the remaining TMTJs without requirement for additional exposure or fixation. The surgeon can then assess the 3rd TMTJ while visualising and palpating its dorsal surface using manipulation of the 3rd metatarsal at the lateral aspect of the approach. If 3rd TMTJ instability is demonstrated, the incision can be extended to allow visualisation of the entire width of the 3rd TMTJ and the same manoeuvres can be applied to the 4th TMTJ while observing its medial aspect and palpating dorsally. Instability can be confirmed with radiographic images during these manoeuvres. Assessment of the lateral column (4th & 5th TMTJ) should not be considered complete however until these manoeuvres have been performed subsequent to stabilisation of the medial column, given the role the potentially stable intermetatarsal ligaments can play in the indirect stabilisation of the lateral column supplied by stabilisation of the medial column.

Attention is now turned to the 1st TMTJ and medial column. It is the authors' experience that in low energy injuries instability of the 1st TMTJ is overdiagnosed and unnecessary fixation of the 1st TMTJ is frequently performed. At the medial aspect of the dorsal approach, the lateral border of the 1st TMTJ can be visualised by retracting Extensor Hallucis brevis and the neurovascular bundle laterally. Although, more limited than the visual assessment for the 3rd TMTJ, the 1st TMTJ

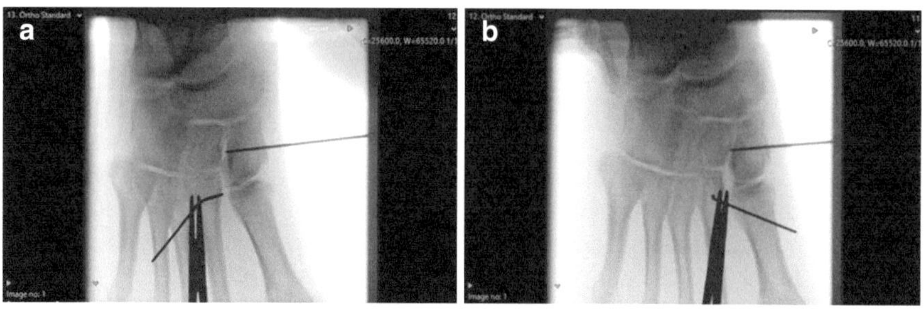

Fig. 20.4 (**a**) Wires inserted percutaneously into medial cuneiform & 2nd metatarsal base for EUA of more subtle injuries (**b**) Diastasis force applied to base of 2nd metatarsal wire while stabilising medial cuneiform wire

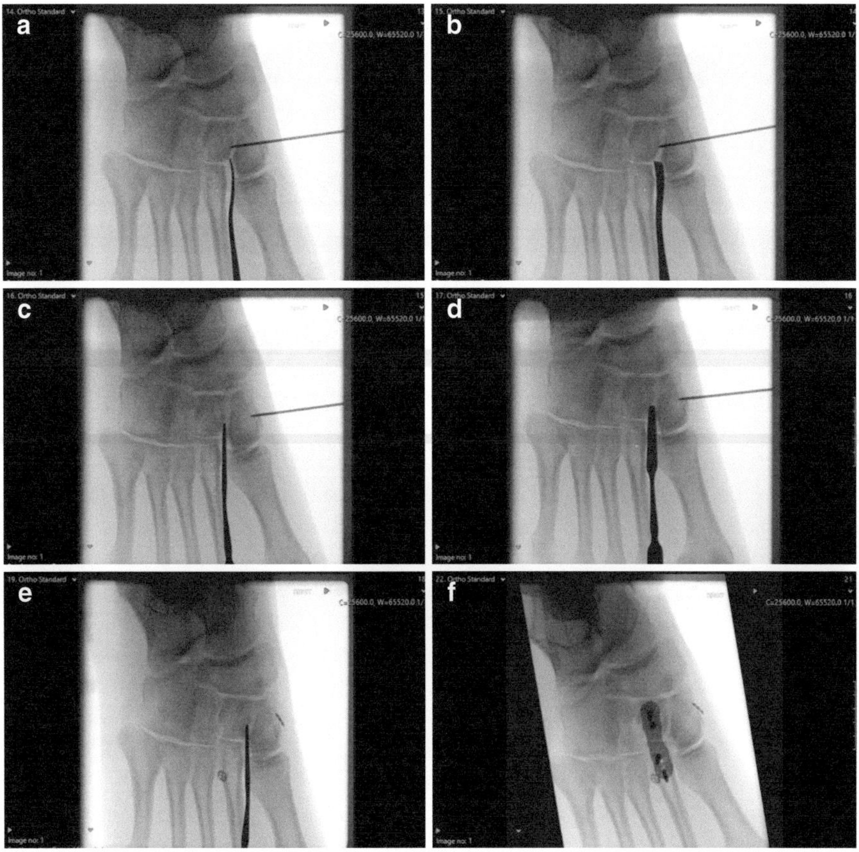

Fig. 20.5 The "Koç twist" test (**a**) periosteal elevator in Lisfranc space, (**b**) twist confirms diastasis at Lisfranc space, (**c**) McDonald elevator in intercuneiform space, (**d**) twist confirms diastasis of intercuneiform space, (**e**) twist test made negative by stabilisation, (**f**) Final fixation construct

can be similarly visualised and dorsally palpated during the application of medial-lateral and dorsal-plantar forces to the 1st metatarsal with the use of a percutaneous threaded K-wire as a joystick or, more commonly, through direct manual manipulation to which the first metatarsal is more amenable compared to the lesser metatarsals. As the entirety of the 1st TMTJ is not visualised yet, intraoperative radiography (dorso-plantar and lateral) is used to identify instability with these manipulations.

If medial column instability is observed, a medial approach centred over the 1st TMTJ is performed taking care to avoid damage to the marginal vein, the dorsal medial branches of the superficial peroneal nerve followed by the tibialis anterior tendon. If instability extends proximally or in the presence of medial cuneiform and/or navicular fractures, the incision is extensile proximally along the course of the medial utility approach to the foot.

If lateral column (4th & 5th TMTJ) instability is observed which is not stabilised by stabilisation of the middle column, a lateral approach may be required based on reducibility. Irreducible subluxation/dislocation will require an open approach. The skin incision is made along the lateral border of the 4th metatarsal. Radiography in the oblique position can be utilised to help localise the incision. After the skin incision, careful attention is made to avoid damaging cutaneous branches of the superficial peroneal and sural nerves. As previously, dissection should be taken to but not through the 4th and 5th TMTJ capsules dorsal injuries can be directly observed and medial-lateral as well as dorsal-plantar stressing can be utilised to assess stability with or without radiographic monitoring as required.

Regardless of the approach(es) taken, meticulous attention should be paid to soft-tissue handling and minimization of disruption to avoid postoperative complications, such as wound healing issues or stiffness [8].

Fixation Sequence

Fixation of Lisfranc injuries follows a systematic assessment of the stability of the individual components of the Lisfranc complex. Given the central role of the 2nd metatarsal base—medial cuneiform interval and, consequently, the middle column, initial assessment and fixation is focused here. Within the middle column, it is the Lisfranc joint, 2nd TMTJ and finally the 3rd TMTJ which are assessed and fixed. Subsequently the medial column is assessed and stabilised if required before the lateral column is addressed. Within each column, provisional fixation of all elements of said column is recommended before application of definitive fixation.

1. Keystone & Second/Third TMT joint: This is the primary focus of fixation as it provides the most stability to the midfoot. The Keystone of the Lisfranc joint (2nd metatarsal base-medial cuneiform articulation) can be fixed (e.g. with a distal to proximal/2nd metatarsal base to medial cuneiform screw) while any dorsal instability of the second TMT joint is stabilised. Studies show that rigid fixation of the second ray is essential to prevent long-term collapse or deformity [9]. The 3rd TMT joint can be fixed similar to the 2nd TMT joint if there is instability.
2. First TMT joint: Fixation of the first TMT joint is often debated. In low-energy injuries, it may not require fixation, but in cases of instability, it should be stabilized. However, recent evidence suggests that over-fixation of the first ray can lead to stiffness, and surgeons should consider this in their decision-making [10].
3. Fourth and Fifth TMT joints: Fixation of the lateral column is generally avoided unless there is significant displacement. Studies have shown that over-fixation of these joints can lead to postoperative stiffness and reduced mobility, particularly in the fourth and fifth TMT joints, which require a degree of motion to accommodate uneven terrain [11].

If the lateral column is reduced but unstable, the authors prefer the use of percutaneously inserted buried K-wires applied to the 5th and/or 4th TMTJs for a period of 6–8 weeks which are removed under local anaesthetic in the outpatient setting. If the lateral column is subluxed/dislocated, and open reduction will be required which provides the option of temporary bridge plating of.

Fixation Techniques

Several fixation techniques have been employed in the management of Lisfranc injuries, with a significant debate surrounding the use of transarticular screws, dorsal plating, and suture-button constructs.

- Transarticular screws: Long considered the gold standard, screws are placed across the TMT joints, providing rigid fixation. However, transarticular screws can damage joint surfaces, leading to post-traumatic arthritis [12].
- Dorsal plating: In contrast, dorsal bridge plating has gained popularity. Extra-articular plating preserves the articular surface yet provides stability. Studies comparing plates to screws suggest that dorsal plating results in less joint stiffness and fewer complications related to hardware [13].
- Suture-button constructs: Recent advancements in fixation include the use of suture-button constructs, which provide dynamic stabilization while allowing some physiological motion at the TMT joints. This technique is particularly effective in ligamentous injuries isolated to the Lisfranc joint, where it offers a balance between stability and preserving motion. Studies indicate favourable outcomes with suture-button fixation, particularly in athletes [14].

Postoperative Care

Postoperative care focuses on protecting the repair while allowing for early mobilization. Most patients are placed in a non-weight-bearing splint for the first 2 weeks to be transitioned to a cast or boot non-weight bearing until 6–8 weeks postoperatively. Gradual weight-bearing is introduced based on radiographic healing and clinical stability, with a transition to full weight-bearing typically by 10–12 weeks.

Mobility in the Lisfranc Joint and TMTJs

Functional Anatomy and Kinematics

The *Lisfranc joint ligaments* are composed of the dorsal, plantar and interosseous ligaments between the 2nd metatarsal base and medial cuneiform. The *Lisfranc joint complex* consists of the five TMT joints, each with distinct functions and degrees of mobility that contribute to the overall biomechanics of the midfoot.

- First TMT joint: The first TMT joint is the most mobile, allowing for significant dorsiflexion and plantarflexion. This mobility is thought to be crucial for shock absorption and propulsion during gait. Disruption to the 1st TMT joint, particularly through over-fixation, can impair these functions and lead to secondary problems in the forefoot and hindfoot [15].
  In vitro testing of the 1st TMTJs has shown that the range of motion is 1.5–3.5 degrees [16]. However, hypermobility of the 1st TMTJ/medial column is well described in the literature, the discussion of which is outside the scope of this text. Therefore in the author's practice, the 1st TMTJ mobility is assessed on both the injured and uninjured side to ascertain discrepancies and guide decision making towards fixation. If Lisfranc joint/Keystone and/or intercuneiform fixation equalises range of motion compared to the uninjured side, the 1st TMTJ is considered stabilised in the absence of obvious bony injury mandating fixation.
- Second TMT joint/2nd metatarsal base-medial cuneiform (Lisfranc) joint: As the keystone of the Lisfranc complex, the second TMT joint is relatively rigid, offering structural stability to the medial and transverse arches. This stability is essential for maintaining foot integrity under load.
- Third TMT joint: Like the second TMT joint, the third is also relatively rigid and adds to the structural stability of the medial longitudinal and transverse arches.
  In vitro testing of the 2nd & 3rd TMT joints has shown that the range of motion is 0.6–2.6 degrees [16]. Therefore in the decision of fixation versus primary arthrodesis in Lisfranc injuries, the 2nd & 3rd TMT joints, given the little physiological range of motion present, selective fusion of these joints may prove to be advantageous in the surgical management of Lisfranc injuries.
- Fourth and Fifth TMT joints: These joints form the lateral column, responsible for accommodating uneven terrain. In vitro testing of the 4th & 5th TMT joints has shown that the range of motion is 9–11 degrees [16]. Given that the fourth and fifth TMT joints exhibit the greatest mobility, fixation should be minimized to avoid compromising their adaptive function [17].

Biomechanical Consequences of Fixation

Over-fixation of the TMT joints, particularly the lateral column but also the 1st ray, can lead to arthrofibrosis and joint stiffness, impacting foot biomechanics and patient function. Studies have highlighted the importance of avoiding unnecessary fixation in low-energy injuries, especially in the lateral TMT joints, where excessive hardware can lead to joint rigidity and discomfort during walking [18].

Controversies in Treatment

Fix or Fuse?

One of the key debates in Lisfranc injuries is whether to fix or fuse. Primary arthrodesis, particularly in primary ligamentous injuries, has shown better outcomes than transarticular screw fixation in terms of preventing arthritis and reducing the need for secondary surgery [12]. However, for low-energy injuries, open reduction and internal fixation (ORIF) is often preferred to preserve joint mobility and avoid over-fixation, with studies demonstrating lower complication rates and better functional outcomes [19]. While many surgeons believe that bridge plating will lead to better outcomes than transarticular screws, there are currently no sufficiently powered randomised trials to prove this.

A critical consideration during TMT fusion should be the meticulous removal of (remaining) cartilage while retaining length through the preservation of subchondral bone which is fenestrated and cross-hatched to provide a larger surface area of subchondral exposed bone. If excessive length is lost through resection, the intermetatarsal ligament attachment to adjacent unfused joints could prevent adequate bony apposition for fusion to occur.

Open vs. Closed Reduction

In cases of low-energy injuries with minimal displacement, closed reduction may be an option if early intervention is possible, though open reduction is typically preferred to ensure accurate anatomical realignment, particularly of the second TMT/Lisfranc joint. Recent literature supports open reduction in most cases, as malalignment is a significant predictor of poor outcomes [20]. Delayed percutaneous fixation can be associated with failure due to intervening soft tissue preventing adequate reduction and/or leading to loss of alignment. Fundamentally, whether open or early closed reduction and stabilisation is performed, anatomic alignment (or near anatomic alignment within 1 mm) should be sought to optimise chances of a good/excellent outcome.

Plates vs. Screws

The debate between dorsal plating and trans-articular screw fixation is ongoing. While screws provide rigid fixation, plates have been shown to cause less damage to the articular surface and offer more consistent long-term outcomes in terms of joint preservation [21].

Suspensory Fixation (Suture-Button)

The use of suture-button fixation has become increasingly popular in the management of lower energy, purely ligamentous Lisfranc injuries. It allows dynamic stabilization of the joint while permitting some physiological motion, which is particularly beneficial in athletes or patients with lower energy injuries [14]. Studies have shown that suture-button constructs offer comparable stability to screws while reducing the risk of post-fixation stiffness.

Hardware Removal

The question of hardware removal remains controversial. Some studies suggest that hardware removal, particularly of screws, is necessary to prevent postoperative stiffness and improve patient comfort, while others recommend leaving hardware in place unless symptomatic. Recent trends favour early removal of screws to prevent complications, particularly in young, active patients [22]. The question of whether bridge plates should be routinely removed remains unresolved, but it is the authors' practice not to perform routine removal of these implants.

Conclusion

Lisfranc injuries, while often subtle, have the potential to cause significant long-term morbidity if not diagnosed and treated promptly. Advances in imaging techniques, including the use of WB X-rays, CT, and MRI, have improved diagnostic accuracy, while newer surgical techniques, including dorsal plating and suture-button constructs, have shifted the treatment paradigm towards preserving joint mobility. However, the debate over fixation vs fusion continues with the evidence suggesting that the results are comparable or favouring fusion. Emerging evidence supports a more nuanced approach, with "more fixations, less fixation"gaining favour in the treatment of low-energy injuries. Ultimately, a patient-specific approach that considers the biomechanics of the foot, the severity of the injury, and the patient's functional demands will lead to the best outcomes.

References

1. Nunley JA, Vertullo CJ. Classification, investigation, and management of midfoot sprains: Lisfranc injuries in the athlete. Am J Sports Med. 2002;30(6):871–8. https://doi.org/10.1177/03635465020300061901. PMID: 12435655.
2. Pourmorteza M, Vosoughi AR. Lisfranc fleck sign: characteristics and clinical outcomes following fixation using a percutaneous position Lisfranc screw. Eur J Trauma Emerg Surg. 2022;48(1):471–9. https://doi.org/10.1007/s00068-020-01415-z. Epub 2020 Jun 19. PMID: 32561962.
3. Sripanich Y, Weinberg MW, Krähenbühl N, Rungprai C, Mills MK, Saltzman CL, Barg A. Imaging in Lisfranc injury: a systematic literature review. Skeletal Radiol. 2020;49(1):31–53. https://doi.org/10.1007/s00256-019-03282-1. Epub 2019 Jul 31. PMID: 31368007.
4. Kitsukawa K, Hirano T, Niki H, Tachizawa N, Mimura H. The diagnostic accuracy of MRI to evaluate acute Lisfranc joint injuries: comparison with direct operative observations. Foot Ankle Orthop. 2022;7(1):24730114211069080. https://doi.org/10.1177/24730114211069080. PMID: 35097492; PMCID: PMC8792696.
5. Raikin SM, Elias I, Dheer S, Besser MP, Morrison WB, Zoga AC. Prediction of midfoot instability in the subtle Lisfranc injury. Comparison of magnetic resonance imaging with intraoperative findings. J Bone Joint Surg Am. 2009;91(4):892–9. https://doi.org/10.2106/JBJS.H.01075. PMID: 19339574.
6. Thomas JL, Kopiec A, Mark K, Chandler LM. Radiographic value of the Lisfranc diastasis in a standardized population. Foot Ankle Spec. 2020;13(6):494–501. https://doi.org/10.1177/1938640019890738. Epub 2019 Dec 2. PMID: 31791155.
7. Myerson MS, Fisher RT, Burgess AR, Kenzora JE. Fracture dislocations of the tarsometatarsal joints: end results correlated with pathology and treatment. Foot Ankle. 1986;6(5):225–42. https://doi.org/10.1177/107110078600600504. PMID: 3710321.
8. Mulier T, de Haan J, Vriesendorp P, Reynders P. The treatment of Lisfranc injuries: review of current literature. Eur J Trauma Emerg Surg. 2010;36(3):206–16. https://doi.org/10.1007/s00068-010-1034-5. Epub 2010 Jun 1. PMID: 26815863.
9. Mayne AIW, Lawton R, Dalgleish S, Harrold F, Chami G. Stability of Lisfranc injury fixation in Thiel cadavers: is routine fixation of the 1st and 3rd tarsometatarsal joint necessary? Injury. 2017;48(8):1764–7. https://doi.org/10.1016/j.injury.2017.04.003. Epub 2017 Apr 11. PMID: 28420541.
10. Stødle AH, Hvaal KH, Brøgger HM, Madsen JE, Husebye EE. Temporary bridge plating vs primary arthrodesis of the first tarsometatarsal joint in Lisfranc injuries: randomized controlled trial. Foot Ankle Int. 2020;41(8):901–10. https://doi.org/10.1177/1071100720925815. Epub 2020 Jun 5. PMID: 32501109; PMCID: PMC7406968.
11. Ward TRW, Boksh K, Airey G, Myatt D, Aamir J, Chapman J, Kyaw H, Jeyaseelan L, Greasley L, Drummond I, Elbannan M, Tanaka H, Mangwani J, Mason L. Lateral column midfoot injury: do they all need fixation? J Orthop. 2024;62:22–6. https://doi.org/10.1016/j.jor.2024.10.010. PMID: 39502676; PMCID: PMC11532135.
12. Ly TV, Coetzee JC. Treatment of primarily ligamentous Lisfranc joint injuries: primary arthrodesis compared with open reduction and internal fixation. A prospective, randomized study. J Bone Joint Surg Am. 2006;88(3):514–20. https://doi.org/10.2106/JBJS.E.00228. PMID: 16510816.
13. Boksh K, Sharma A, Grindlay D, Divall P, Mangwani J. Dorsal bridge plating versus. Transarticular screw fixation for Lisfranc injuries: a systematic review and meta-analysis. J Clin Orthop Trauma. 2020;11(3):508–13. https://doi.org/10.1016/j.jcot.2020.03.019. Epub 2020 Apr 3. PMID: 32581491; PMCID: PMC7303533.
14. Chona DV, Park CN, Kim BI, Lau BC. Clinical and biomechanical outcomes of suture button fixation for ligamentous Lisfranc injury: a systematic review and meta-analysis. Orthop J Sports Med. 2023;11(8):23259671231186387. https://doi.org/10.1177/23259671231186387. PMID: 37538534; PMCID: PMC10395171.

15. Tashiro T, Ikuta Y, Maeda N, Arima S, Morikawa M, Kaneda K, Ishihara H, Tsutsumi S, Kawai M, Brand A, Nakasa T, Adachi N, Komiya M, Urabe Y. First tarsometatarsal joint mobility in hallux valgus during gait: A synchronized ultrasound and three-dimensional motion capture analysis. J Med Ultrason. 2001;51(2):331–9. https://doi.org/10.1007/s10396-024-01414-2. Epub 2024 Mar 28. PMID: 38546904; PMCID: PMC11098882.
16. Ouzounian TJ, Shereff MJ. In vitro determination of midfoot motion. Foot Ankle. 1989;10(3):140–6. https://doi.org/10.1177/107110078901000305. PMID: 2613125.
17. van Hoeve S, Stollenwerck G, Willems P, Witlox MA, Meijer K, Poeze M. Gait analysis and functional outcome in patients after Lisfranc injury treatment. Foot Ankle Surg. 2018;24(6):535–41. https://doi.org/10.1016/j.fas.2017.07.003. Epub 2017 Jul 18. PMID: 29409269.
18. Moracia-Ochagavía I, Rodríguez-Merchán EC. Lisfranc fracture-dislocations: current management. EFORT Open Rev. 2019;4(7):430–44. https://doi.org/10.1302/2058-5241.4.180076. PMID: 31423327; PMCID: PMC6667981.
19. Ahn BJ, Quinn M, Zhao L, He EW, Dworkin M, Naphade O, Byrne RA, Molino J, Blankenhorn B. Statistical fragility analysis of open reduction internal fixation vs primary arthrodesis to treat Lisfranc injuries: a systematic review. Foot Ankle Int. 2024;45(4):298–308. https://doi.org/10.1177/10711007231224797. Epub 2024 Feb 8. PMID: 38327213.
20. Stavrakakis IM, Magarakis GE, Christoforakis Z. Percutaneous fixation of Lisfranc joint injuries: a systematic review of the literature. Acta Orthop Traumatol Turc. 2019;53(6):457–62. https://doi.org/10.1016/j.aott.2019.08.005. Epub 2019 Sep 28. PMID: 31575479; PMCID: PMC6939019.
21. Kirzner N, Zotov P, Goldbloom D, Curry H, Bedi H. Dorsal bridge plating or transarticular screws for Lisfranc fracture dislocations: a retrospective study comparing functional and radiological outcomes. Bone Joint J. 2018;100-B(4):468–74. https://doi.org/10.1302/0301-620X.100B4.BJJ-2017-0899.R2. PMID: 29629578; PMCID: PMC6503757.
22. Rhodes AML, McMenemy L, Connell R, Elliot R, Marsland D. A systematic review of outcomes following Lisfranc injury fixation: removal vs retention of metalwork. Foot Ankle Orthop. 2022;7(4):24730114221125447. https://doi.org/10.1177/24730114221125447. PMID: 36247414; PMCID: PMC9558891.

Chapter 21
Talus and Calcaneal Fracture Fixation

Callum Clark and Shilpa Jha

Talus Fractures

Introduction

Fractures involving the talus are an uncommon yet potentially devastating injury; surgical management is complicated by a unique three-dimensional anatomy with extensive cartilaginous cover leading to tenuous blood supply and limited surface for fixation.

The talus is anatomically divided into the body, neck, head and lateral and posterior processes. Of these areas, the neck is the most commonly injured accounting for 50% of all talar fractures [1]. This likely relates to the sharp change in trabecular direction at the junction of the body and neck creating susceptibility to fracture; the usual mechanism is excessive ankle dorsiflexion and axial loading combined with hindfoot supination leading to dorsomedial impact of the talar neck against the medial malleolus. This results in dorsomedial comminution with the classical displacement pattern of varus and extension at the talar neck.

The blood supply to the talus is predominantly extraosseous given there are no muscular attachments and extensive cartilage cover. The posterior tibial artery contributes most of the blood supply to the talar body and medial neck via the deltoid branches and tarsal canal artery. Branches of the perforating peroneal artery and

C. Clark (✉)
Trauma & Orthopaedic Department, Heatherwood & Wexham Park Hospitals, Frimley Health NHS Foundation Trust, Ascot, UK
e-mail: Callum.clark2@nhs.net

S. Jha
Trauma & Orthopaedic Department, University Hospitals of Leicester NHS Trust, Leicester, UK
e-mail: Shilpa.jha@uhl-tr.nhs.uk

M. Bhatia (ed.), *Surgical Techniques of the Foot and Ankle*,
https://doi.org/10.1007/978-3-031-93742-2_21

anterior tibial artery supply the neck and form the sinus tarsi artery. The tarsal canal and sinus tarsi arteries anastomose at the inferior talar neck. Displaced talar neck fractures lead to significant disruption of this network; the deltoid branches are the often the only remaining supply and consideration must be made to this when planning surgical approaches. The extent of displacement and associated dislocations correlate with risk of avascular necrosis. The commonest complication overall is post-traumatic arthrosis with rates ranging 50–100% reported.

Classically it has been considered that talar neck fracture dislocations require emergent reduction (which may need to be open) to minimise the risk of avascular necrosis. However recent data suggests no difference between rates of AVN in Hawkins II, III and IV injuries which were reduced within 6 h compared to those reduced after 6 h up to 7 days [2]. Anatomic reduction is the key to optimising outcome, with even 2 mm malalignment leading to significant change in subtalar contact pressures and subsequent risk of arthrosis [3]. This would suggest that waiting for the availability of specialists experienced in this type of surgery and able to perform a single definitive operation with anatomic reduction may well be preferable to emergent surgery performed by a generalist (which often requires a specialist to perform definitive fixation in a second stage).

Set-up and Intra-operative Imaging

The majority of talar fracture surgery is performed supine under tourniquet with a sandbag under the ipsilateral buttock to neutralise rotation of the limb (particularly helpful when using dual approaches). A femoral distractor can be a useful reduction aid in talar neck fracture dislocations.

Intra-operative standard AP views of the ankle are useful in assessing talar body fractures whilst lateral views of the ankle are useful for assessing the correction of extension malalignment and posterior facet reduction.

When operating on talar neck fractures it is extremely useful to obtain a 'dorso-plantar' or 'Canale' view (as described by Canale and Kelly [4]). To obtain this view the foot is placed on the table with the ankle in maximum equinus. The foot is angled to 15° of pronation. The C-arm is then angled at 75° from the horizontal and centres over the hindfoot. This view provides a useful evaluation of the talar neck to properly assess comminution as well as reduction of varus angulation and shortening.

Approaches

General Considerations

As with all approaches in the foot it is important to develop full thickness flaps and avoid undermining tissue to prevent wound complications. A combination of approaches is often required; when using dual approaches, it is important to plan incisions to maximise skin bridges and avoid excessive dissection adjacent to the deltoid and sinus tarsi to protect the vascular supply. Dual approaches should be used judiciously and only when required as they have been associated with significantly increased risk of AVN compared to single approaches [2]. However this observation may be confounded by the tendency for their use in more displaced and complicated fracture patterns.

During the fixation of talar neck fractures it is important to properly visualise the subtalar joint (usually through the anterolateral incision) and to identify and remove any loose bone fragments which may impede reduction.

Approaches to the Neck

Anterolateral

This approach is routinely used in talar neck fractures and may be combined with a medial approach to aid exposure and fixation. Surface landmarks are the fourth metatarsal shaft and lateral malleolus (see Fig. 21.1). This is an extensile approach in continuity with the anterolateral approach to the ankle. The incision begins 2 cm anterior to the anterior border of the lateral malleolus continuing distally in line with the fourth metatarsal. Careful subcutaneous dissection is required as the superficial peroneal nerve may cross in the proximal part of the incision. The extensor digitorum brevis muscle belly is subsequently identified and split longitudinally to gain

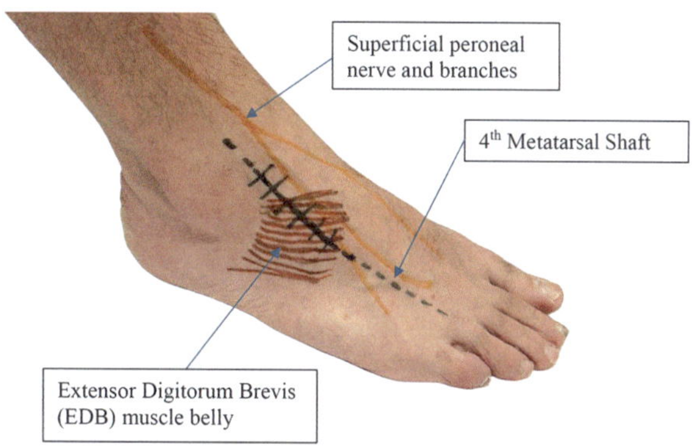

Fig. 21.1 Surface anatomy anterolateral approach to talar neck

access to the lateral talar neck and subtalar joint. Excessive inferior dissection should be avoided to prevent damage to the sinus tarsi artery.

Anteromedial

This approach is often performed alongside the anterolateral approach in talar neck fractures; a dual approach is frequently required in order to obtain accurate reduction, especially in the presence of significant medial comminution. Surface landmarks are the tibialis posterior tendon coursing over the ankle joint into the navicular, as well as the anteromedial aspect of ankle joint ('soft spot') (see Fig. 21.2). A longitudinal incision is made just inferior/medial to the tibialis anterior tendon extending towards the navicular. Care should be taken to avoid starting the proximal incision more postero-inferior as this will be directly over the deltoid ligament; it is vital to preserve the deltoid arterial branches as this may be the last remaining blood supply to the talar neck. Similarly care must be taken to ensure deep dissection down to the medial neck remains distal to the deltoid ligament. If this approach does not provide enough exposure a medial malleolar osteotomy should be considered.

Medial Malleolar Osteotomy

The distal incision is similar to the above anteromedial approach but proximally the incision is curved posteriorly directly over the medial malleolus. The medial malleolus is exposed and the tibialis posterior tendon must be retracted and protected throughout. The osteotomy should exit just beyond (lateral) to the medial shoulder of the plafond in order to ensure optimal talar exposure. A chevron osteotomy is often utilised as this affords more stability after fixation as well as a useful reference for reduction. The osteotomy is usually fixed with two partially threaded cannulated screws which are pre-drilled prior to making the osteotomy to ensure accurate reduction when the malleolus is re-attached. This is a useful approach in talar neck fractures with proximal extension as well as medial talar dome/body injuries.

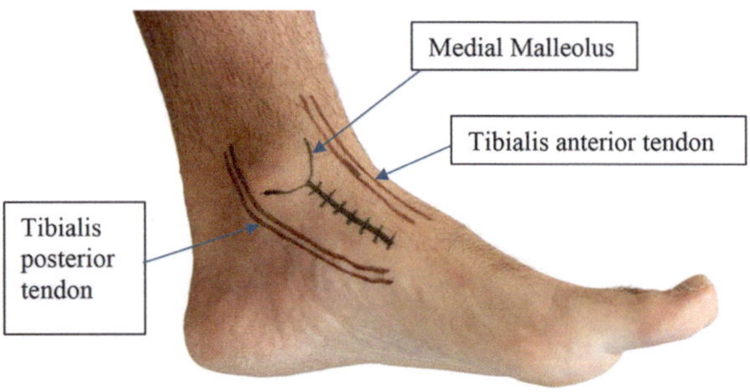

Fig. 21.2 Surface anatomy anteromedial approach to talar neck

Approaches to the Body/Dome

Medial talar body fractures can be approached using the medial malleolar osteotomy technique above. Lateral talar body fractures can either be approached through a fibular osteotomy or alternatively a lateral transligamentous approach. An incision is made at the anterolateral ankle and the anterior talofibular ligament and calcaneofibular ligament are incised (and later reconstructed at the end of the procedure). A bone lever is then placed behind the lateral talus to rotate the talar dome; over 75% of the talar dome is accessible through this approach [5].

Approaches to the talar Processes

Lateral Process Fractures

Lateral talar process fractures ('Snowboarder's fractures') which occur with forced dorsiflexion and eversion can be approached with a direct lateral approach should they require surgery. A longitudinal incision is made distal to the fibula just anterior to the peroneal tendons. The lateral process lies directly beneath the deep fascia here and can be accessed for fixation or for excision.

Posterior Process Fractures

The FHL tendon lies between the posterolateral and posteromedial tubercles of the posterior talar process. Generally one tubercle is fractured in isolation and can be approached using either a posteromedial or posterolateral approach accordingly.

In the posteromedial approach to the talus a longitudinal incision is made at the level of the subtalar joint adjacent to the medial border of the achilles tendon. The interval between FHL and the achilles is utilised with the neurovascular bundle retracted medially. The posterolateral approach to the talus involves a longitudinal incision between the achilles tendon and the peroneal tendons at the level of the subtalar joint. The FHL muscle belly (and tendon distally) are retracted medially. Screw fixation is with 1.5 mm, 2 mm or 2.7 mm lag screws depending on the size of the fragment [6].

Fixation Strategies

Talar Neck fractures (See Fig. 21.3—Schematic/Algorithm for fixation Strategies)

The mechanism of injury in talar fractures leads to varus and hyper-extension displacement at the talar neck with varying degrees of medial comminution.

The lateral neck is generally less comminuted and therefore provides a useful cortical read for the purposes of reduction.

Optimal definitive surgery in talar neck fractures requires fixation into both the medial and lateral talar neck. Depending on fracture type and the extent of medial comminution, this may be with two screws only, a lateral plate and medial screw, or both medial and lateral plating in the most comminuted cases; this may require augmentation with bone graft medially if there is significant bone loss.

Where possible titanium implants should be utilised to minimise MRI artefact should this imaging be required in future to assess for avascular necrosis.

In less comminuted fractures a single anterolateral approach can be performed to utilise the lateral cortical read. A lateral neck screw running anterior to posterior (A-P) is inserted in compression mode (4 mm partially threaded cancellous screw);

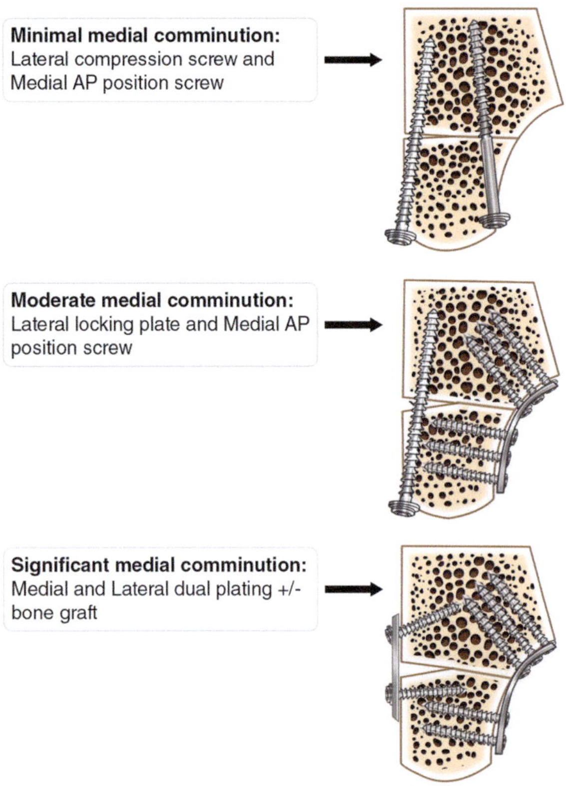

Fig. 21.3 Schematic (representing canale view of talus) of suggested algorithm for talar neck fracture fixation

the entry point is non-articular just proximal to the lateral talo-navicular joint. In general compression screws should be avoided on the medial side due to risk of displacement secondary to medial comminution. A fully threaded cancellous screw can be applied anterior to posterior (A-P). In this case the head needs to be countersunk as the entry point for the screw lies in the medial edge of the talonavicular joint. An alternative is to apply a posterior-to-anterior (P-A) screw entering at the posterolateral tubercle. Classically this has been performed with a percutaneous approach however cadaveric studies have shown a 27.2% incidence of damage to the sural nerve [7]; a formal posterolateral approach to identify the and protect the sural nerve is therefore recommended. Furthermore, if this P-A screw is aimed into the inferior half of the talar head there is a risk of vascular injury to the vessels in the roof of the sinus tarsi. If using a P-A medial screw this should therefore be aimed into the superior half of the talar head.

In more comminuted fracture patterns plating provides a length-stable bridging construct. Talar neck site-specific locking plates are available from manufacturers; alternatively mini-fragment locking plates (2.0/2.4/2.7 mm) can be cut to size and contoured appropriately.

The lateral talar neck provides greater surface area for plate application; the curved plate is applied in the area between the lateral talar process and the lateral head which allows screws placed distally into the head/neck and proximally into the body. For moderate comminution a lateral plate with medial A-P or P-A screws may be sufficient.

For significant comminution dual plating may be utilised. The medial neck provides very limited surface area for plate application; often 1–2 screws in each fragment is the maximum achieved. Care must be taken with proximal plate position as this can lead to medial tibiotalar impingement; a burr can be utilised to create a small recessed bed in the talus for the plate to minimise this.

In fractures with significant comminution and bone loss medially, cancellous bone graft may be applied (the calcaneus and distal tibia provide easily accessible autograft harvest sites) to minimise the risk of non-union.

Talar Body Fractures

Fixation in talar body fractures generally consists of screws given the lack of surface area for plate applications; screws must be therefore headless or countersunk and are utilised in compression mode (commonly 3.5 or 4 mm). Posterior to Anterior screws are biomechanically advantageous with large posterior body fragments.

Talar Process Fractures

Small or comminuted process fragments are not amenable to fixation and therefore surgically excised. Where fixation is performed this requires mini-fragment cannulated compression screws (2.0/2.4/2.7 mm).

Post-operative Management

A below knee splint is applied for 2 weeks postoperatively to promote wound healing, with patients advised on the importance of strict elevation in the early post-op phase.

After 2 weeks, depending on the intraoperative stability of fixation and the fracture pattern, a further period in lightweight cast may be required (up to 6 weeks), alternatively patients may be given a removable boot to allow commencement of ROM exercises and physiotherapy (2–6 weeks).

Plain radiographs are performed at 6 and 12 weeks. Weight Bearing is progressed accordingly and should be commenced at the lates by 12 weeks. Hawkin's sign does not always appear and furthermore is not always a reliable indicator of vascularity of the talar body; as such it should not be relied upon to determine when the patient can start bearing weight [8]. CT and MRI are useful imaging adjuncts to assess for union and talar viability correspondingly.

Calcaneal Fractures

Introduction

Calcaneal fractures account for approximately 60% of all tarsal bone fractures. The fracture may be non-displaced or isolated to the sustentaculum tali, tuberosity or anterior process, but high energy axial loads (most commonly from falls from a height or road traffic accidents) result in a high degree of comminution. This comminution often "depresses" the posterior facet of the subtalar joint and changes the alignment of the heel. Unless these displacements are adequately reduced, there are significant deleterious effects on the motion of both the subtalar and ankle joints, the pulley functions of the malleoli and tubercles, and the heel strike function of the calcaneal body. Calcaneo-cuboid joint congruity can also be disrupted by anterior extension of the fracture, meaning that an isolated calcaneal fracture can potentially affect the function of three joints. The soft tissue swelling and bony comminution secondary to the high energy of the injury, and the critical weight-bearing and articular function of the calcaneus combine to make management difficult. Isolated sustentacular, tuberosity and process fractures will not be discussed further in this chapter.

Brief History of Calcaneal Fracture Management

Even after the invention of X-rays at the turn of the twentieth Century, Cotton commented "the man who breaks his heel bone is "done" so far as his industrial future is concerned" [9]. In 1952 Essex-Lopresti was the first to successfully classify his large series of fractures, and to outline a treatment algorithm and surgical technique. There was a step-change in treatment with the advent of CT scanning in the 1970s and the development of the Extensile/Extended Lateral Approach (ELA) and dedicated plating systems, but treatment has remained controversial with conflicting evidence in support of ORIF and non-operative management [10]. Minimally invasive techniques of reduction and external or percutaneous fixation have therefore remained lower-risk alternatives, but there has been a significant increase in their popularity in the twenty-first Century. Most common is the "Sinus tarsi approach" (STA), similar in many ways to the surgical technique originally described by Essex-Lopresti.

Emergent Treatment and Decision-Making

Calcaneal fractures which are associated with vascular compromise or open fractures, whether with or without soft tissue loss, require emergent reduction and/or debridement. Displaced tongue type fractures and tuberosity avulsion fractures can cause critical ischaemia of the posterior heel skin (see Fig. 21.4), leading to subsequent skin necrosis unless reduced and fixed immediately. If delayed, the skin defect resulting from posterior heel necrosis renders further management very challenging.

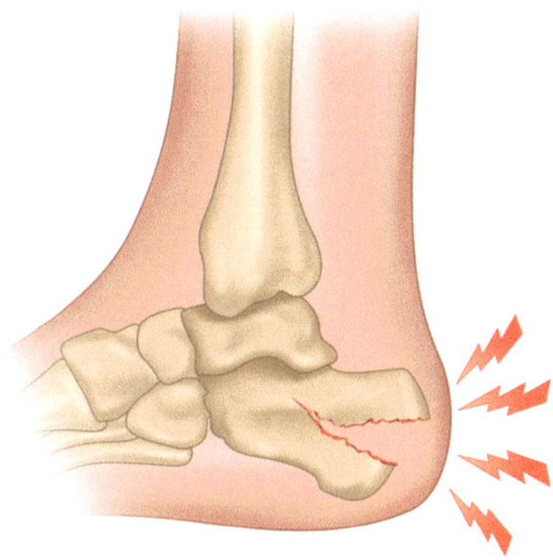

Fig. 21.4 Morphology of displaced tongue type fracture leading to critical ischaemia of skin of posterior heel

Emergent management for all other calcaneal fractures involves splintage, elevation and surgical decision-making. Non-displaced fractures are managed nonoperatively, but in all displaced fractures, both patient and fracture factors need to be weighed against the potential for complications from nonoperative and operative treatment.

Comorbidities, drug/alcohol abuse, smoking and poor compliance are associated with increased risk of wound necrosis and infection, and for patients with low functional demand these risks may outweigh the benefits of surgery [11]. Bruising and skin blistering are also risk factors, so surgery often needs to be delayed until this has reduced sufficiently—specifically until the skin is wrinkling and any blisters have epithelialized. There is therefore controversy over the relative merits of operative and non-operative management. Minimally invasive reduction and fixation has a lower rate of associated wound complications, meaning surgery can potentially be undertaken in higher risk patients and with less delay [12].

If surgical treatment is planned, then the timing of surgery will therefore depend on the state of the soft tissues and the surgical approach to be used. With both open and minimally invasive approaches, adequate reduction and fixation of the fracture are the major determinants of long-term outcome.

Fracture Classification

Understanding the type and morphology of the calcaneal fracture is essential for planning the appropriate surgical approach. There are several systems, but the two most widely used classification systems are:

1. **The Essex-Lopresti Classification** [13]: This X-ray classification into types of fracture remains relevant:
   - Intra-articular "joint depression type"—the posterior facet joint fragment is separated from the body fragment
   - "Tongue type"—the body fragment remains attached to the articular segment, which can require emergent reduction due to posterior heel skin compromise.
2. **The Sanders Classification** [14]: This system divides intra-articular calcaneal fractures into four types based on the number and location of posterior facet articular fragments on the coronal CT scan slices:
   - Type I: All non-displaced fractures.
   - Type II: Two-part fractures.
   - Type III: Three-part fractures.
   - Type IV: Highly comminuted facet.

When the calcaneus fractures under axial load, the lateral process of the talus is driven downwards into the angle of Gissane and creates a fracture line extending posteriorly and medially through the posterior facet, and secondary fracture line(s) depending on the position of the foot and direction of the force. Although no two fractures are the same, there are certain constant fragments and patterns [15].

The sustentacular fragment is usually the constant fragment and remains attached to the talus. The body fragment is usually driven laterally, upwards (proximally) and into varus. The lateral joint fragment (or fragments) is "depressed" or driven down (distally) and rotated posteriorly. The lateral wall is displaced laterally or "blown out", and the anterior process is driven upwards and may be comminuted.

Goals of Operative Treatment

The surgical goals are to both restore congruity to the subtalar joint posterior facet and to restore the morphology of the calcaneus—the height, width, length and coronal alignment. It is therefore important to have a good understanding of the normal and fracture anatomy. Specifically, the body fragment must be moved distally, medially and rotated out of excessive varus, the joint fragment(s) must be elevated, and the lateral wall and anterior process fragments reduced. Stable fixation is required to hold the reduction.

Radiographically, the goals are to restore the crucial angle of Gissane (see Fig. 21.5) and Bohler's angle (see Fig. 21.6), the posterior facet joint congruity (seen on lateral and Broden fluoroscopic views) and the calcaneal body alignment (seen on axial fluoroscopic view). In the case of primary subtalar arthrodesis, the morphology of the calcaneus must be restored in addition to preparation and fixation of the subtalar joint posterior facet.

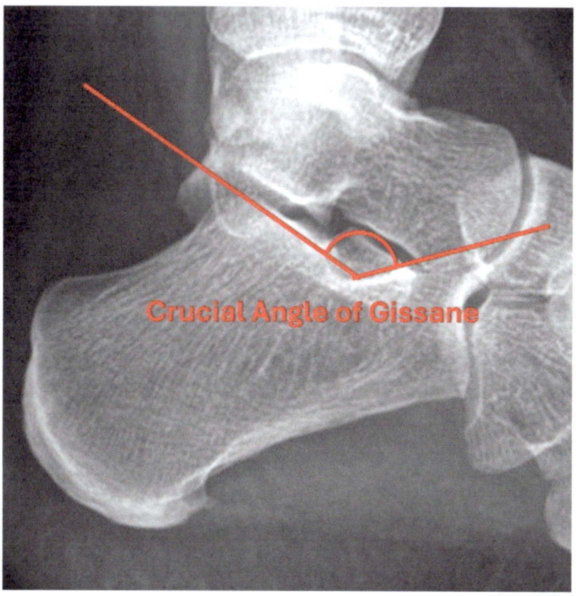

Fig. 21.5 Crucial Angle of Gissane

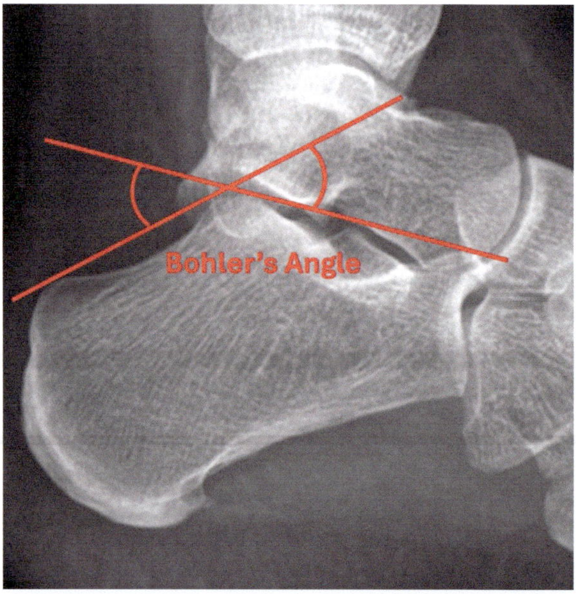

Fig. 21.6 Bohler's angle

Preparation and Positioning (See Fig. 21.7)

As with any operation, operating theatre set-up and patient positioning are key to enabling an efficient procedure. The suggested set-up is similar for both ELA and STA. The patient should be positioned in the full lateral position, with slight flexion of the knee to reduce the pull of the Achilles tendon. A foam block or pillow should be placed under the injured lower leg and ankle. A thigh tourniquet should be applied but need not be inflated, depending on surgeon preference and patient factors.

The suggested theatre set-up allows for a surgeon, assistant and scrub nurse to perform the operation with minimal disruption caused by introduction of the fluoroscope. With this set-up, lateral and dorsal-plantar foot, Broden and axial calcaneal views (the latter by rotating the C-arm parallel to the floor) can be obtained without altering the position of the patient.

Extensile Lateral Approach

This approach is based on the blood supply of the skin of the lateral heel from the peroneal artery. The incision is planned in the watershed area between the lateral calcaneal branch (which supplies the elevated flap) and the posterior calcaneal branch of this artery and the medial calcaneal branch of the posterior tibial artery, which supply the posterior and inferior skin margins. A large L-shaped incision is optimal, but extreme care must be taken with elevation n of the flap, as the corner of the flap is at extreme risk of necrosis if the skin is handled or crushed. For this

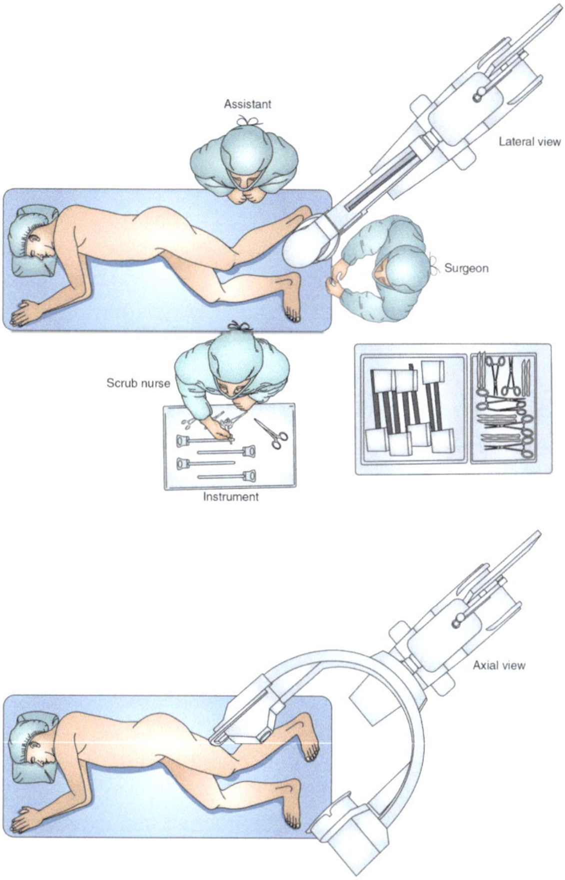

Fig. 21.7 Diagram of suggested pre-operative positioning and set-up for calcaneal fracture fixation

reason, a 95–100° angle is also preferred to a “right angle”, and the author prefers a single cut down to bone when performing the corner part of the incision, in order to raise a full-thickness flap. Care is also needed in the distal part of the horizontal limb of the incision, as the sural nerve is at risk here [16].

The flap should then be elevated from the underlying calcaneus by sharp dissection and “pushing” the flap upwards from deep, instead of “pulling” on the superficial layers and skin. As the flap is elevated, the calcaneo-fibular ligament (CFL) and inferior peroneal retinaculum and peroneus longus and brevis tendons are elevated from the bone with the flap. When the talar inferior articular surface of the posterior facet of the subtalar joint is visualised, the large flap will need to be secured in a retracted position. This can be achieved either by temporary suture of the flap onto the lateral ankle skin, or more commonly by two or three 1.6 mm K wires inserted from distal to proximal in into the fibula and/or talus, which are then bent over to hold the flap in place.

The intra-articular fracture can then be fully visualised by retracting or removing the lateral wall fragment(s). The body, joint and anterior process fragments can then be reduced directly in sequence:

1. If necessary, the lateral joint fragment(s) can be removed entirely to facilitate reduction. Throughout fracture reduction, an image intensifier is used to check reduction after temporary fixation, so that adjustments can be made prior to definitive fixation as required.
2. A MacDonald elevator or periosteal elevator can be passed through the primary fracture line between the sustentacular and body fragments to dis-impact the body and to lever it distally, medially and back into slight valgus. Using a Steinman or Schanz pin inserted from lateral to medial in the centre of the body fragment as a "joystick" can also help with this manoeuvre. Temporary fixation of this fragment, with one or more 1.6 or 1.2 mm K wires from distal to proximal medially, engaging the sustentacular fragment, can be helpful.
3. The lateral joint fragment(s) are replaced / reduced, checking visually and by palpation with an elevator that the articular surface covering the fragments aligns with the remaining intact surface on the sustentacular fragment. Once reduced, fixation is from lateral to medial, usually with 1–2 cannulated screws of 4 mm diameter or less.
4. The lateral joint fragment(s) usually have hard cortical bone attached anteriorly, forming part of the crucial angle of Gissane, and this needs to be "keyed" in with the anterior process fragment(s) to recreate the angle.
5. The anterior process can be fractured through to its articular surface with the cuboid, and it is also important to reduce and fix this element of the fracture, usually with further cannulated screws.
6. Due to the dis-impaction involved with fracture reduction, there is usually a "dead space" under the reduced lateral joint fragment, which some authors prefer to fill with bone graft or graft substitutes. The author does not routinely do this.
7. The final step in reduction is replacement of the lateral wall fragment(s), after which the lateral calcaneal plate is applied. There are multiple designs of plate available, but screws should always be inserted through the lateral joint fragment(s) into the sustentacular fragment (in addition to the separate cannulated screws), the body fragment and the anterior process.

Tongue type fractures require a different sequence of reduction but can also be accessed via this approach. In these fractures, the lateral joint fragment is still attached to the superior part of the body fragment (the "tongue") and so a Schanz pin can be inserted through the fragment from the posterior heel anteriorly. By pulling the pin distally, not only is the body fragment dis-impacted, but the joint fragment is also elevated back into position. In addition to the usual lateral to medial articular fragment cannulated screws, a dorso-plantar screw(s) is also important to hold reduction in addition to the lateral plate.

It is important to exercise care with closure of the lateral heel flap, avoiding pinching the skin edges with forceps and instead holding the deep dermis or deeper layers. There may be some tension, which can usually be dealt with by interrupted deep dermal sutures inserted in sequence. It is important that epidermal closure is tension-free, and the author prefers 3/0 Nylon sutures. A plaster of Paris below-knee splint or similar is applied and the leg elevated for 2 weeks until wound healing.

Sinus Tarsi Approach

The skin incision used for this approach is similar to that used for open subtalar joint arthrodesis or arthroereisis screw insertion. The direction of the incision is from the tip of the fibula towards the base of the fourth metatarsal, but only 3–4 cm is usually required. The deeper approach is dorsal/anterior to the peroneal tendons and sural nerve and directly onto the sinus tarsi and posterior facet of the subtalar joint. The CFL can be spared, but it may need to be divided or elevated for access. If plate fixation is preferred then the peroneal tendons and inferior retinaculum are elevated from the lateral wall fragment posteriorly to allow access to the upper part of the body fragment.

The same basic sequence of reduction is followed, and the lateral joint fragment, sustentacular fragment and angle of Gissane can be reduced under direct vision, but the body and lateral wall fragment reduction manoeuvres are indirect. The author's preferred technique for both Tongue type and Joint Depression fractures is:

1. Insert a Schanz pin from the posterior heel towards and just below the joint depression fragment. The pin is then levered distally, which dis-impacts the body and joint depression fragments.
2. An elevator is inserted via the sinus tarsi incision through the primary fracture line, either under or through the joint fragment(s) and under the sustentacular fragment, to reduce the body in the coronal plane. This can be aided by manipulation of the body and/or a second Schanz pin from lateral to medial, as with the ELA.
3. The lateral joint fragment, angle of Gissane and anterior process are reduced as with the ELA and temporary fixation wires are inserted from body and lateral joint fragments to sustentaculum as above.
4. The lateral wall fragment is reduced by manipulation, and definitive fixation is by 4 mm cannulated screws or similar from lateral to medial though the lateral joint fragment(s). If required the anterior process is also fixed with cannulated screws as above.
5. The author prefers to fix the body fragment with two cannulated screws of 6.5-8 mm size (preferably fully- or long-threaded to avoid compression) from the posterior heel through to anterior process, as these often also pass under the joint fragment and act as a "raft". There are several bespoke sinus tarsi approach plates available, which offer better fixation of the body fragment in particular, but which involve dissection underneath the peroneal tendons and can cause tendon irritation [17]. A bespoke calcaneal nail is a further option, which is inserted from posterior to anterior and is bridged by locking bolts into the major fragments [18], but these can be technically demanding to insert.
6. Closure of the wounds is much easier than the ELA.

Post-operative and Non-operative Management

Immobilisation and rehabilitation must both allow optimal healing without risking loss of reduction and allow mobilisation of the ankle and hindfoot joints as rapidly as possible to reduce post-traumatic stiffness. This can be particularly challenging as compliance is often lower in this patient group due to a higher incidence of multiple trauma, drug and alcohol abuse and psychiatric illness.

The author's preferred method is a fixed padded splint for 2 weeks to allow wound healing/reduction of oedema, followed by mobilisation without weight-bearing in a removable splint (which can be removed to mobilise the ankle and foot) for 2–4 weeks. Finally, a period of protected weight-bearing in a removable boot continues for another 4–6 weeks and physiotherapy commences. Post-operative radiographs are performed before protected weight-bearing and prior to removal of the boot.

References

1. Summers NJ, Murdoch MM. Fractures of the talus: a comprehensive review. Clin Podiatr Med Surg. 2012;29(2):187–203, vii. https://doi.org/10.1016/j.cpm.2012.01.005. Epub 2012 Feb 21. PMID: 22424484.
2. Alley MC, Vallier HA, Tornetta P 3rd. Orthopaedic trauma research consortium. Identifying risk factors for osteonecrosis after talar fracture. J Orthop Trauma. 2024;38(1):25–30. https://doi.org/10.1097/BOT.0000000000002706.
3. Sangeorzan BJ, Benirschke SK, Mosca V, Mayo KA, Hansen ST Jr. Displaced intra-articular fractures of the tarsal navicular. J Bone Joint Surg Am. 1989;71(10):1504–10. PMID: 2592390.
4. Canale ST, Kelly FB Jr. Fractures of the neck of the talus. Long-term evaluation of seventy-one cases. J Bone Joint Surg Am. 1978;60(2):143–56. PMID: 417084.
5. Lambert LA, Mangwani J, Davies MB, Molloy AP, Mason LW. The lateral transligamentous approach to the talar dome. Foot Ankle Surg. 2021;27(7):767–71. https://doi.org/10.1016/j.fas.2020.10.003. Epub 2020 Oct 12. PMID: 33153917.
6. Majeed H, McBride DJ. Talar process fractures: an overview and update of the literature. EFORT Open Rev. 2018;3(3):85–92. https://doi.org/10.1302/2058-5241.3.170040. PMID: 29657849; PMCID: PMC5890124.
7. Roberts LE, Pinto M, Staggers JR, Godoy-Santos A, Shah A, de Cesar NC. Soft tissue structures at risk with percutaneous posterior to anterior screw fixation of the talar neck. Foot Ankle Int. 2018;39(10):1237–41. https://doi.org/10.1177/1071100718777771. Epub 2018 Jun 2. PMID: 29860866.
8. Griffin JT, Landy DC, Mechas CA, Nazal MR, Foster JA, Moghadamian ES, Srinath A, Aneja A. The Hawkins sign of the talus: the impact of patient factors on prediction accuracy. J Bone Joint Surg Am. 2024;106(11):958–65. https://doi.org/10.2106/JBJS.23.00906. Epub 2024 Mar 21. PMID: 38512980.
9. Cotton F, Henderon F. Results of fractute of the Os Calcis. JBJS Am. 1916;s2–14:290–8.
10. Buckley R, Tough S, McCormack R, Pate G, Leighton R, Petrie D, Galpin R. Operative compared with nonoperative treatment of displaced intra-articular calcaneal fractures a prospective, randomized, controlled multicenter trial. JBJS. 2002;84-A(10):1733–44.

11. Gougoulias N, McBride D, Maffulli N. Outcomes of management of displaced intra-articular calcaneal fractures. The Surgeon. 2021;19(5):e222–9.
12. Attenasio A, Heiman E, Hong I, Bhalla A, Jankowski J, Yoon R, Liporace F, Dziadosz D. Postoperative wound complications in extensile lateral approach versus sinus tarsi approach for calcaneal fractures: Are we improving? Updated meta-analysis of recent literature. Injury. 2024;55(6).
13. Essex-Lopresti P. The mechanism, reduction technique, and results in fractures of the os calcis. Br J Surg. 1952;39(157):395–419.
14. Sanders R. Current concepts review – displaced intra-articular fractures of the calcaneus. JBJS. 2000;82:225–50.
15. Eastwood DM, Langkamer VG, Atkins RM. Intra-articular fractures of the Calcaneum (parts I and II). JBJS(Br). 1993;75-B:189–95.
16. Rammelt S, Zwipp H. Calcaneus fractures: facts, controversies and recent developments. Injury. 2004;35:443–61.
17. Pitts C, Almaguer A, Wilson J, Quade J, Johnson M. Radiographic and post-operative outcomes of plate versus screw constructs in open reduction and internal fixation of calcaneus fractures via the sinus tarsi. Foot Ankle Int. 2019;40(8):929–35.
18. Zwipp H, Pasa L, Zilka L, Amlang M, Rammelt S, Pompach M. Introduction of a new locking nail for treatment of intraarticular calcaneal fractures. J Orthop Trauma. 2016;30(3):e88–92.

Chapter 22
Fifth Metatarsal Fractures: Fixation Techniques

Amr Eldessouky and Maneesh Bhatia

Introduction

Fifth metatarsal fractures are one of the most common foot injuries. The optimal approach to treating these fractures remains controversial among surgeons due to the unique blood supply to the base of the fifth metatarsal. Factors influencing treatment choices include not only the fracture location but also the patient's age, activity level, and bone health. Inadequate treatment of these injuries can substantially impact a patient's overall quality of life.

Anatomy

A strong understanding of the anatomy of the fifth metatarsal plays a crucial role in the management plan. The blood supply to the fifth metatarsal consists of the metaphyseal, periosteal, and nutrient arteries. When a fracture occurs at the proximal diaphysis, it can compromise the nutrient artery, potentially resulting in delayed or non-union due to reduced blood flow [1]. Additionally, the sural nerve and its lateral dorsal cutaneous branch, which lie close to the base of the fifth metatarsal, are vulnerable during fixation procedures [2].

A. Eldessouky
Royal Orthopaedic Hospital, Birmingham, UK

M. Bhatia (✉)
Consultant Orthopaedic Foot Ankle Surgeon, University Hospitals Leicester, Spire Hospital Leicester and Nuffield Health Leicester, Leicester, UK

Associate Professor, University of Leicester, Leicester, UK

Professor, DeMontfort University Leicester, Leicester, UK

M. Bhatia (ed.), *Surgical Techniques of the Foot and Ankle*,
https://doi.org/10.1007/978-3-031-93742-2_22

Classification

Lawrence and Botte introduced their classification for proximal fifth metatarsal fractures in 1993 and it remains widely used today [3]. This classification categorizes fractures into three zones.

A summary of the characteristics and treatment methods for each zone of injury is shown in (Table 22.1) [4].

Table 22.1 Summary of the characteristics and treatment methods for each zone of injury

Zone of injury	Description	Mechanism of injury	Union rates	Treatment methods
Zone 1	Avulsion fracture of the tuberosity	Forceful contraction of the peroneus brevis or lateral band of the plantar fascia during foot inversion	Non-union is uncommon	**Functional treatment**: Suitable for most cases
				Surgical treatment: Recommended for severely displaced fractures and symptomatic non-union. (options include excision, IM screw, hook plate, tension band wire)
Zone 2 (Jones fracture)	Fracture at the metaphyseal-diaphyseal junction	Forced forefoot adduction while the hindfoot is in plantar flexion	Increased risk of delayed and non-union	**Functional treatment**: For low demand patients
	Involves the fourth and fifth metatarsal articulation			**Surgical treatment:** For high demand patients. (options include IM screw, plantar plate, tension band wire)
Zone 3	-Proximal diaphyseal fracture	Repetitive overloading	Increased risk of delayed and non-union	**Conservative treatment**: For low demand patients (Cast immobilisation, ESWT)
	Distal to the fourth and fifth metatarsal articulation			-**Surgical treatment:** For high demand patients. (options include IM screw, plantar plate with or without bone grafting)

IM Intramedullary, *ESWT* Extracorporeal Shock Wave Therapy

Fixation Techniques

The choice of fixation method depends on the fracture's location and age, as well as the surgeon's familiarity with the technique.

Intramedullary Screw Fixation

Set up: The patient is positioned in a semi-lateral position with sandbags under the ipsilateral buttock. Towels are placed under the lower leg to elevate the foot off the table, facilitating easier wire or screw insertion. Alternatively, the patient can be positioned supine with the knee flexed at 90°. A thigh tourniquet may be used, although the procedure can be performed without it in cases of percutaneous fixation. The C-arm is positioned opposite the operating side.

Approach: A 1 cm longitudinal stab incision is made 15 mm proximal to the base of the fifth metatarsal, exposing the insertion of the peroneus brevis tendon (Fig. 22.1). Caution is essential to prevent injury to the lateral dorsal cutaneous nerve (LDCN), a branch of the sural nerve, which runs close to the incision site. Blunt dissection and the use of tissue protectors are vital to safeguarding the nerve and its branches. If open reduction is needed, a lateral approach over the fracture site is used.

Fixation: The entry point for the guide wire is identified under fluoroscopy in both anteroposterior and lateral views, a critical step given the unique curvature of the fifth metatarsal (Fig. 22.2). After inserting the guide wire, a reamer of appropriate size is selected based on the screw diameter. Some studies recommend that intramedullary (IM) screws be at least 4.5 mm in diameter. A headless compression screw of the appropriate size and length is inserted, ensuring that all distal threads cross the fracture line to achieve maximum compression (Fig. 22.3). Alternatively, conventional partially threaded screw may be used though it can cause soft tissue irritation.

Pitfalls:

- Improper positioning of the entry point in the sagittal or coronal planes may require selecting a shorter screw length to prevent the screw tip from breaching the cortex, which could lead to fracture distraction.
- The screw diameter is crucial. Smaller-diameter screws are associated with a higher risk of failure, delayed union, or non-union. However, excessively large IM screws may cause stress shielding and additional fractures.

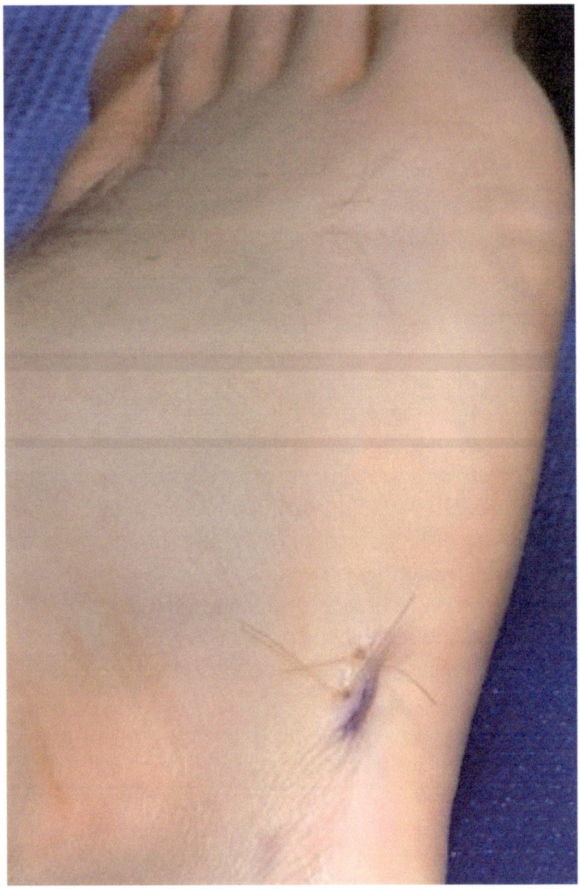

Fig. 22.1 Incision for IM screw insertion, 15 mm proximal to the base of the fifth metatarsal

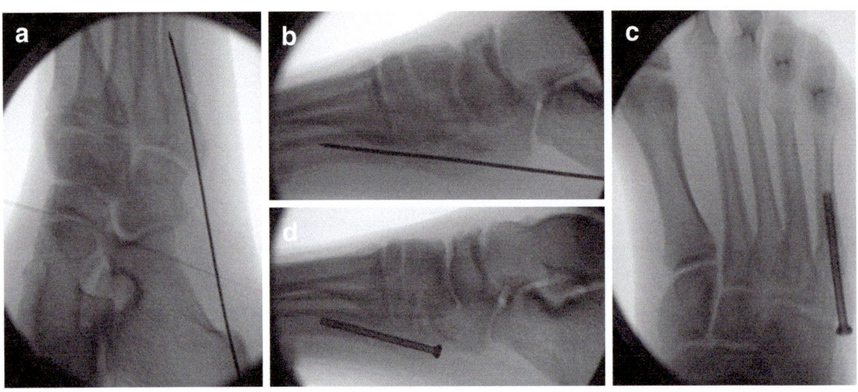

Fig. 22.2 Intra-operative radiographs showing the position of the guide wire in oblique (**a**) and lateral (**b**) views. Anteroposterior (**c**) and lateral (**d**) radiographs after screw insertion

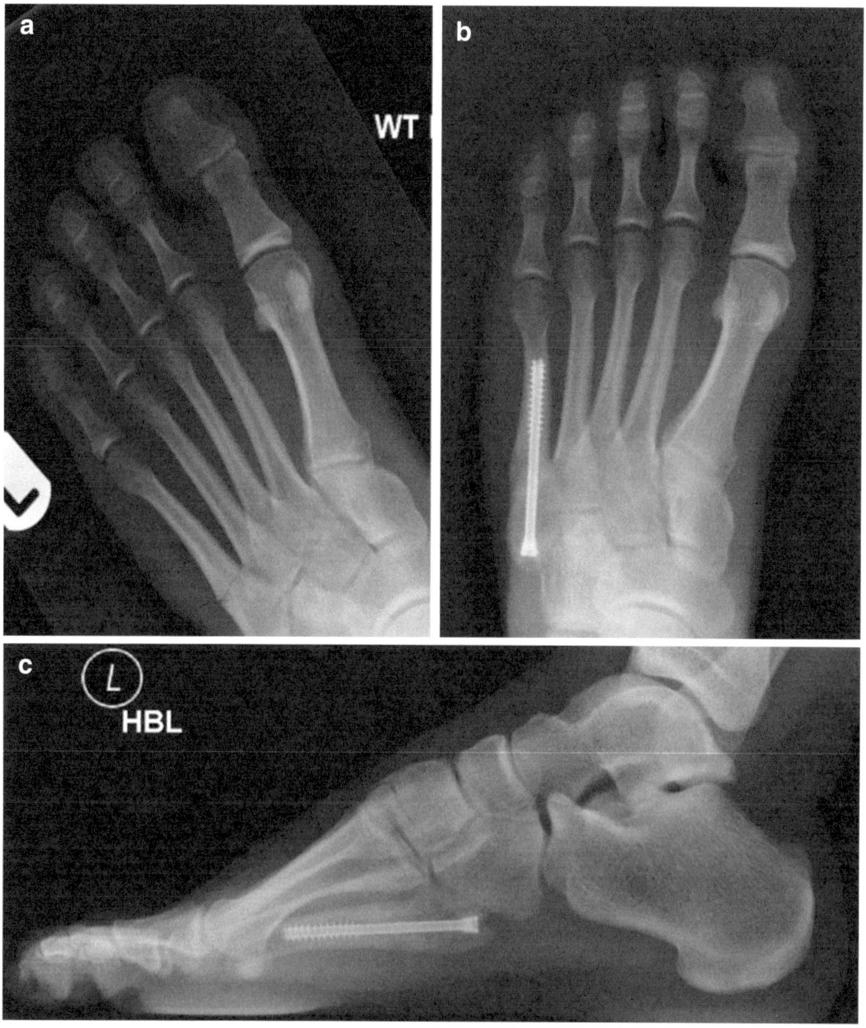

Fig. 22.3 Anteroposterior radiograph (**a**, **b**) showing Jones fracture. Anteroposterior (**a**) and lateral (**c**) radiographs 10 weeks later showing full union [4]

Plantar Plate Fixation

Set up: The patient is positioned in a semi-lateral position with sandbags under the ipsilateral buttock. Towels are placed under the lower leg to elevate the foot off the table, facilitating easier access to the bone. A thigh tourniquet is used. The C-arm is positioned opposite the operating side.

Approach: A 4 cm incision is made along the lateral-plantar surface of the fifth metatarsal, centred over the fracture. Dissection is performed carefully using blunt techniques to avoid damaging the sural nerve branches while exposing the bone. The abductor digiti minimi muscle is gently retracted downward to fully visualize the fracture. If needed, the fracture edges are refreshed, and cancellous bone graft from the calcaneus can be inserted into the fracture site to promote healing.

Fixation: A pointed reduction clamp is used to reduce and compress the fracture. Alternatively, compression can be achieved using the plate's dynamic compression option. A plate of appropriate length is selected, which can be contoured if needed to sit flush on the plantar aspect of the bone. The plate is secured with a cortical screw proximal to the fracture site, followed by insertion of a second proximal locking screw. Next, a distal cortical compression screw is placed eccentrically in the plate's compression slot. Fill the remaining screw holes as appropriate.

Hook Plate Fixation

Set up: Similar to the plantar plate fixation.

Approach: Similar to plantar plate fixation. The incision will need to be extended 15 mm proximal to the tuberosity.

Fixation: Temporarily stabilize the fracture using a K-wire, ensuring the wire does not interfere with plate application. Position the plate so that the plate hook engages the proximal fragment. Once the plate position is satisfactory, place a distal cortical compression screw eccentrically in the plate's compression slot. Before fully tightening the screw, use a suitable impactor to compress the fracture site by impacting the plate hooks. The screw can then be fully tightened. Fill the remaining plate screw holes as needed. Optionally, a cross screw may be inserted through a hole between the hooks on the tuberosity (Fig. 22.4).

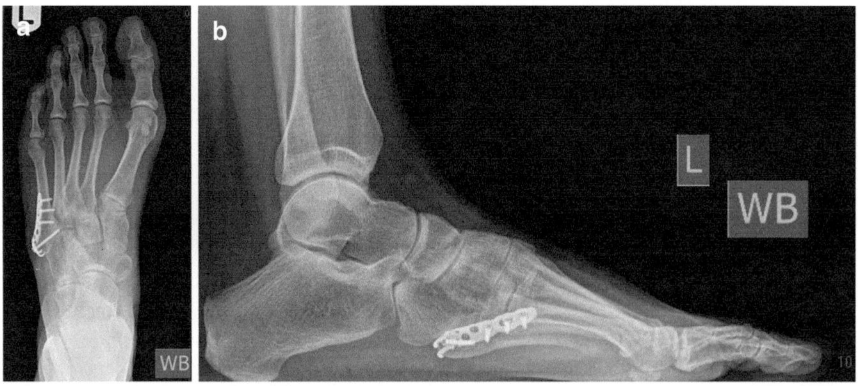

Fig. 22.4 Anteroposterior (**a**) and lateral (**b**) radiographs showing hook plate fixation for avulsion tuberosity fracture [4]

Wound Closure

The subcutaneous tissue is closed with 2-0 Vicryl®, and the skin is closed with 4-0 Monocryl®. A nonadherent dressing is applied, followed by a compressive, well-padded dressing.

Postoperative Care

- Elevate the leg.
- Mobilize the patient as non-weight-bearing in a walker boot for 6 weeks, encouraging ankle movements.
- Check the wound in 2 weeks.
- Perform an X-ray at 6 weeks to confirm satisfactory union. Once the fracture has united, the boot may be gradually discontinued.
- Return to sports can begin once the fracture is fully united, both clinically and radiologically, usually after 3 months.

Management of Specific Cases

Delayed / Non-union Stress Fractures

Fracture site debridement, followed by bone grafting or bone morphogenetic proteins (BMPs), is typically combined with fixation, most often using an intramedullary screw [5]. In contrast, other studies have shown that full union can be achieved within 3 months using only percutaneous screw fixation, without the need for fracture site debridement [6] (Fig. 22.5).

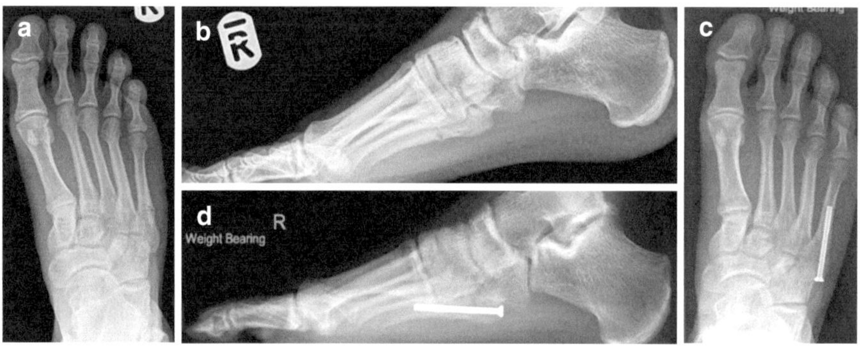

Fig. 22.5 Anteroposterior (**a**) and lateral (**b**) radiographs of 19 tears old footballer showing non-united stress fracture. Anteroposterior (**c**) and lateral (**d**) radiographs showing full union 6 weeks later following fixation

Revision

For the revision of previous screw fixation, re-reaming of the medullary canal and the use of a screw with a larger diameter are performed [5].

Os Vesalianum Pedis

Os Vesalianum pedis (OVP) is an uncommon accessory bone that lies within the peroneus brevis tendon and can be mistaken for non-united fracture (Fig. 22.6). Diagnosis is confirmed by x-raying both feet as it typically presents bilaterally [7]. Surgical management involves partially detaching the peroneus brevis tendon to allow for bone excision, followed by reattachment of the tendon using suture anchors.

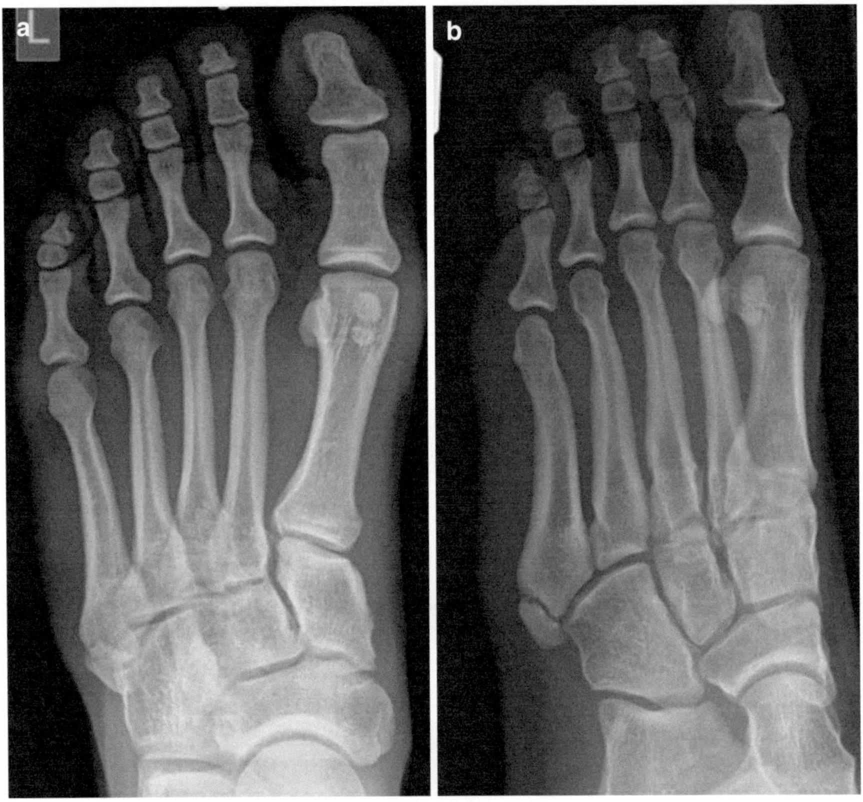

Fig. 22.6 Anteroposterior (**a**) and oblique (**b**) radiographs showing os vesalianum pedis [4]

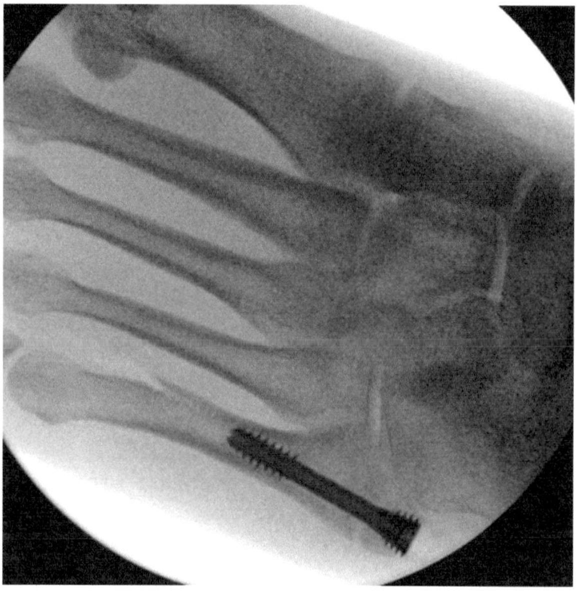

Fig. 22.7 Intraoperative radiograph showing iatrogenic fracture in the fifth metatarsal shaft following fixation with intramedullary screw [4]

Complications

Complications specific to surgical fixation include wound infection, sural nerve injury, refracture (8.6%), delayed and non-union (6.8%), hardware irritation/failure and iatrogenic fracture (Fig. 22.7) [8].

References

1. Smith JW, Arnoczky SP, Hersh A. The intraosseous blood supply of the fifth metatarsal: implications for proximal fracture healing. Foot Ankle. 1992;13(3):143–52.
2. Fansa AM, Smyth NA, Murawski CD, Kennedy JG. The lateral dorsal cutaneous branch of the sural nerve: clinical importance of the surgical approach to proximal fifth metatarsal fracture fixation. Am J Sports Med. 2012;40(8):1895–8.
3. Lawrence SJ, Botte MJ. Jones' fractures and related fractures of the proximal fifth metatarsal. Foot Ankle. 1993;14(6):358–65.
4. Eldessouky A, Bhatia M. Fifth metatarsal fractures: review of the current concepts. J Arthrosc Surg Sports Med. 2025; https://doi.org/10.25259/JASSM_34_2024.
5. Hunt KJ, Anderson RB. Treatment of Jones fracture nonunions and refractures in the elite athlete: outcomes of intramedullary screw fixation with bone grafting. Am J Sports Med. 2011;39(9):1948–54.

6. Grant MJ, Molloy AP, Mason LW. The use of percutaneous screw fixation without fracture site preparation in the treatment of fifth metatarsal base nonunion. J Foot Ankle Surg. 2020;59(4):753–7.
7. Kalbouneh H, Alajoulin O, Shawaqfeh J, Abu-Hassan D, Al-Juboori S, Jaber S, et al. The anatomical variations of the lateral sesamoid bones of the foot: a retrospective radiographic analysis. Folia Morphol (Warsz). 2022;81(4):983–90.
8. Goodloe JB, Cregar WM, Caughman A, Bailey EP, Barfield WR, Gross CE. Surgical management of proximal fifth metatarsal fractures in elite athletes: a systematic review. Orthop J Sports Med. 2021;9(9):23259671211037647.

Index

M. Bhatia (ed.), *Surgical Techniques of the Foot and Ankle*,
https://doi.org/10.1007/978-3-031-93742-2

MIX
Papier aus verantwortungsvollen Quellen
Paper from responsible sources
FSC® C105338

FSC
www.fsc.org

If you have any concerns about our products,
you can contact us on
ProductSafety@springernature.com

In case Publisher is established outside the EU,
the EU authorized representative is:
Springer Nature Customer Service Center GmbH
Europaplatz 3, 69115 Heidelberg, Germany

Printed by Libri Plureos GmbH
in Hamburg, Germany